Atlas of GENODERMATOSES

Atlas of GENODERMATOSES

Ruggero Caputo **Gianluca Tadini**

Institute of Dermatological Sciences
University of Milan
IRCCS Ospedale Policlinico
Mangiagalli e Regina Elena
Milan, Italy

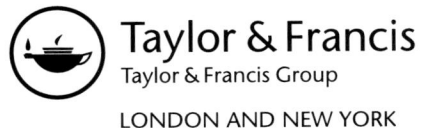

Taylor & Francis
Taylor & Francis Group

LONDON AND NEW YORK

© 2006 Taylor & Francis, an imprint of the Taylor & Francis Group

First published in the United Kingdom in 2006
by Taylor & Francis,
an imprint of the Taylor & Francis Group,
2 Park Square, Milton Park
Abingdon, Oxon OX14 4RN, UK

Tel.: +44 (0) 20 7017 6000
Fax.: +44 (0) 20 7017 6699
E.mail: info.medicine@tandf.co.uk
Website: www.tandf.co.uk/medicine

All rights reserved. No part of this publication may be reproduced, stored in a retrieval system, or transmitted, in any form or by any means, electronic, mechanical, photocopying, recording, or otherwise, without the prior permission of the publisher or in accordance with the provisions of the Copyright, Designs and Patents Act 1988 or under the terms of any licence permitting limited copying issued by the Copyright Licensing Agency, 90 Tottenham Court Road, London W1P 0LP.

Although every effort has been made to ensure that all owners of copyright material have been acknowledged in this publication, we would be glad to acknowledge in subsequent reprints or editions any omissions brought to our attention.

British Library Cataloguing in Publication Data

Data available on application

Library of Congress Cataloging-in-Publication Data

Data available on application

ISBN10: 1-84184-251-6
ISBN13: 9-78-1-84184-251-6

Distributed in North and South America by

Taylor & Francis
2000 NW Corporate Blvd
Boca Raton, FL 33431, USA

Within Continental USA
Tel.: 800 272 7737; Fax.: 800 374 3401
Outside Continental USA
Tel.: 561 994 0555; Fax.: 561 361 6018
E-mail: orders@crcpress.com

Distributed in the rest of the world by
Thomson Publishing Services
Cheriton House
North Way
Andover, Hampshire SP10 5BE, UK
Tel.: +44 (0) 1264 332424
E-mail: salesorder.tandf@thomsonpublishingservices.co.uk

Composition by C&M Digitals (P) Ltd., Chennai, India
Printed and bound by T.G. Hostench S.A., Spain

Contents

Preface xi
Foreword – Rudolf Happle xiii
Illustration credits xv

1 **Epidermolysis bullosa**
   Epidermolytic epidermolysis bullosa (EEB) 1
   Junctional epidermolysis bullosa (JEB) 5
   Dermolytic epidermolysis bullosa 9

2 **Epidermolytic hyperkeratoses**
   'Classical' epidermolytic hyperkeratosis 15
   Ichthyosis bullosa of Siemens 19
   Ichthyosis Curth–Macklin 20
   'Stellate' epidermolytic hyperkeratosis 22

3 **Acantholytic diseases**
   Darier's disease 25
   Acrokeratosis verruciformis 29
   Hailey–Hailey disease 30
   Peeling skin syndrome 32

4 **Ichthyoses**
   Dominant ichthyosis 35
   X-linked ichthyosis 38
   Self-healing collodion baby 40
   Lamellar ichthyosis 42
   Harlequin fetus 48
   Pityriasis rotunda 50
   Congenital reticular ichthyosiform erythroderma (CRIE) 51

5 **Syndromic ichthyoses**
   Netherton syndrome 53
   Sjögren–Larsson syndrome 57
   Refsum syndrome 58
   Trichothiodystrophy 59
   Dorfman–Chanarin syndrome 63

v

6 Erythrokeratodermas
Erythrokeratoderma variabilis — 65
Symmetric progressive erythrokeratoderma — 67

7 Palmoplantar keratodermas
Epidermolytic palmoplantar keratoderma — 69
Unna–Thost palmoplantar keratoderma — 70
Keratoderma hereditaria mutilans — 72
Greither's disease — 74
Olmsted's syndrome — 75
Papillon–Lefevre syndrome — 77
Huriez's syndrome — 79
Mal de Meleda — 80
Punctate palmoplantar keratoderma — 82
Striate keratoderma — 84
Richner–Hanhart syndrome — 85
Painful callosities — 87
Pachydermoperiostosis — 88
Akrokeratoelastoidosis — 89
Naxos syndrome — 90

8 Other disorders of keratinization
Porokeratoses — 93
Kyrle's disease — 97
CHILD syndrome — 98
X-linked dominant chondrodysplasia punctata — 100
KID syndrome — 102
Pityriasis rubra pilaris — 104

9 Poikilodermas and aging syndromes
Kindler's syndrome — 107
Xeroderma pigmentosum — 110
Rothmund–Thomson syndrome — 113
Naegeli–Franceschetti syndrome — 114
Werner's syndrome — 116
Hutchinson–Gilford syndrome — 117
Kitamura–Dowling–Degos disease — 119
Cockayne's syndrome — 121

10 Hair diseases
Alopecias
  Marie–Unna hypotrichosis — 123
  Hypotrichosis simplex of the scalp — 124
  Ichthyosis follicularis with atrichia and photophobia — 125
  Alopecia areata — 127
  Ulerythema ophryogenes — 128
  Triangular alopecia — 130

Hirsutism
  Hypertrichosis congenita — 131
  Localized hypertrichosis — 133

Hair shaft abnormalities
  Monilethrix — 134
  Pili annulati — 136
  Pili torti — 137

	Woolly hair	139
	Elejalde's syndrome	140
	Griscelli's syndrome	141
	Uncombable hair syndrome	143
	Menkes' kinky hair syndrome	144
	Trichorhinophalangeal syndrome	145
	Atrichia with papular lesions	146
	Loose anagen syndrome	148
	Keratosis follicularis spinulosa decalvans	149

11 Nail disorders
Pachyonychia congenita	151
Nail–patella–elbow syndrome	154
Twenty-nail dystrophy	156
Malalignment of the great toenails	157
Leukonychia	158
Pterygium inversum of nails	159
Iso-Kikuchi syndrome	160

12 Sebocystomatosis   161

13 Oral mucosa
White sponge nevus	165
Dyskeratosis congenita	166
Oral-facial-digital syndrome type I	169

14 Neurocutaneous syndromes
Neurofibromatosis type 1	171
Neurofibromatosis type 2	178
Noonan's syndrome	179
Tuberous sclerosis complex	180
Cardiofacio-cutaneous syndrome	187
Phakomatosis pigmentokeratotica	188
Epidermal nevi and epidermal nevus syndromes	192
Waxy keratosis of childhood	196
Papular epithelial hamartomas and neurologic abnormalities syndrome	198
Proteus syndrome	200

15 Ectodermal dysplasias and related disorders
15.1 Ectodermal dysplasias
Hypohidrotic ectodermal dysplasia	203
Rapp–Hodgkin–AEC, EEC syndrome, limb–mammary disease, adult-spectrum ectodermal dysplasia	208
Tricho-dento-osseous syndrome	212
Witkop's syndrome	213
Ellis–Van Creveld–Weyers acrodental dysostosis complex	214
Cleft lip–palate with ectodermal dysplasia syndrome	216
Clouston's disease	217
Ectodermal dysplasia–skin fragility syndrome	219
Pure hair–nail ectodermal dysplasia	220
Incontinentia pigmenti	222

15.2 'Ectomesodermal' dysplasias
Goltz's syndrome	227
MIDAS syndrome	231

16 Fatty tissue anomalies
Launois–Bensaude syndrome — 233
Total lipodystrophy — 234
Partial lipodystrophy — 236

17 Disorders of connective tissue
Ehlers–Danlos syndromes — 239
Cutis laxa — 247
Pseudoxanthoma elasticum — 249
Marfan's syndrome — 251
Connective tissue nevi and Buschke–Ollendorff syndrome — 253
Elastosis perforans serpiginosa — 255
Costello's syndrome — 256
Michelin tire baby — 257
Juvenile hyaline fibromatosis — 258
Cutaneous mastocytosis — 260
Cutaneous leiomyomatosis — 261
Restrictive dermopathy — 262
Dermochondrocorneal dystrophy — 263
Progressive osseous heteroplasia — 264
Cutis verticis gyrata — 266

18 Aplasia cutis — 269

19 Disorders of pigmentation
Oculocutaneous albinisms — 275
Hermansky–Pudlak syndrome — 279
Hypomelanosis of Ito — 280
Piebaldism — 281
Waardenburg's syndrome — 283
McCune–Albright syndrome — 284
Linear and figurated hypo- and hyperpigmented nevi — 286
Segmental lentiginosis — 289
Leopard syndrome — 292
Ota nevus — 294
Cutis tricolor — 295
Dyschromatosis symmetrica hereditaria — 296

20 Vascular disorders
Complex of Sturge–Parkes–Weber, Klippel–Trénaunay and Cobb's syndromes — 297
Sturge–Weber syndrome — 297
Klippel–Trénaunay syndrome — 300
Cobb's syndrome — 302
Von Hippel–Lindau syndrome — 303
Ataxia telangiectasia — 304
Hemorrhagic telangiectasia — 306
Cutis marmorata telangiectatica congenita — 308
Maffucci syndrome — 311
Blue rubber bleb nevus syndrome — 312
Diffuse benign telangiectasia and port-wine stains complex — 314
Unilateral nevoid and generalized 'essential' telangiectasia — 315
Nevus anemicus — 318
Phakomatosis pigmentovascularis — 319

	Lymphedema	321
	Generalized cyanosis, phlebectases and soft skin syndrome	322
	Glomuvenous malformation	324
21	**Metabolic disease**	
	Porphyria cutanea tarda and hepatoerythropoietic porphyria	327
	Erythropoietic protoporphyria	330
	Erythropoietic porphyria	332
	Acrodermatitis enteropathica	334
	Fabry's disease	335
	Sea-blue histiocytosis	337
	Cerebrotendinous xanthomatosis	339
	Prolidase deficiency	341
	Methylmalonic aciduria	342
22	**Immunodeficiency disorders**	
	Omenn's syndrome	345
	Hyper IgE syndrome	347
	C1q esterase inhibitor deficiency	348
	Chediak–Higashi syndrome	349
23	**Complex malformative syndromes with distinctive cutaneous signs**	
	Rubinstein–Taybi syndrome	351
	Cornelia de Lange syndrome	353
	Cohen's syndrome	355
	Branchio-oculofacial syndrome	356
	Barber–Say syndrome	358
	Turner's syndrome	359
	Pallister–Killian syndrome	361
	Encephalocraniocutaneous lipomatosis	363
	GAPO syndrome	364
24	**Genodermatoses related to malignancy**	
	Nevoid basal cell carcinoma syndrome	367
	Muir–Torre syndrome	369
	Cowden's syndrome	371
	Gardner syndrome	373
	Bloom's syndrome	374
	Howel–Evans syndrome	376
	Multiple endocrine neoplasia syndrome, type 2b	377
	Peutz–Jeghers syndrome	378
	Birt–Hogg–Dubé syndrome	380
	Carney's complex	382
	Bazex–Dupré–Christol syndrome	383
	Epidermodysplasia verruciformis	385
	Brooke–Spiegler syndrome	386
	Progressive mucinous histiocytosis	388
	Degos' disease	389
	Rombo syndrome	391
25	**Cutaneous mosaicism**	393
Index		407

Preface

Professor Ferdinando Gianotti founded the Pediatric Dermatology Unit in Milan in the early 1970s and since then one of its major interests and goals has been to classify and investigate genodermatoses. During these years, many ultrastructural studies have been performed by our team of investigators to elucidate the causes and to better understand the pathogenesis of these diseases. However, we had to wait until 1988 when Dr Vincenzo Nazzaro, who had studied in France, founded the Center for Inherited Cutaneous Diseases of the University of Milan. This resulted at last in a special consultation center devoted exclusively to clinical assistance for and investigations of genetic diseases of the skin, becoming the first Italian reference center. From that period until the present we have enrolled more than 3000 patients who are now in follow-up.

The year 1988 was also a time of tremendous effort from the scientific community to define the genes and mutations related to each genetic skin disease, and now only a few genetically determined diseases remain to be elucidated.

The past 15 years of specific practice have prompted us to collect in an atlas our clinical photographs in order to share with students, fellows and colleagues our experience in this field, which is traditionally difficult to commit to memory. In planning this project, we have made some editorial choices that could appear somewhat 'alternative', and which we try to explain in the following notes.

This is an 'atlas' and not simply a 'textbook', because figures obviously have an impact on students and readers.

We have included figures from our own files and from the best cases that we were not able to see in Italy, obtained from leading authors from all over the world, to ensure extensive coverage.

We have chosen only high-quality slides, trying to obtain an overview of the particular signs of each disorder.

This is a concise but complete text for both beginners and experts.

There are no legends to the figures, only references in the text, to avoid repetition and to force the reader to adhere to the concise lecture of the text.

The focus is on genetics and pathogenesis (molecular biology).

An effort has been made to classify diseases following new examples, but at the same time an almost classical subdivision of categories remains.

Rapid practical diagnostic notes (appropriate examinations and tests) are included.

A few notes regarding management are also included.

There are personal views and classifications of many diseases (ichthyoses and ectodermal dysplasias and 'vascular' genetic skin diseases).

There is particular 'devotion' given to mosaicism, following Happle's indications and with some personal insight.

We have also chosen to use a few histopathological images, but only when essential, and some ultrastructural specimens when relevant, leaving as much space as possible for the clinical images.

Special insight is gained into complex genetic syndromes with minor cutaneous signs, and a chapter is devoted to cancer-related genodermatoses.

The rarest genetically determined 'metabolic' diseases with non-specific cutaneous signs are excluded.

Selected references from the recent literature are included, in particular on genetic aspects.

Making choices perhaps means creating both friends and enemies, but we are sure to have the comprehension of the reader.

ACKNOWLEDGEMENTS

We would like to thank first our colleagues from the Institute of Dermatological Sciences of the University of Milan, and especially our masters and friends Professor Gianotti and Dr Nazzaro, who died prematurely in the joy and the peace of Christ, as well as the patients and their families to whom the atlas is dedicated.

We also acknowledge colleagues from Italy and outside who have provided us 'promptly' with their knowledge, and in particular Professor Rudolph Happle from Marburg, Professor José Mascarò from Barcelona, Dr Claudine Blanchet-Bardon from Paris and Professor Amy S. Paller from Chicago. We are grateful to the entire staff of the Pediatric Dermatology Unit, who have supported our efforts during the past 2 years, represented by our colleague and friend Professor Carlo Gelmetti.

In particular, we wish to thank Dr Stefano Cambiaghi, 'probably the best genodermatologist in the world', and Dr Riccardo Cavalli, the 'master of immunofluorescence', with whom we have shared 10 constructive and dialectic years, and we cannot forget the contribution of Dr Alberto Brusasco, the 'poet of electron microscopy'.

Finally, we would like to thank our young colleagues and fellows of the Postgraduate School of Dermatology of Milan, especially one of them who has supported us with her joy and brightness, Dr Alessandra Di Benedetto, who has revised slides and chapters, and also the Secretary of the Department, Mrs Giuliana Siena, who has provided technical assistance in management of the project and compiling the figures.

We also acknowledge, Robert Peden, Martin Lister and the staff of Taylor & Francis for their patience and technical advice.

Ruggero Caputo
Gianluca Tadini
Milan, Italy

Foreword

During the past years, our knowledge on genodermatoses has undergone dramatic changes. In the light of the present molecular research, the vehement discussions regarding nosological categories that prevailed in the past century are now coming to an end, and new avenues of thinking have been opened. In these revolutionary times, Gianluca Tadini and Ruggero Caputo, two internationally known experts in this discipline, have undertaken the great task of presenting a comprehensive *Atlas of Genodermatoses* in which the clinical features of the various phenotypes are presented together with their molecular basis. In this way, the authors are successfully bridging the gap between clinical practice and molecular genetics.

The working group lead by Ruggero Caputo has created a center for hereditary skin diseases in Milan. Here, the clinical observations of these Italian genodermatologists are brought together, enhancing the progress of our understanding of hereditary skin diseases. This center has a paradigmatic function, and I hope that other European countries will follow this model.

In principle, all dermatologists should be eidetics. According to Butterworths Medical Dictionary, the term *eidetic* means '1, referring to the power of exact visual reproduction of anything previously seen or imaged; 2, an individual who is able to call up at will a clear picture of any object or event he has seen or imagined'. This Atlas will help all of us to improve our eidetic skills.

In particular, I should like to thank Gianluca Tadini for his continuous enthusiasm in carrying out missionary work regarding the various theories of cutaneous mosaicism, in particular, the classification of pigmentary patterns, twin spotting, paradominant inheritance, and the type 2 segmental involvement of autosomal dominant skin disorders.

Making a correct diagnosis of a rare hereditary skin disorder is of utmost importance for genetic counseling. Unfortunately, we are today far from the ultimate goal – to develop a practically available gene therapy, at least for the most devastating hereditary skin disorders such as xeroderma pigmentosum or the dystrophic and junctional types of epidermolysis bullosa. For the time being, a refined and improved prenatal diagnosis is the only measure that can be offered by scientific progress. Prenatal diagnosis is today no longer based on morphological techniques but on molecular analysis. Hence, the correlation between clinical features and molecular data as presented in this Atlas will be of increasing importance for affected families and their physicians.

This Atlas reflects the tremendous progress in the field of genodermatology. I should like to congratulate the authors with this comprehensive and timely work. The book will certainly be of great value for dermatologists, pediatricians, and clinical geneticists in their daily practice.

Rudolf Happle
Marburg, Germany

Illustration credits

The authors are grateful to the following colleagues for their kind permission to reproduce the following illustrations in the Atlas.

Dr Lucia Brambilla and Dr Vinicio Boneschi, II Department of Dermatology, Milan, Italy: 7.32, 24.8, 24.9, 24.10

Dr Michel Janier, Hôpital S. Louis, Paris, France: 7.46

Professor Marcel Jonkman, Department of Dermatology, Groningen, The Netherlands: 1.12, 25.32, 25.33

Professor Giovanni Borroni, Department of Dermatology, Pavia, Italy: 23.19, 23.20, 23.21

Dr Bernard Ackerman, New York, USA: 1.41, 1.42, 2.02, 4.9, 14.28, 14.30, 14.35, 14.45, 15.52, 17.38, 19.33

Dr Claudine Blanchet-Bardon, Hôpital S. Louis, Paris, France: 2.9, 7.10, 7.26, 7.27, 7.28, 7.29, 7.30, 7.31, 7.33, 7.36, 7.37, 7.38, 7.39, 7.47, 8.08, 8.09, 8.24, 8.26, 8.27, 10.44, 10.45, 14.47, 14.48, 15.38, 24.28, 24.29, 24.30

Professor William Bacon, Department of Dentofacial Orthopedics, Strasbourg, France: 23.30, 23.31

Professor Enrico Nunzi, Department of Dermatology, Genes, Italy: 19.4, 19.5

Professor Robin Eady and Professor John McGrath, Department of Dermatology, St. John's Institute of Dermatology, London, UK: 15.41, 15.42, 15.43

Dr Carmelo Schepis, Department of Dermatology, Oasi Troina, Italy: 17.37, 19.17

Professor Rudolph Happle, University Hospital Marburg, Germany: 8.15, 8.16, 8.17, 8.18, 8.19, 8.20, 8.21, 8.22, 8.23, 20.56, 20.57, 20.60, 25.17, 25.18, 25.19, 25.23

Professor K. Naritomi, Nishihara, Okinawa, Japan: 25.15

Professor José Maria Mascarò, Department of Dermatology, Barcelona, Spain: 21.1, 1.22

Dr Jorge L. Sanchez, Hato Rey, San Juan, Puerto Rico: 19.6

Dr Angelo Gobello, IDI, Rome, Italy: 14.70, 14.71, 14.72

Dr Angelo Selicorni, Department of Pediatrics, Milan, Italy: 10.42, 10.43, 14.21, 14.23, 14.24, 17.27, 17.28, 17.29, 23.5, 23.6

Dr Marco Somaschini, Department of Pediatrics, Seriate, Italy: 17.16

Professor Ramon Ruiz-Maldonado, Mexico City, Mexico: 10.15, 10.16, 10.17, 10.36, 10.37, 22.9

Professor Annalisa Patrizi, Department of Dermatology, Bologna, Italy: 10.13, 10.14, 10.46, 10.47, 10.48, 23.16, 23.17, 23.18

Dr Sylvia Schauder, Department of Dermatology, University of Göttingen, Germany: 14.68

Dr Siranoush Manoukian, Institute of Cancer, Milan, Italy: 24.17, 24.18, 24.19

Professor Rino Cavalieri and Dr Mauro Paradisi, IDI, Rome, Italy: 9.13, 9.14, 9.19, 9.20, 14.49, 15.31, 15.32, 15.33

Professor Mario Pippione, Department of Dermatology, Turin, Italy: 21.29, 21.30, 21.31

Professor H. Honigsmann, Department of Dermatology, Vienna, Austria: 9.9

Professor Antonella Tosti, Department of Dermatology, Bologna, Italy: 7.49, 7.50, 7.51, 7.52, 10.45, 11.09, 11.10, 11.11, 20.15, 20.19

Dr A. De Moor, Department of Dermatology, University of Antwerp, Belgium: 17.47, 17.48, 17.49

Istituto Neurologico Besta, Milan, Italy: 20.14, 20.18

Professor Hugo Cabrera and Dr Della Giovanna, Department of Dermatology, University of Buenos Aires, Argentina: 17.57, 21.40, 21.41, 21.42, 21.43, 21.44

Professor Yukio Tomita, Department of Dermatology, Nagoya University Graduate School of Medicine, Showa-ku, Japan: 19.45, 19.46

Professor Nelida Pizzi de Parra, Department of Dermatology, Universitad de Cuyo, Mendoza, Argentina: 11.19, 11.20

Michaelson G, Olsson, Westermark P. The Rombo syndrome: a familial disorder with vermiculate atrophoderma, milia, hypotrichosis, trichoepitheliomas, basal cell carcinomas and peripheral vasodilation with cyanosis. Acta Dermatovener (Stockholm) 1981; 61: 497–503: 24.52, 24.53

CHAPTER 1

Epidermolysis bullosa

Definition

Epidermolysis bullosa (EB) consists of a heterogeneous group of mechanobullous diseases due to mutations on at least ten different genes.

Table 1.1 gives a classification of hereditary epidermolysis bullosa.

As can be seen, the old denominations are commonly used, but we prefer to define EB regarding simply the site of the cleavage, abandoning the denomination of 'simple' and 'dystrophic' that are, in our opinion 'old'.

Epidemiology

In Italy there are 700 EB patients among 58 000 000 inhabitants.

EPIDERMOLYTIC EPIDERMOLYSIS BULLOSA (EEB)

Genetics and pathogenesis

This group of EB is, in the vast majority, transmitted as an autosomal dominant trait, and encompasses 40% of EB patients. Fewer than 1% of cases are inherited recessively.

Three genes are involved in the pathogenesis of the disease, encoding, respectively, keratin 5 (K5), keratin 14 (K14) and plectin. In one pedigree, the collagen COLAXVII gene also causes epidermolytic EB.

Table 1.1 Classification of hereditary epidermolysis bullosa (EB)

Major EB type	Major EB subtype	Protein/gene systems involved
EBS ('epidermolytic EB')	EBS-WC	K5, K14
	EBS-K	K5, K14
	EBS-DM	K5, K14
	EBS-MD	Plectin
JEB	JEB-H	Laminin 5*
	JEB-Nh	Laminin 5, type XVII collagen
	JEB-PA†	$\alpha6\beta4$ integrin‡
DEB ('dermolytic EB')	DDEB	Type VII collagen
	RDEB-HS	Type VII collagen
	RDEB-nHS	Type VII collagen

EBS, EB simplex; JEB, junctional EB; DEB, dystrophic EB; DDEB, dominant dystrophic EB; EBS-DM, EBS, Dowling–Meara; EBS-K, Köbner; EBS-MD, EBS with muscular dystrophy; EBS-WC, EBS, Weber–Cockayne; JEB-H, JEB, Herlitz; JEB-nH, JEB, non-Herlitz; JEB-PA, JEB with pyloric atresia; RDEB-HS, recessive dystrophic EB, Hallopeau–Siemens

*Laminin 5 is a macromolecule composed of three distinct ($\alpha3$, $\beta3$, $\gamma2$) laminin chains; mutations in any of the encoding genes result in a JEB phenotype

†Some cases of EB associated with pyloric atresia may have intraepidermal cleavage or both intralamina lucida and intraepidermal clefts

‡$\alpha6\beta4$ integrin is a heterodimeric protein; mutations in either gene have been associated with the JEB-PA syndrome

Clinical cutaneous and extracutaneous findings

PPEEB, GEEB, EEBDM (genes: K5, K14)

Bullae may involve mainly palmoplantar sites (PPEEB) (Figures 1.1 and 1.2) or be more widely distributed

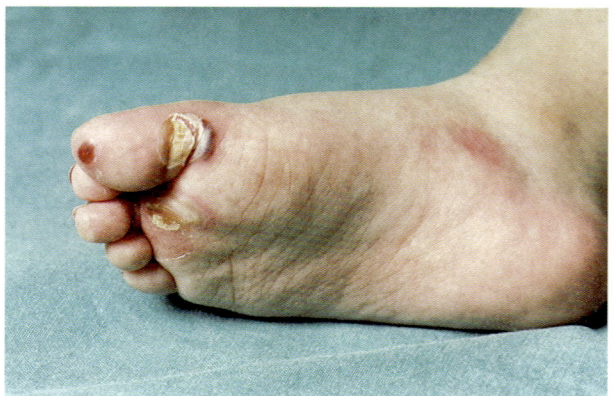

Figure 1.1

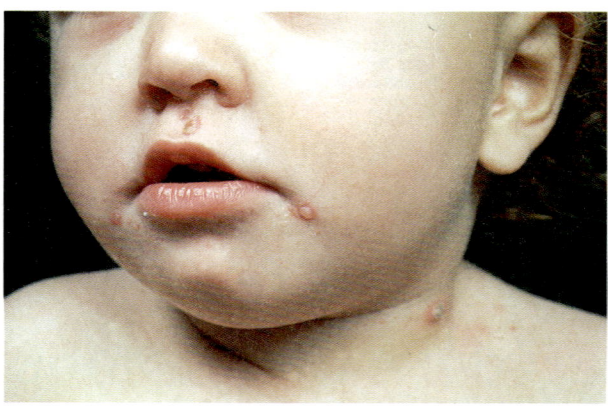

Figure 1.4

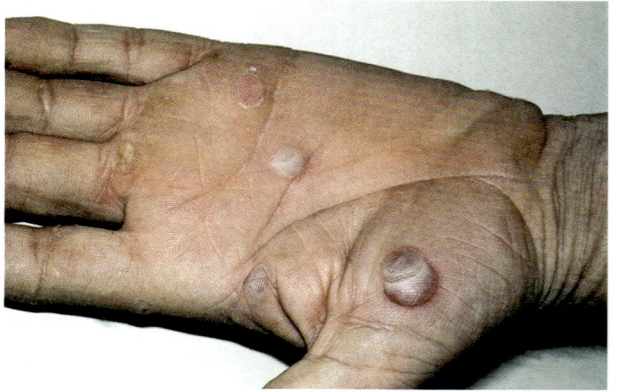

Figure 1.2

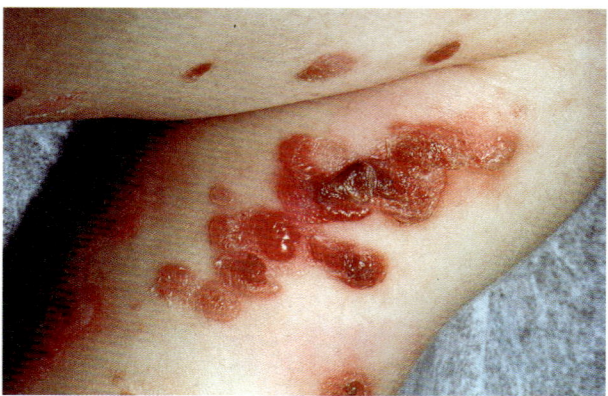

Figure 1.5

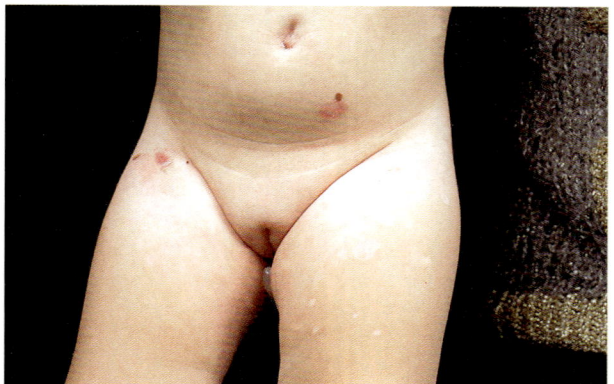

Figure 1.3

(general, GEEB) (napkin areas, folds) (Figures 1.3 and 1.4). Normally the disease is not severe, except in some cases with herpetiform distribution and hemorrhagic bullae (EEBDM, Dowling–Meara (Figures 1.5 and 1.6). In these cases blisters involve palmoplantar areas and are rapidly recurrent, causing palmoplantar keratodermas (Figures 1.7 and 1.8). A few fatal cases are reported in the perinatal period due to the extreme severity of the disease. These children reach milestones of physical development, such as the ability to walk and run (and hence attend school), later, partly because of the palmoplantar lesions and partly because of the frequent oral lesions (Figure 1.9) that impair food consumption.

In these patients nails are frequently absent (Figure 1.10) and alopecic areas may be detected as well as milia on the dorsa of the hands.

At around 8–10 years of age the situation tends to improve, and in adulthood EEB is restricted to occasional mechanically involved sites such as feet, elbows and knees.

Symptoms in all the EEB subgroups tend to worsen during the summer and in hot and humid weather.

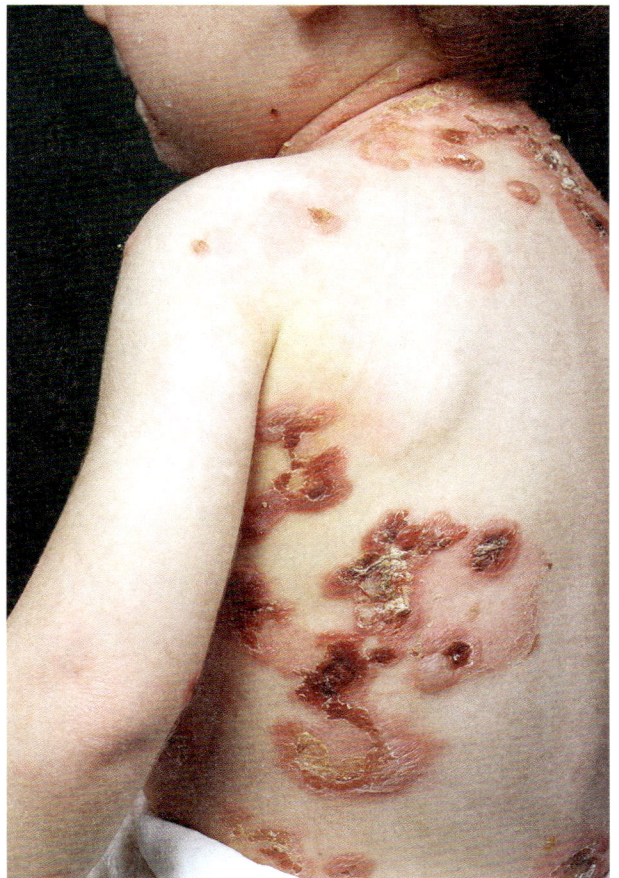

Figure 1.6

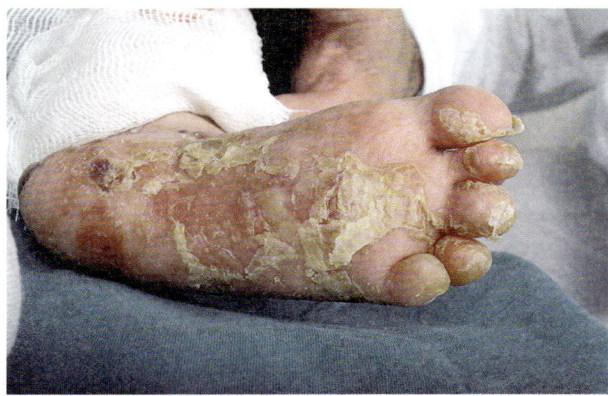

Figure 1.8

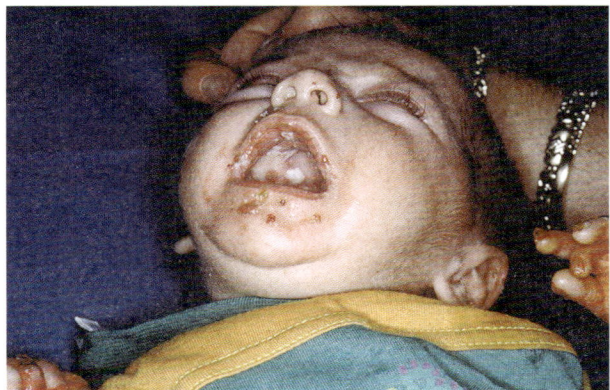

Figure 1.9

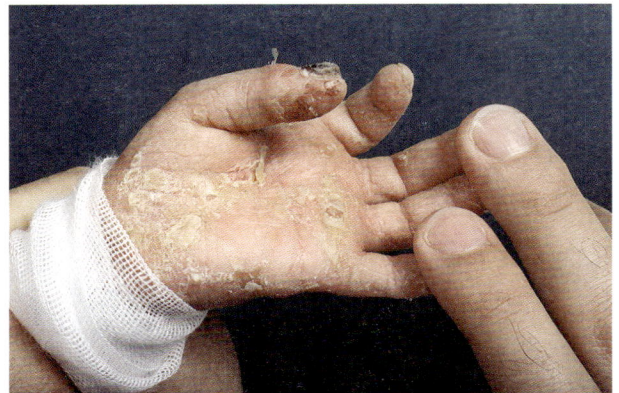

Figure 1.7

In the few described EEB families with the recessive mode of inheritance (1%), lesions are in general more severe (Figures 1.11 and 1.12) than in families with dominant inheritance.

EEB with muscular dystrophy (gene plectin)

In some families, a clinical picture of GEEB is accompanied by a late onset weakness of muscular origin (7–10 years) (Figure 1.13). Obviously, muscular dystrophy tends to overwhelm skin lesions regarding the course and prognosis of the disease.

In Norway, in a large group of families with EEB without signs of muscular involvement, formerly described as the Ogna subgroup, the disease has been found to be related to mutations in the same gene as in EEB with muscular dystrophy (plectin).

Laboratory findings

Skin biopsies, taken at the peribullous areas, are necessary to perform electron microscopy that demonstrates intraepidermal cleavage with

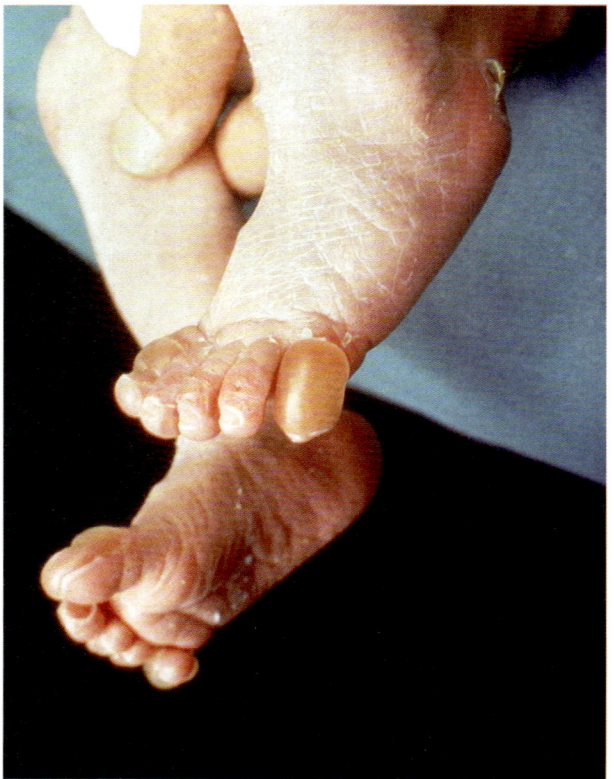

Figure 1.10

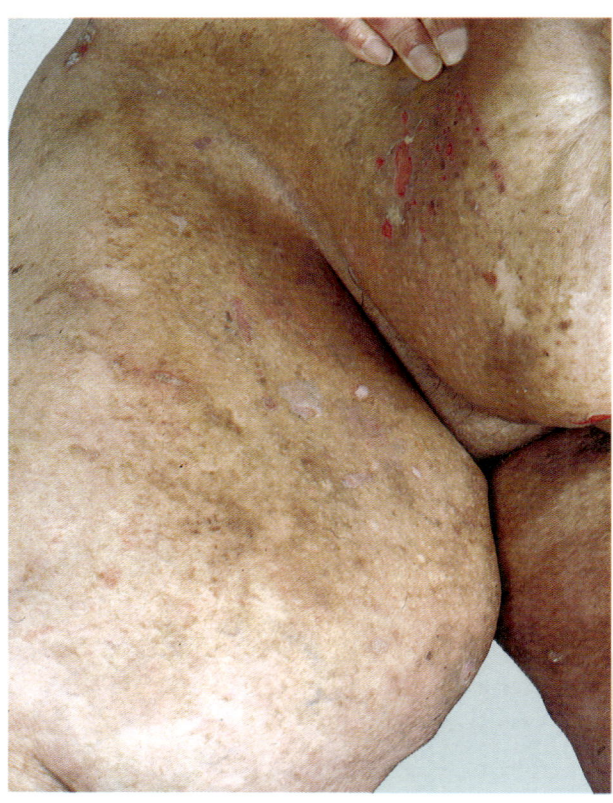

Figure 1.12

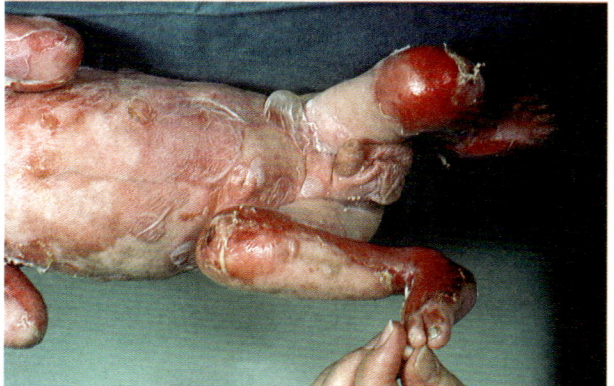

Figure 1.11

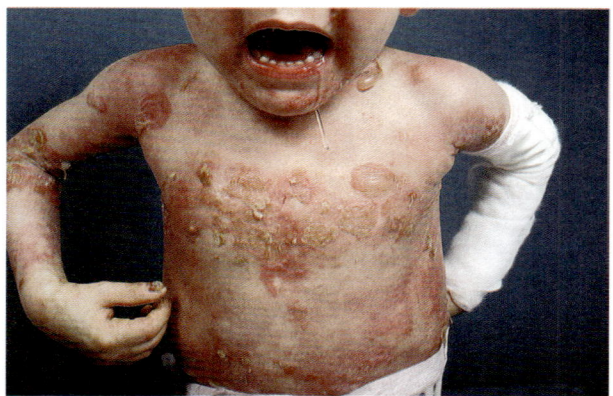

Figure 1.13

cytolysis and clumping of tonofilaments in the basal layers.

In large dominant pedigrees, as well as for recessive inherited EEB, molecular studies are performed with keratinocyte cultures, or blood samples are made available, in order to detect mutations in the K5 and K14 genes or the plectin gene for EEB with muscular dystrophy and the former Ogna subgroup.

Follow-up and therapy

Fortunately, for the majority of patients, EEB does not represent an obstacle to a normal life. In contrast, the more severe patients (EEBDM) have to be frequently checked during preschool age in order to maintain normal food intake and growth centiles.

Orthopedic advice is mandatory to assess devices and physiotherapy for normal walking and development.

JUNCTIONAL EPIDERMOLYSIS BULLOSA (JEB)

Genetics and pathogenesis

JEB is a heterogeneous subgroup of EB due to mutations in several genes encoding the major constituent of the hemidesmosomes, and represents usually fewer than 10% of EB patients.

The involved genes are the following:

- Laminin 5, for Herlitz JEB (lethal variant or very severe generalized disease)
- Laminin 5 for non-Herlitz JEB (non-lethal variants, but moderately severe generalized involvement with particularly severe pretibial localizations)
- Collagen XVII gene (non-lethal variants with moderately severe generalized involvement, with alopecia and major dental defects)
- Integrin α6 and β4 for JEB with pyloric atresia (lethal and non-lethal cases)

Clinical cutaneous and extracutaneous findings

Herlitz JEB

The extreme severity of the disease is already noticeable at birth (Figure 1.14).

Bullae present spontaneously even with a gentle touch. After the eruption, blisters lose their roof and remain visible as erosions that do not heal (Figure 1.15). In particular, granulomatous and easily bleeding lesions (Figure 1.16) arise on such eroded epithelium.

The general condition is very poor, with characteristic laryngeal stridor and cry.

Pulmonary involvement is frequent, and recurrent, very severe episodes with bronchiolitis and pneumonia are detected and require permanent hospitalization in a neonatal pathology unit.

Oral mucosa is heavily involved as well as the mucosa of the upper respiratory tract. In contrast, the esophageal epithelium is less involved.

Nails are involved and are often absent.

Characteristically, eroded lesions begin at the face, in the zygomatic areas (Figure 1.17) and can progressively reach large dimensions (Figures 1.18 and 1.19). Usually these patients die within the first year of life, but some, rare, patients with generalized cutaneous and internal disease reach the age of 10–15 years.

Non-Herlitz JEB

This subgroup is composed of two distinct clinical pictures that diverge in terms of some particular aspects.

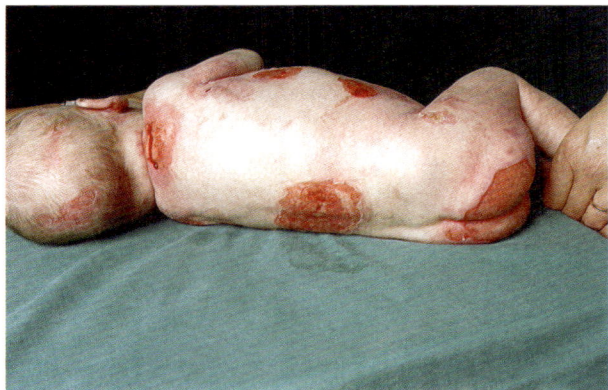

Figure 1.14

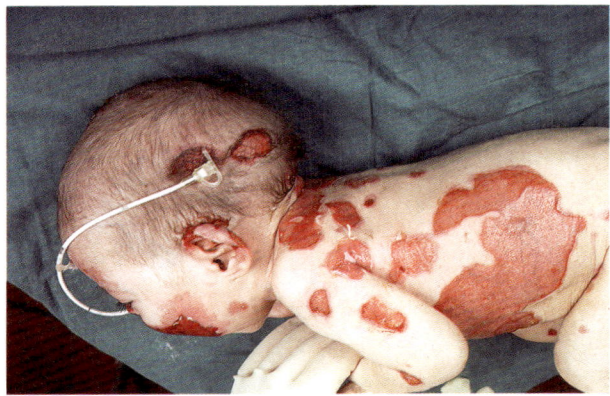

Figure 1.15

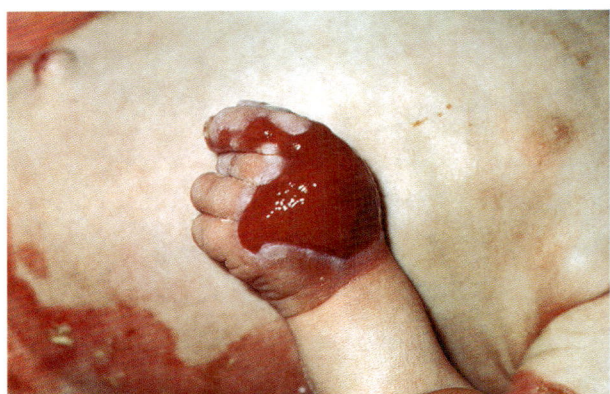

Figure 1.16

The first (related to a non-lethal defect on the laminin 5 (LAM5) gene) has generalized involvement, and the bullae are smaller and tend to heal within days (Figures 1.20–1.21). The nails are always involved and dystrophic. In particular, patients develop large ulcerated lesions on pretibial areas, due to continuous recurrence of the bullae (Figures 1.22–1.23). There is a high risk of cancer in these areas (Figure 1.23). Sudden eruptions of small

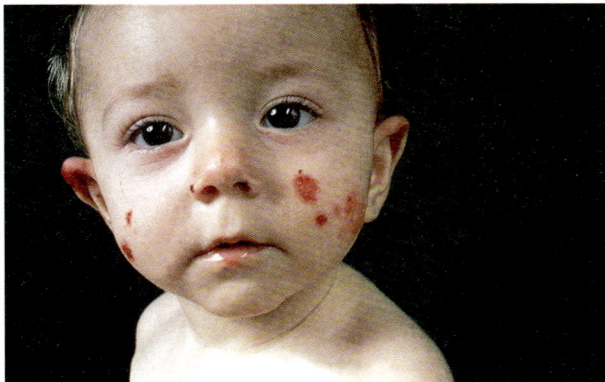

Figure 1.17

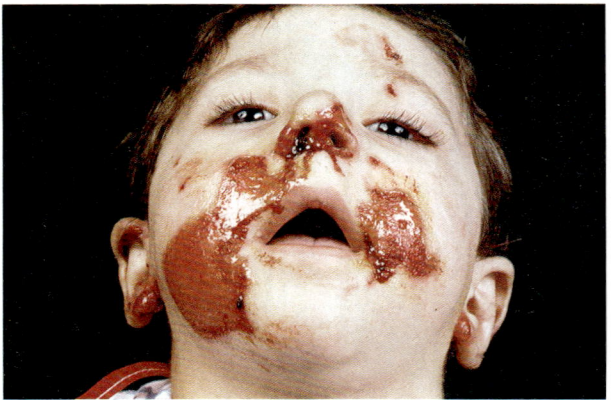

Figure 1.18

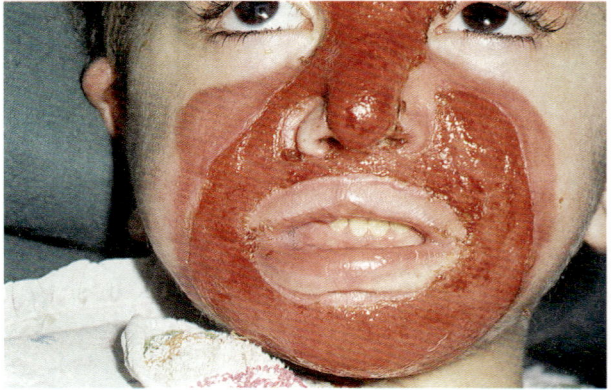

Figure 1.19

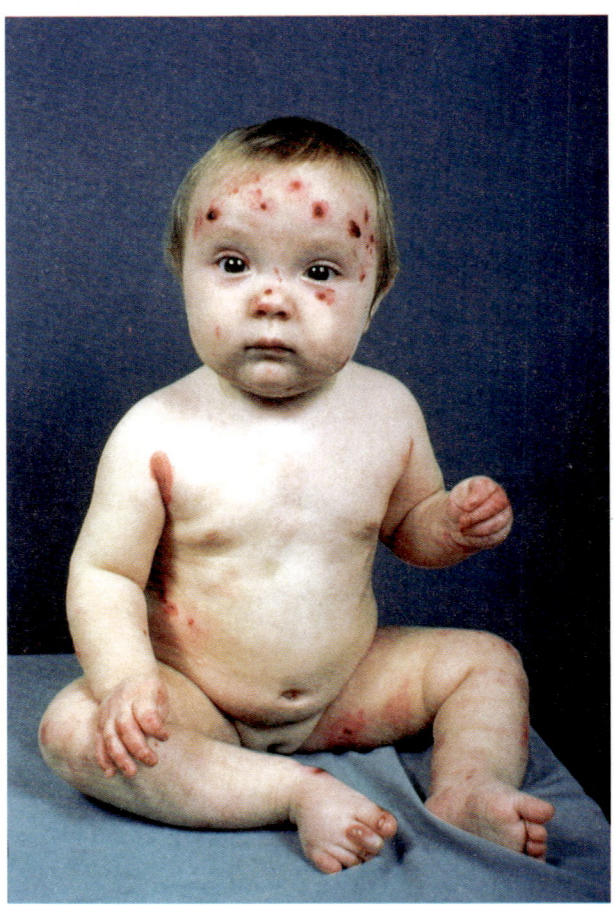

Figure 1.20

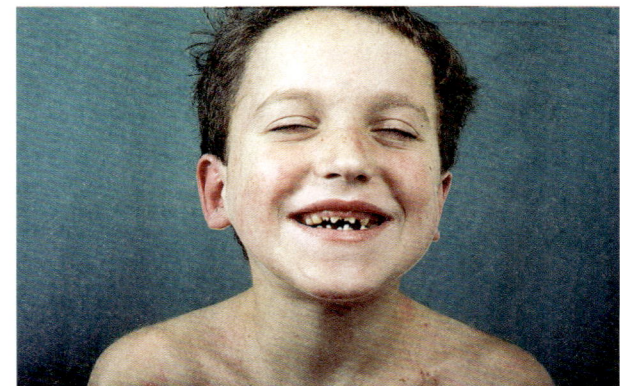

Figure 1.21

follicular blisters are possible during adolescence (Figure 1.24), as well as the development of pigmented post-bullous lesions that, at the epidiascopicic examination, are diagnosed as true melanocytic nevi. These latter may be less frequently visible in epidermolytic and dermolytic EB also (Figure 1.25).

The second group (related to mutations on the BPAG2 gene) is characterized by generalized and severe involvement (Figures 1.25–1.27) with oral mucosa and very severe dental anomalies (Figure 1.28), and especially by male-pattern-like alopecia visible in both sexes (Figure 1.29). Hands and feet are thin and long, with dystrophic or absent nails (Figure 1.30).

Despite the risk of cancer, in these patients the disease allows an almost normal life span.

Epidermolysis bullosa

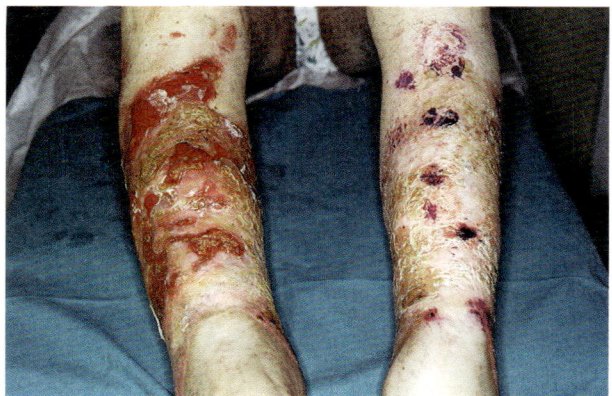

Figure 1.22

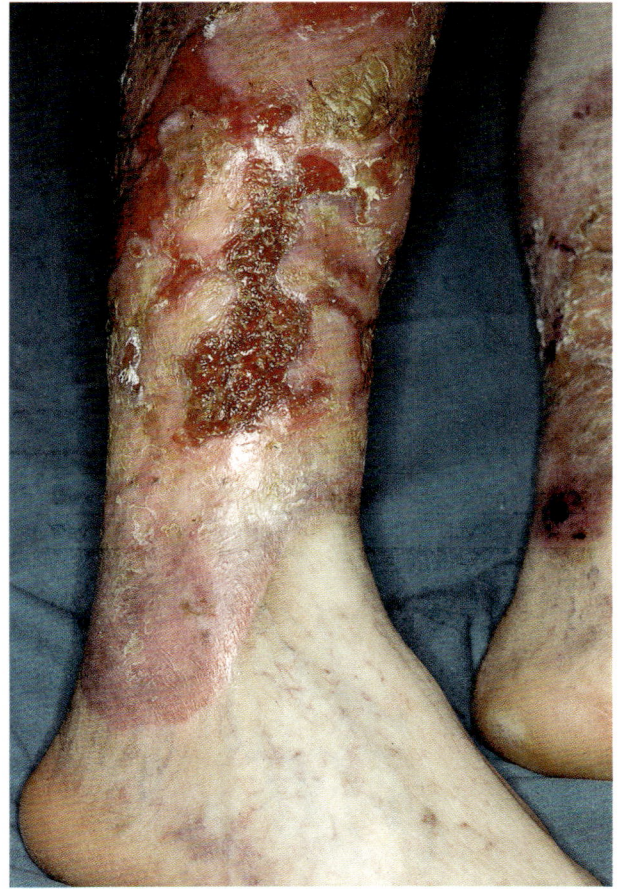

Figure 1.23

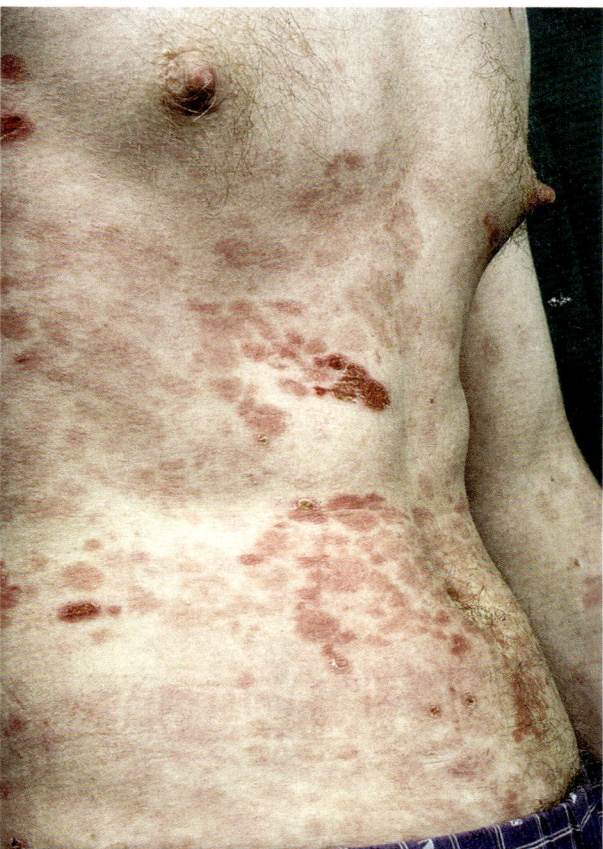

Figure 1.24

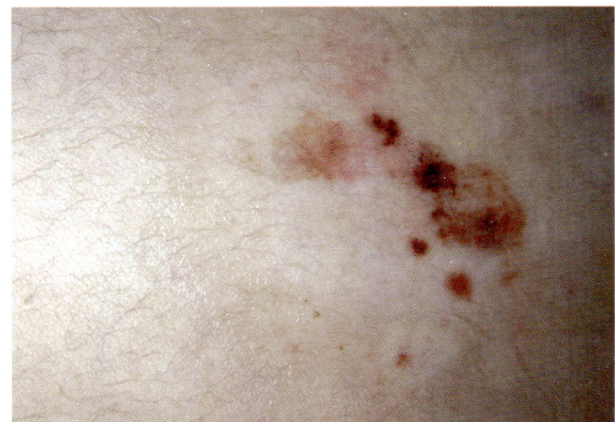

Figure 1.25

JEB with pyloric atresia

Pregnancy may be complicated by polyhydramnios. Patients are severely involved at birth (Figure 1.31) as in Herlitz JEB, and suddenly develop gastrointestinal symptoms such as intractable vomiting. X-rays without contrast demonstrate enlargement of the stomach (Figure 1.32). Pyloric reconstruction is mandatory in the first days of life. In some patients, cutaneous involvement is not so deep, allowing the recanalized patient to reach a normal life span, but usually these babies die within the first months of life.

Follow-up and therapy

- Neonatal pathology units for severely affected patients
- Antibiotics for pulmonary infections

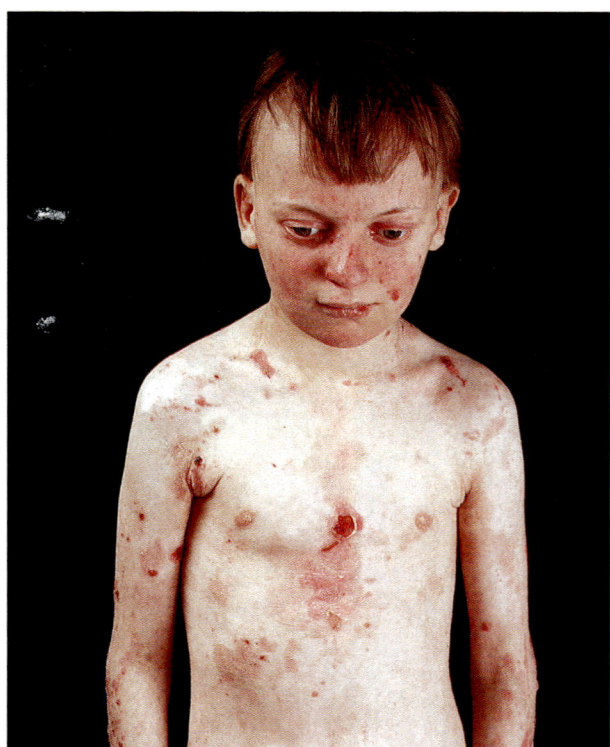

Figure 1.26

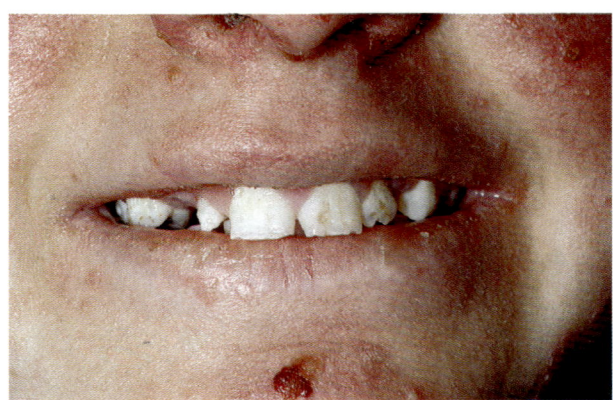

Figure 1.28

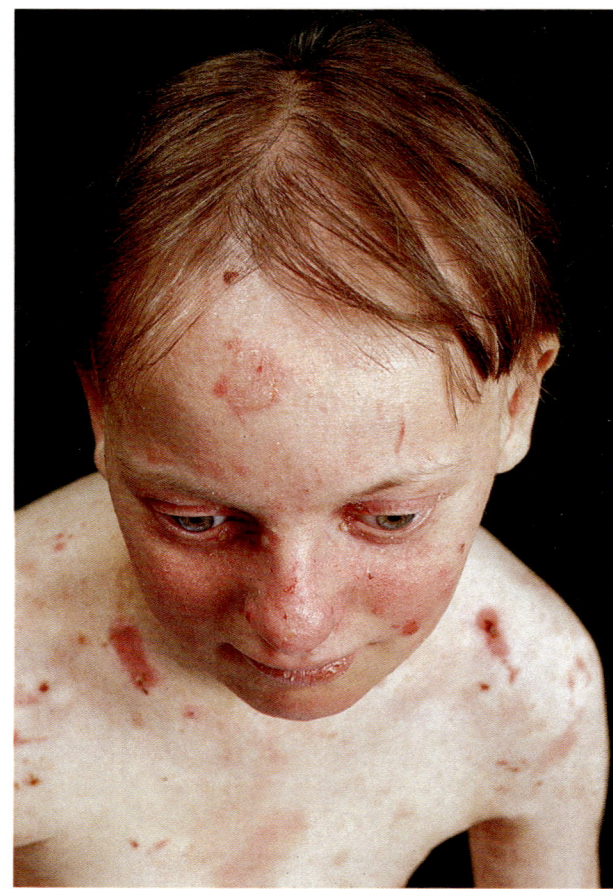

Figure 1.29

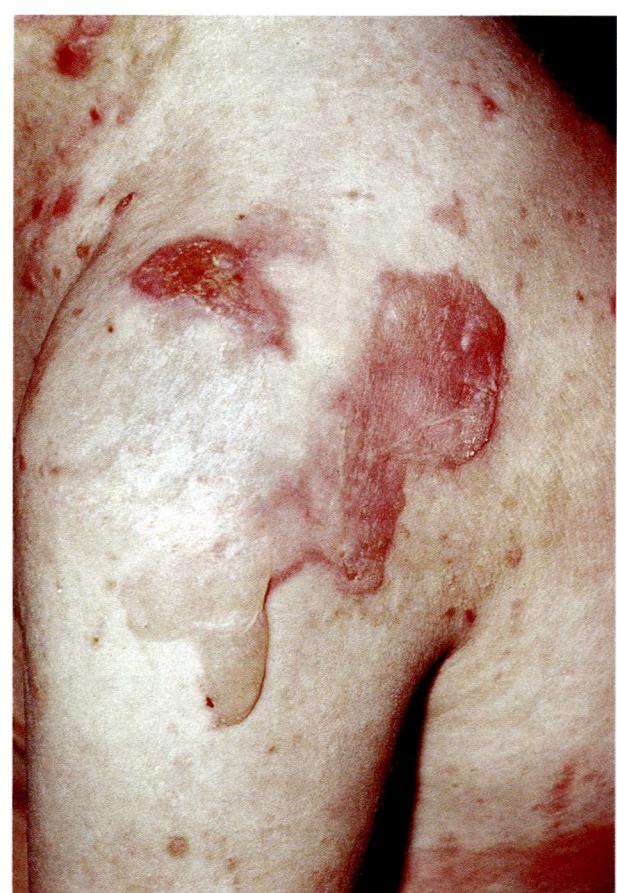

Figure 1.27

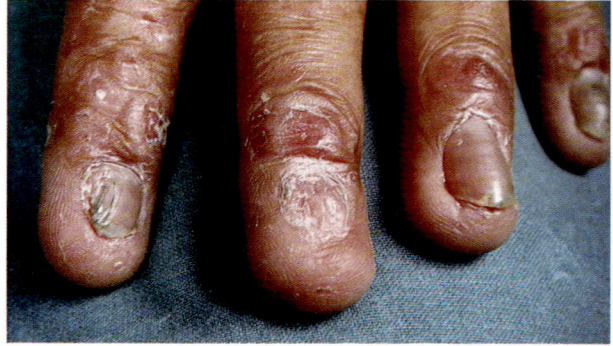

Figure 1.30

Epidermolysis bullosa

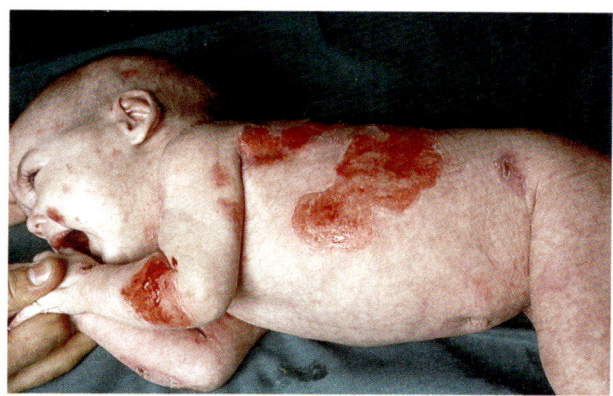

Figure 1.31

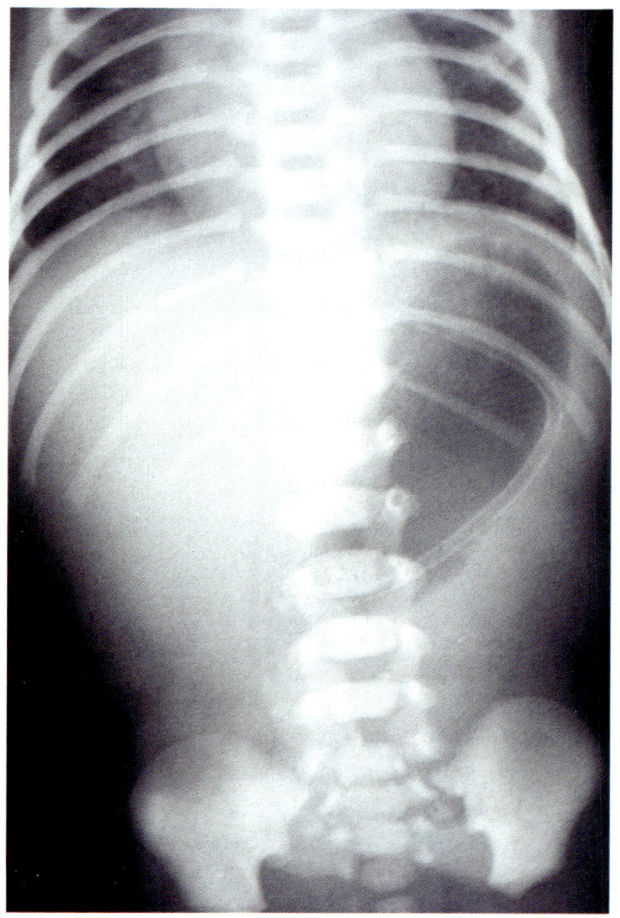

Figure 1.32

- Local antisepsis for slowly healing lesions
- Specific dressing
- Periodic (3–6 months) day-hospital for general examination
- Psychological support for patients and families
- Surgery for pyloric obstruction

DERMOLYTIC EPIDERMOLYSIS BULLOSA

Genetics and pathogenesis

Dermolytic EB can be inherited in both dominant and recessive fashion and account for more than a half of EB patients.

The underlying molecular defect is unique and is related to the COLAVII1 gene, encoding for collagen type VII, the major constituent of the anchoring fibers. The wide spectrum of severity in dermolytic EB is determined by the type of mutation in the COLAVII1 gene.

Clinical findings

Dominant inherited type

Lesions are visible at birth and are related to friction areas, especially on hands and feet, where fingers and nails are always involved (Figures 1.33–1.35). Blisters invariably cause scars and milia (Figures 1.36). During infancy and childhood, blisters are visible on the extensor surface of the hands, elbows, knees and shoulders, where they heal assuming an onion-like appearance (Figure 1.37). Nails are seldom healthy and mucosae can be heavily affected (Figure 1.38), especially in the esophageal tract, where severe strictures are possible, often in sharp contrast with the scarce cutaneous involvement. Usually, fingers and toes are not affected by major cicatricial retractions (Figure 1.39). The former albopapuloid Pasini–Pierini variant defines only a particular healing pattern of these patients (Figure 1.40).

To be defined as dominant, each dermolytic EB patient must have confirmation in the pedigree, in order to avoid the false parallelism: 'mild case = dominant, severe case = recessive' that in the past led to wrong genetic counseling.

Recessive inherited types

In the current classification two types are described as Hallopeau–Siemens type and 'non'-Hallopeau–Siemens type, indicating, respectively, the 'very severe' cases and the 'severe' cases. As previously described, the underlying different genetic defect (mutation) defines the clinical picture of the single patient, and theoretically these two types of recessive dermolytic EB are considered as a unique group of patients with a wide spectrum of phenotypes (Figures 1.41–1.48).

The 'non-Hallopeau–Siemens' subtype is defined by some related mutations leading to a 'milder'

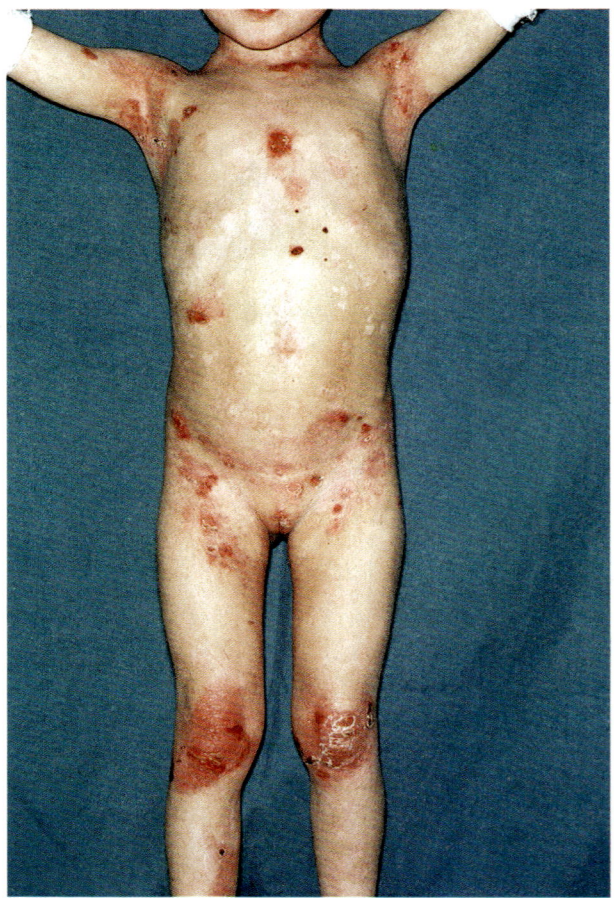

Figure 1.33

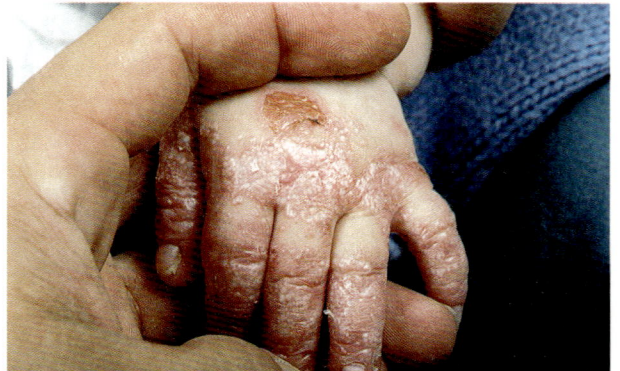

Figure 1.34

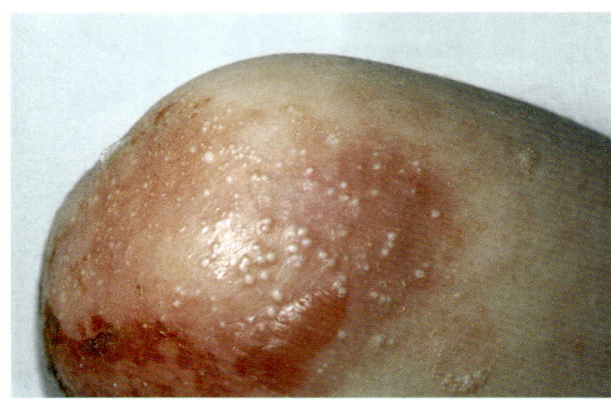

Figure 1.35

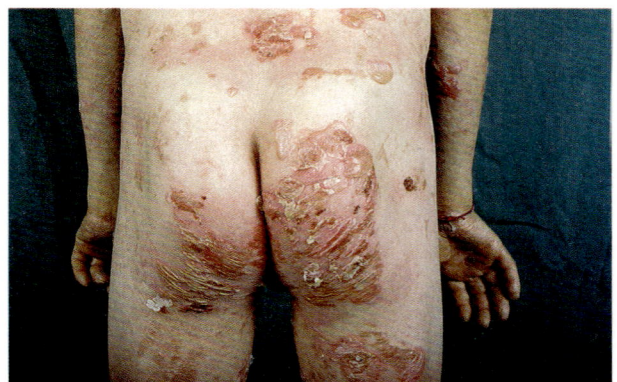

Figure 1.36

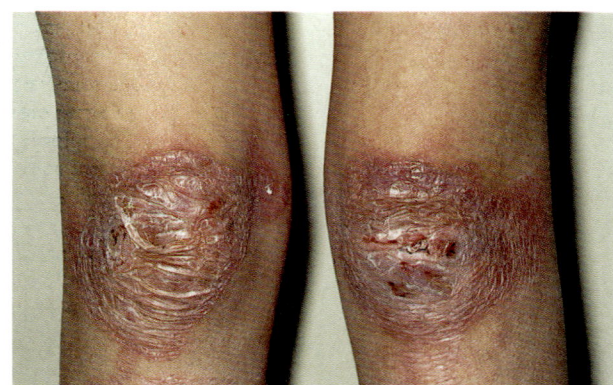

Figure 1.37

phenotype, with generalized cutaneous involvement and esophageal strictures with or without cicatricial pseudosyndactyly of the hands and feet. Cutaneous involvement and esophageal lesions allow the patients to grow following the lower centiles, and with minor food intake problems.

'Hallopeau–Siemens' patients are often linked to homozygous premature stop codon mutations, leading to a phenotype characterized by generalized cutaneous blisters and erosions that, during early infancy, lead to retractive scars of the hands and feet (pseudosyndactyly), and, later, retractions of the major joints

Epidermolysis bullosa

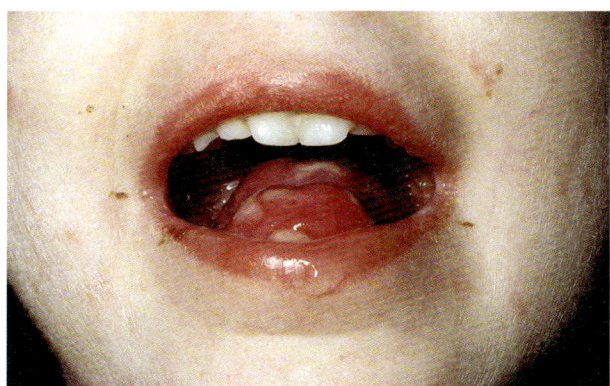

Figure 1.38

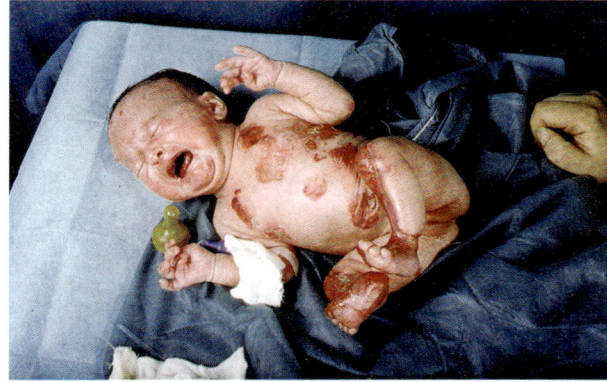

Figure 1.41

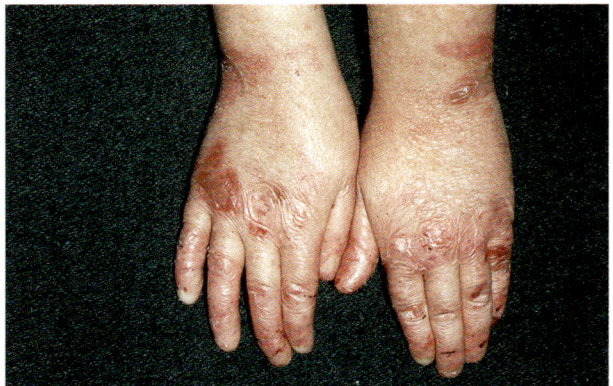

Figure 1.39

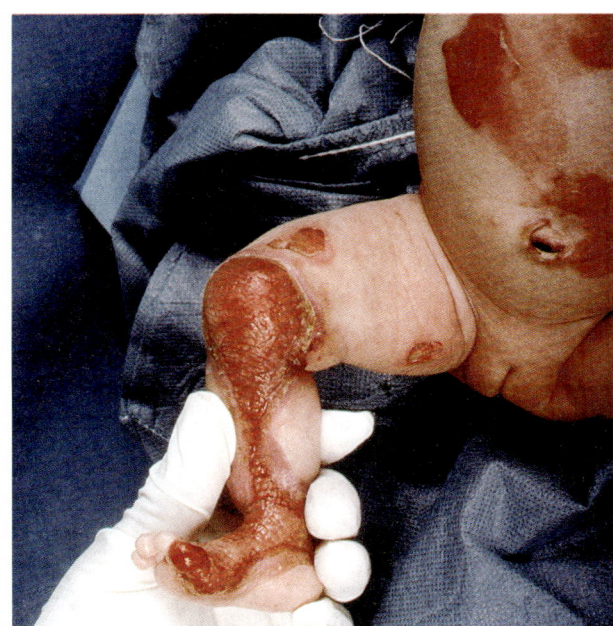

Figure 1.42

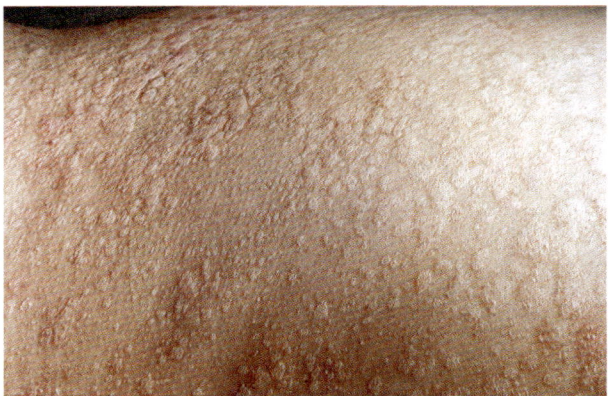

Figure 1.40

of the arms and legs that cause, in adolescence, an almost complete inability to stand up correctly. The hands are deeply affected, and in extreme cases resemble a bag or a pouch.

Mucosae are heavily involved, with oral, pharyngeal and esophageal scarring leading to dramatic strictures and related low capacity for food intake that, together with chronic blood loss from the erosions and ulcers, cause severe anemia. Usually these patients have hemoglobin levels ranging from 4 to 8 g/100 ml.

The risk of cancer is very high, and squamocellular carcinoma is the major cause of death in these patients who have an expectancy of life to around the third–fourth decade (Figure 1.49).

Less frequently patients may develop a clinical picture with a 'nodular prurigo' pattern, associated with severe itching, especially on the lower trunk and legs (Figures 1.50 and 1.51). This presentation is rare, and may be related to the presence of autoantibodies against collagen VII protein.

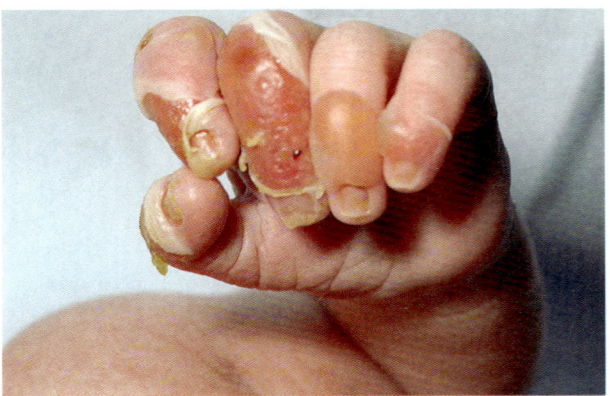

Figure 1.43

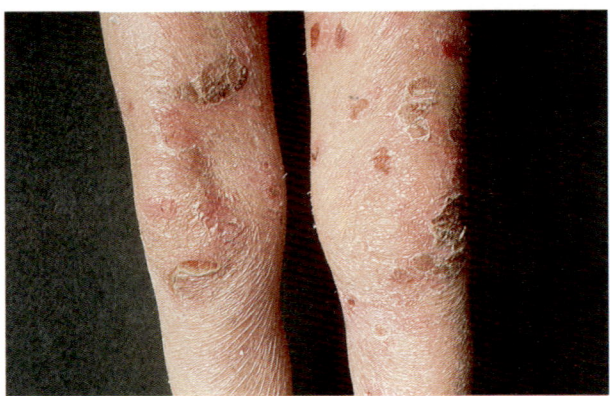

Figure 1.45

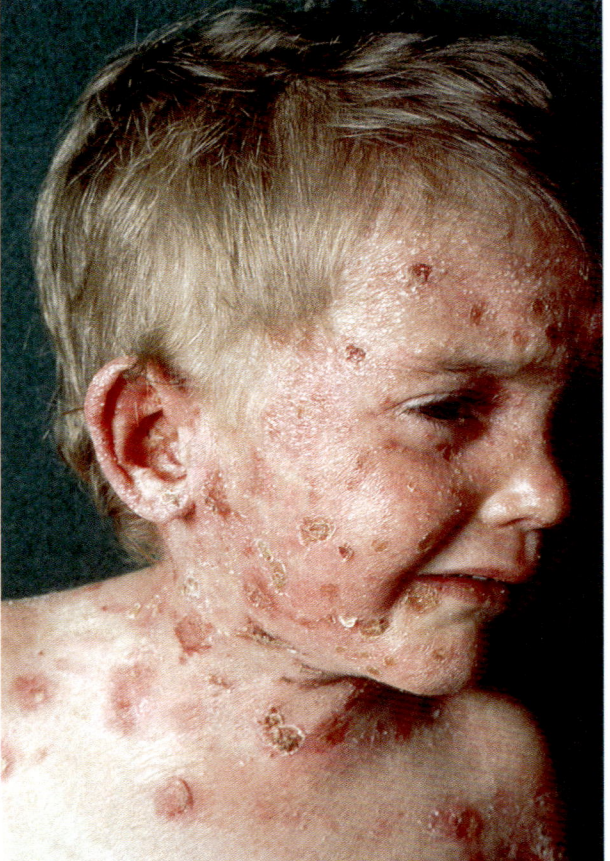

Figure 1.44

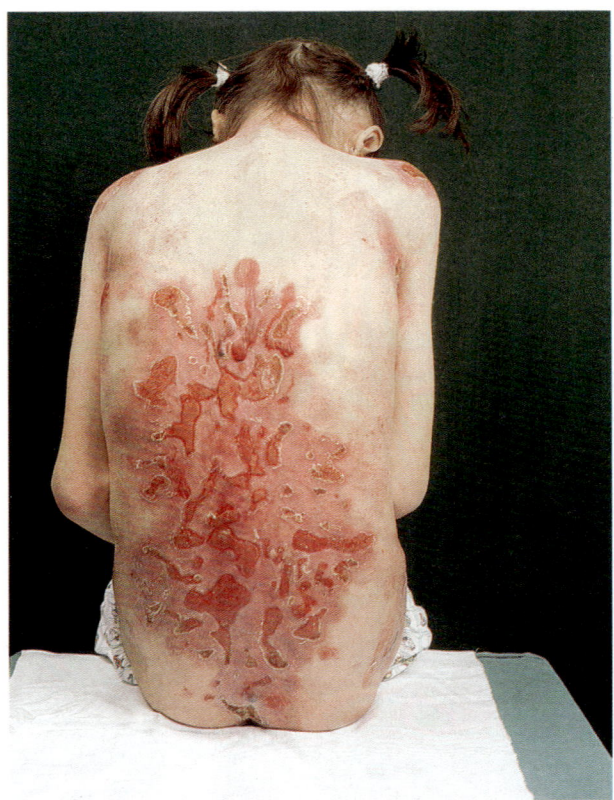

Figure 1.46

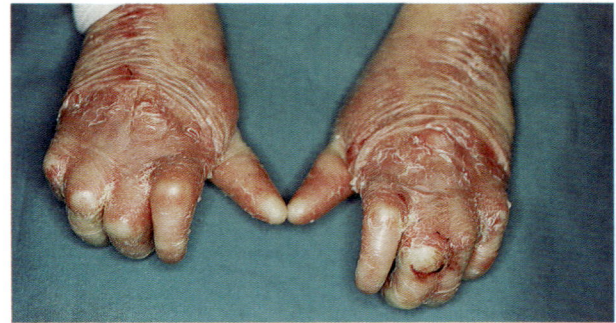

Figure 1.47

Follow-up

- Check every 3–6 months for clinical status (especially for skin cancer)
- Blood examinations for hemoglobin and electrolytes and proteins
- Bacteriological samples for infections
- Radiography for hands and feet deformities

Epidermolysis bullosa

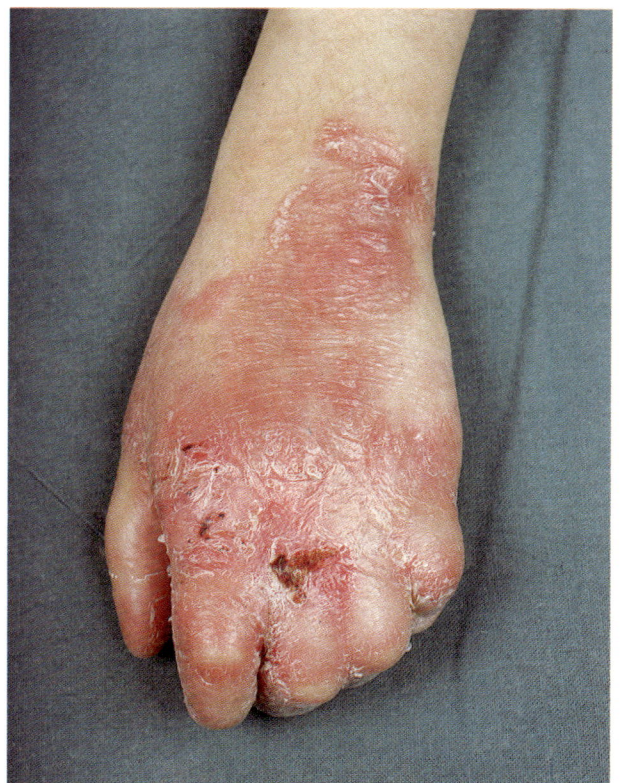

Figure 1.48

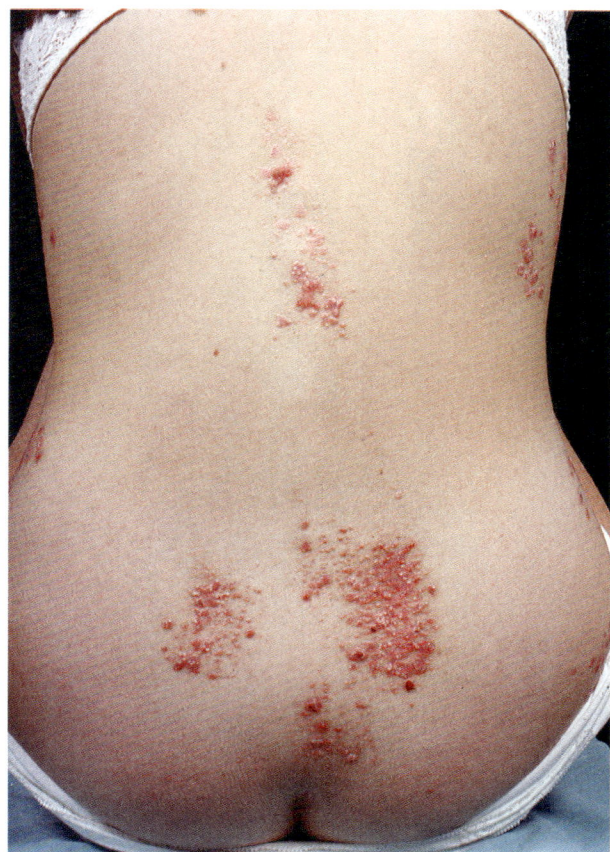

Figure 1.50

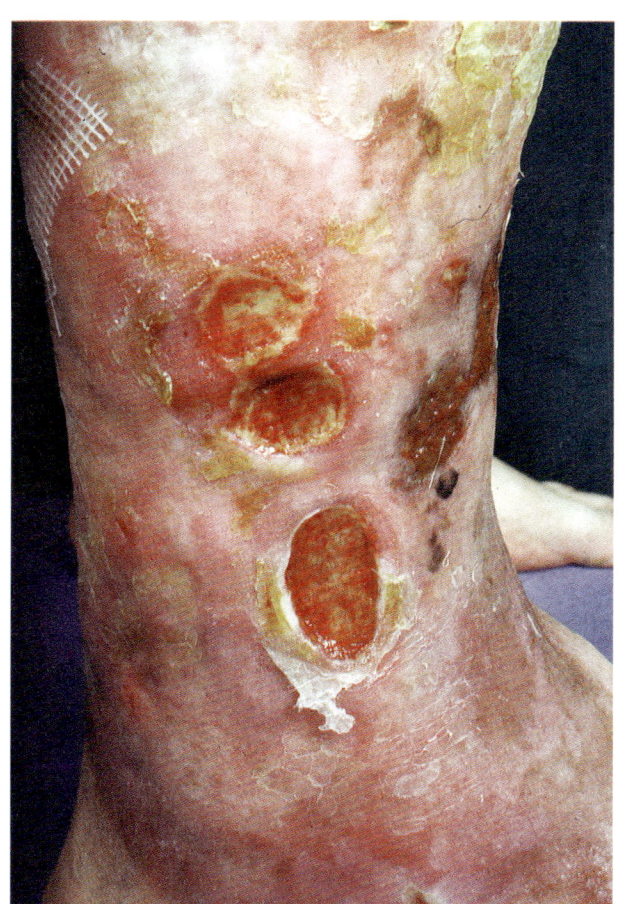

Figure 1.49

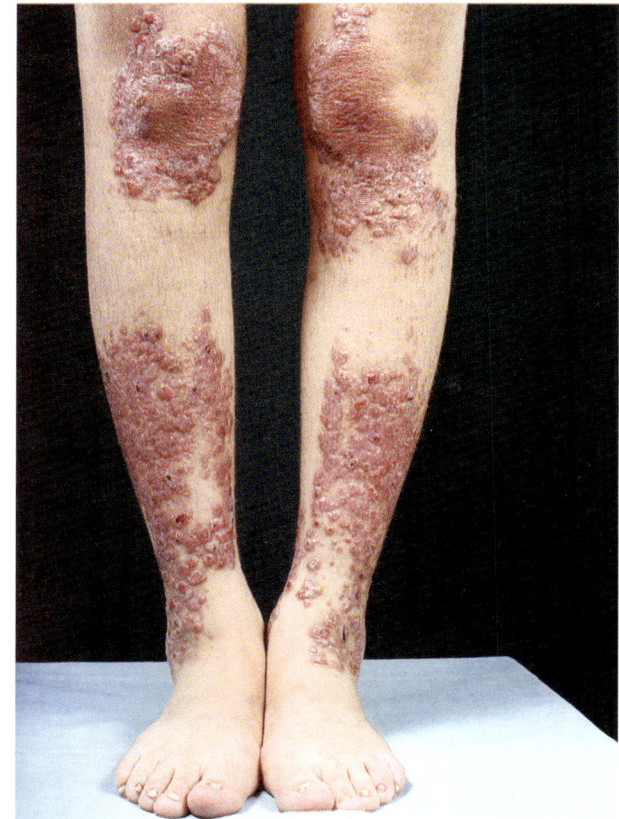

Figure 1.51

- Radiography for esophageal strictures
- Multidisciplinary approach:
  - odontostomatology for caries and oral erosions
  - pediatrics for anemia, renal insufficiency and nutrition
  - physiotherapy for hands, feet and joints
  - plastic and hand surgeons for correction of pseudosyndactyly
  - urologist and gynecologist for urethral and vulvar restrictions
  - thoracic surgeon for esophageal dilatation

Therapy

- Antiseptic local therapy
- Special dressings and gauzes
- Antibiotic therapy, local and systemic
- Human recombinant erythropoietin and iron for anemia
- Vaccines (especially for varicella and measles)
- Surgical treatment for scars on hands (and feet)
- Surgical treatment for skin tumors
- Genetic therapy

Differential diagnosis of all types of hereditary EB

- Kindler's syndrome
- Epidermolytic hyperkeratosis
- Congenital syphilis
- Congenital bullous autoimmune disease

REFERENCES

Baudoin C, Miquel C, Cagnoux-Palacios L, et al. A novel homozygous nonsense mutation in the LAMC2 gene in patients with the Herlitz junctional epidermolysis bullosa. Hum Mol Genet 1994; 3: 1909–10

Brown TA, Gil SG, Sybert VP, et al. Defective integrin alpha 6 beta 4 expression in the skin of patients with junctional epidermolysis bullosa and pyloric atresia. J Invest Dermatol 1996; 107: 384–91. Erratum in J Invest Dermatol 1997; 108: 237

Cambiaghi S, Brusasco A, Restano L, et al. Epidermolysis bullosa pruriginosa. Dermatology 1997; 195: 65–8

Chavanas S, Gache Y, Tadini G, et al. A homozygous in-frame deletion in the collagenous domain of bullous pemphigoid antigen BP180 (type XVII collagen) causes generalized atrophic benign epidermolysis bullosa. J Invest Dermatol 1997; 109: 74–8

Fine JD, Eady RA, Bauer EA, et al. Revised classification system for inherited epidermolysis bullosa: report of the Second International Consensus Meeting on diagnosis and classification of epidermolysis bullosa. J Am Acad Dermatol 2000; 42: 1051–66

Gardella R, Barlati S, Zoppi N, et al. A-96C→T mutation in the promoter of the collagen type VII gene (COL7A1) abolishing transcription in a patient affected by recessive dystrophic epidermolysis bullosa. Hum Mutat 2000; 16: 275

Gardella R, Castiglia D, Posteraro P, et al. Genotype–phenotype correlation in Italian patients with dystrophic epidermolysis bullosa. J Invest Dermatol 2002; 119: 1456–62

Gardella R, Nuytinck L, Barlati S, et al. Characterization of mutations leading to recessive dystrophic epidermolysis bullosa and Marfan syndrome in a single patient. Clin Exp Dermatol 2001; 26: 710–13

Gardella R, Zoppi N, Ferraboli S, et al. Three homozygous PTC mutations in the collagen type VII gene of patients affected by recessive dystrophic epidermolysis bullosa: analysis of transcript levels in dermal fibroblasts. Hum Mutat 1999; 13: 439–52

Tadini G, Ermacora E, Cambiaghi S, et al. Positive response to 5TH-2 antagonists in a family affected by epidermolysis bullosa Dowling–Meara type. Dermatology 1993; 186: 80

Tadini G, Kanitakis J, Cavalli R, et al. Altered expression of a new antigen of the dermal–epidermal junction (NU-T2 DEJ Ag) in junctional epidermolysis bullosa. Arch Dermatol Res 1995; 287: 699–704

Turco AE, Peissel B, Rossetti S, et al. Prenatal testing in a fetus at risk for autosomal dominant polycystic kidney disease and autosomal recessive junctional epidermolysis bullosa with pyloric atresia. Am J Med Genet 1993; 47: 1225–30

CHAPTER 2

Epidermolytic hyperkeratoses

'CLASSICAL' EPIDERMOLYTIC HYPERKERATOSIS

Synonym

- Bullous ichthyosiform erythroderma

Age of onset

- At birth

Epidemiology

Even though it is a well-known and established disease, there is no accurate study of incidence and prevalence. The estimated prevalence is 1 : 200 000–300 000.

Clinical findings

A collodion baby presentation at birth is frequent but the film is rarely complete and fades within a few hours or days, leaving an erythematous and fine scaling pattern with superficial bullae and erosions (Figure 2.1). Nevertheless, the number of blisters is low, owing to the fragility of the blister roof (Figure 2.2). Bullae are visible in the first years of life, leading to a picture with bright erythema, superficial erosions and desquamation (Figure 2.3). As years go by the hyperkeratosis prevails, showing a peculiar pattern of enhancement of the cutaneous ridges with a particular seborrheic-yellowish aspect especially visible on major folds (axillary pillars, neck) (Figures 2.4–2.6).

In some rare cases the hyperkeratosis becomes grayish (Figures 2.7 and 2.8) and in some cases black and vegetant, covering the whole body with a thick, papillomatous shell, leading to a pattern known in the past as 'ichthyosis hystrix' (Figure 2.9).

In adulthood there is a sort of evolutive polymorphism that includes, in the same subject, hyperkeratosis, erosions and erythema, while bullae are absent.

Patients have a characteristic acute and unpleasantly sweetish smell due to fermentation of the bacteria

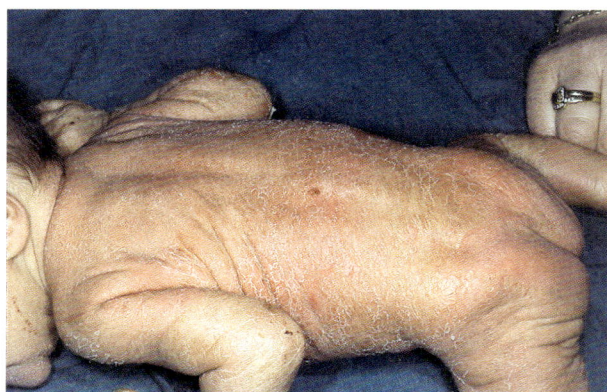

Figure 2.1

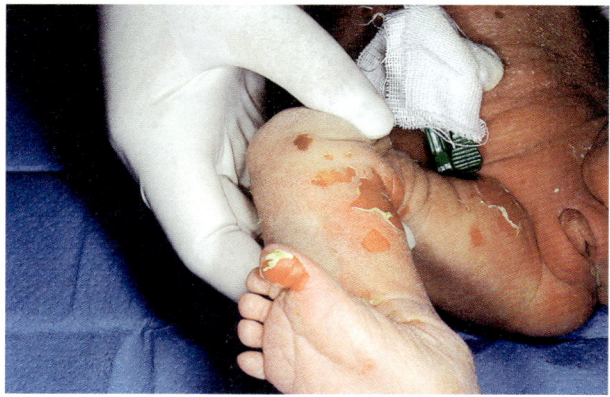

Figure 2.2

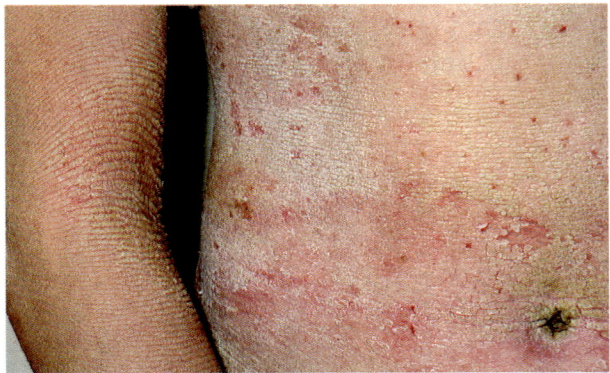

Figure 2.3

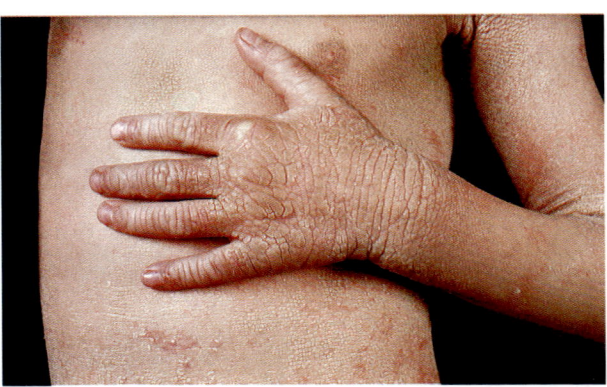

Figure 2.6

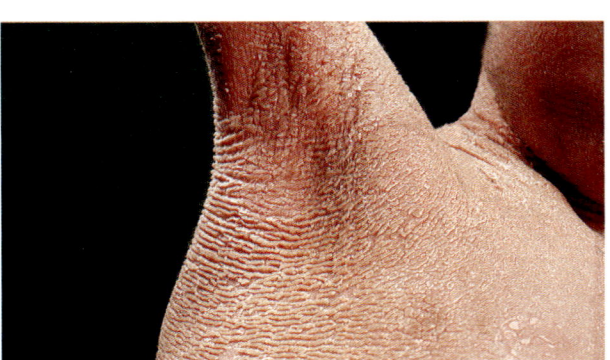

Figure 2.4

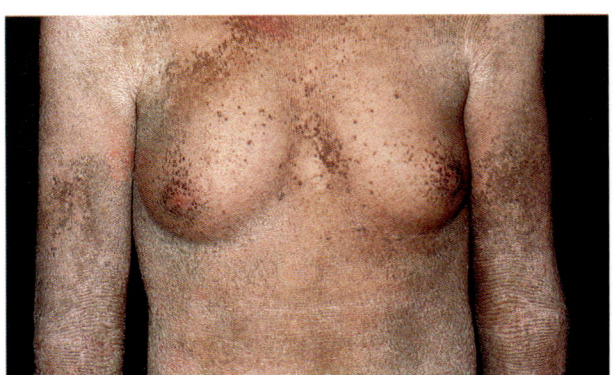

Figure 2.7

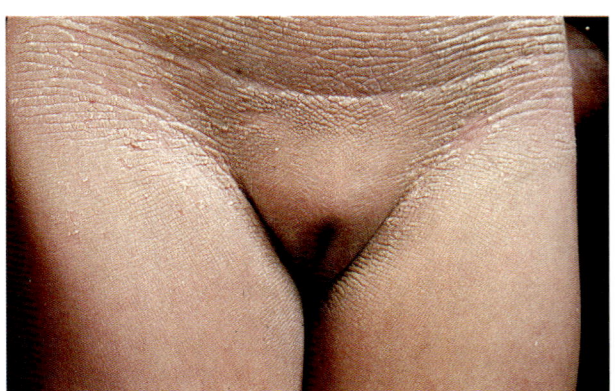

Figure 2.5

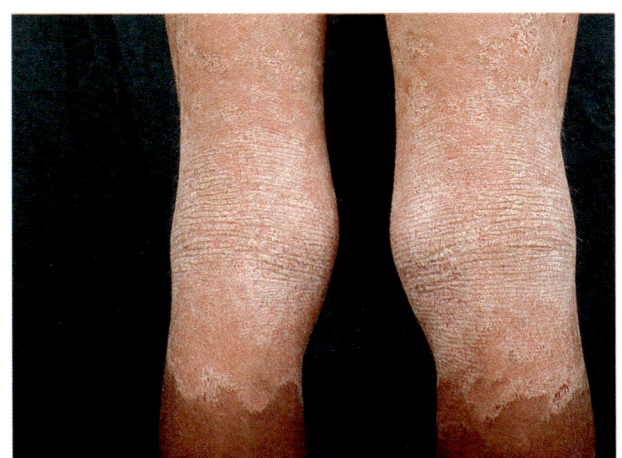

Figure 2.8

in such a pabulum. The scalp is always involved (Figure 2.10), but in contrast the palms and soles appear less affected (Figures 2.11 and 2.12).

Epidermolytic hyperkeratosis (EH) is present also in a mosaic pattern as 'epidermolytic (acantholytic) nevus', and may be isolated or diffuse (Figures 2.13 and 2.14). In the latter case gonadic involvement is possible, leading to a rare pedigree in which a parent with diffuse linear EH gives birth to a child affected by epidermolytic hyperkeratosis (see cutaneous mosaicism, Chapter 25).

Epidermolytic hyperkeratoses

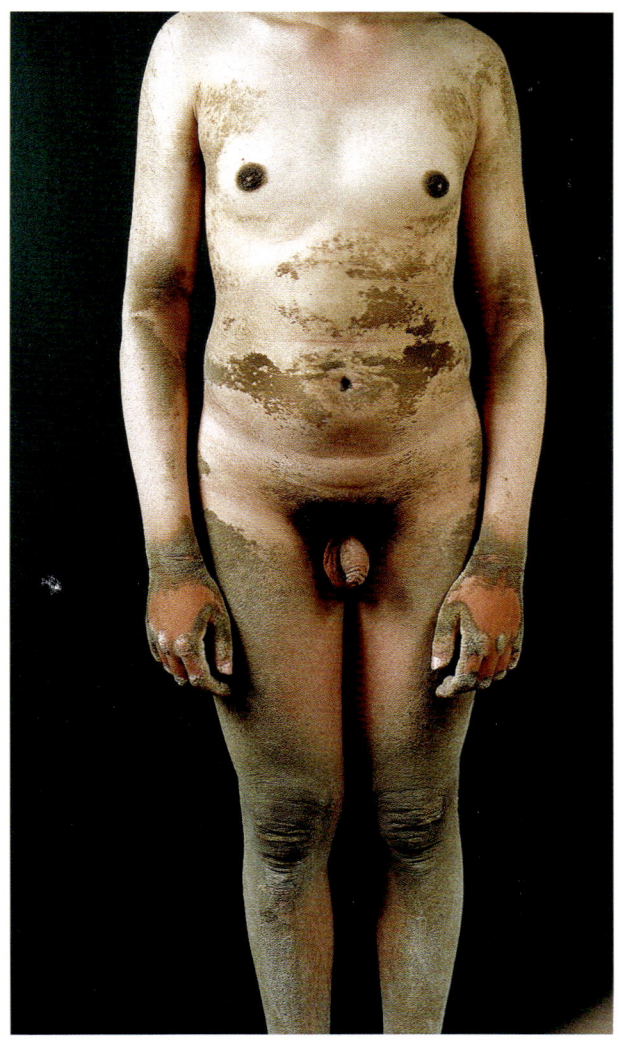

Figure 2.9

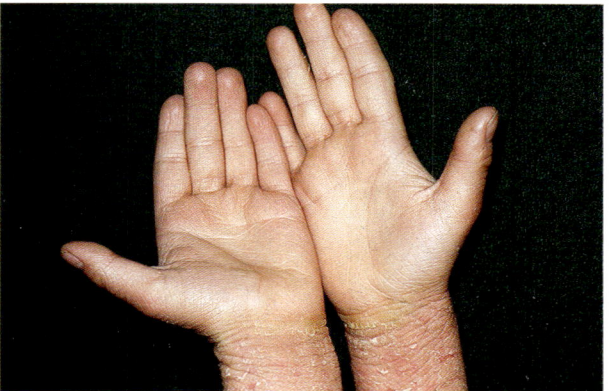

Figure 2.11

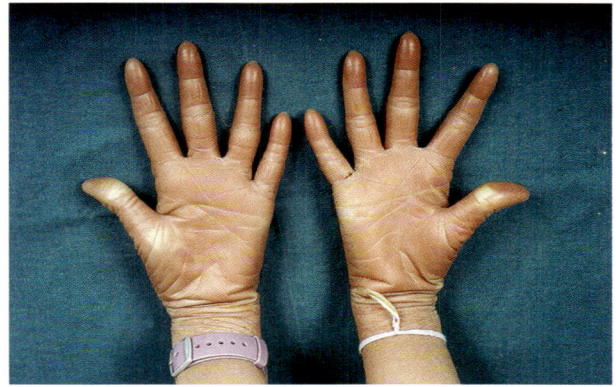

Figure 2.12

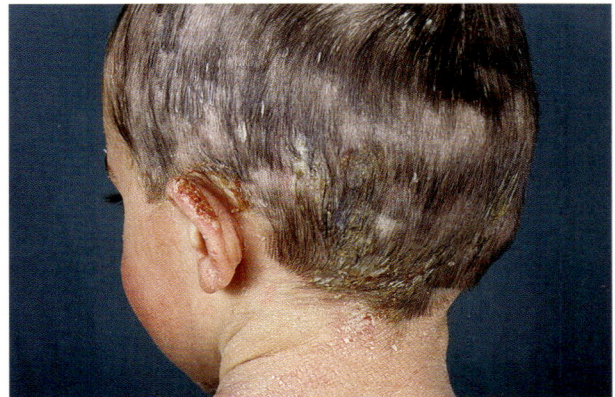

Figure 2.10

Extracutaneous symptoms and complications

- Pyogenic infections
- Sepsis
- Impaired thermoregulation
- Social discomfort

Course

- Lifelong and steady

Laboratory findings

Histologically there is a pattern, including acantholysis in the stratum spinosum, with hyperkeratosis and a 'gothic church' aspect. Ultrastructurally, cytolysis and filament clumping are visible in the suprabasal layers, with an increased number of corneocyte sheets.

Genetics and pathogenesis

EH is due to mutations in two differentiation keratins, namely K1 and K10.

There is some hot-spot in these genes for the more frequent mutations causing EH.

Mutated keratins are not able to polymerize and to create the ultimate keratin filaments.

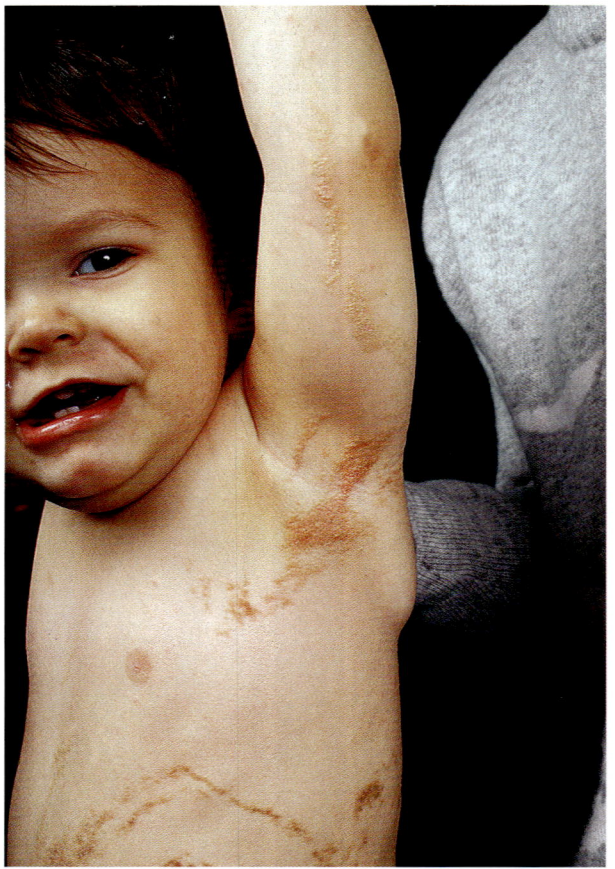

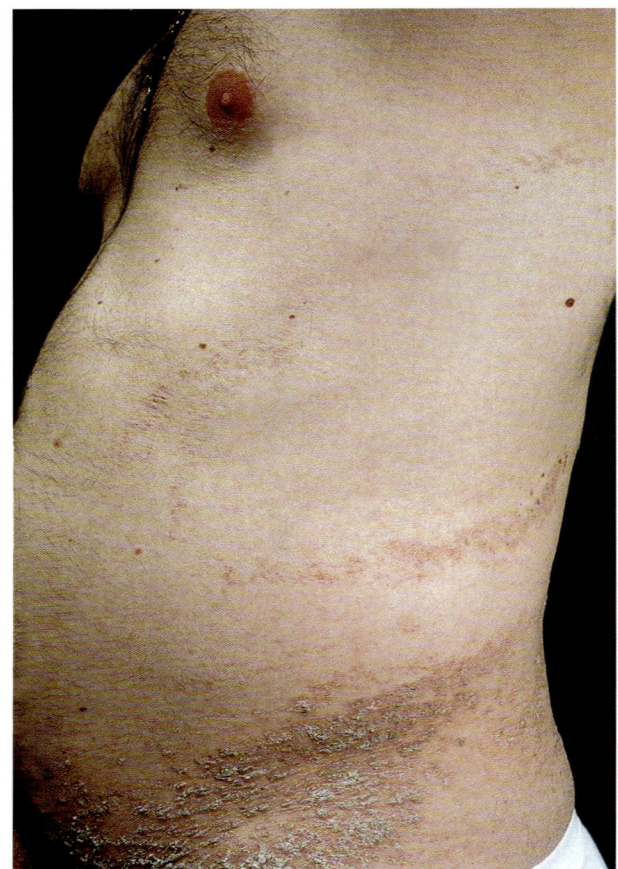

Figure 2.13

Figure 2.14

Keratins appear as 'balls' or 'clumps' that are dynamically unable to cope with mechanical stress, leading to blister formation and erosions.

In the same way, an abnormal keratin substrate does not allow the formation of a physiological stratum corneum.

Differential diagnosis

- Lamellar ichthyosis
- Ichthyosis bullosa of Siemens
- Epidermolysis bullosa
- Netherton's disease
- Omenn's disease

Follow-up

- Assessment for topical therapy
- Periodic bacteriological examination with antibiogram to detect infections

Therapy

- Emollients and mild keratolytic agents
- Antibiotics for cutaneous infections
- Retinoids may be useful in some cases

REFERENCES

Paller AS, Syder AJ, Chan YM, et al. Genetic and clinical mosaicism in a type of epidermal nevus. N Engl J Med 1994; 331: 1408–15

Porter RM, Lane EB. Phenotypes, genotypes and their contribution to understanding keratin function. Trends Genet 2003; 19: 278–85

Vahlquist A, Ganemo A, Pigg M, et al. The clinical spectrum of congenital ichthyosis in Sweden: a review of 127 cases. Acta Derm Venereol (Stockh) 2003; 213 Suppl: 34–47

Virtanen M, Smith SK, Gedde-Dahl T Jr, et al. Splice site and deletion mutations in keratin (KRT1 and KRT10) genes: unusual phenotypic alterations in Scandinavian patients with epidermolytic hyperkeratosis. J Invest Dermatol 2003; 121: 1013–20

ICHTHYOSIS BULLOSA OF SIEMENS

Age of onset

- At birth

Epidemiology

There are no available data. The estimated prevalence is 1 : 500 000.

Clinical findings

At birth, a collodion-like presentation is possible.

Ichthyosis bullosa of Siemens (IBS) is defined by a picture of superficial hyperkeratosis and erosions with rare bullae in the first years of life. The pattern of diffuse, fine scaling and the contemporaneous presence of desquamative ovalar ridges is called 'mauserung', and is typical of IBS (Figures 2.15–2.17).

Palmoplantar keratoderma is always present, as well as involvement of the scalp.

Nails can be dystrophic.

These patients may have a discomfiting, sweetish macerative odor.

Extracutaneous symptoms and complications

- Infections by pyogenes bacteria
- Osseous remodeling in severe palmoplantar keratoderma

Course

A progressive amelioration of symptoms with age is reported.

Laboratory findings, genetics and pathogenesis

The disease is due to mutations in the keratin 2e gene and is autosomal dominant.

Keratin 2e is expressed in the final steps of differentiation. These mutations cause instability of the keratin network and abnormalities in the formation of the corneocyte envelope.

Differential diagnosis

- Epidermolytic hyperkeratosis
- Ichthyoses

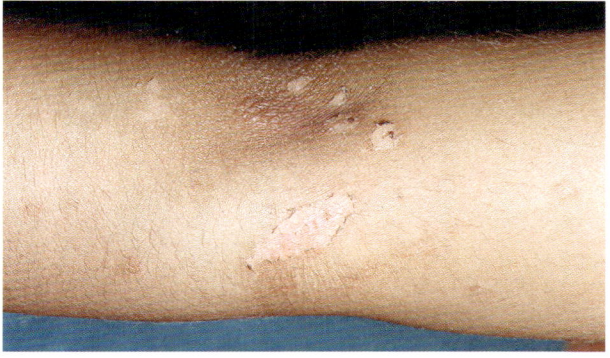

Figure 2.15

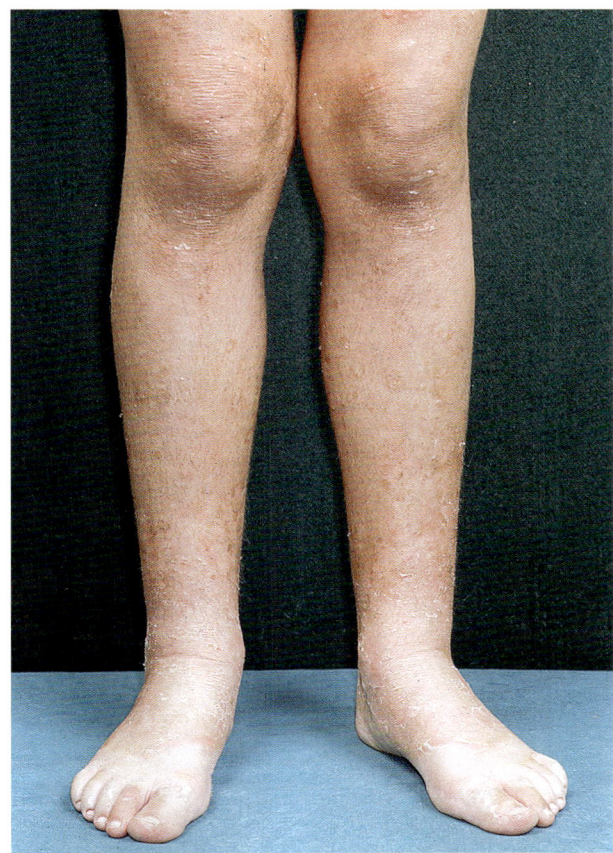

Figure 2.16

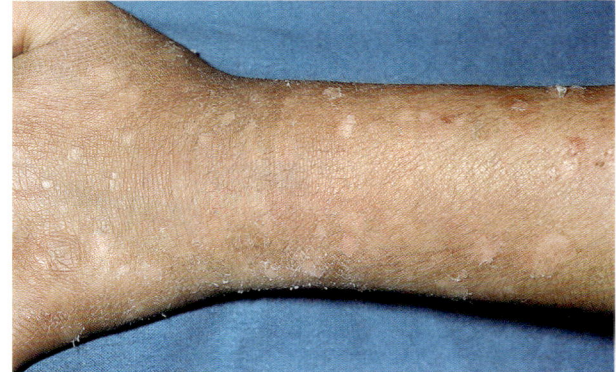

Figure 2.17

Follow-up and therapy

- Assessment for cutaneous infections
- Topical emollients and keratolytics
- In severe cases oral retinoids are advised

REFERENCES

Kremer H, Zeeuwen P, McLean WH, et al. Ichthyosis bullosa of Siemens is caused by mutations in the keratin 2e gene. Invest Dermatol 1994; 103: 286–9

McLean WH, Morley SM, Lane EB, et al. Ichthyosis bullosa of Siemens – a disease involving keratin 2e. J Invest Dermatol 1994; 103: 277–81

Smith F. The molecular genetics of keratin disorders. Am J Clin Dermatol 2003; 4: 347–64

ICHTHYOSIS CURTH–MACKLIN

Synonym

It has been described as and confused with ichthyosis hystrix, which, on the contrary, is associated with severe cases of EH.

Epidemiology

The disease is very rare, with an estimated prevalence of 1 : 500 000–1 : 1 000 000

Clinical findings

True Curth–Macklin (CM) cases have diffuse fine scaling with brown-grayish cerebriform hyperkeratotic plaques on extensor surfaces, especially on elbows and knees (Figures 2.18–2.21).

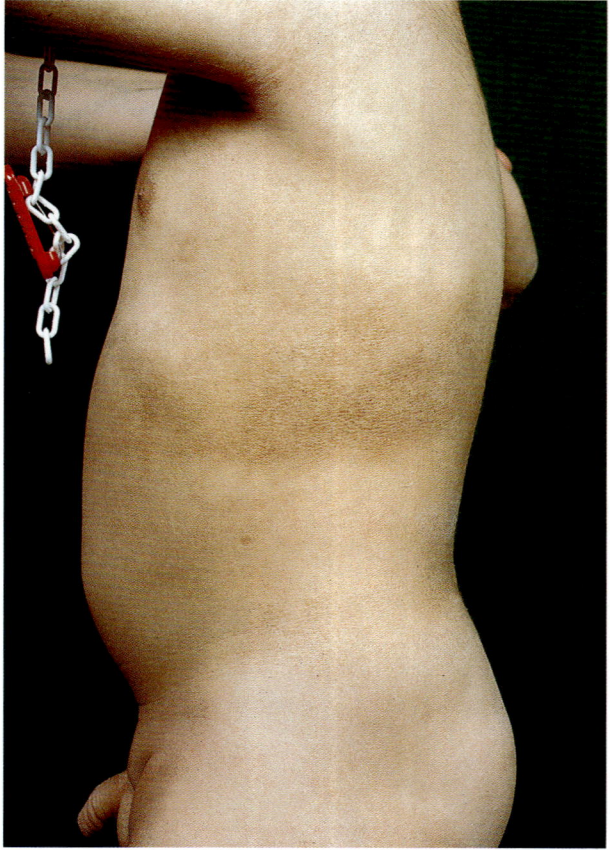

Figure 2.18

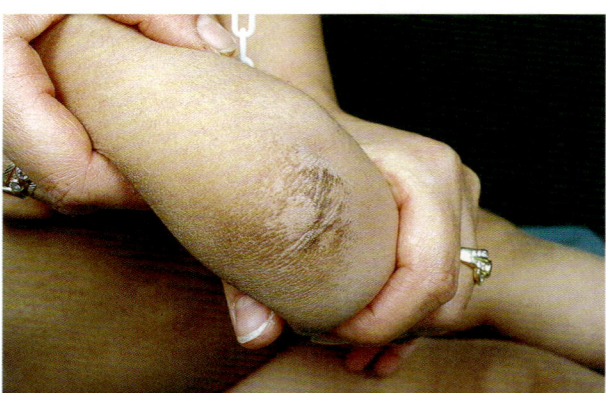

Figure 2.19

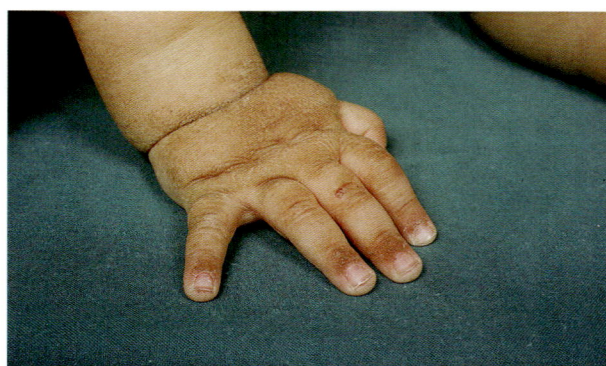

Figure 2.20

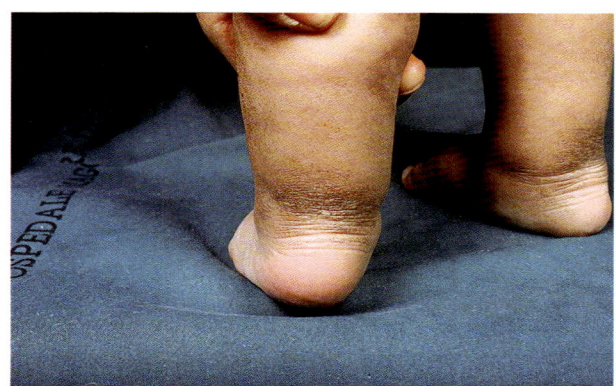

Figure 2.21

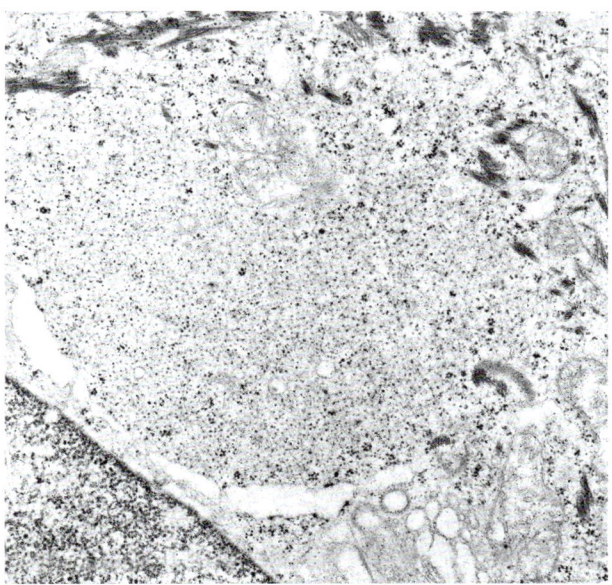

Figure 2.22

Palmoplantar areas and scalp are involved, and nails may be thickened.

The face may be erythematous.

Extracutaneous symptoms and complications

Rarely, these patients may experience cutaneous infections.

Course

- Lifelong

Laboratory findings

The ultrastructure defines the diagnosis, showing binucleated cells and perinuclear shells that are pathognomonic (Figure 2.22).

Genetics and pathogenesis

CM is inherited as an autosomal dominat trait. Keratin 1 gene mutations are responsible in the pathogenesis of the disease, making Curth–Macklin disease a mere variant of classic epidermolytic hyperkeratosis.

Differential diagnosis

- Epidermolytic hyperkeratosis
- Ichthyoses

Follow-up and therapy

- Emollients and keratolytics are needed

REFERENCES

Brusasco A, Cavalli R, Cambiaghi S, et al. Ichthyosis Curth–Macklin: a new sporadic case with immunohistochemical study of keratin expression. Arch Dermatol 1994; 130: 1077–9

Ishida-Yamamoto A, Richard G, Takahashi H, Iizuka H. In vivo studies of mutant keratin 1 in ichthyosis hystrix Curth–Macklin. J Invest Dematol 2003; 120: 498–500

Ishida-Yamamoto A, Takahashi H, Iizuka H. Lessons from disorders of epidermal differentiation-associated keratins. Histol Histopathol 2002; 17: 331–8. Review

'STELLATE' EPIDERMOLYTIC HYPERKERATOSIS

Epidemiology

Fewer than five reports in the literature tend to separate this entity from classic EH.

Age of onset

- At birth

Clinical findings

- Collodion presentation
- Generalized erythema
- In antecubital fossae and cavi poplitei progressive eruption of 'stellate' grouping of hyperkeratotic streaks (Figures 2.23 and 2.24)
- Cerebriform appearance of knees and elbows (Figure 2.25)
- Marked erythema and thickening on the dorsa of hands (Figure 2.26) and feet

Extracutaneous findings

- None

Course and prognosis

- The disease is slowly progressive

Laboratory findings

Upon ultrastructural examination there are small foci of acantholysis, but without massive clumping or perinuclear shells as evident in classic EH or Curth–Macklin disease.

Genetics and pathogenesis

The disease is autosomal dominant. Mutations on K1 or K10 genes are probable.

Follow-up and therapy

Emollients and keratolytic agents may be useful, as well as calcipotriol.

Retinoid therapy can be used as an alternative.

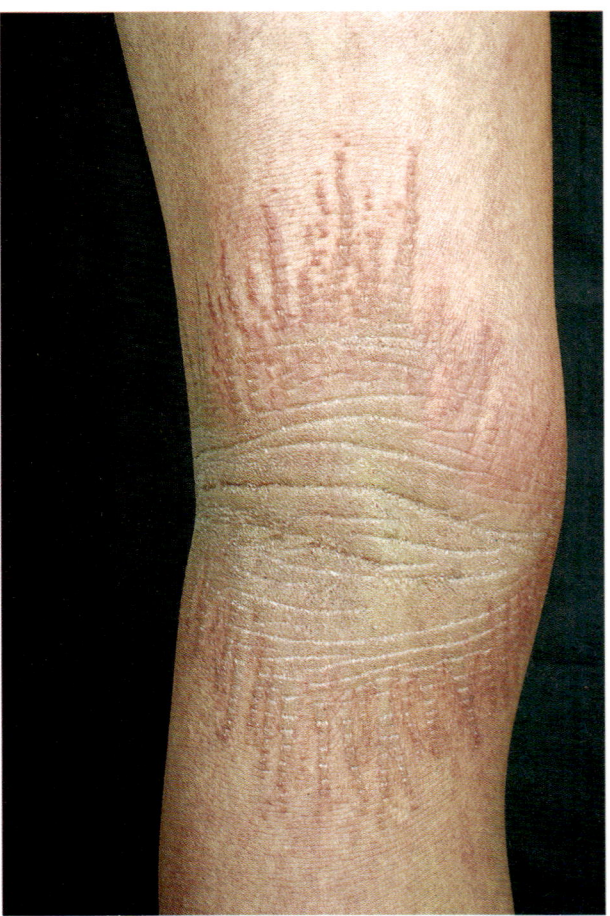

Figure 2.23

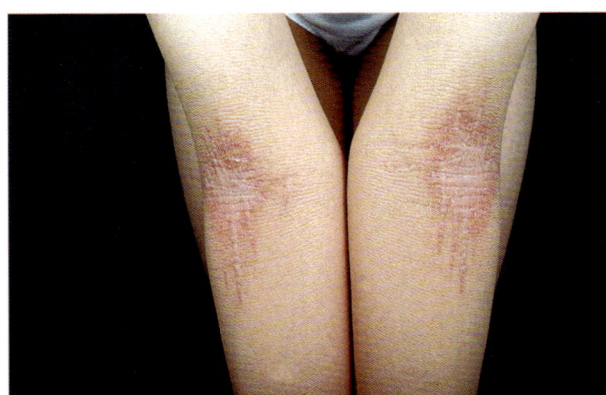

Figure 2.24

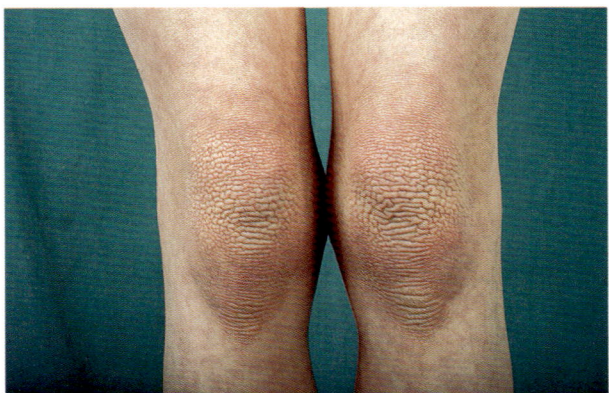

Figure 2.25

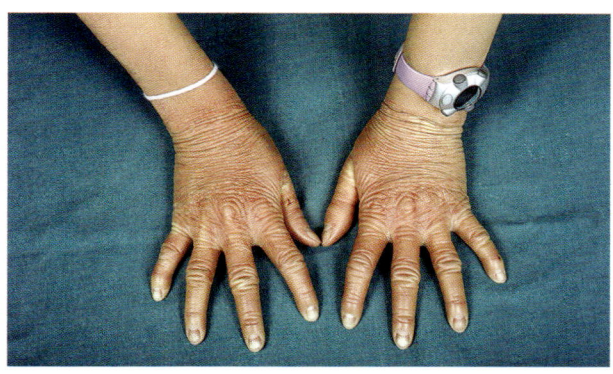

Figure 2.26

Differential diagnosis

(This disease may represent a mere variant of classic EH.)

- Diseases with collodion presentation
- Curth–Macklin disease

REFERENCE

Vahlquist A, Ganemo A, Pigg M, et al. The clinical spectrum of congenital ichthyosis in Sweden: a review of 127 cases. Acta Derm Venereol (Stockh) 2003; 213 Suppl: 34–47

CHAPTER 3

Acantholytic diseases

DARIER'S DISEASE

Synonym

- Darier–White disease

Age of onset

Usually during the teenage years, but earlier onset is not rare (Figure 3.1).

Clinical findings

Skin and mucosal lesions

- Rough, brownish keratotic papules on the face and upper part of the trunk (seborrheic areas) coalescing to form plaques (Figures 3.2–3.5)
- Flat, wart-like papules on the dorsa of the hands and feet (Figure 3.6)
- Palmoplantar punctate keratoses (pits) (Figures 3.7 and 3.8)
- Guttate leukodermatous macules
- Nail plate involvement: longitudinal splits, V-shaped notches of the distal part, subungual hyperkeratosis (Figure 3.9)
- Less frequently major folds are involved (Figure 3.10)
- Oral, vaginal, anal involvement: white papules clustered in a 'cobblestone' pattern
- Lesions in a mosaic linear pattern are frequent (Figures 3.11 and 3.12)

Extracutaneous symptoms

- Epilepsy and mental retardation
- Corneal, bone, pulmonary, urogenital abnormalities
- Thyroiditis

Course and complications

There is increased susceptibility to widespread cutaneous infections, both bacterial (Figure 3.13) and

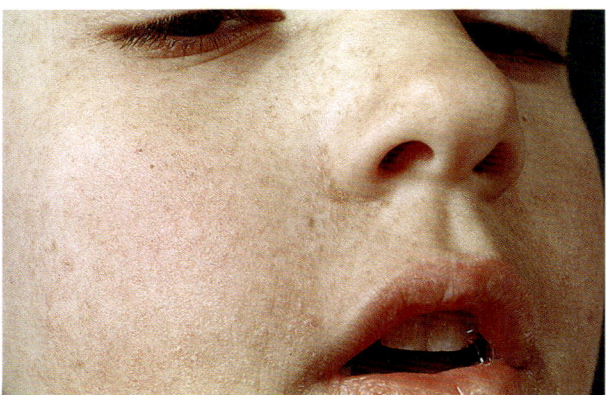

Figure 3.1

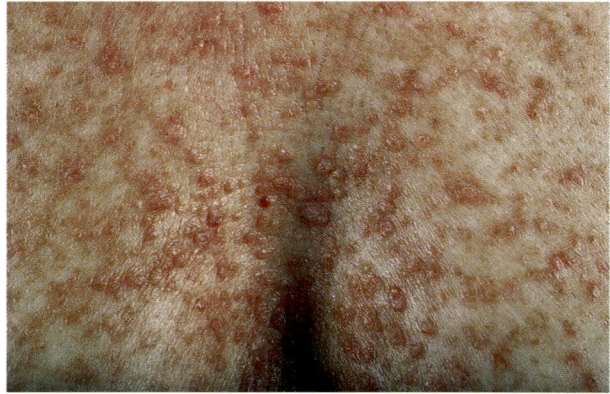

Figure 3.2

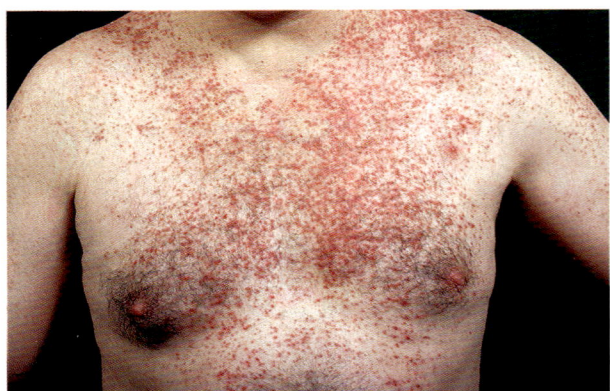

Figure 3.3

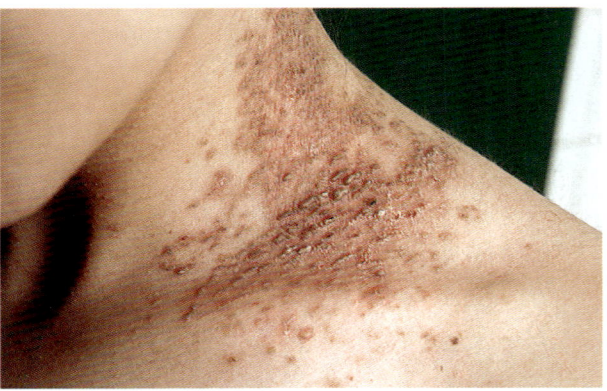

Figure 3.4

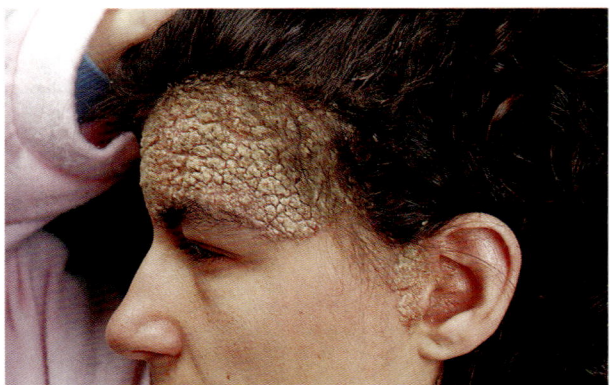

Figure 3.5

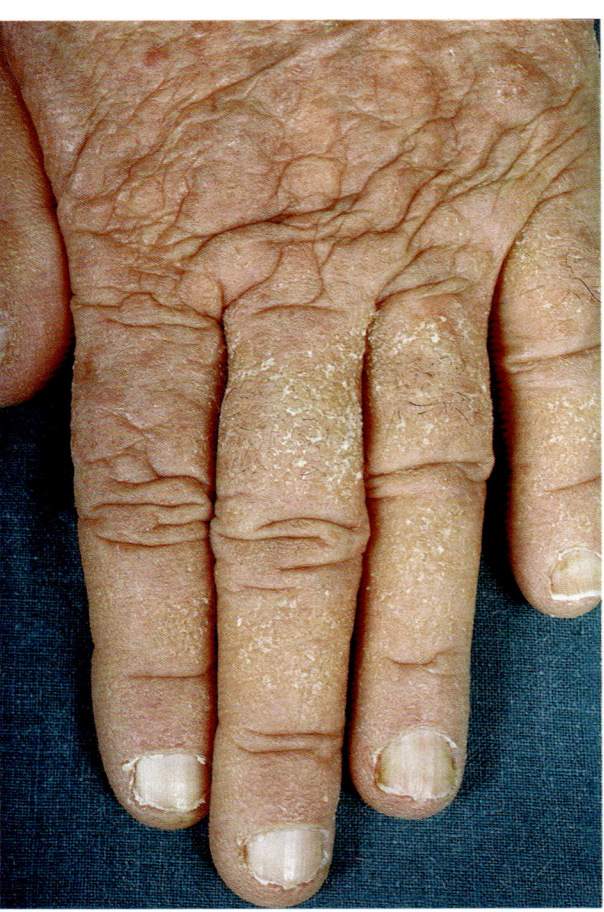

Figure 3.6

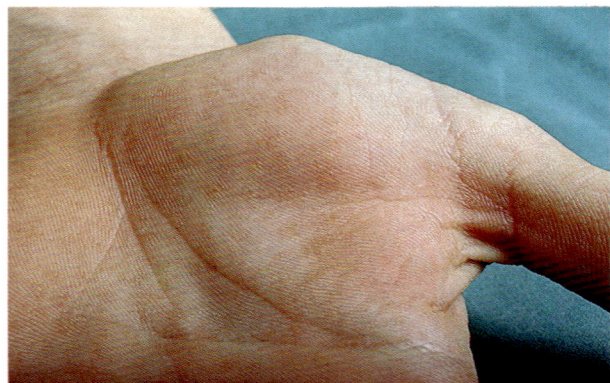

Figure 3.7

herpetic (Figure 3.14). It is a persistent and long-standing disease.

Laboratory findings

Histopathologic features include foci of suprabasal clefts, and acantholytic dyskeratotic cells in the spinous and granular layers.

Genetics and pathogenesis

This is an autosomal dominant disease related to mutations of a gene ATP2A2 encoding a specific keratinocyte Ca^{2+} pump. These mutations are responsible for an impaired formation of desmosomes and for the subsequent increased acantholysis.

Acantholytic diseases 27

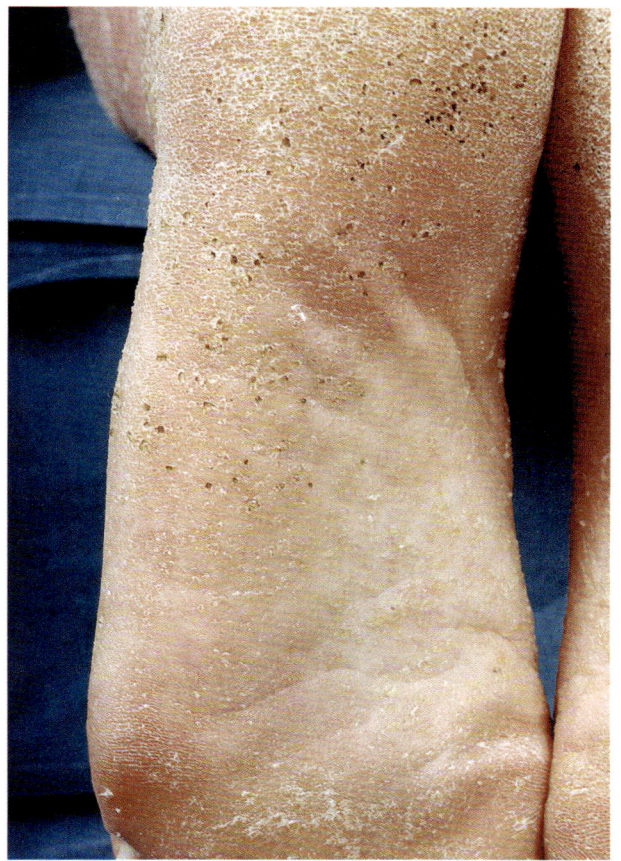

Figure 3.8

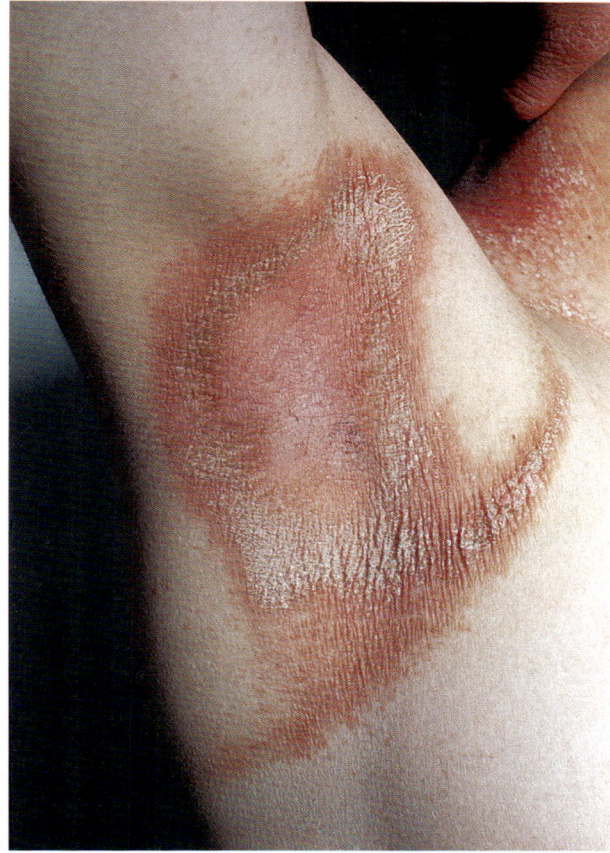

Figure 3.10

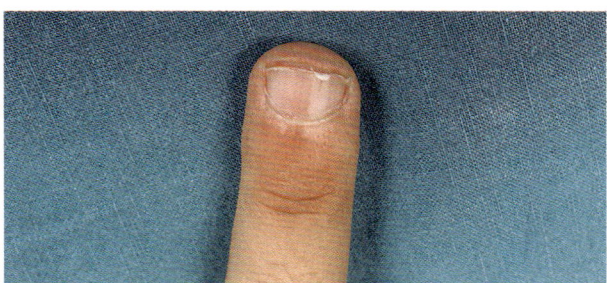

Figure 3.9

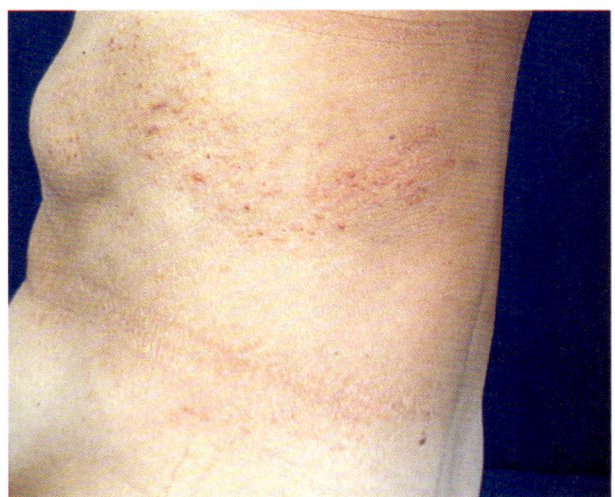

Figure 3.11

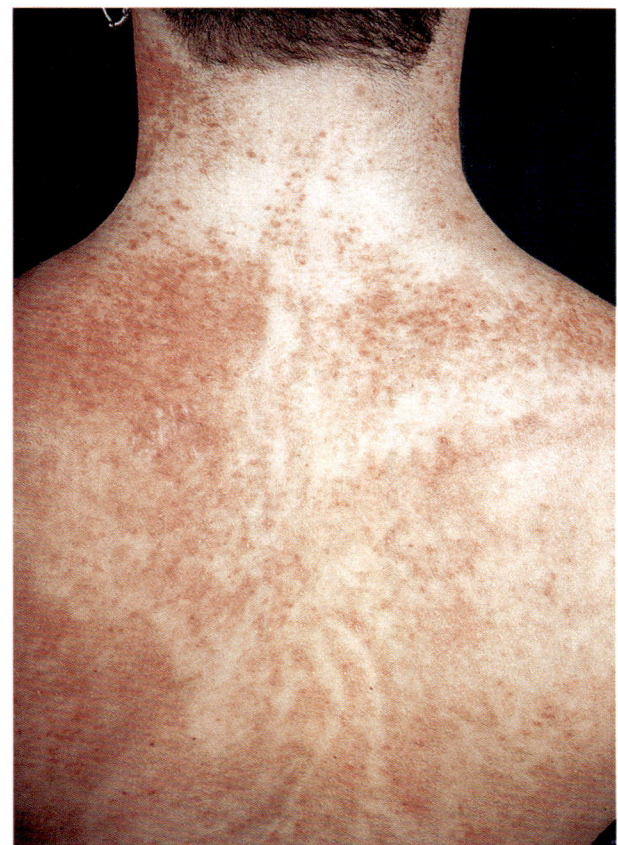

Figure 3.12

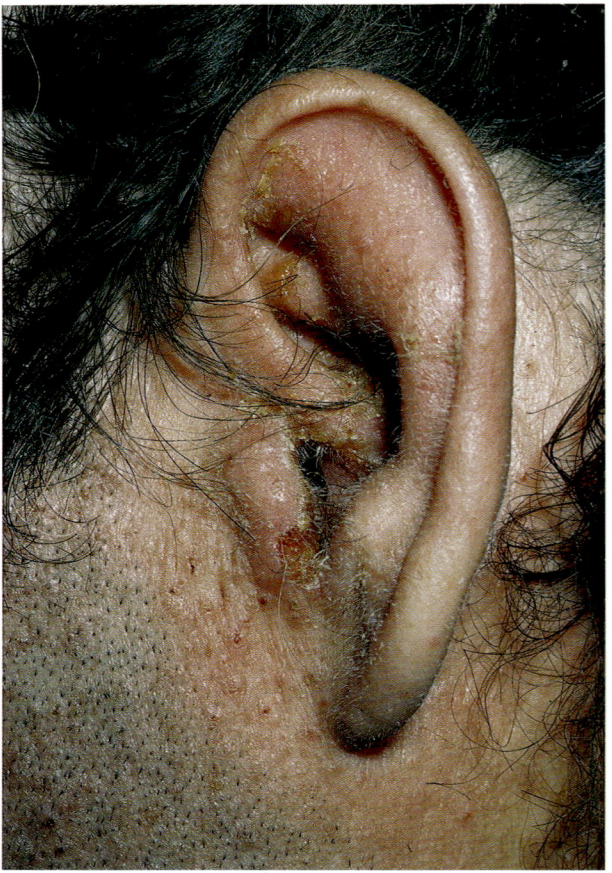

Figure 3.13

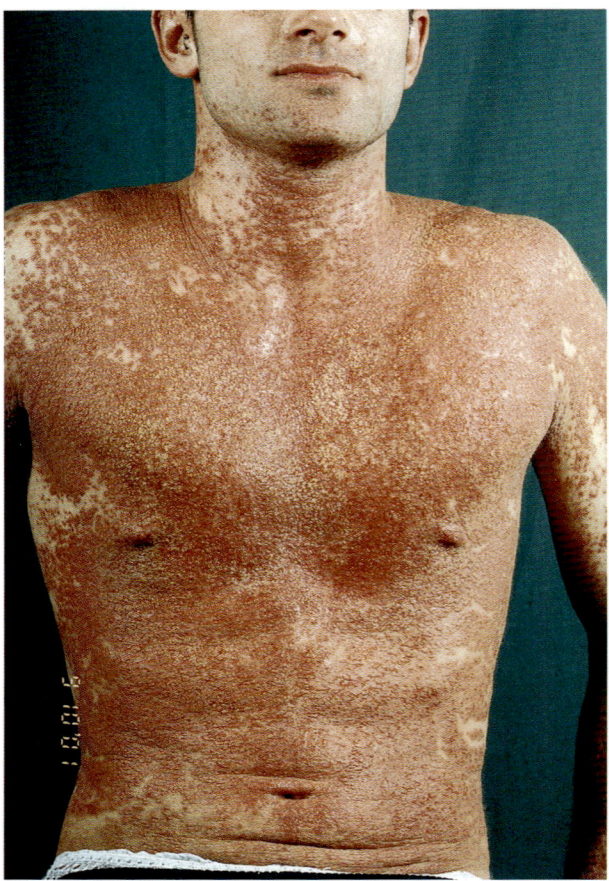

Figure 3.14

Differential diagnosis

- Seborrheic dermatitis
- Hailey–Hailey disease
- Keratosis pilaris
- Grover's disease

Follow-up and therapy

General health remains usually unaffected; there are exacerbations during summer, sun exposure and lithium carbonate treatment.

- Topical emollients and keratolytic ointments (retinoids, tacalcitol, 5-fluorouracil)
- Etretinate (0.5 mg/kg/day: good results)
- Sun protection

REFERENCES

Ahn W, Lee MG, Kim KH, Muallem S. Multiple effects of SERCA2b mutations associated with Darier's disease. J Biol Chem 2003; 278: 20795–801

Dhitavat J, Dode L, Leslie N, et al. Mutations in the sarcoplasmic endoplasmic reticulum Ca^{2+} ATPase isoform cause Darier's disease. J Invest Dermatol 2003; 121: 486–9

Ikeda S, Mayuzumi N, Shigihara T, et al. Mutations in ATP2A2 in patients with Darier's disease. J Invest Dermatol 2003; 121: 475–7

Shull GE, Okunae G, Liu LH, et al. Physiological functions of plasma membrane and intracellular Ca^{2+} pumps revealed by analysis of null mutants. Ann NY Acad Sci 2003; 986: 453–60

ACROKERATOSIS VERRUCIFORMIS

Synonym

- Acrokeratosis verruciformis of Hopf

Age of onset

- Childhood

Clinical findings

Cutaneous manifestations

- Convex to flat-topped, warty, flesh-colored papules a few millimeters in diameter on the dorsal aspects of the hands and feet (Figure 3.15), forearms, wrists and knees
- Punctate pits covered by horny pearls on palms and soles
- Whitish thickened nails with longitudinal ridges
- Sparing of seborrheic areas

Course

The disease is persistent without seasonal changes.

Laboratory investigations

Histopathologic findings include hyperkeratosis, hypergranulosis, achanthosis and papillomatosis ('gothic church' aspect).

Genetics and pathogenesis

There is autosomal dominant inheritance. It is considered a variant or a part of Darier's disease.

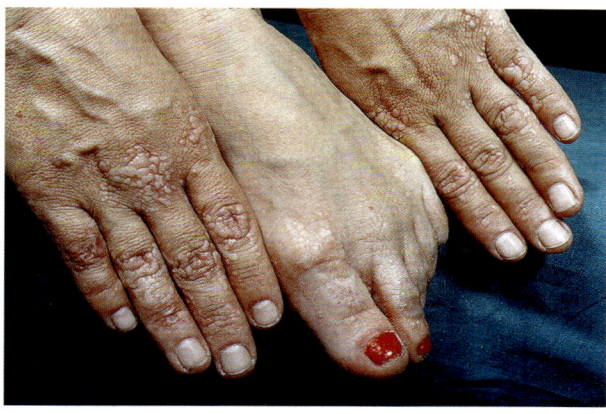

Figure 3.15

Differential diagnosis

- Epidermodysplasia verruciformis
- Darier's disease
- Flat warts

Therapy

- Keratolytic agents
- Topical retinoids

REFERENCES

Panja R. Acrokeratosis verruciformis (Hopf): a clinical entity? Br J Dermatol 1977; 96: 643–52

Rook A, Stevanovic D. Acrokeratosis verruciformis. Br J Dermatol 1957; 69: 450–1

Schuller WA. Acrokeratosis verruciformis of Hopf. Arch Dermatol 1972; 106: 81–3

HAILEY–HAILEY DISEASE

Synonym

- Benign familial chronic pemphigus

Age of onset

- Adolescence

Clinical findings

- Recurrent eruptions of vesicles and blisters on an erythematous background located on the main folds (axillae, groins, neck) (Figures 3.16–3.18)
- Erosion, crusts and vegetant lesions may occur (Figures 3.19–3.21)
- Unpleasant odor arising from diseased areas
- Rare mucosal erosions (mouth and vulva)

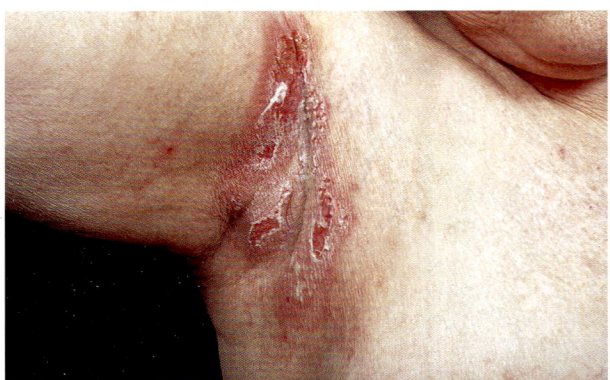

Figure 3.16

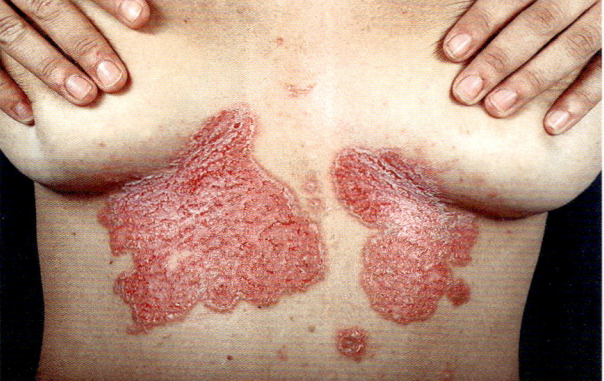

Figure 3.17

Complications

- Secondary infections are very common

Course

- Chronic with periods of remission and recurrence
- Summer exacerbations

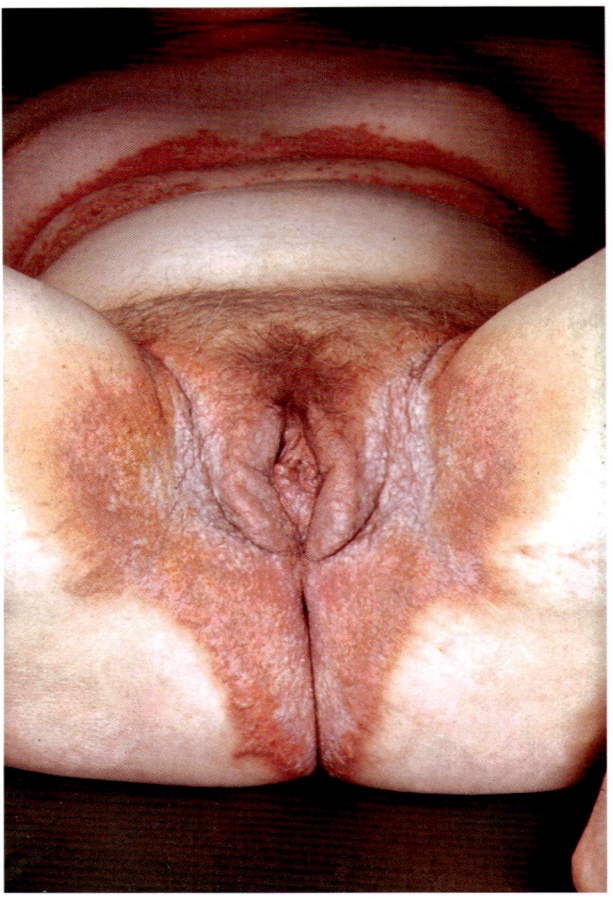

Figure 3.18

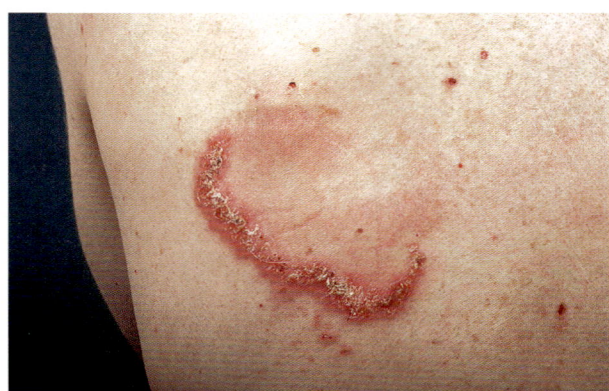

Figure 3.19

Laboratory findings

Histopathologic features include suprabasal cleavage, intercellular edema and acantholysis with the appearance of a 'dilapidated brick wall'.

Direct and indirect immunofluorescence shows negative findings.

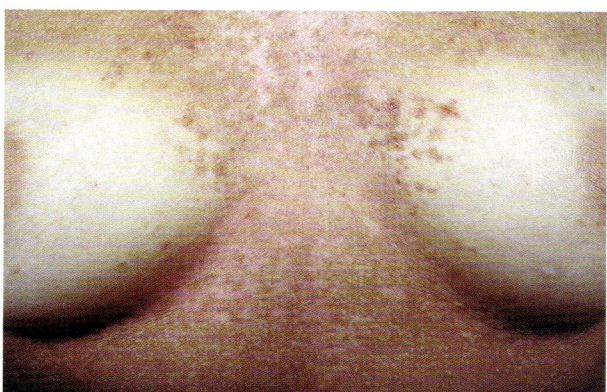

Figure 3.20

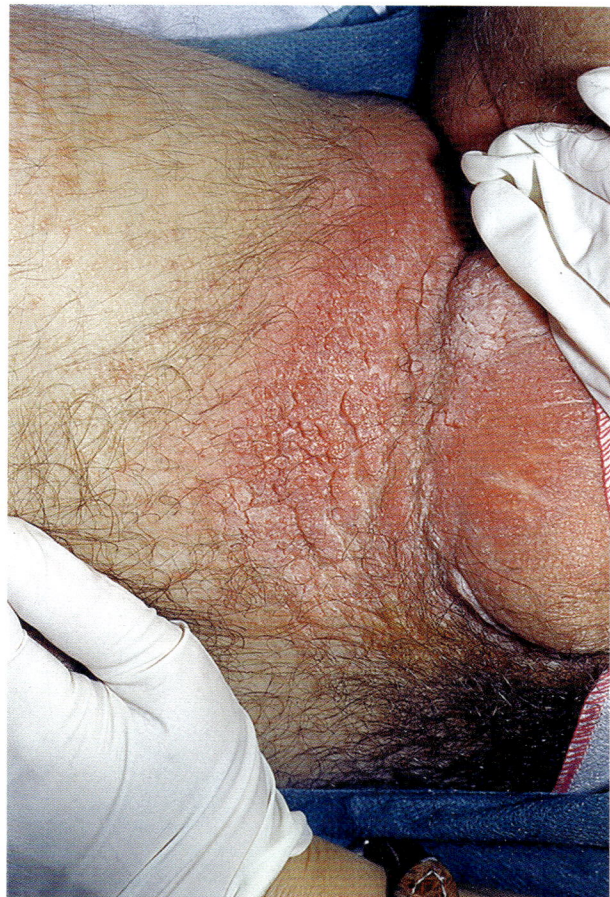

Figure 3.21

Genetics and pathogenesis

This is an autosomal dominant disease.
The disease is due to mutations of a gene encoding for a Ca^{2+} pump, called ATAC2; impairment of this energy provider may cause imbalance of desmosomal component synthesis, causing acantholysis.

Differential diagnosis

- Bacterial and fungal infections
- Pemphigus vulgaris and vegetans
- Transient acantholytic dermatosis of Grover
- Darier's disease

Follow-up

- Normal life span with significant discomforts
- Decrease of severity with age

Therapy

- Topical antibacterial and antimycotic agents
- Topical cortisteroids
- Tacalcitol
- Oral antibiotics and antimycotic drugs
- Ciclosporin
- Dapsone
- Surgical excisions and grafting
- Dye laser

REFERENCES

Behne MJ, Tu CL, Aronchik I, et al. Human keratinocyte ATP2C1 localizes to the Golgi and controls Golgi Ca^{2+} stores. J Invest Dermatol 2003; 121: 688–94

Burge S. Hailey-Hailey disease: the clinical features, response to treatment and prognosis. Br J Dermatol 1992; 126: 275–82

Burge SM, Millard PR, Wonjnarowska F. Hailey-Hailey disease: a widespread abnormality of cell adhesion. Br J Dermatol 1991; 124: 329–32

Quitadamo MJ, Spencer SK. Surgical management of Hailey-Hailey disease. J Am Acad Dermatol 1991; 25: 342–3

PEELING SKIN SYNDROME

Synonyms

- Keratolysis exfoliativa congenita
- Idiopathic deciduous skin

Epidemiology

Few reports in the literature. Personal observation of three families in a 15-year survey.

Age of onset

- At birth or during infancy

Clinical findings

Cutaneous manifestations

- Type A (non-inflammatory): continuous, asymptomatic, generalized non-inflammatory exfoliation of stratum corneum
- Type B (inflammatory): generalized erythematous scaling with seasonal variations (worsening in summer) and pruritus
- Type C (localized): strictly localized areas of desquamation well demarcated by a red border mainly involving the palms and soles (Figures 3.22–3.24); lesions may extend to the dorsa of hands and feet (Figure 3.25)
- Onychodystrophies and hair changes

Extracutaneous findings

- Short stature
- Sexual infantilism
- Eosinophilia

Course

- Lifelong

Laboratory investigations

- Occasionally aminoaciduria and low plasma tryptophan levels
- Histopathologic findings: subcorneal separation without or with (inflammatory form) psoriasiform epidermal hyperplasia and dermal inflammation

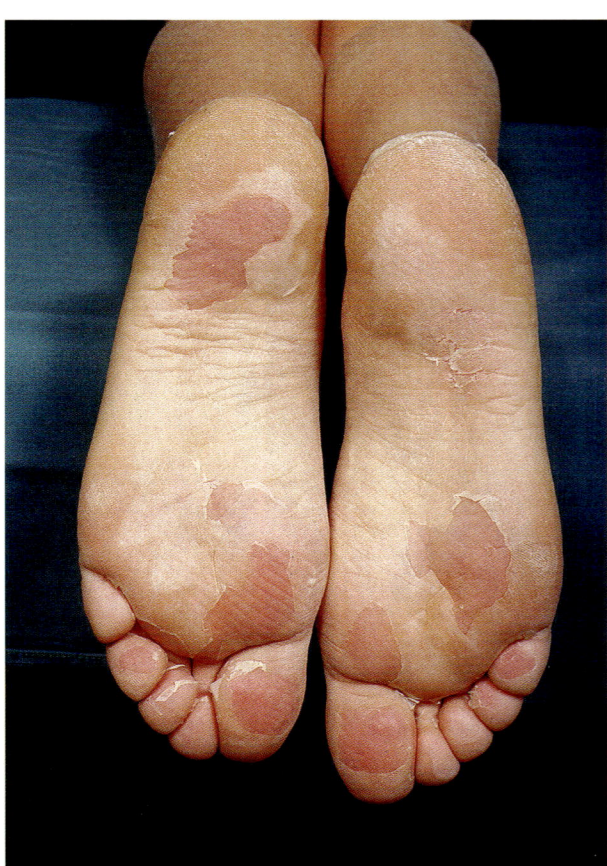

Figure 3.22

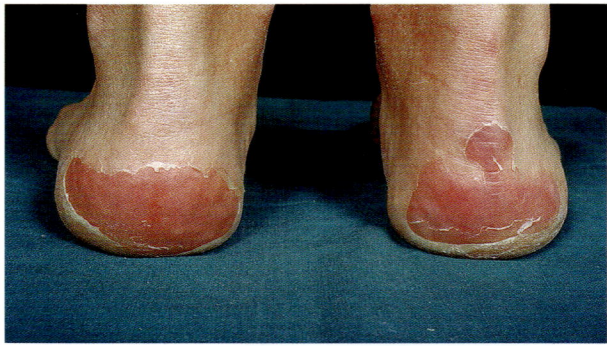

Figure 3.23

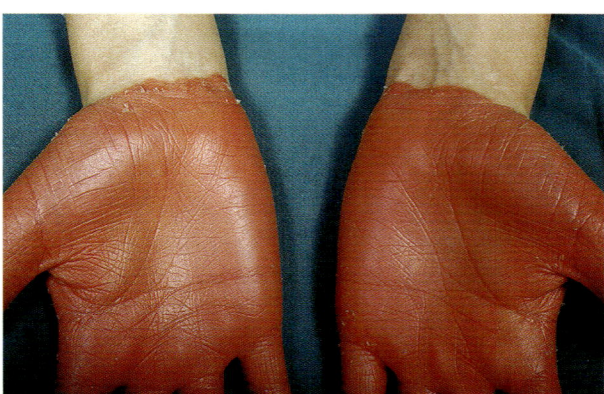

Figure 3.24

Acantholytic diseases

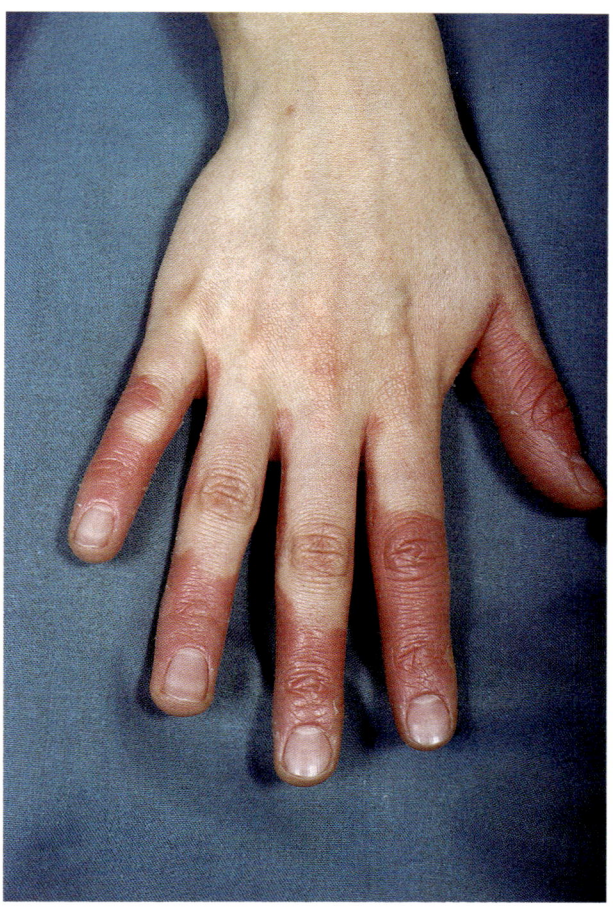

Figure 3.25

Genetics and pathogenesis

- Autosomal recessive inheritance
- Pathogenesis unknown; a keratin gene or a keratin-related gene is strongly suspected

Differential diagnosis

- Ichthyosis linearis circumflexa
- Epidermolytic epidermolysis bullosa

Therapy

- Keratolytic agents
- Oral retinoids occasionally useful

REFERENCES

Brusasco A, Veraldi S, Tadini G, et al. Localized peeling skin syndrome: case report with ultrastructural study. Br J Dermatol 1988; 139: 492–5

Hashimoto K, Hamzavi I, Tanaka K, Shwayder T. Acral peeling skin syndrome. J Am Acad Dermatol 2000; 43: 1112–19

Mevorah B, Orion E, de Viragh P, et al. Peeling skin syndrome with hair changes. Dermatology 1998; 197: 373–6

Tasan HB, Akar A, Gur AR, Deveci S. Peeling skin syndrome. Int J Dermatol 1999; 38: 208–10

CHAPTER 4

Ichthyoses

DOMINANT ICHTHYOSIS

Synonym

- Ichthyosis vulgaris

Epidemiology

This is the most frequent disease in the group of ichthyoses, with a prevalence rising from 1 : 500 to 1 : 3000.

Age of onset

It may be visible shortly after birth, but more frequently the clinical picture is more easily seen during the first year of life.

Clinical findings

Dominant ichthyosis (DI) is characterized by very different clinical presentations that vary from slightly visible xerotic itchy skin to very severe pictures similar to those of lamellar ichthyoses (Figures 4.1–4.3).

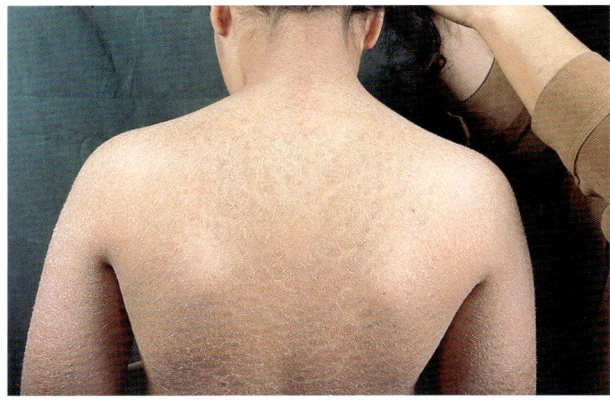

Figure 4.1

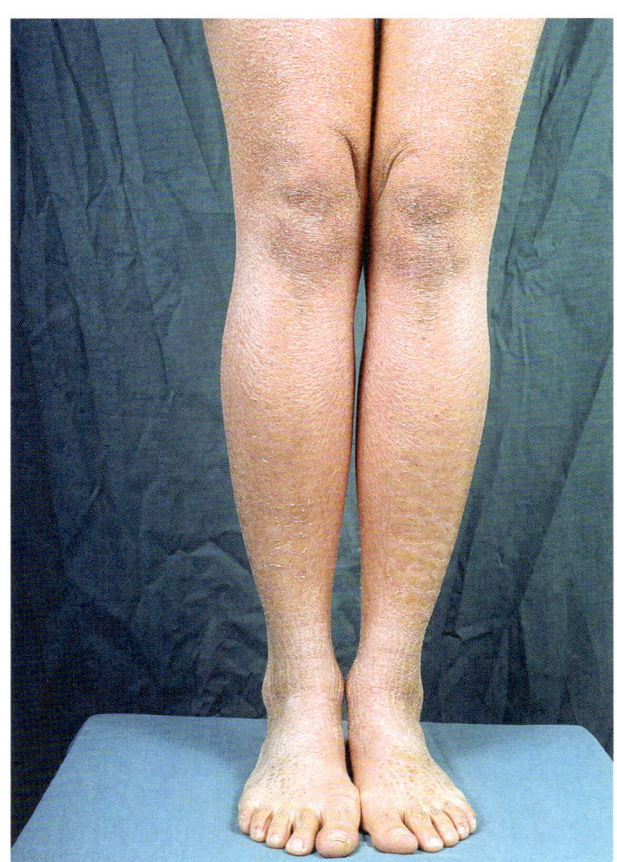

Figure 4.2

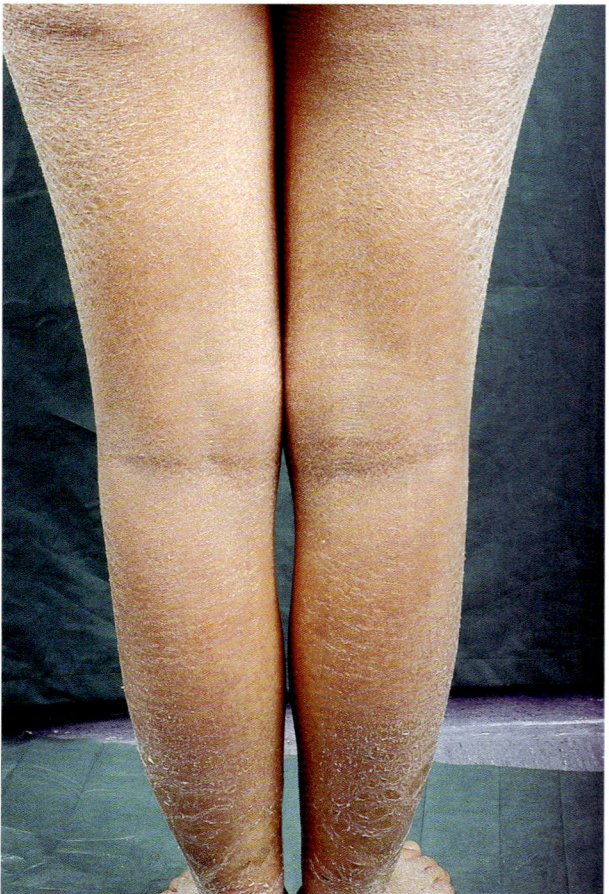

Figure 4.3

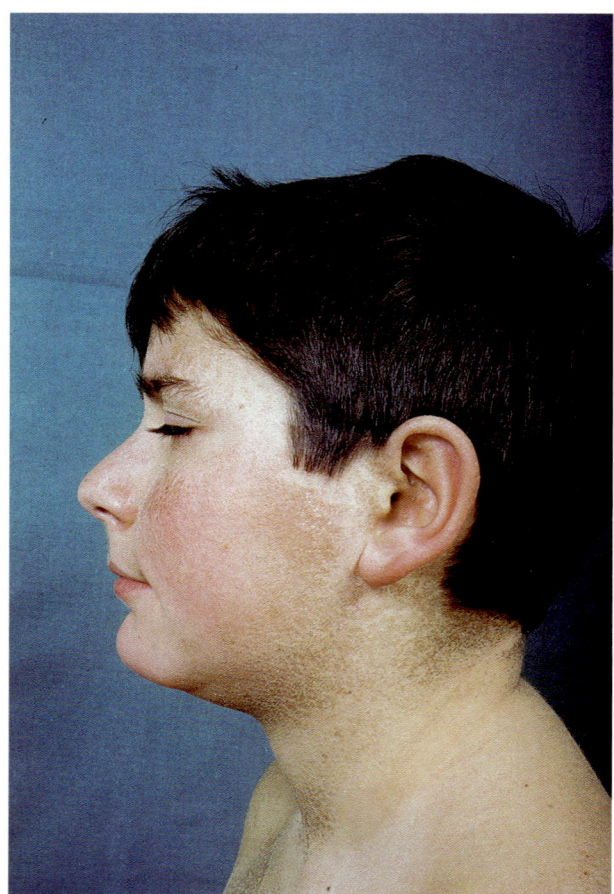

Figure 4.4

The particular presentation is a combination of erythematous scaly cheeks and face (Figure 4.4), small gray to brownish scales covering all of the body including folds, follicular hyperkeratosis and hyperlinearity of the palms and soles (Figures 4.5 and 4.6).

Extracutaneous symptoms

- Atopic dermatitis and diathesis (Figure 4.6)

Course

This is a lifelong disease with seasonal changes due to humidity and sun exposure.

Laboratory findings

Histology shows a decrease of stratum granulosum; the ultrastrucure shows anomalies of keratohyaline granules.

Allergy testing shows frequent positivity to nickel.

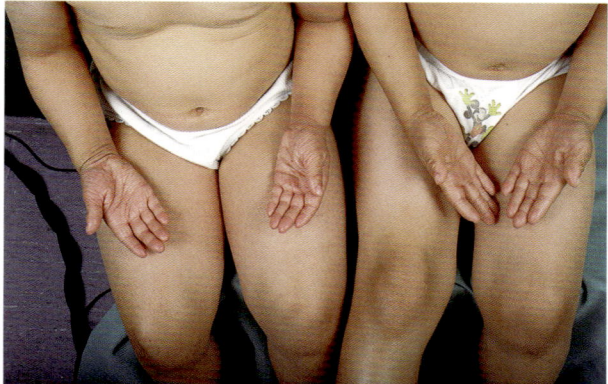

Figure 4.5

Genetics and pathogenesis

Ichthyosis vulgaris is inherited as an autosomal dominant trait.

The disease is related to anomalies in the synthesis of filaggrin, but, even if the gene structure is well known, no genetic defects have been demonstrated to date.

Ichthyoses

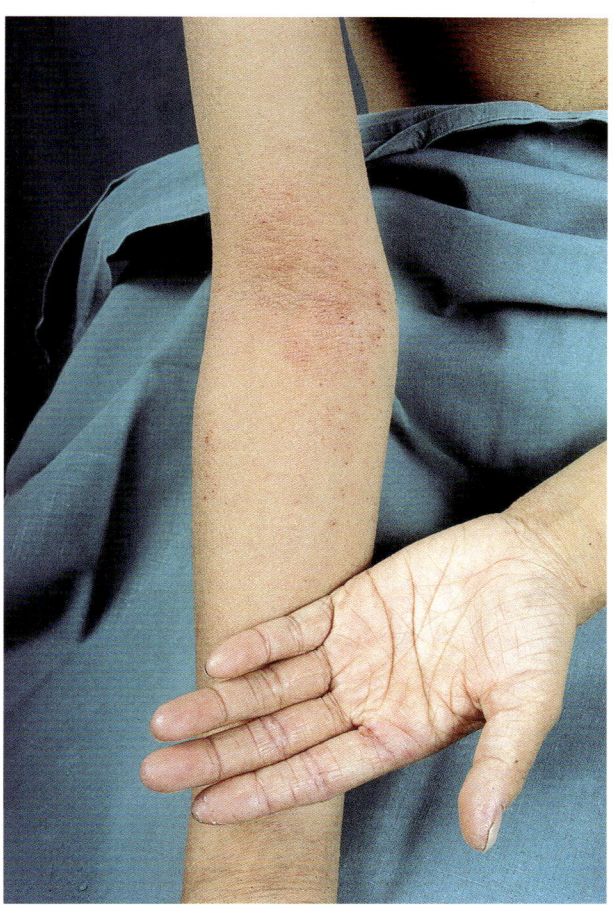

Figure 4.6

Differential diagnosis

Severe DI must be differentiated from mild lamellar ichthyosis.

Follow-up

During childhood, allergologic evaluation is mandatory in severe atopic patients.

Therapy

Local therapy must be individualized, but mild keratolytic agents and emollients are recommended.

REFERENCES

Candi E, Oddi S, Paradisi A, et al. Expression of transglutaminase 5 in normal and pathologic human epidermis. J Invest Dermatol 2002; 119: 670–7

Compton JG, DiGiovanna JJ, Johnston KA, et al. Mapping of the associated phenotype of an absent granular layer in ichthyosis vulgaris to the epidermal differentiation complex on chromosome 1. Exp Dermatol 2002; 11: 518–26

Fleckman P, Brumbaugh S. Absence of the granular layer and kerotohyalin define a morphologically distinct subset of individuals with ichthyosis vulgaris. Exp Dermatol 2002; 11: 327–36

Zhong W, Cui B, Zhang Y, et al. Linkage analysis suggests a locus of ichthyosis vulgaris on 1q22. J Hum Genet 2003; 48: 390–2

X-LINKED ICHTHYOSIS

Age of onset

- Third to sixth month of life

Clinical findings

Dark discrete medium-sized scales, especially visible on the extensor surface (cobblestone appearance), are the hallmark of the disease (Figures 4.7 and 4.8).

All surfaces are involved.

At the site of major folds the skin appears lighter in contrast to the 'nigricant' aspect of the surrounding skin, implying false 'disease-free' areas (Figures 4.9 and 4.10).

In severe cases the face shows dark, fine desquamation with underlying erythema (Figure 4.11). The scalp is covered by fine, dandruff-like scales.

(There is no hyperlinearity of palms and soles or follicular hyperkeratosis.)

Extracutaneous findings

- Cryptorchidism
- Corneal opacities
- Hypoanosmy (Kallmann's syndrome)

Complications

- Slow growth during childhood

Course

The disease is present lifelong but dramatic amelioration during summer or after ultraviolet (UV) light exposure is highly characteristic of this disease.

Laboratory findings

Steroid sulfatase enzyme deficiency can be detected in female carriers.

Genetics and pathogenesis

Large deletions of the gene encoding steroid sulfatase cause X-linked ichthyosis.

This enzyme plays a key role in the metabolism of membrane-related steroids, causing anomalies in formation of the cornified envelope.

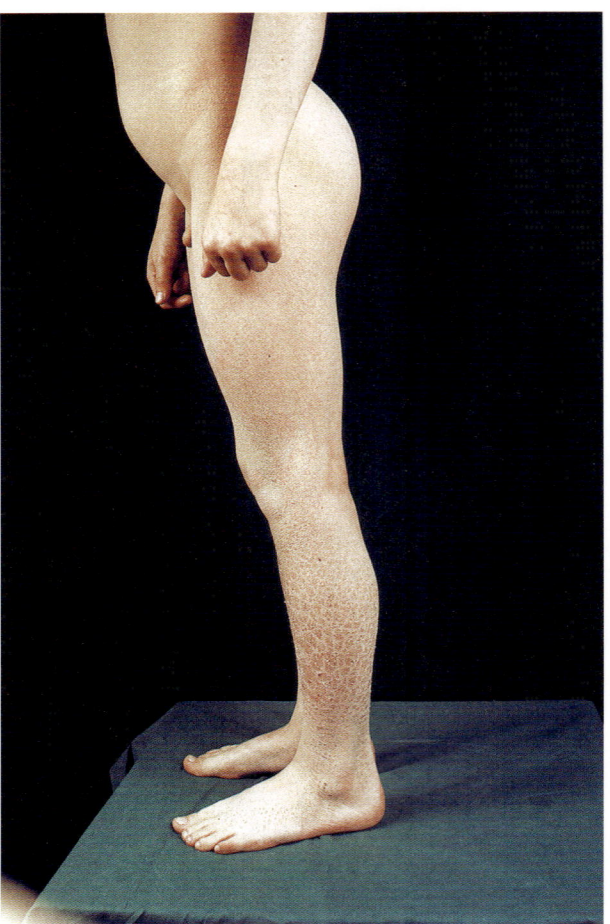

Figure 4.7

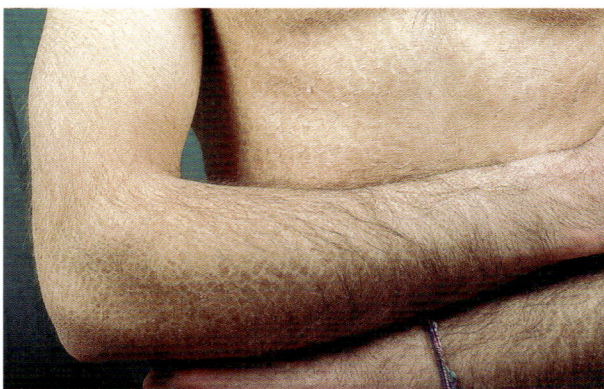

Figure 4.8

Differential diagnosis

X-linked ichthyosis must be differentiated from the mild 'nigricans' lamellar ichthyoses due to transglutaminase-1 gene mutations, which can have a similar presentation but have larger scales, and from DI in patients with dark skin.

Ichthyoses

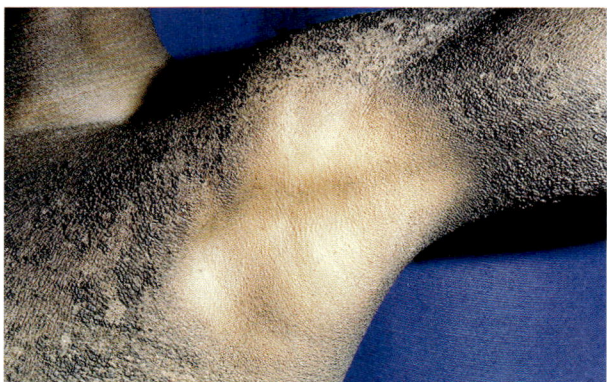

Figure 4.9

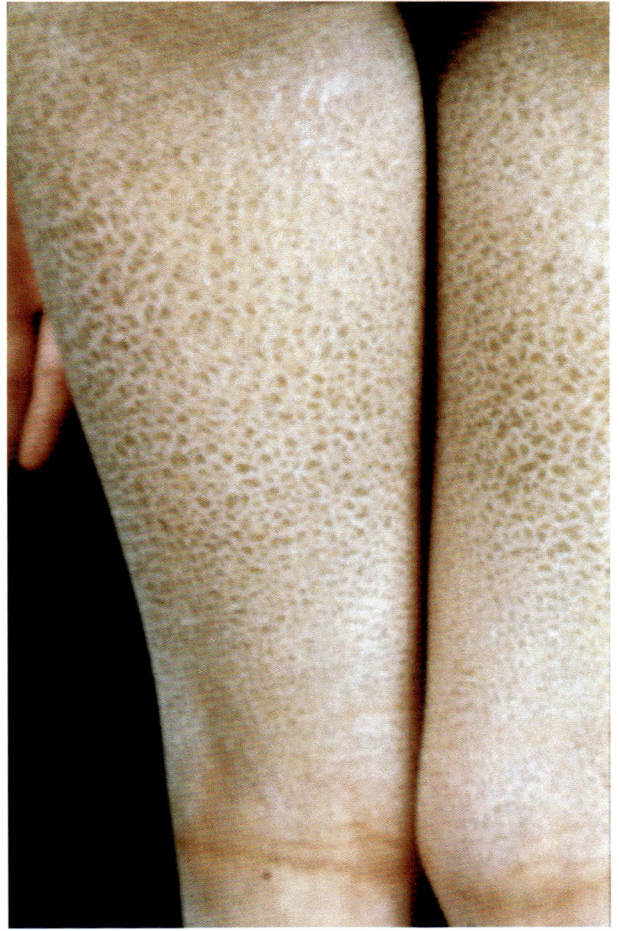

Figure 4.10

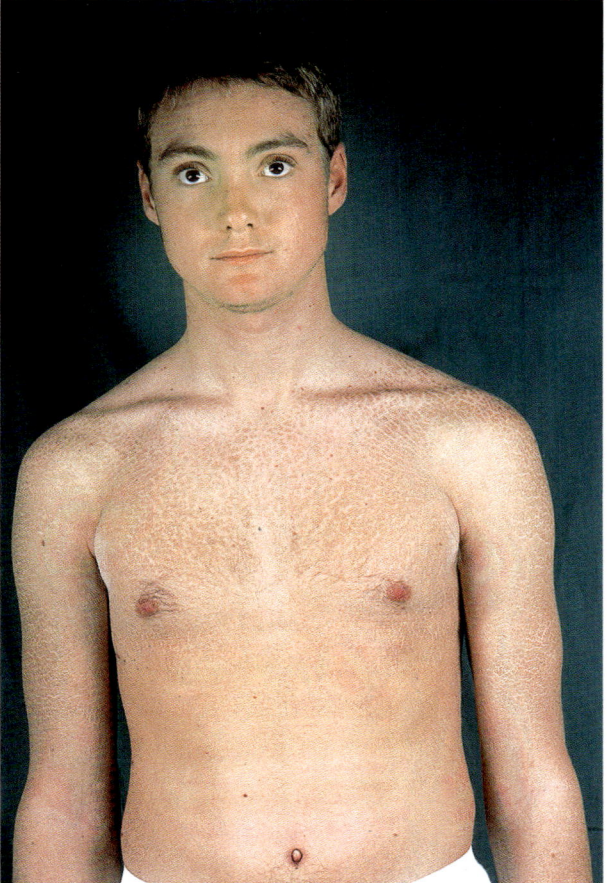

Figure 4.11

Therapy

- UV radiation, natural or lamp-originated
- Mild keratolytic agents (urea)
- Emollients

REFERENCES

Cuevas-Covarrubias SA, Jimenez-Vaca AL, Gonzalez-Huerta LM, et al. Somatic and germinal mosaicism for the steroid sulfatase gene deletion in a steroid sufatase deficiency carrier. J Invest Dermatol 2002; 119: 972–5

Rudolf M, Grosch S, Geerling G. Recurrent bilateral corneal erosions and opacities in corneal stroma. Pre-Descement dystrophy in X chromosome recessive ichthyosis. Opthalmologe 2002; 99: 962–3

Valdes-Flores M, Kofman-Alfaro SH, Vaca AL, Cuevas-Covarrubias SA. Deletion of exons 1–5 of the STS gene causing X-linked ichthyosis. J Invest Dermatol 2001; 116: 456–8

Follow-up

- Cryptorchidism must be monitored and cured when necessary
- Ophthalmological examination is advised when corneal anomalies are detected; rarely, corneal transplantation is necessary
- Genetic counseling for female carriers

SELF-HEALING COLLODION BABY

Age of onset

- At birth

Clinical findings

After a premature birth, babies are totally and firmly covered by a translucent, parchment-like film, 1–2 mm deep, that involves all of the body (Figure 4.12). There is ectropion and coarctation of the external ears.

The underlying epidermis may be erythematous.

Extracutaneous findings

- Respiratory distress
- Electrolyte imbalance
- Fever due to impaired temperature control

Course and complications

The membrane begins a slow, progressive detachment in large lamellae (Figures 4.13–4.15 same patient) that continues until the scales are very small. This process takes 1–6 months to conclude, leaving an appearance of normal skin.

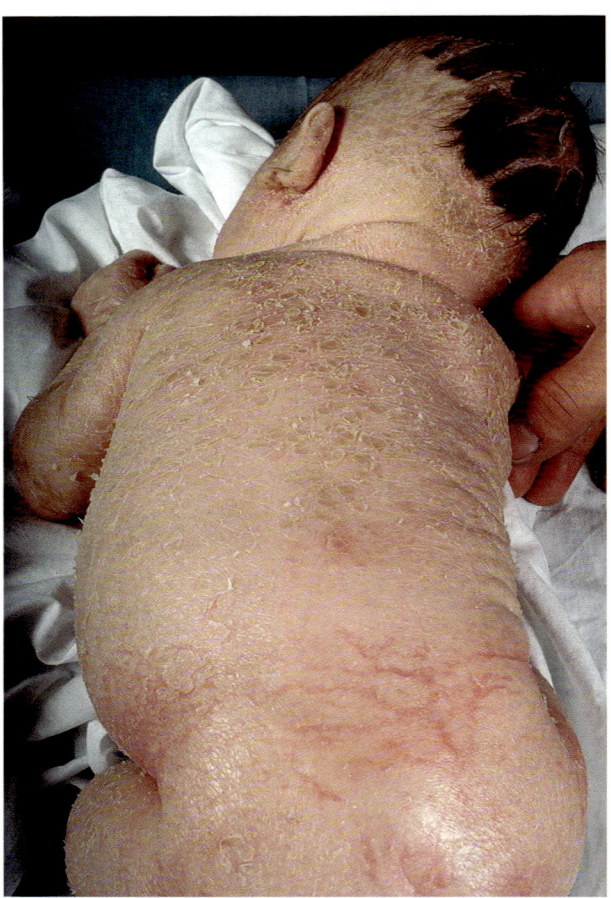

Figure 4.14

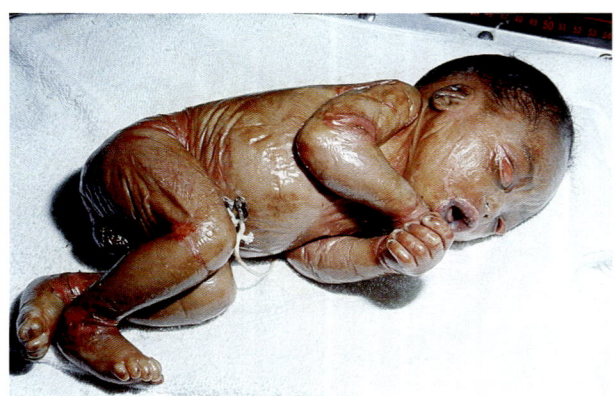

Figure 4.12

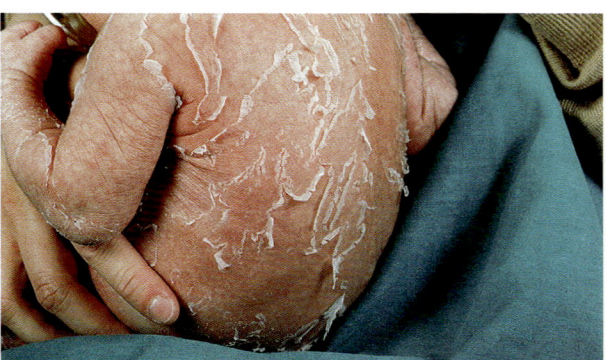

Figure 4.13

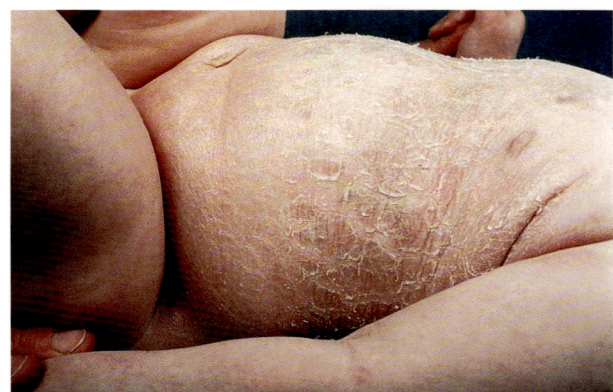

Figure 4.15

Infections and sepsis occur at perinatal and neonatal ages.

Laboratory findings

Ultrastructural studies demonstrate only an increase of the stratum corneum, without specific markers.

Genetics and pathogenesis

In some cases consanguinity has been reported.

Also in some cases certain transglutaminase-1 gene mutations are related to this clinical picture. The phenomenon is related to activation of this enzyme after birth. Transglutaminase-1 seems to be blocked in some way by heat or pressure of the amniotic fluid during pregnancy, causing a pathological differentiation and the related clinical presentation at birth ('dynamic phenotype').

Differential diagnosis

Despite the description of these cases as a self-healing disease, collodion baby is to be considered a symptom and not a disease, owing to the fact that many other diseases at birth may have a collodion-baby presentation:

- Lamellar ichthyosis
- Epidermolytic hyperkeratosis
- Hypohidrotic ectodermal dysplasia
- Omenn's syndrome
- Netherton's disease

Follow-up

Hospitalization in the neonatal period is necessary to avoid major complications.

Therapy

- Sterile paraffin oil and control of the temperature and humidity in neonatal equipment
- Ointments and creams to allow detachment of scales in a short period

REFERENCE

Raghunath M, Hennies HC, Ahvazi B, et al. Self-healing collodion baby: a dynamic phenotype explained by a particular transglutaminase-1 mutation. J Invest Dermatol 2003; 120: 224–8

LAMELLAR ICHTHYOSIS

Synonyms

- Congenital ichthyosis
- Recessive ichthyosis

Age of onset

- At birth

Epidemiology

This recessively inherited group of diseases is very rare. In a 10 year survey in Italy, we found only 150 cases.

Clinical findings

Classification: There are two ways to classify this group of diseases according the current literature.

Clinical

- ('True') lamellar ichthyosis (LI)
- 'Non-bullous' congenital ichthyosiform erythroderma (CIE)

(These two categories were known some years ago as erythrodermic LI (ELI) and non-erythrodermic LI (NELI).)

In our opinion, the term 'non-bullous CIE' is incorrect. In fact, 'bullous CIE' is not an ichthyosis and is better defined as 'epidermolytic hyperkeratosis'. Hence, we think that the above term is confusing.

Ultrastructural

- Type I: vesicular bodies in corneocytes without any other specific marker (Figure 4.16a)
- Type II: electronlucent brick-shaped crystals in corneocytes (Figure 4.16b)
- Type III: membranes and laminar structures in the granulosum and corneum and vescicular keratinosomes (Figure 4.16c)
- Type IV: folded membranes in stratum granulosum (Figure 4.16d)

The above two categories should be replaced in the near future by a genetic–functional classification, according to recent progress made in molecular genetics that has linked two clinical pictures to two different genes.

Findings

Patients can have a severe erythematous and scaling disease, deriving always from a collodion-baby presentation, with ectropion, eclabion, and everted and deformed ears.

The scalp and adnexae are involved. The rare dominant inherited pedigrees show this 'clinical pattern' (type I of ultrastructural classification) (Figures 4.17–4.24).

Milder or slightly affected patients are born as collodion babies with slight erythema and mild, whitish scale that may resemble ichthyosis vulgaris, giving to the skin the highly characteristic 'translucency' (type I of ultrastructural classification) (Figures 4.25 and 4.26).

Patients can be born as collodion babies but with a brown 'nigricans' presentation, having large lamellae with or without erythematous underlying areas, accompanied by severe ectropion and scalp involvement. Palmoplantar keratoderma is present (type II of ultrastructural classification) (Figures 4.27–4.29).

Patients may be born collodion with a reticulate pattern on the trunk end major folds, mild erythema and involvement of the scalp and palmoplantar areas (type III of ultrastructural classification) (Figures 4.30–4.32).

Babies may be born prematurely as collodion of average severity with severe respiratory distress, prominent Darier's sign and itching. Collodion baby fades in a few months leaving a follicular hyperkeratosis especially visible on the arms and legs (type IV of ultrastructural classification) (Figures 4.33 and 4.34).

Extracutaneous symptoms and complications

- Nystagmus
- Neurologic abnormalities
- Failure to thrive
- Phalangeal malformations and reabsorption in severe cases

Laboratory findings

Ultrastructural observations are cited above.

Molecular biology is performed in the majority of patients, searching for the three established loci (transglutaminase-1 gene, lipo-oxygenase gene and ABCA genes).

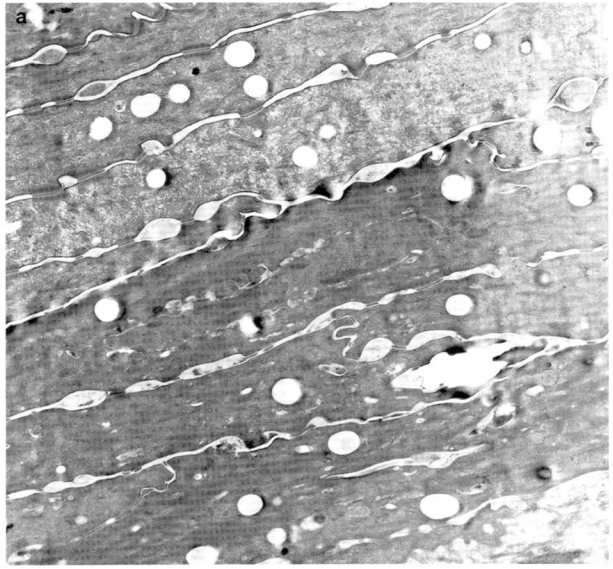
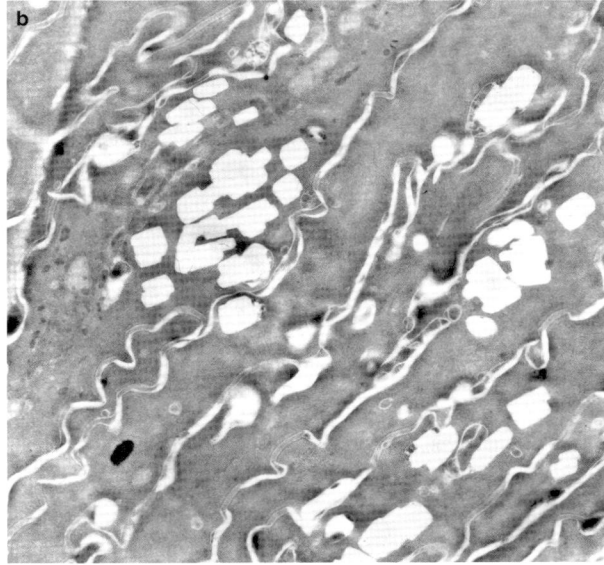
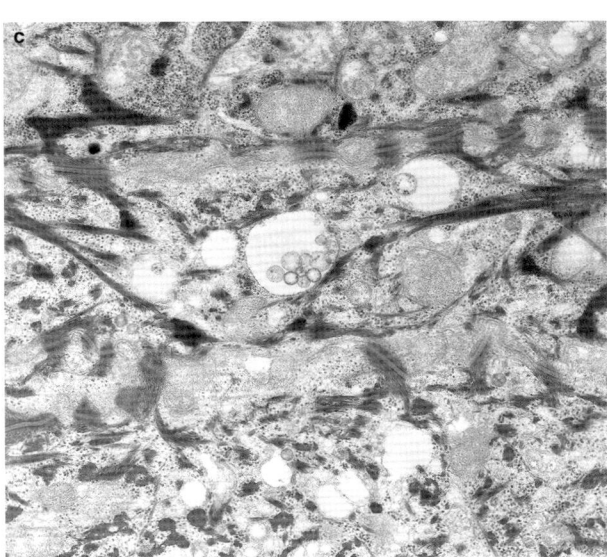
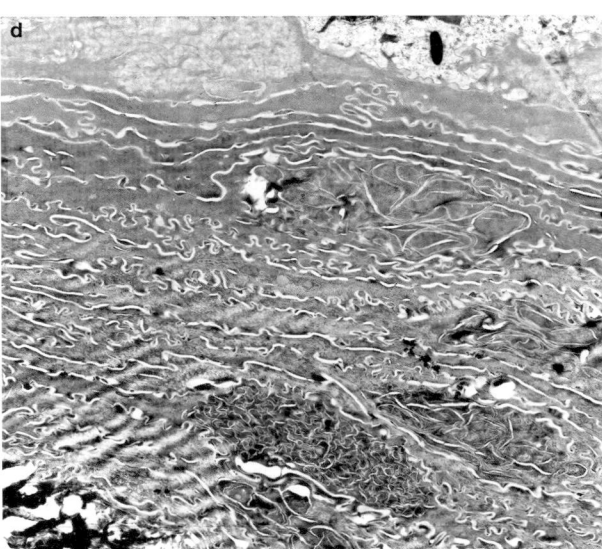

Figure 4.16

Genetics and pathogenesis

The group of LI is autosomal recessive, except for several established autosomal dominant pedigrees.

Three genes have been discovered to cause LI:

- The lipo-oxygenase gene is mutated in some patients with an erythematous and severe scaling pattern
- The transglutaminase-1 gene has been described to cause LI characterized by a large, blackish lamellae pattern (type II)
- ABCA12 gene in few pedigrees of LI type II

Other genes are described to be linked with LI, but no specific mutations have been found.

Lipo-oxygenase, transglutaminase-1 and ABCA are enzymes that allow correct stratification of the complex lipid molecules to form the corneocyte envelope, the final step of the differentiation process.

Differential diagnosis

- Epidermolytic hyperkeratosis
- Self-healing collodion baby

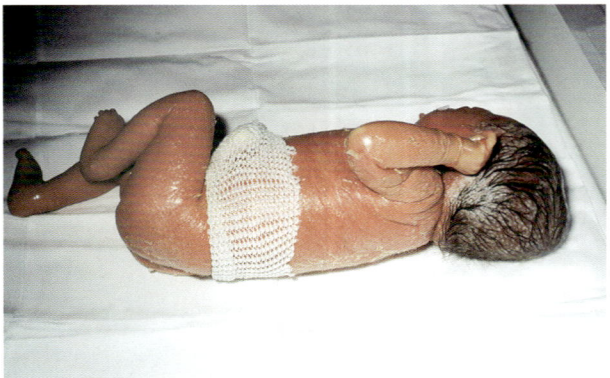

Figure 4.17

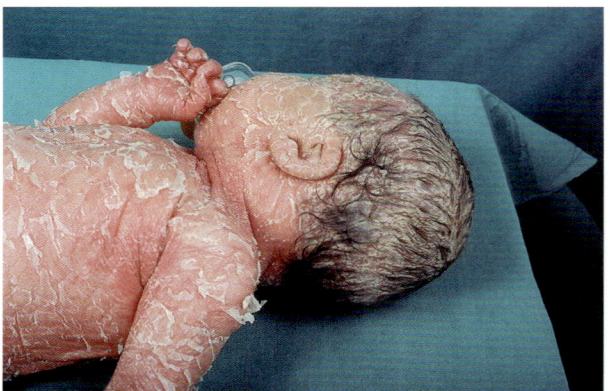

Figure 4.18

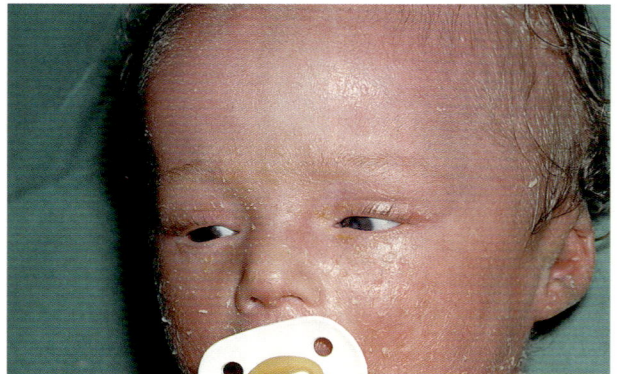

Figure 4.19

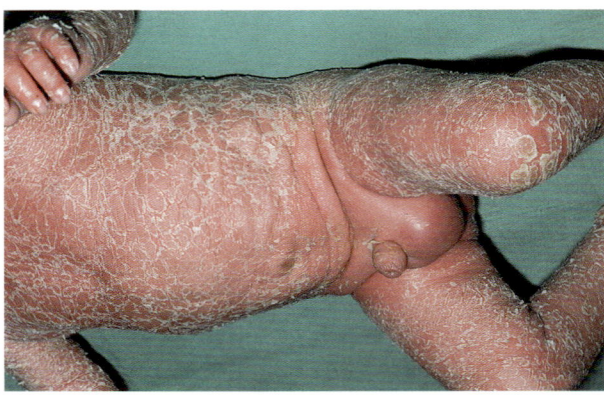

Figure 4.20

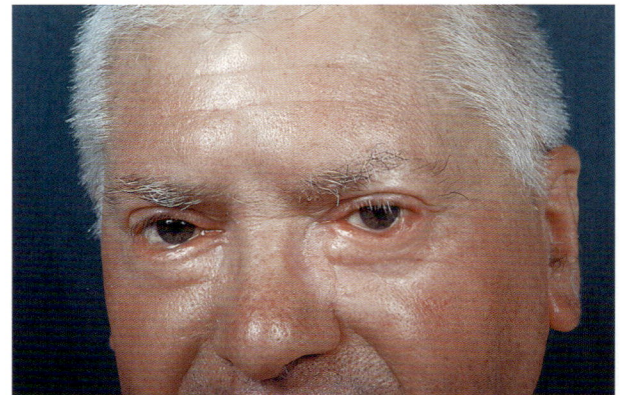

Figure 4.21

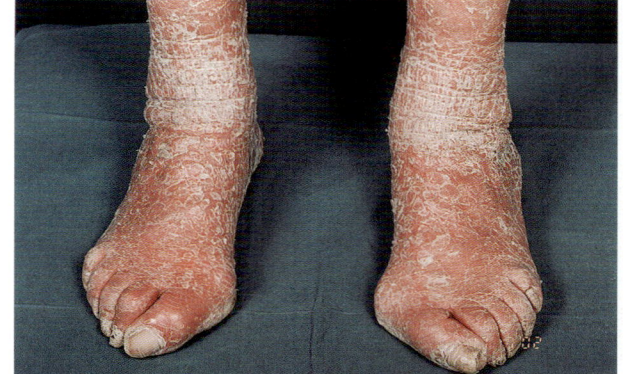

Figure 4.22

- Dorfman–Chanarin disease
- Trichothiodystrophy
- Netherton's syndrome
- Severe dominant 'ichthyosis vulgaris'
- Initial phases of hypohidrotic ectodermal dysplasia
- Syndromic ichthyoses

Follow-up

- Routine dermatological assessment for local keratolytic therapy and retinoid therapy
- Psychological consultation for the patient and family
- Ophthalmologist for follow-up of ectropion

Ichthyoses 45

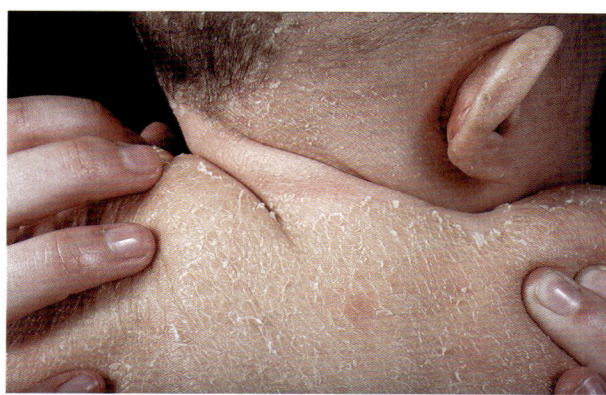

Figure 4.23

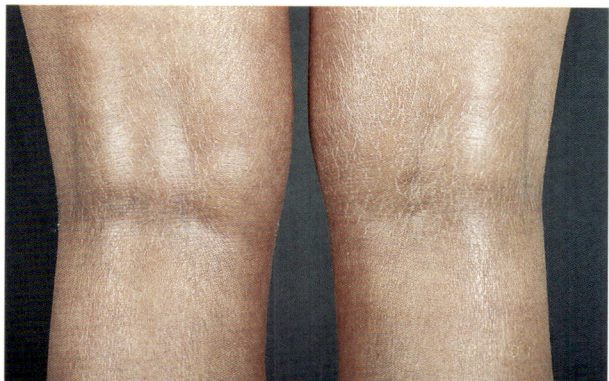

Figure 4.25

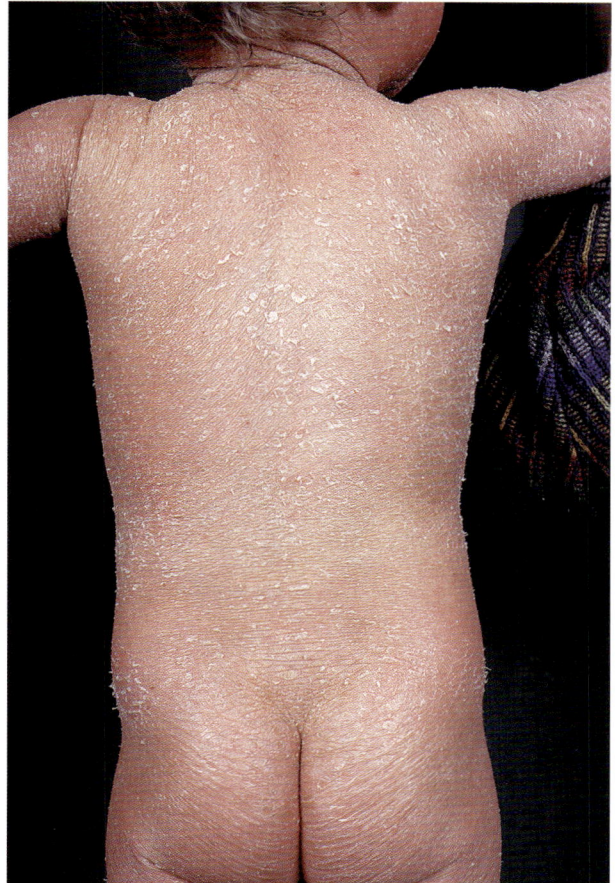

Figure 4.24

- Blood testing and radiography for oral retinoid therapy

Therapy

- Emollients
- Keratolytic agents (urea)

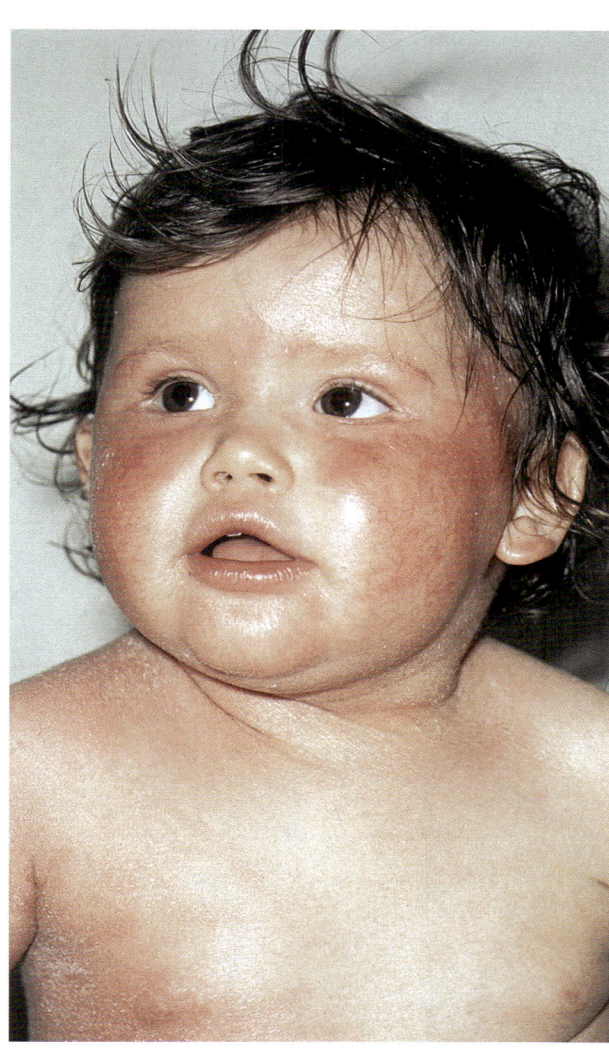

Figure 4.26

- Salicylic acid for palmoplantar sites
- Calcipotriol
- Oral retinoids (0.4–0.8 mg/kg/day)

46 Atlas of Genodermatoses

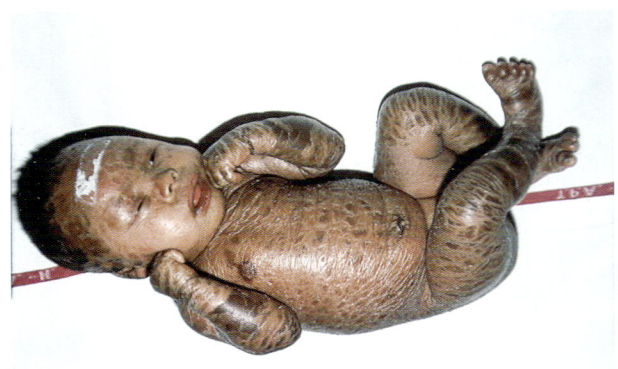

Figure 4.27

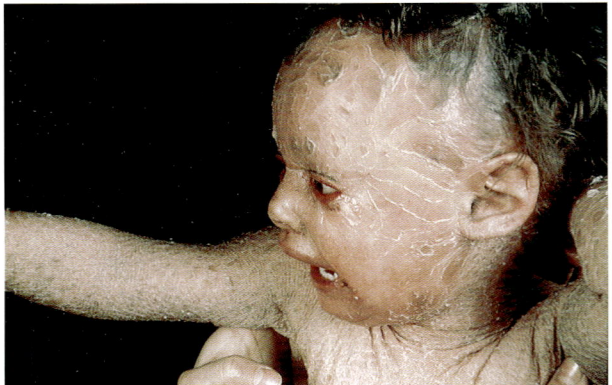

Figure 4.28

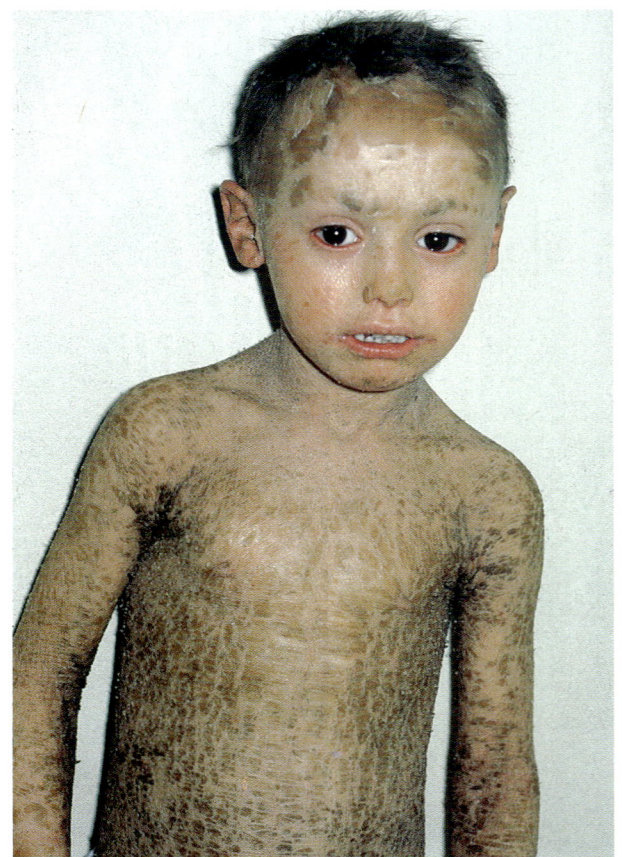

Figure 4.29

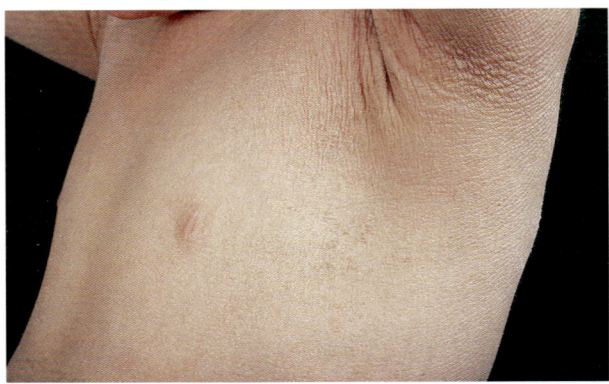

Figure 4.30

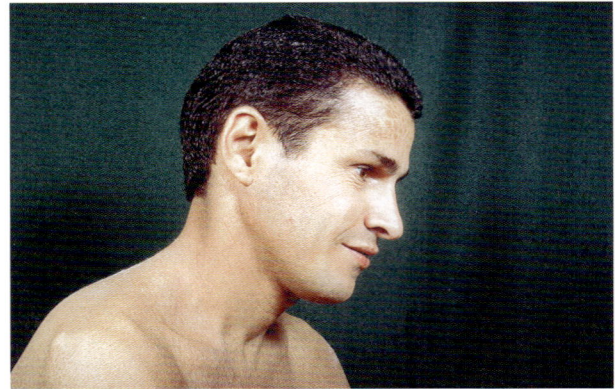

Figure 4.31

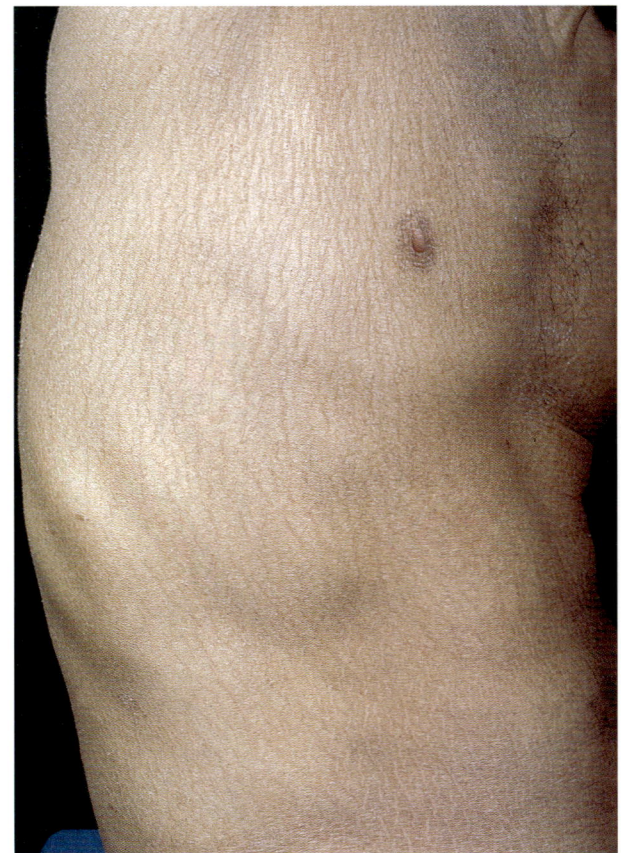

Figure 4.32

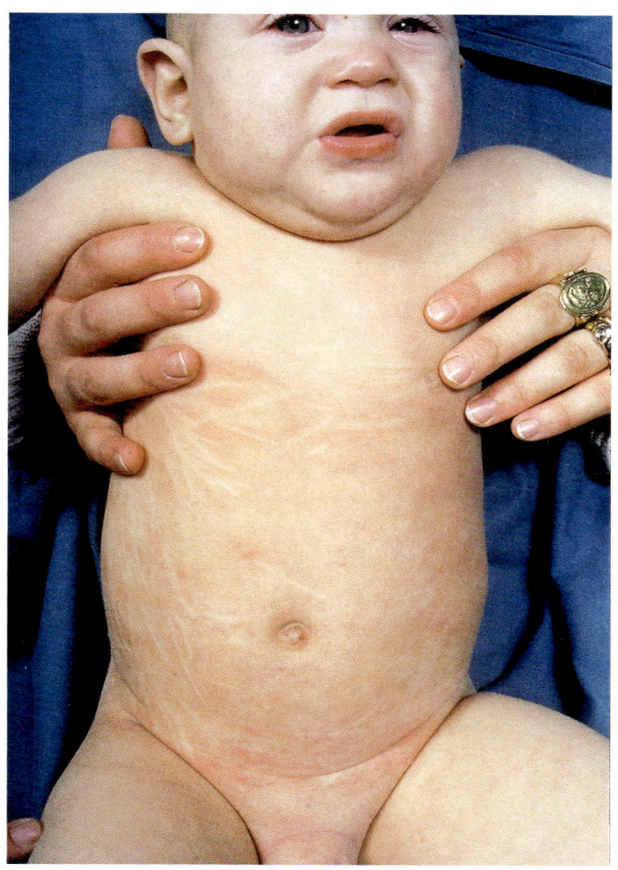

Figure 4.33

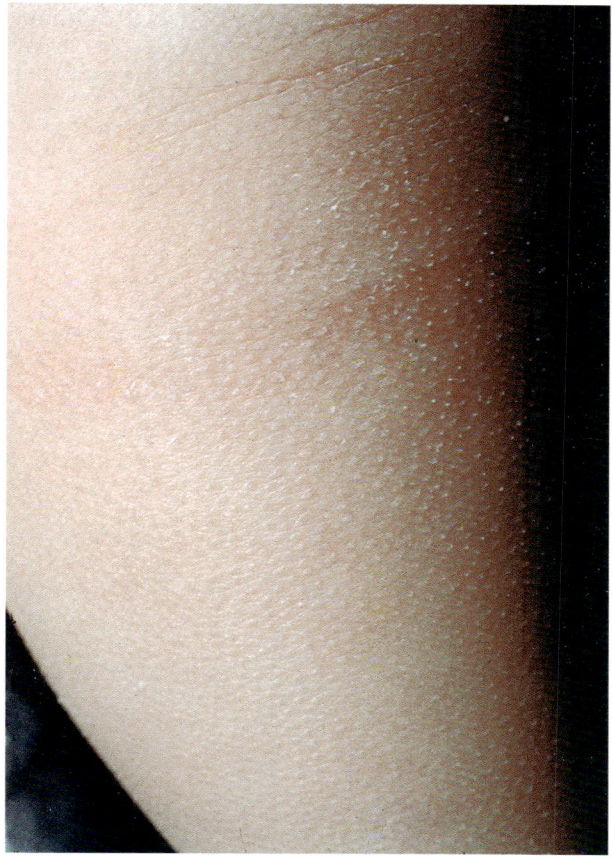

Figure 4.34

REFERENCES

Akiyama M, Takizawa Y, Kokaji T, Shimizu H. Novel mutations of TGM1 in a child with congenital ichthyosiform erythroderma. Br J Dermatol 2001; 144: 401–7

Akiyama M, Takizawa Y, Suzuki Y, et al. Compound heterozygous TGM1 mutations including a novel missense mutation L204Q in a mild form of lamellar ichthyosis. J Invest Dermatol 2001; 116: 992–5

Annilo T, Shulenin S, Chen ZQ, et al. Identification and characterization of a novel ABCA subfamily member, ABCA12 located in the lamellar ichthyosis region on 2q34. Cytogenet Genome Res 2002; 98: 169–76

DiGiovanna JJ, Robinson-Bostom L. Ichthyosis: etiology, diagnosis, and management. Am J Clin Dermatol 2003; 4: 81–95

Jobard F, Lefevre C, Karaduman A, et al. Lipoxygenase-3 (ALOXE3) and 12(R)-lipoxygenase (ALOX12B) are mutated in non-bullous congenital ichthyosiform erythroderma (NCIE) linked to chromosome 17p13.1. Hum Mol Genet 2002 1; 11: 107–13

Lefevre C, Audebert S, Jobard F, et al. Mutations in the transporter ABCA12 are associated with lamellar ichthyosis type 2. Hum Mol Genet 2003; 12: 2369–78. Epub 2003 Jul 15

HARLEQUIN FETUS

Synonym

- Harlequin ichthyosis

Age of onset

- At birth

Epidemiology

This disease is very rare; fewer than 100 cases have been described worldwide.

Clinical findings

This shows a dramatic pattern represented by a thick (0.5–1 cm), compact white-grayish shell that covers the entire body (Figure 4.35).

This 'cuirass' is fixed, and divided into irregular quadrangular plates that mimic grotesquely the dress of the traditional Italian character named Harlequin (Figure 4.36).

Extreme ectropion, eclabion and an 'O'-shaped mouth are visible, together with very severe auricular malformations.

The hair is enveloped by the cornified shell. The nails are deformed.

The whole body is so strongly enveloped that the baby is forced to lie in a flexed position.

Extracutaneous symptoms and complications

- Nystagmus and corneal opacities
- Distal phalanges may be necrotic owing to strictures
- Osseous malformations of fingers
- Xerostomia
- Neurologic abnormalities and malformations
- Superinfections and sepsis that are the more frequent cause of death of these patients

Course

Without therapy the disease is invariably lethal.

When high-dose oral retinoid therapy is correctly administered, 50% of patients may survive. The 'cuirass' of the survivors fades within 2 months and they develop an erythematous, scaly, severe ichthyosis pattern with ectropion (Figures 4.37 and 4.38). Hands and feet are largely malformed, with osseous reabsorption (Figures 4.39 and 4.40).

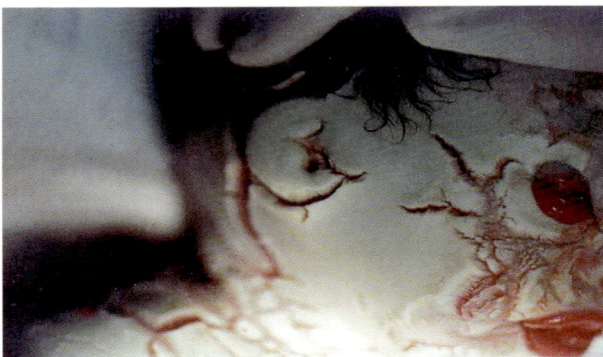

Figure 4.35

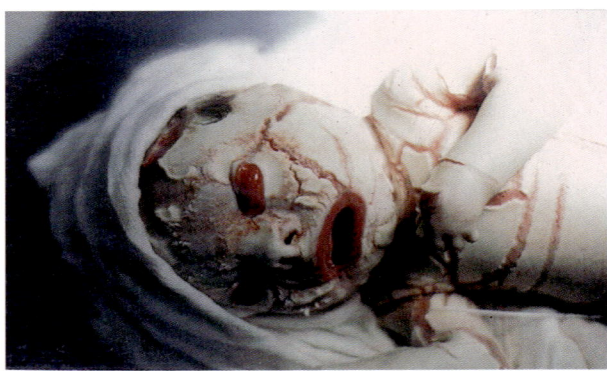

Figure 4.36

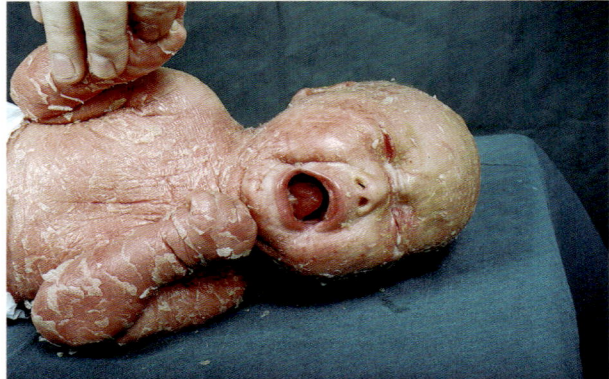

Figure 4.37

Laboratory findings, genetics and pathogenesis

The condition has a recessive pattern of inheritance. Recently, ABCA12 gene-mutations have been found in ten unrelated patients.

Differential diagnosis

- Restrictive dermopathy

Ichthyoses

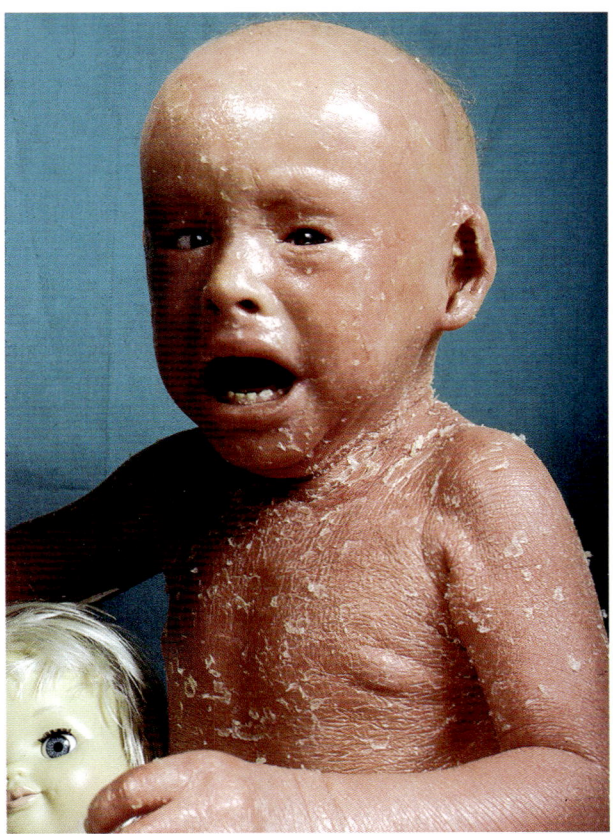

Figure 4.38

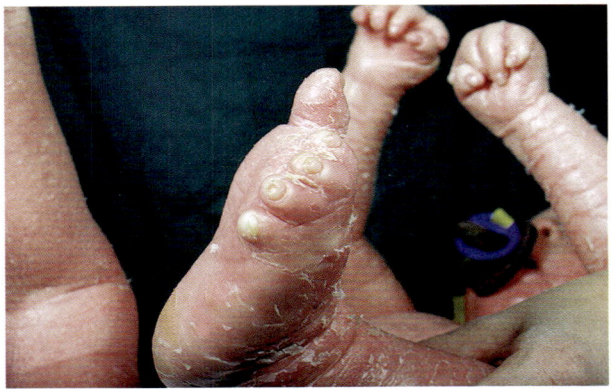

Figure 4.39

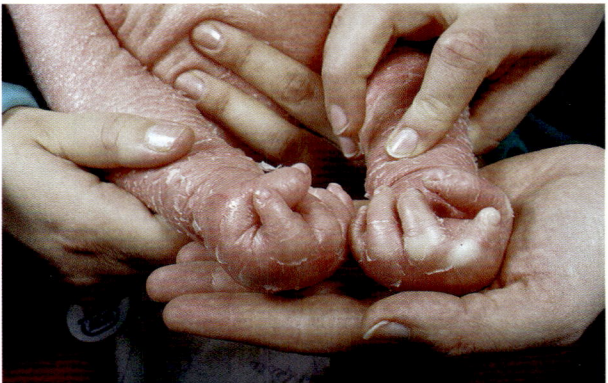

Figure 4.40

Follow-up and therapy

A multidisciplinary approach is advised to cope with related problems, but the ophthalmologist, orthopedic specialist and neurologist play key roles in the first years of life. Physiotherapy may help for the correct development of posture and walking.

The dermatologist is essential for the assessment of local emollients and for the management of oral retinoids.

- Oral retinoids at an initial dose of 1–2 mg/kg/day
- Surgery for ectropion and hands and feet malformation
- Emollients and keratolytic ointments

REFERENCES

Bianca S, Ingegnosi C, Bonaffini F. Harlequin foetus. J Postgrad Med 2003; 49: 81–2

Kelsell DP, Norgett EE, Unsworth H, et al. Mutations in ABCA12 underlie the severe congenital skin disease harlequin icththyosis. AM J Hum Genet 2005; 76: 794–803

Laranjeira JR, Macedo JL, Costa JN, et al. Harlequin fetus. J Pediatr (Rio J) 1996; 72: 184–6

PITYRIASIS ROTUNDA

Synonym

- Pityriasis rotunda type II

Age of onset

- Infancy to childhood

Clinical findings

Cutaneous manifestations

- Multiple, asymptomatic, circular hypopigmented and scaly patches, varying in size from 0.5 to about 30 cm; the lesions are sharply demarcated, tend to merge giving a characteristic geometric appearance and involve the trunk and limbs (Figures 4.41 and 4.42)
- Not associated with systemic diseases and malignancies
- Diffuse xerosis

Course

The duration of the disease varies from several months to a few years, and then tends to spontaneous resolution. Summer remissions and winter exacerbations may occur.

Laboratory investigation

Histopathologic findings include laminar orthokeratosis associated with a thinned granular layer.

Genetics and pathogenesis

This is an autosomal dominant disease involving almost exclusively Sardinian and Japanese populations.

Differential diagnosis

- Tinea versicolor
- Dermatomycoses
- Leprosy
- Pityriasis alba
- Parapsoriasis in plaques

Therapy

- Topical keratolytic agents

REFERENCES

Aste N, Pau M, Aste N, et al. Pityriasis rotunda: a survey of 42 cases observed in Sardinia – Italy. Dermatology 1997; 194: 32–5

Ena P, Cerimele D. Pityriasis rotunda in childhood. Pediatr Dermatol 2002; 19: 200–3

Grimalt R, Gelmetti C, Brusasco A, et al. Pityriasis rotunda: report of a familial occurrence and review of the literature. J Am Acad Dermatol 1994; 31: 866–71

Hashimoto Y, Suga Y, Chikenji T, et al. Immunohistological characterization of a Japanese case of pityriasis rotunda. Br J Dermatol 2003; 149: 196–8

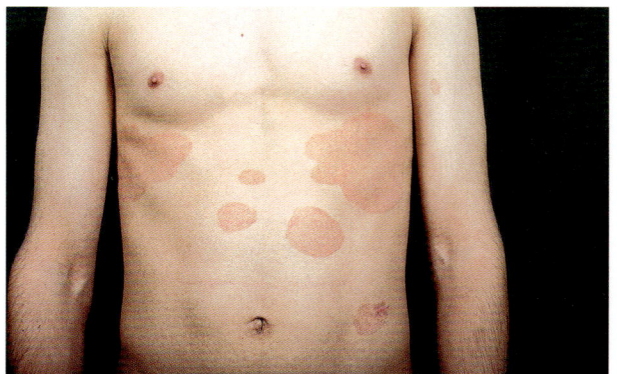

Figure 4.41

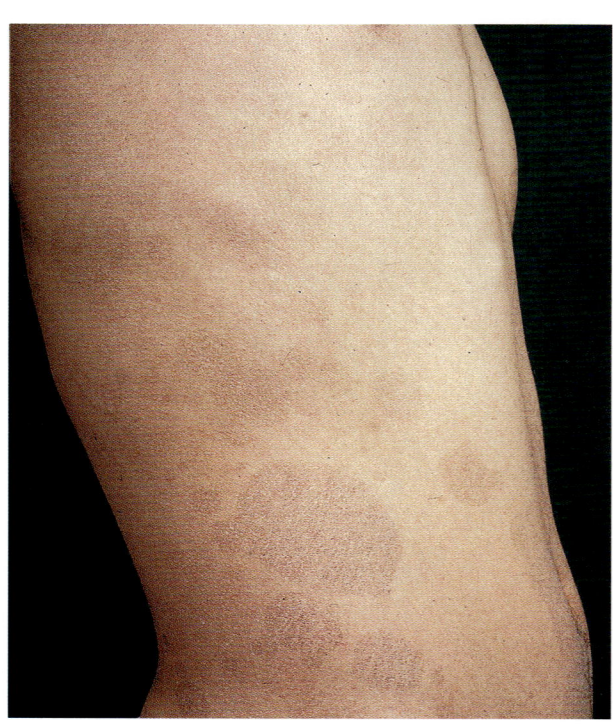

Figure 4.42

Ichthyoses 51

CONGENITAL RETICULAR ICHTHYOSIFORM ERYTHRODERMA (CRIE)

Synonyms

- Ichthyosis 'en confettis'
- 'Ichthyosis variegata'

Epidemiology

Fewer than ten cases are reported in the literature.

Clinical findings

The condition presents with a bright, erythematous, collodion baby at birth, with subsequent lamellar ichthyosis during infancy and childhood.

At puberty or shortly thereafter, 'dots' of whitish, non-ichthyotic skin arise, especially on the face and upper trunk, becoming larger in size and number, reaching hundreds of whitish, slightly scaling macules intermingled in the ichthyotic erythema, 0.5–1 cm wide (Figures 4.43 and 4.44).

Late in the second decade, hypertrichosis appears on the arms and legs, becoming a prominent feature (Figure 4.45). Contemporaneously, brown-grayish hyperpigmented macules appear on the lower third of the legs and less frequently on the arms (Figure 4.46). There can be severe hyperhidrosis and pruritus; ectropion and auricle deformities are present; hair and nails are normal.

Extracutaneous findings

- Severe psychological discomfort

Course and complications

As already stated, this syndrome has a particular course with dramatic changes at the end of the first decade. These features (white macules, hypertrichosis and hyperpigmented macules) are unpredictable at birth.

These patients complain of severe hyperhidrosis and pruritus later in life. There is normal life expectancy.

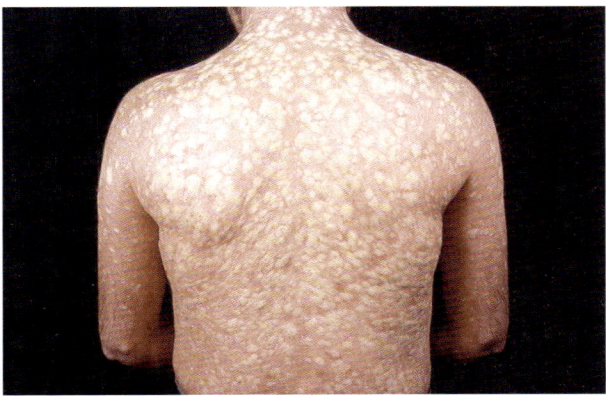

Figure 4.43

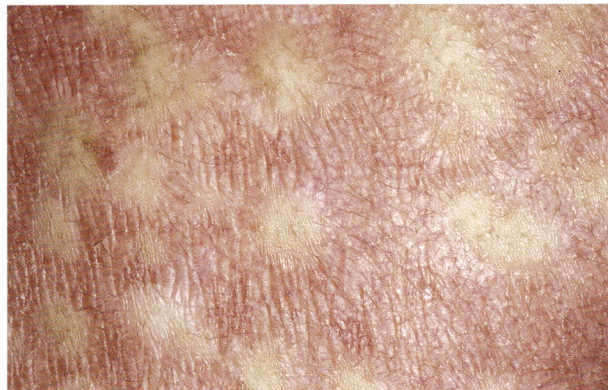

Figure 4.44

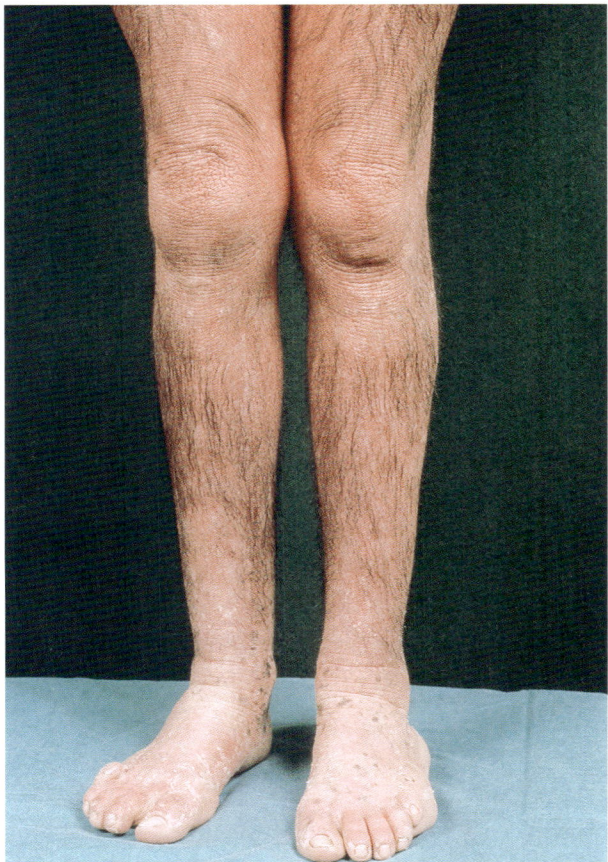

Figure 4.45

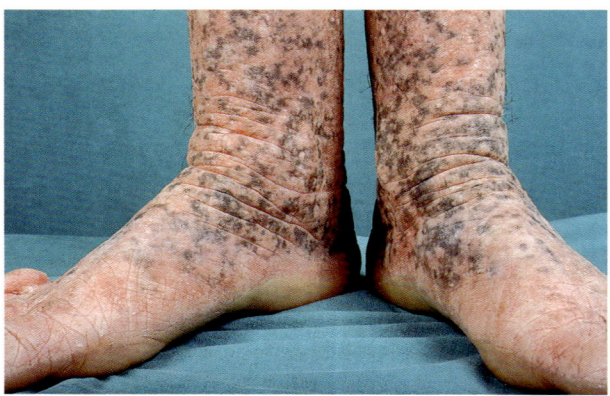

Figure 4.46

- Cutaneous infections due probably to scratching, especially on the lower legs
- Ectropion-related conjunctivitis and corneal ulcerations

Laboratory findings

Electron microscopy shows the feature of fine granular perinuclear shells in the keratinocytes.

Genetics and pathogenesis

To date, there has been no locus found for this disease.

In order to explain the progressive occurrence of macules, it is hazardous but intriguing to hypothesize that some stem cells could survive without the mutations, or that a mosaic stem cell could be postzygotically mutated and become visible when, for example, hormonal stimuli trigger proliferation.

Differential diagnosis

- Lamellar ichthyosis with erythema and collodion presentation

Follow-up and therapy

- Patients must be psychologically supported
- Keratolytic agents may be helpful
- Oral retinoids are suggested
- Antibiotics for superinfections

REFERENCES

Brusasco A, Cambiaghi S, Tadini G, et al. Unusual hyperpigmentation developing in congenital reticular ichthyosiform erythroderma (ichthyosis variegata). Br J Dermatol 1998; 139: 893–6

Brusasco A, Tadini G, Cambiaghi S, et al. A case of congenital reticular ichthyosiform erythroderma – ichthyosis 'en confettis'. Dermatology 1994; 188: 40–5

Marghescu S, Anton-Lamprecht I, Rudolph PO, Kaste R. [Congenital reticular ichthyosiform erythroderma.] Hautarzt 1984; 35: 522–9

CHAPTER 5

Syndromic ichthyoses

NETHERTON SYNDROME

Synonym

- Netherton–Comel Syndrome

Age of onset

This can be at birth as collodion baby or during the first months of life as ichthyosis lineariss circumflexa or ichthyosiform dermatosis.

Clinical findings

The disorder is characterized by the triad ichthyosiform dermatosis, hair shaft defects and atopic diathesis.

Ichthyosiform dermatosis

Two phenotypes of ichthyosis may be expressed:

- Ichthyosis linearis circumflexa: slowly migrating, erythematous, scaling, serpiginous lesions with a distinctive double-edged desquamation at the periphery (Figures 5.1–5.3)

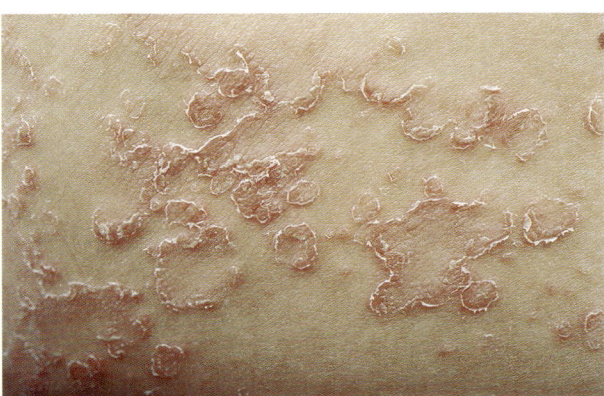

Figure 5.2

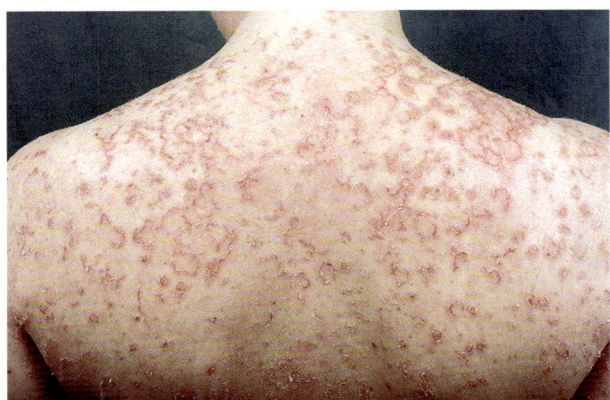

Figure 5.1

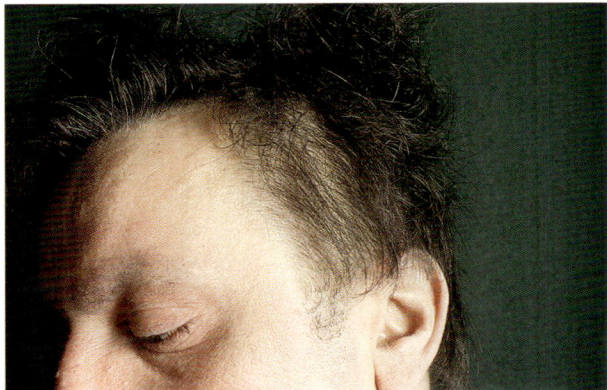

Figure 5.3

- Generalized erythroderma and erythematous collodion baby presentation at birth (Figures 5.4 and 5.5)

Patients present a characteristic facies and, during adolescence and in adult life, flexural, malodorous lichenifications (Figures 5.6–5.10).

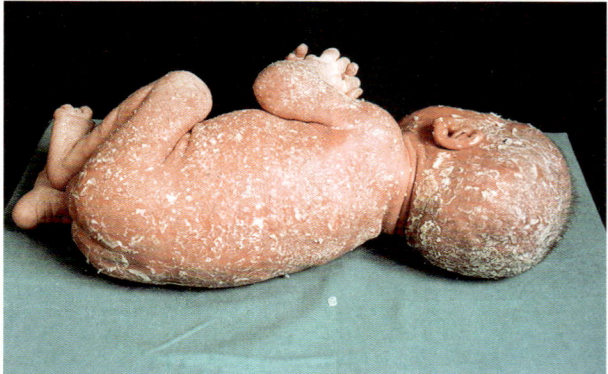

Figure 5.4

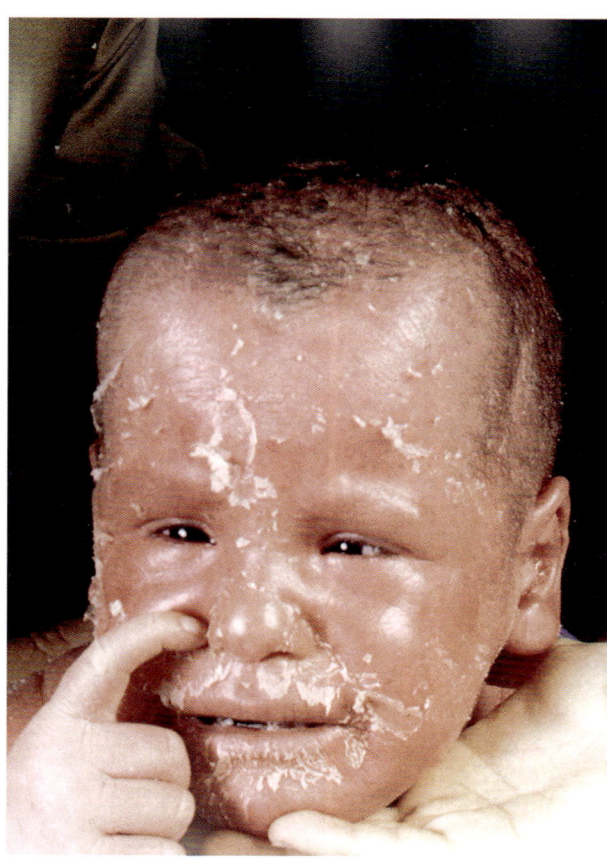

Figure 5.5

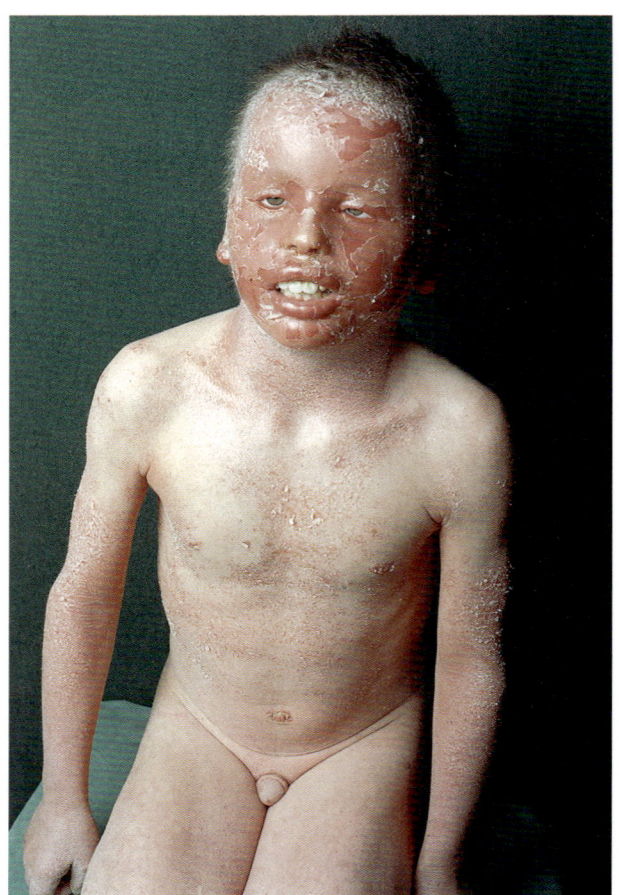

Figure 5.6

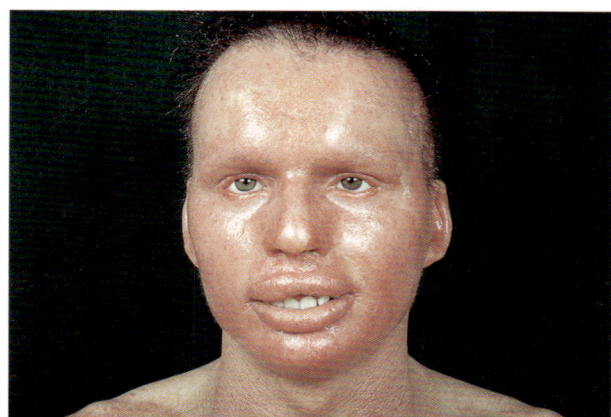

Figure 5.7

Atopic diathesis

Itching eczematous lesions are present in 30–60% of patients, and frequently overlap the ichthyosiform manifestations.

Syndromic ichthyoses 55

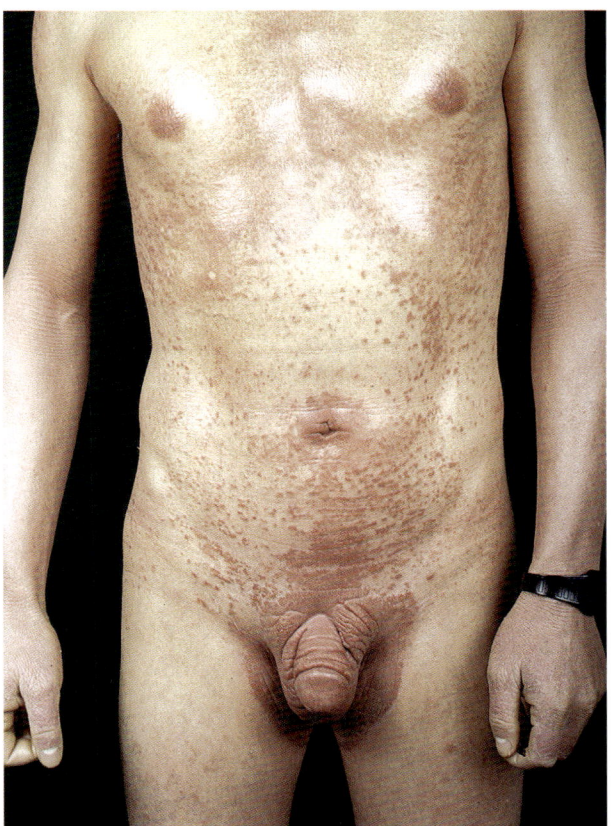

Figure 5.8

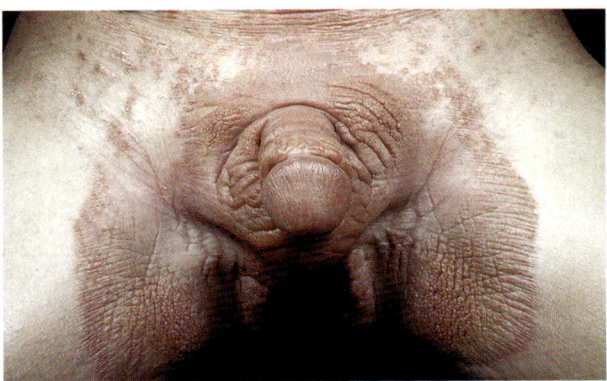

Figure 5.9

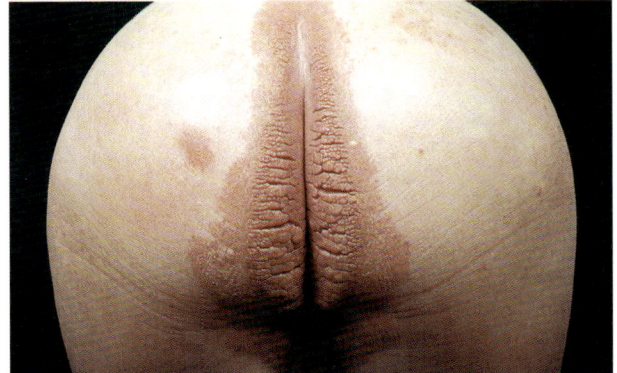

Figure 5.10

Hair shaft defects

The hair is sparse, short and brittle. The distinctive microscopic feature is trichorrhexis invaginata (bamboo hair), more easily seen on eyebrow hairs (Figures 5.11 and 5.12).

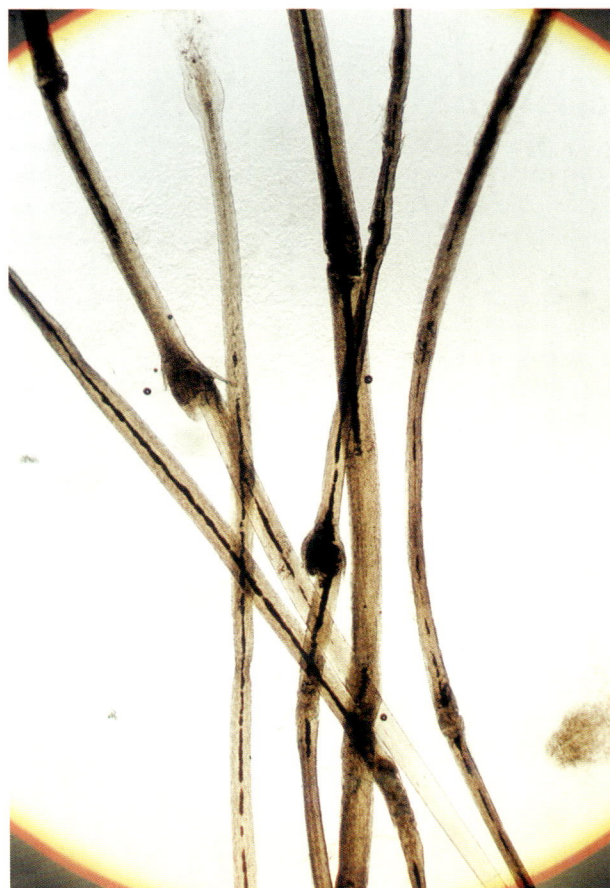

Figure 5.11

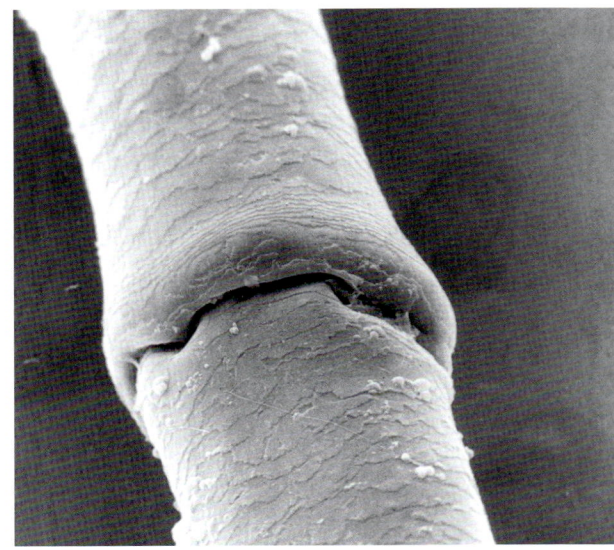

Figure 5.12

Association

- Anaphylactoid reactions (25% of patients) after ingestion of nuts, peanuts, eggs, milk or fish
- Increased incidence of asthenia
- Delayed growth and body development
- Mental deficiency
- Recurrent infections

Course

The disease may improve with age and the hair abnormalities may disappear. However the erythrodermic form is usually persistent. Life span is reduced owing to recurrent infections.

Laboratory findings

- Elevated level of serum immunoglobulin E
- Moderate eosinophilia
- Inconstant aminoaciduria

Genetics and pathogenesis

- Autosomal recessive disease, consanguinity in about 10%
- Mutation of the gene SPINK5 encoding the serine protease inhibitor LEKTI

Differential diagnosis

- Erythrodermic ichthyosis
- Leiner's disease
- Acrodermatitis enteropathica
- Erythrokeratodermia variabilis

Follow-up

- Microbiological cultures to detect superinfections
- Allergological examinations to prevent severe manifestations of atopy
- Psychological assessment

Therapy

- Emollients and keratolytic preparation
- The use of aromatic retinoids is controversial: worsening of atopic manifestations during treatment

REFERENCES

Bitoun E, Micheloni A, Lamant L, et al. LEKTI proteolytic processing in human primary keratinocytes, tissue distribution and defective expression in Netherton syndrome. Hum Mol Genet 2003; 12: 2417–30

Chavanas S, Bodemer C, Rochat A, et al. Mutations in SPINK5, encoding a serine protease inhibitor, cause Netherton syndrome. Nature Genet 2000; 25: 141–2

Judge MR, Morgan G, Harper JI. A clinical and immunological study of Netherton's syndrome. Br J Dermatol 1994; 131: 615–21

Krasagakis K, Ioannidou DJ, Stephanidou M, et al. Early development of multiple epithelial neoplasms in Netherton syndrome. Dermatology 2003; 207: 182–4

Van Gysel D, Koning H, Baert MRM, et al. Clinico-immunological heterogeneity in Comel–Netherton syndrome. Dermatology 2001; 202: 99–107

Walden M, Kreutz P, Drogemuller K, et al. Biochemical features, molecular biology and clinical relevance of the human 15-domain serine proteinase inhibitor LEKTI. Biol Chem 2002; 383: 1139–41

SJÖGREN–LARSSON SYNDROME

Age of onset

This is at birth in many cases, but may be postponed for several months of life.

Epidemiology

This is a very rare disease. There is no study on prevalence available.

Clinical findings

There is a diffuse, moderate, non-erythematous ichthyosiform presentation with a tendency to become darker during infancy, especially on the trunk and legs (Figures 5.13 and 5.14).

Patients complain of pruritus, and scratching signs are often visible. The scalp is involved and mild palmoplantar hyperkeratosis may be present. Nails, hair and sweat glands are normal.

Extracutaneous findings

- Spastic dyplegia or tetraplegia leading to severe disability (Figure 5.15)
- Non-progressive moderate to severe mental retardation from early infancy
- Seizures in about 40% of patients
- Retinal abnormalities ('whitish macular dots') and, in about half of cases, corneal opacities and vision impairment with photophobia
- Short stature

Course and complications

Although immune deficiency is not a characteristic feature of Sjögren–Larsson syndrome, there is an increased risk of premature death from pulmonary infections, related to tetraplegic conditions.

The ichthyosis and mental retardation are non-progressive. Early death is related to severe mental retardation and spastic conditions.

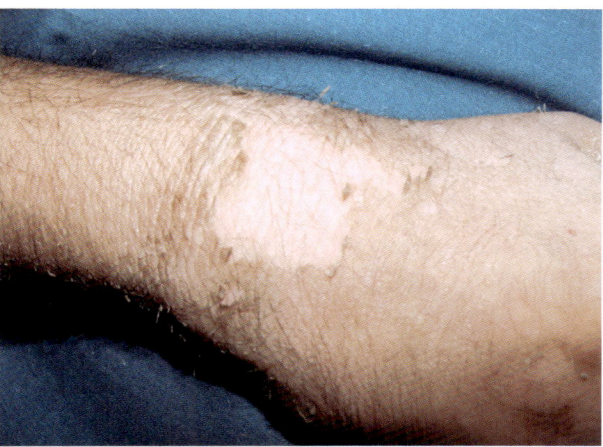

Figure 5.13

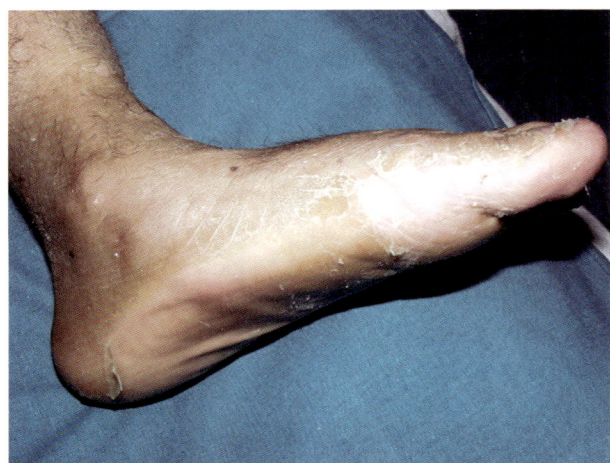

Figure 5.14

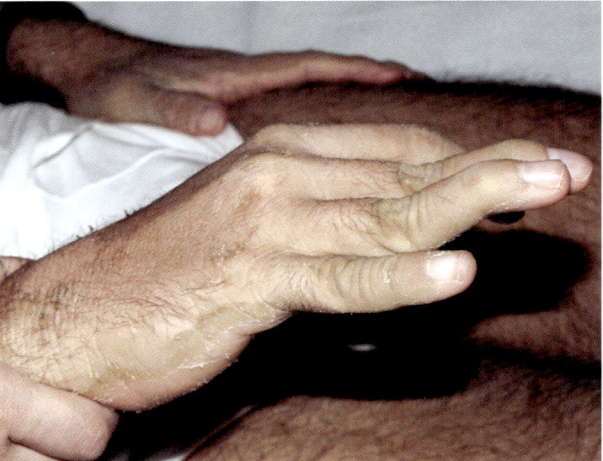

Figure 5.15

Laboratory findings, genetics and pathogenesis

The disease is autosomal recessive. The causative gene is called FALDH and encodes for the enzyme fatty aldehyde dehydrogenase that produces accumulations of long chain fatty alcohols in skin and the central nervous system. Mutations have been found in patients and carriers.

Differential diagnosis

Lamellar and X-linked ichthyosis may be compared for skin features, but early severe mental retardation and retinal abnormalities are not features of either.

Trichothiodystrophy (TTD) may show ichthyosiform features and severe mental retardation, but hair changes in TTD are diagnostic.

Other rarer syndromes associated with ichthyosis, metabolic defects with neurological abnormalities as in Gaucher's disease.

Follow-up and therapy

- Keratolytic ointments may be helpful
- Prevention of decubitus ulcers
- Pharmacological control of seizures
- Prevention and care of pulmonary infections

REFERENCES

Auada MP, Taube MB, Collares EF, et al. Sjögren–Larsson syndrome: biochemical defects and follow up in three cases. Eur J Dermatol 2002; 12: 263–6

Wells RS, Kerr CB. Genetic classification of ichthyosis. Arch Dermatol 1965; 92: 1–6

Willemsen MA, Iklst L, Steijlen PM, et al. Clinical, biochemical and molecular genetic characteristics of 19 patients with the Sjögren–Larsson syndrome. Brain 2001; 124: 1426–37

REFSUM SYNDROME

Synonym

- Phytanic acid deficiency

Age of onset

- Late childhood or adolescence

Clinical findings

- Generalized desquamative disorder resembling dominant ichthyosis vulgaris (Figures 5.16 and 5.17)
- Palmoplantar hyperlinearity is reported

Extracutaneous findings

- Progressive ataxia and peripheral neuropathy
- Late-onset retinitis pigmentosa
- Anosmia
- Central hearing loss
- Cardiac arrhythmias
- Long bone defects at the extremities

Course and complications

Characteristically, the extracutaneous symptoms are of late onset and may worsen with age.

Laboratory findings

Under the electron microscope, keratinocytes contain cytoplasmic lipid droplets.

Genetics and pathogenesis

The disease is autosomal recessive.
There is a defect of the α-oxidation of phytanic acid.
The involved genes are the phytanoil-CoA hydroxylase (PHYH) and PTS2 receptor (PEX7).

Differential diagnosis

- Lamellar and syndromic ichthyoses
- Other syndromic ichthyoses with neurological abnormalities

Follow-up and therapy

- Multidisciplinary approach for eye and neurological symptoms
- Emollients and keratolytic agents for ichthyosis

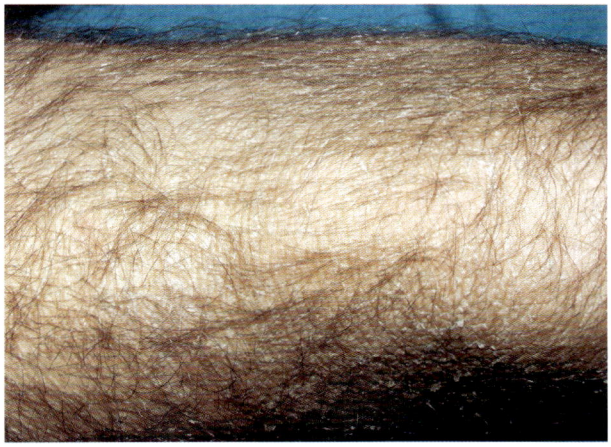

Figure 5.16

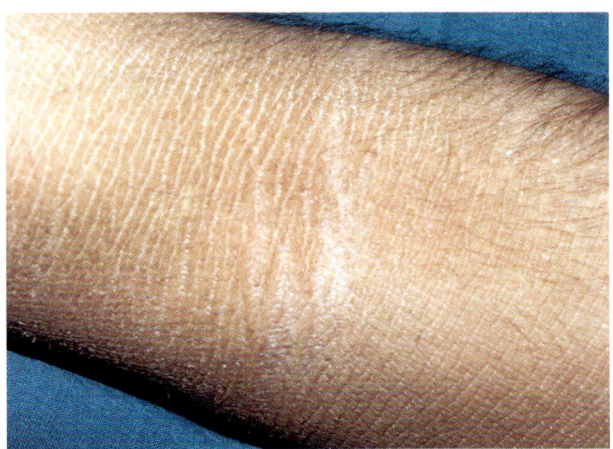

Figure 5.17

REFERENCES

Gootjes J, Schmohl F, Mooijer PA, et al. Identification of the molecular defect in patients with peroxisomal mosaicism using a novel method involving culturing of cells at 40 degrees C: implications for other inborn errors of metabolism. Hum Mutat 2004; 24: 130–9

Jansen GA, Waterham HR, Wanders RJ. Molecular basis of Refsum disease: sequence variations in phytanoyl-CoA hydroxylase (PHYH) and the PTS2 receptor (PEX7). Hum Mutat 2004; 23: 209–18. Review.

Wanders RJ, Jansen GA, Lloyd MD. Phytanic acid alpha-oxidation, new insights into an old problem: a review. Biochim Biophys Acta 2003; 631: 119–35

TRICHOTHIODYSTROPHY

Synonym

- Sulfur-deficient brittle hair syndrome

Epidemiology

We have personally diagnosed five families (seven patients) with TTD in a 12-year survey. About 200 cases are described in the literature.

Age of onset

- At birth

Clinical findings

Cutaneous manifestations

- Collodion baby presentation possible
- Dry, dull, brittle, unruly, broken hair (Figures 5.18–20)
- Partial or total alopecia of the scalp, eyelashes and eyebrows and subsequently of the secondary sexual hair (Figure 5.20)
- Ichthyosis (Figure 5.21), eczema, follicular keratosis, photosensitivity (Figure 5.22), cheilitis (Figure 5.23), telangiectasia, hypohidrosis, freckles, atopic dermatitis in 30%
- Dystrophic nails (Figure 5.24) with koilonychia, ridging, lamellar splitting and spotted leukonychia

Extracutaneous manifestations

- Neurologic symptoms: mental retardation, spasticity, paralysis, motor control impairment, pyramidal signs, hyperreflexia and 'party-behavior' appearance, with wide spectrum of severity
- Morphologic changes and dysmorphia: growth retardation with short stature, microcephaly, cranial dysplasia, micrognathia, protruding ears, dental abnormalities, high arched palate
- Ocular lesions: cataract, conjunctivitis, nystagmus, photophobia, retinal dystrophy, ectropion
- Genital hypoplasia, cryptorchidism, hypospadia
- Bone lesions
- Recurrent (pulmonary) infections due to severe immunodeficiency
- Failure to thrive

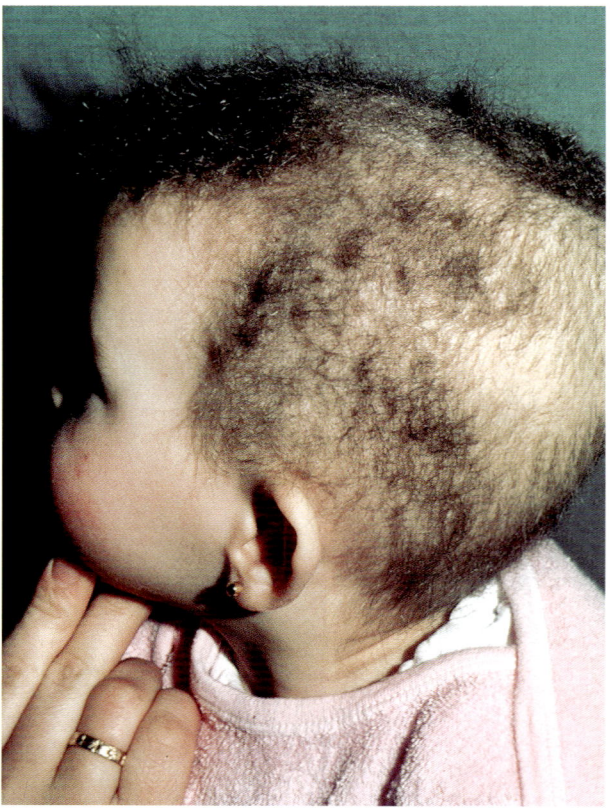

Figure 5.18

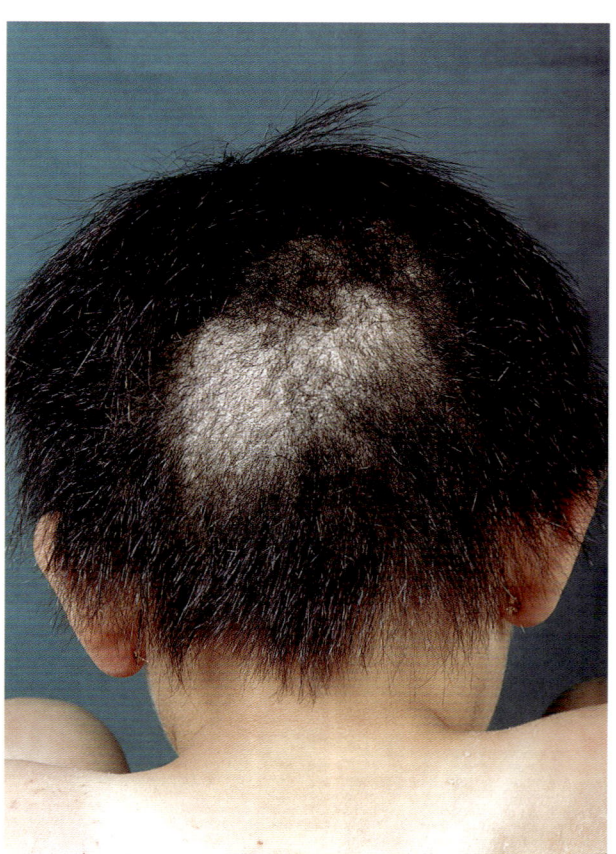

Figure 5.19

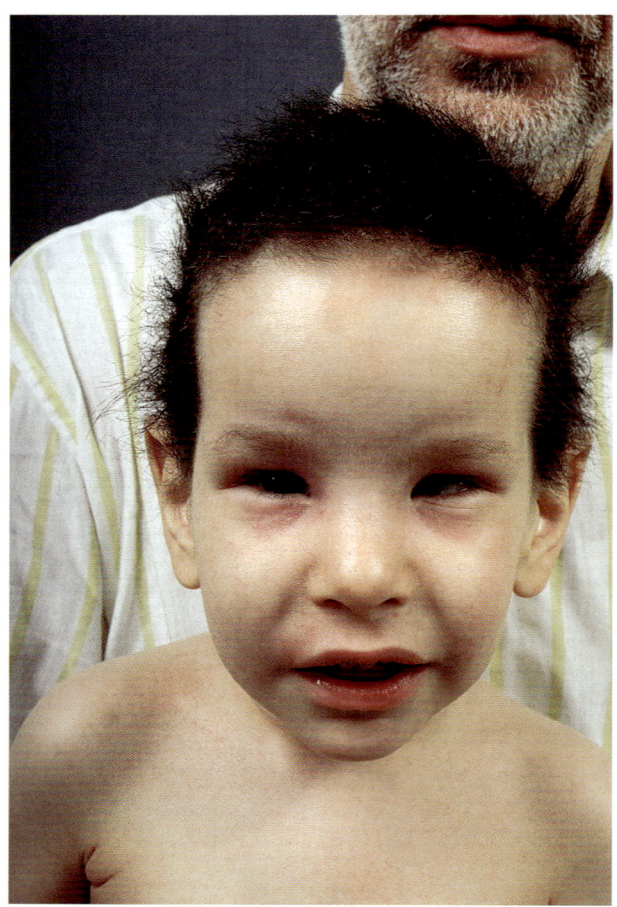

Figure 5.20

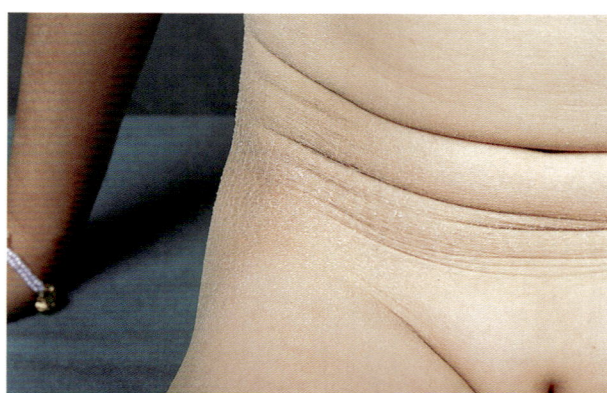

Figure 5.21

In the literature can be found all the following clinical forms that are TTD-related:

- Brittle hair + mental retardation = Sabonis' syndrome
- Brittle hair, intellectual impairment, decreased fertility, short stature = BIDS syndrome

Syndromic ichthyoses

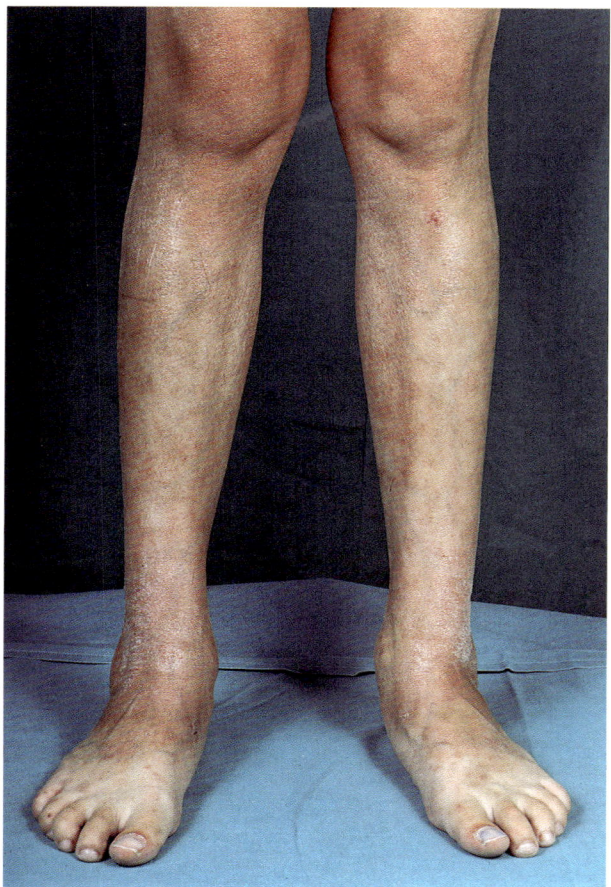

Figure 5.22

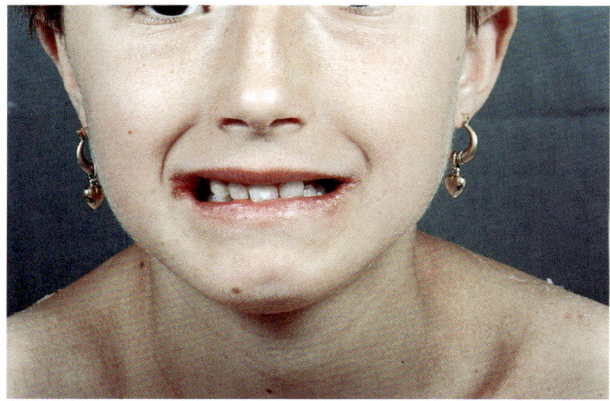

Figure 5.23

- Ichthyosiform + BIDS = IBIDS syndrome = Tay's syndrome
- Photosensitivity + IBIDS = PIBIDS syndrome
- Osteosclerosis + IBIDS = SIBIDS syndrome
- Brittle hair, mental retardation, immunodeficiency
- Brittle hair + intrauterine growth restriction

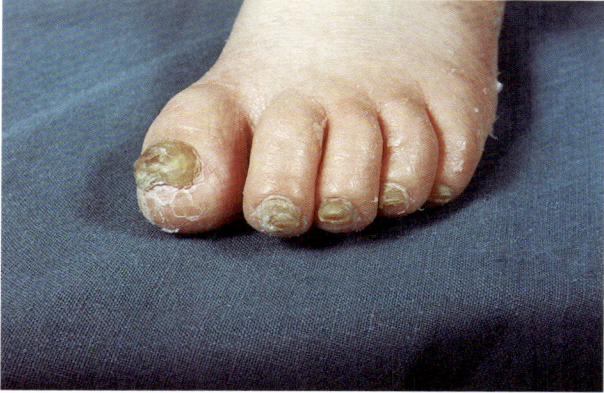

Figure 5.24

- Cerebellar ataxia, oligophrenia, bilateral cataracts, short stature, TTD = Marinesco–Sjögren syndrome

We strongly support, on the basis of molecular genetics findings, that TTD should be described as a single entity, and that older terms are seen as an attempt to clarify the different phenotypes at a time when molecular and functional genetics were not available.

Course and prognosis

- Lifelong
- Strictly dependent on severity of neurological manifestations and immune deficiency, but life expectancy is reduced

Laboratory investigations and data

- Aminoacid analysis of the hair shaft: decrease in cystine and cysteine content
- Light microscopy and electron microscopy: trichoschisis (transverse fractures through the hair shaft) and absence of cuticle (Figure 5.25)
- Polarizing microscopy: presence of alternating light and dark bands (tiger-tail pattern) (Figure 5.26), that may be absent in the first year or two of life
- Phototesting

Genetics and pathogenesis

- Autosomal recessive inheritance
- TTD is due to genetic defects shared by xeroderma pigmentosum, a disease characterized by DNA repair anomalies. At least two genes that are responsible for two forms of XP also cause TTD phenotypes

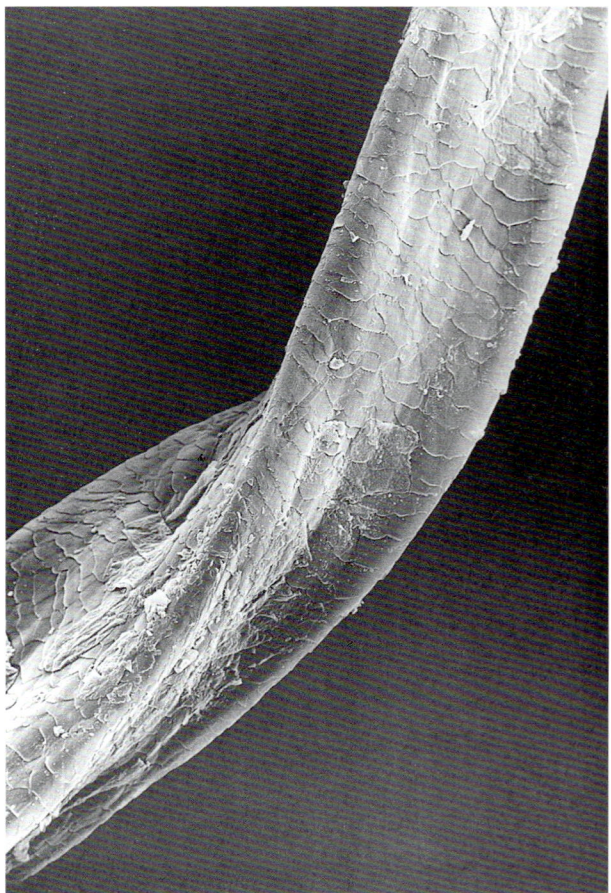

Figure 5.25

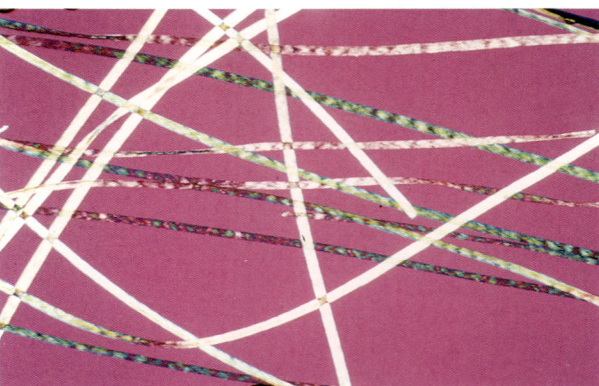

Figure 5.26

- The XP-D and XP-B genes have been found to be mutated in the majority of patients affected by TTD
- A third recent finding allows a genetic defect called TTD-A to be defined

Mutations that cause XP and TTD are different, demonstrating that a single gene can (by different mutation, different loci in the same gene) cause different diseases.

In fact, TTD patients do not show any susceptibility to cancer, and XP patients do not display a sulfur content deficit in their structural proteins.

TTD and XP only share photosensitivity.

XPD and XPB are subunits of the TFIIH factor complex which is a multiprotein complex involved in gene transcription, demonstrating that XPD and XPB play a double role in cell biology, the first being the DNA-repair system and the second the gene transcription – the first step that changes genetic information in proteins.

Different TTD phenotypes (severity of the disease) are related to the residual function of the XPD-B-TFIIH complex and are all mutations that can cause partial interference with the DNA repair system (the 'photosensitivity' of TTD), but are not enough to cause susceptibility to cancer as occurs in the XP mutations that conversely do not interfere with the formation of a normal transcriptional complex. TFIIH complex may be relevant in particular compartments such as skin and CNS development genes, explaining the clinical features of hair anomalies, ichthyosis and mental retardation.

Differential diagnosis

The diagnosis of TTD, compared with Sjögren–Larsson, Menkes' and Netherton's, is based on:

- Hairs with low sulfur content
- Trichoschisis
- Tiger-tail pattern of hairs on polaroscopy

Follow-up and therapy

- Photoprotection
- Symptomatic: prevention of pulmonary infections, application of emollients, physiotherapy, etc.

REFERENCES

Giglia-Mari G, Coin F, Ranish JA, et al. A new, tenth subunit of TFIIH is responsible for the DNA repair syndrome trichothiodystrophy group A. Nature Genet 2004; 36: 714–9. Epub 2004 Jun 27.

Masson C, Menaa F, Pinon-Lataillade G, et al. Global genome repair is required to activate KIN17, a UVC-responsive gene involved in DNA replication. Proc Natl Acad Sci USA 2003; 100: 616–21

Nishiwaki Y, Kobayashi N, Imoto K, et al. Trichothiodystrophy fibroblasts are deficient in the repair of ultraviolet-induced cyclobutane pyrimidine dimers and (6–4)photoproducts. J Invest Dermatol 2004; 122: 526–32

Sperling LC, Di Giovanna JJ. 'Curly' wood and tiger tails: an explanation for light and dark banding with polarization in trichothiodystrophy. Arch Dermatol 2003; 139: 1189–92

Zhou NY, Bates SE, Bouziane M, et al. Efficient repair of cyclobutane pyrimidine dimmers at mutational hotspots is restored in complemented xeroderma pigmentosum group C and trichothiodystrophy/xeroderma pigmentosum group D cells. J Mol Biol 2003; 332: 337–51

DORFMAN–CHANARIN SYNDROME

Synonym

- Neutral lipid storage disease with ichthyosis

Epidemiology

This is very rare, and no data are available on prevalence. We have personally observed a single case in a cohort of more than 250 lamellar ichthyoses.

Age of onset

- At birth

Clinical findings

- Possible collodion baby presentation
- Diffuse ichthyosiform erythroderma with small to medium whitish-gray scales (Figures 5.27 and 5.28)

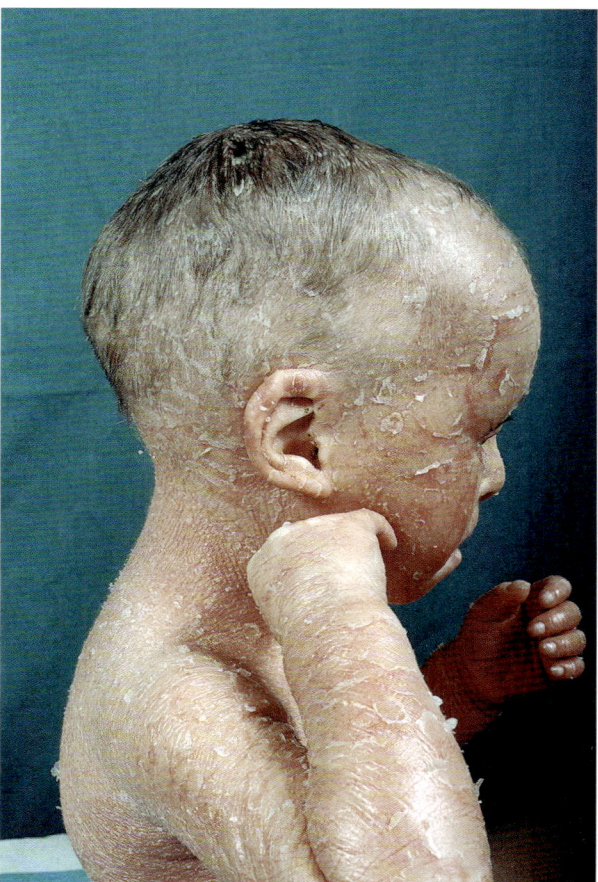

Figure 5.27

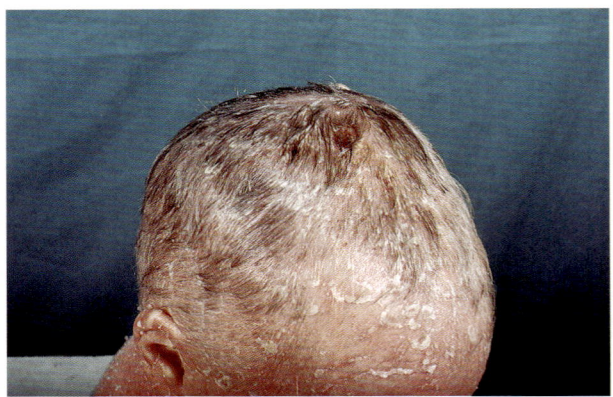

Figure 5.28

- Ectropion is possible
- Indistinguishable from erythrodermic lamellar ichthyosis

Extracutaneous findings

- Mental retardation of variable severity in one-third of patients
- Nystagmus is frequent
- Cataracts and deafness are possible
- Ataxia and myopathy reported in a small percentage of patients
- Hepatic involvement

Complications and course

Extracutaneous signs are of delayed onset, as usually seen in neutral lipid storage disease.

Laboratory findings

The disease is easily diagnosed with lipid droplets in white cells in blood smears. Also, upon electron microscopy, lipids are seen in the cytoplasm of white cells series in many tissues.

Genetics and pathogenesis

This is an autosomal recessive disease. The gene underlying the disease, encoding CGI-58 protein, causes malformation of cytoplasmic lamellar granules and abnormal formation of the cornified envelope.

Differential diagnosis

- Lamellar ichthyosis (type I)

Follow-up and therapy

- Assessment for nystagmus and mental retardation
- Oral retinoids
- Keratolyic agents

REFERENCES

Akiyama M, Sawamura D, Nomura Y, et al. Truncation of CGI-58 protein causes malformation of lamellar granules resulting in ichthyosis in Dorfman–Chanarin syndrome. J Invest Dermatol 2003; 121: 1029–34

Kaassis C, Ginies JL, Berthelot J, Verret JL. [Dorfman–Chanarin syndrome.] Ann Dermatol Venereol 1998; 125: 317–19

Wollenberg A, Schaller M, Roschinger W, et al. [Dorfman–Chanarin syndrome – a neutral lipid storage disease.] Hautarzt 1997; 48: 753–8

CHAPTER 6

Erythrokeratodermas

ERYTHROKERATODERMA VARIABILIS

Synonyms

- Mendes da Costa's disease
- Genodermatosis 'en cocarde'

Age of onset

- At birth (30% of cases) or during the first years of life

Clinical findings

The figurate, sharply demarcated patches of erythema and hyperkeratosis vary in size, shape and distribution within hours or days. The common sites of involvement are the face (Figures 6.1 and 6.2), buttocks and limbs (Figures 6.3 and 6.4). Mucous membranes, hair and nails are not involved. General health is good.

Course

The course is chronic with many exacerbations and remissions.

Laboratory findings

Histopathologic features include mamillated epidermal hyperplasia of compact and basket-woven orthokeratosis. The number of keratinosomes is decreased.

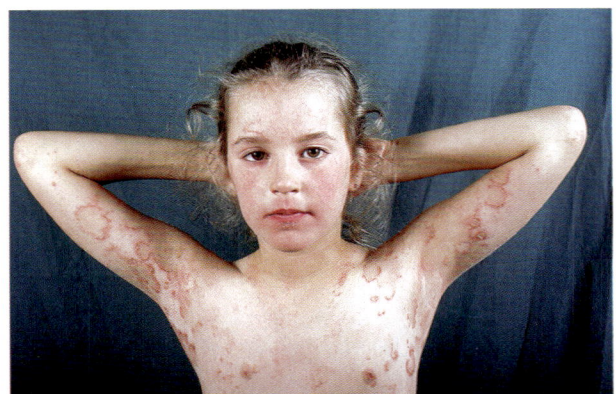

Figure 6.1

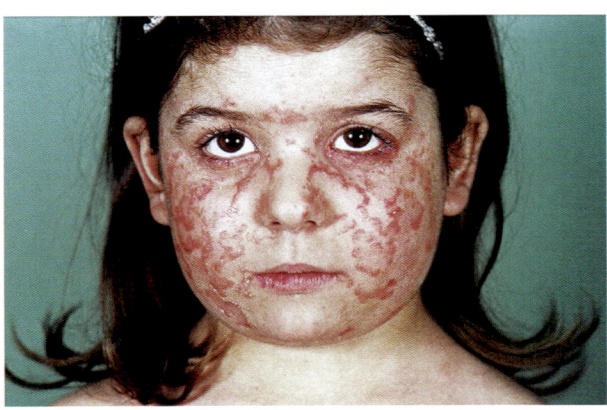

Figure 6.2

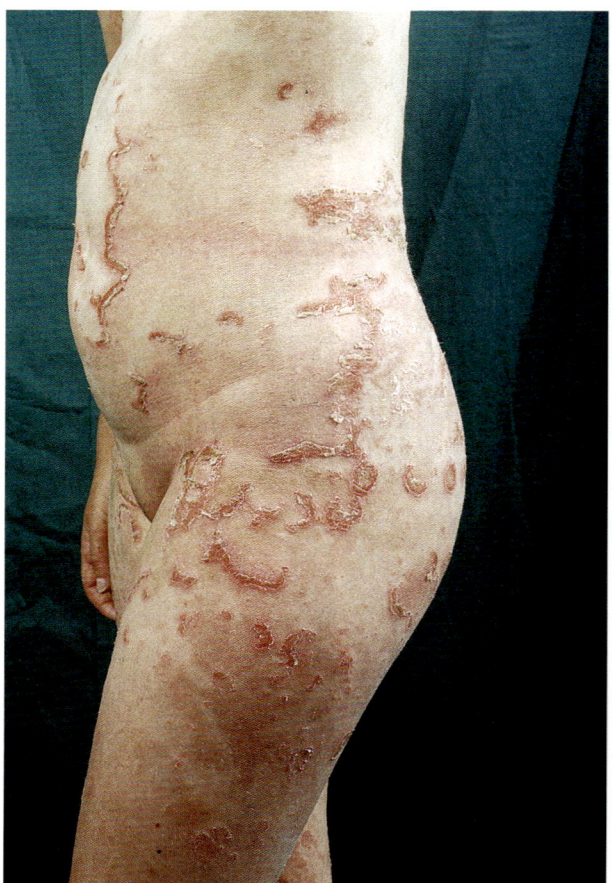

Figure 6.3

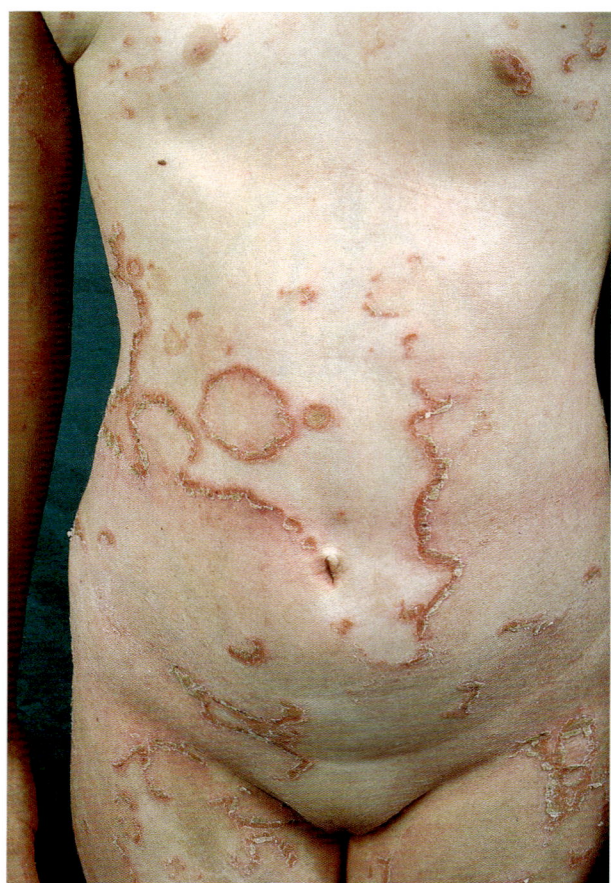

Figure 6.4

Genetics and pathogenesis

- Autosomal dominant disease
- Mutations in connexin 30.3, connexin 31 and in the gap junction-associated protein β-3

Differential diagnosis

- Netherton–Comel syndrome
- Symmetric progressive erythrokeratoderma

Follow-up

- Life span is unaffected. The erythematous lesions may improve with age

Therapy

- Topical treatments with ointments and keratolytic agents
- Oral retinoids may be used with favorable results

REFERENCES

Artia K, Akiyama M, Tsuji Y, et al. Erythrokeratoderma variabilis without connexin 31 or connexin 30.3 gene mutation: immunohistological, ultrastructural and genetic studies. Acta Dermatol Venereol 2003; 83: 266–70

Di WL, Monypenny J, Common JE, et al. Defective trafficking and cell death is characteristic of skin disease-associated connexin 31 mutations. Hum Mol Genet 2002; 11: 2005–14

Papadavid E, Koumantaki E, Dawler RPR. Erythrokeratoderma variabilis: case report and review of the literature. J Eur Acad Dermatol 1998; 11: 180–3

Wilgoss A, Leigh IM, Barnes MR, et al. Identification of a novel mutation R42P in the gap junction protein beta-3 associated with autosomal dominant erythrokeratoderma variabilis. J Invest Dermatol 1999; 113: 1119–22

Erythrokeratodermas

SYMMETRIC PROGRESSIVE ERYTHROKERATODERMA

Synonym

- Gottron's syndrome

Age of onset

- During the first years of life

Clinical findings

Sharply defined, slowly progressive, erythemato-hyperkeratotic plaques are symmetrically distributed on the extremities, the buttocks and the head (Figures 6.5–6.10).

Pruritus may occasionally be present.

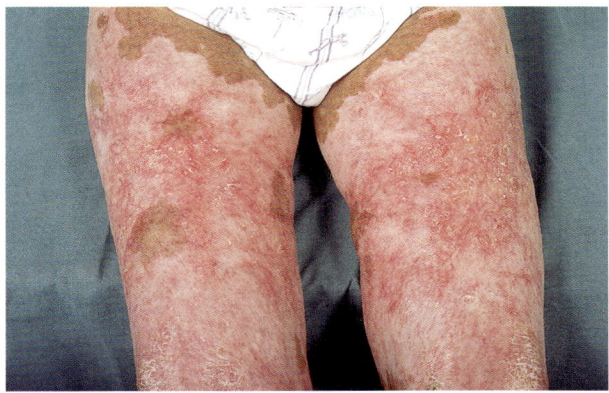

Figure 6.6

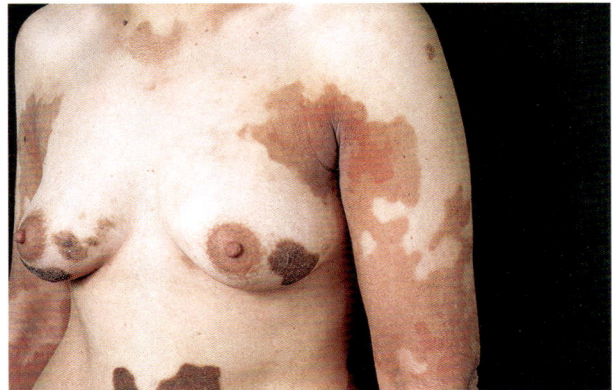

Figure 6.7

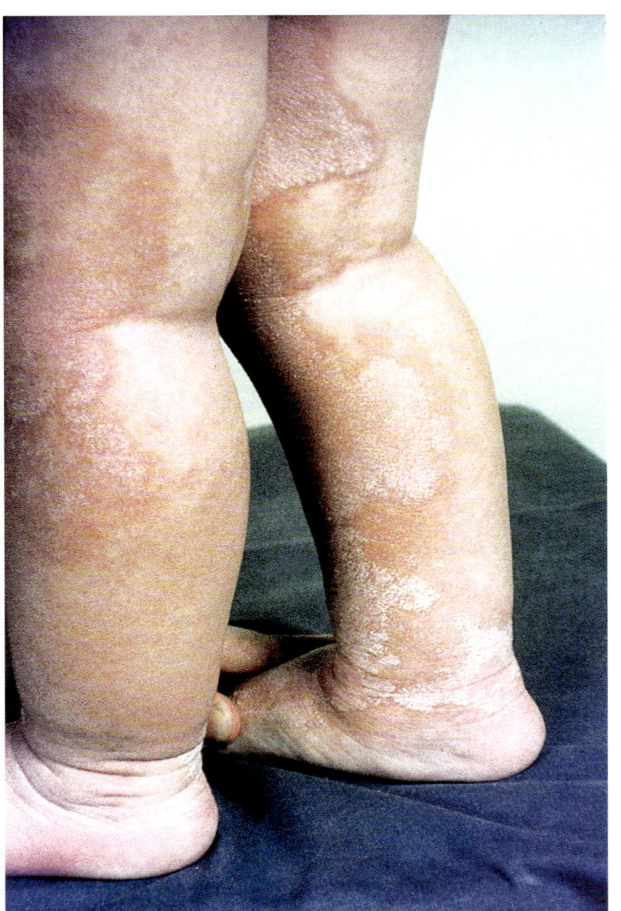

Figure 6.5

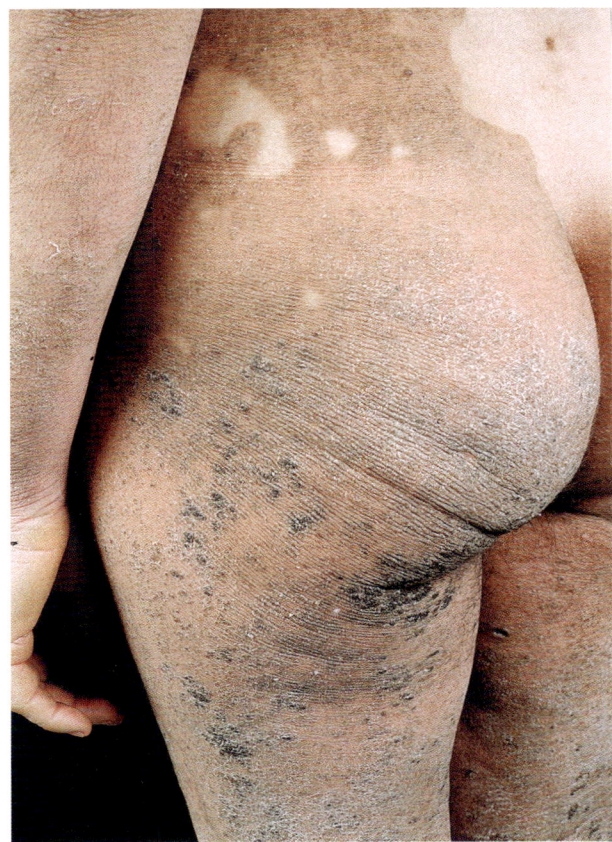

Figure 6.8

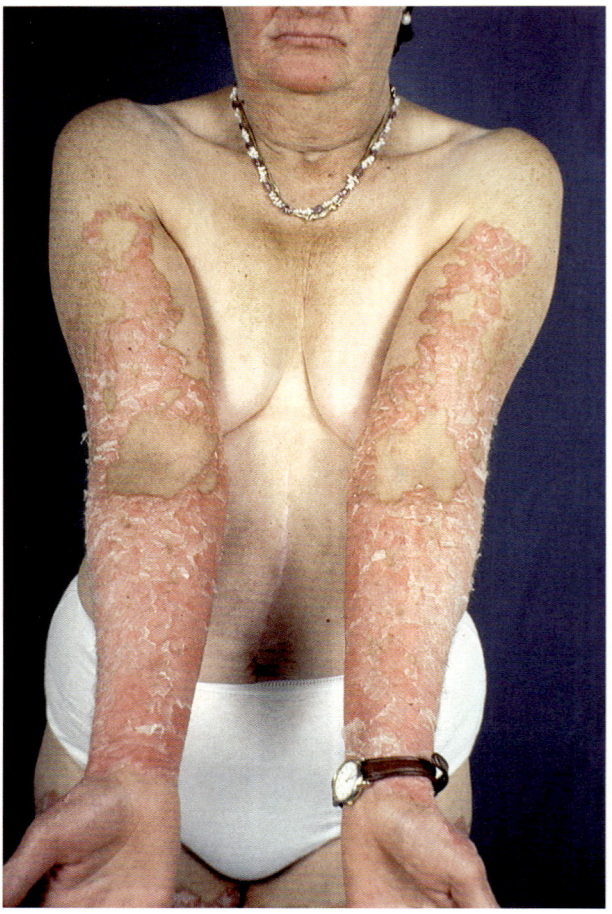

Figure 6.9

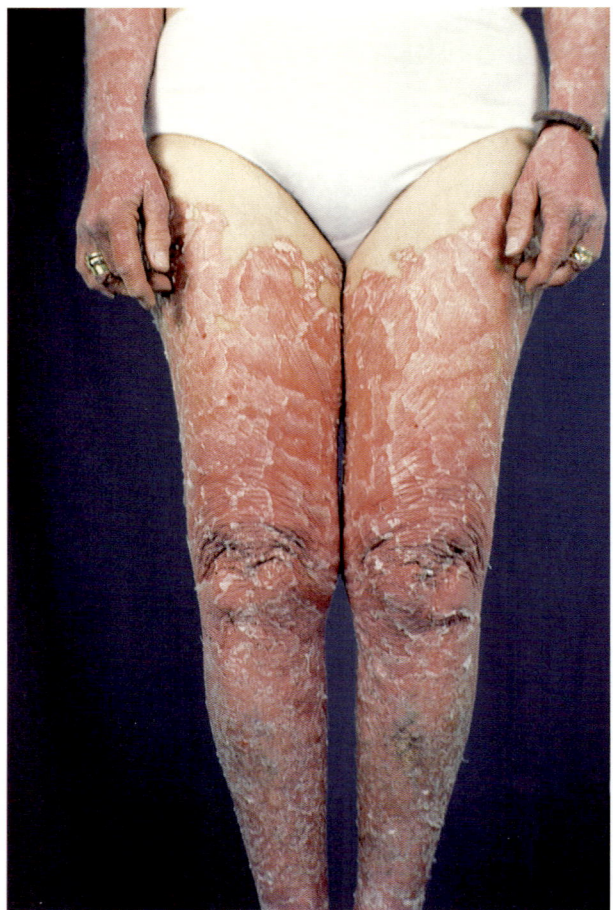

Figure 6.10

Course

The lesions are usually most severe in infancy and may improve after puberty.

Laboratory findings

Histopathologically there is psoriasiform epidermal hyperplasia with focal areas of parakeratosis.

Genetics and pathogenesis

The disease is inherited as an autosomal dominant trait. Mutations in the loricrin gene have been established in some pedigrees.

Follow-up

The life span is unaffected.

Treatment

- Ointments and keratolytic agents as topical treatments
- Oral retinoids have been used with good results
- In adolescents psoralen and ultraviolet A (PUVA) treatment may be effective

REFERENCES

Nazzaro V, Blanchet-Bardon C. Progressive symmetric erythrokeratoderma: histological and ultrastructural study of patient before and after treatment with etretinate. Arch Dermatol 1986; 122: 434–40

Ruiz-Maldonado R, Tamayo L, del Castillo V, et al. Erythrokeratoderma progressive symmetrica: report of 10 cases. Dermatologica 1982; 164: 133–41

Suga Y, Jarnik M, Attar PS, et al. Transgenic mice expressing a mutant form of loricrin reveal the molecular basis of the skin diseases, Vohwinkel syndrome and progressive symmetric erythrokeratoderma. J Cell Biol 2000; 151: 401–12

CHAPTER 7

Palmoplantar keratodermas

EPIDERMOLYTIC PALMOPLANTAR KERATODERMA

Synonym

- Vörner's disease

Age of onset

- At birth or during the first months of life

Clinical findings

Cutaneous manifestations

- Thick, yellow-brown, parchment-like hyperkeratosis involving palms and soles, well demarcated by an erythematous ring (non-transgrediens form resembling Unna–Thost disease) (Figures 7.1–7.3)
- Decreased resistance to physical trauma resulting in blisters and erosions
- Hyperhidrosis

Course

There is a stable course, with difficulty in walking and social discomfort.

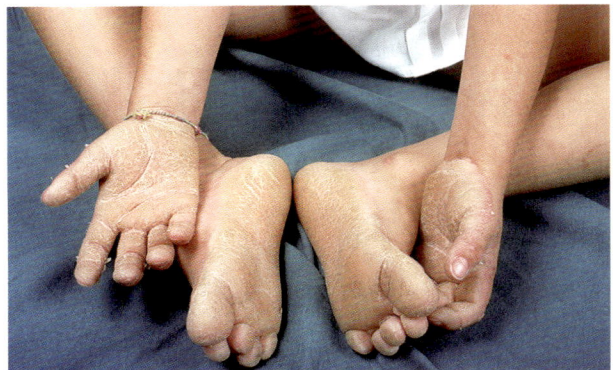

Figure 7.1

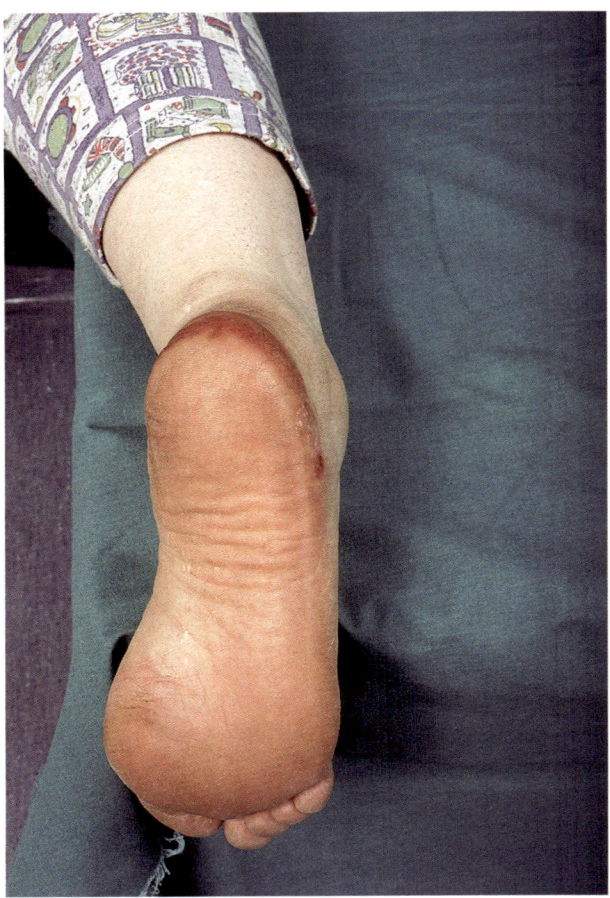

Figure 7.2

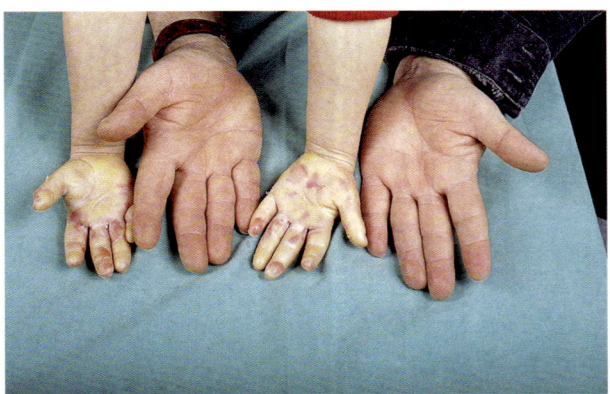

Figure 7.3

Laboratory investigations and data

Histopathologic findings include typical features of epidermolytic hyperkeratosis.

Genetics and pathogenesis

- Autosomal dominant inheritance
- The disease is caused by mutations in the highly conserved coil 1A domain of the keratin 9 gene KRT9

Differential diagnosis

- Unna–Thost disease

Therapy

- Keratolytics
- Oral retinoids

REFERENCES

Coleman CM, Munro CS, Smith FJD, et al. Epidermolytic palmoplantar keratoderma due to a novel type of keratin mutation, a 3 bp insertion in the keratin 9 helix termination. Br J Dermatol 1999; 140: 486–90

Kanitakis J, Tsoitis G, Kanitakis C. Hereditary epidermolytic palmoplantar keratoderma (Vörner type). J Am Acad Dermatol 1997; 17: 414–22

Mofid MZ, Costarangos C, Gruber SB, et al. Hereditary epidermolytic palmoplantar keratoderma (Vörner type) in a family with Ehlers-Danlos syndrome. J Am Acad Dermatol 1998; 38: 825–30

UNNA–THOST PALMOPLANTAR KERATODERMA

Synonyms

- Diffuse palmoplantar keratoderma (PPK)
- Non-acantholytic PPK
- Keratin 1-associated PPK

Age of onset

- First months of life

Clinical findings

Cutaneous manifestations

- Diffuse, non transgrediens, very thick yellow-waxy hyperkeratosis of the palms and soles (Figures 7.4 and 7.5)
- Well circumscribed with an erythematous halo
- Usual marked hyperhidrosis
- Occasional nail thickening and dystrophy

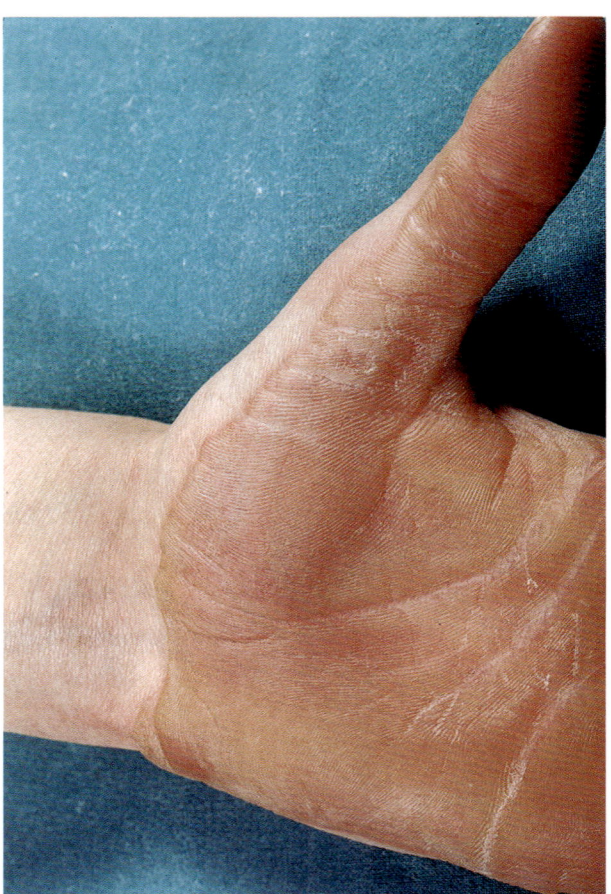

Figure 7.4

Palmoplantar keratodermas

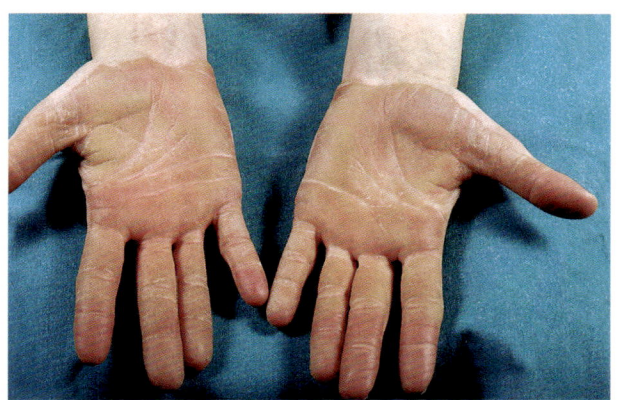

Figure 7.5

Complications

- Frequent dermatophyte infections
- Painful fissuring

Associations

- Mental retardation
- Acro-osteolysis
- Clubbing of fingers
- Clinodactyly

Course

- Keratoderma increases gradually up to the third decade
- Winter worsening

Laboratory investigations

Histopathologic findings include diffuse orthokeratotic thickening of the horny layer, acanthosis and papillomatosis.

Genetics and pathogenesis

- Autosomal dominant inheritance
- Mutations of keratin 1 (V1 end domain)

Differential diagnosis

Other forms of palmoplantar keratoderma are mainly of the Vörner type.

Therapy

- Topical keratolytics
- Oral retinoids
- Biotin administration

REFERENCES

Kimonis V, DiGiovanna JJ, Yang JM, et al. A mutation in the V1 end domain of keratin 1 in non-epidermolyic palmarplantar keratoderma. J Invest Dermatol 1994; 103: 764–9

Lucker GPH, Van de Kerkhof PCM, Steylen PM. The hereditary palmoplantar keratoses: an updated review and classification. Br J Dermatol 1994; 131: 1–14

Menni S, Saleh F, Piccinno R, et al. Palmoplantar keratoderma of Unna–Thost: response to biotin in one family. Clin Exp Dermatol 1992; 17: 337–8

Ratnavel RC, Griffiths WAD. The inherited palmoplantar keratodermas. Br J Dermatol 1997; 137: 485–90

KERATODERMA HEREDITARIA MUTILANS

Synonym

- Vohwinkel's syndrome

Age of onset

- Infancy

Clinical findings

Skin lesions

- Hyperkeratosis of the palms and soles with a characteristic 'honeycomb' appearance (Figures 7.6–7.8)
- 'Star-shaped' keratotic plaques on the dorsa of the hands and feet, elbows, knees and knuckles (Figure 7.9)
- Constricting fibrous bands (pseudoainhum) encircling digits of hands and feet with possible auto-amputation (Figures 7.9 and 7.10)
- Occasional scarring alopecia
- An 'ichthyotic' presentation is possible (related to loricrin gene mutations)

Extracutaneous findings

- Hearing loss (related to 'non-ichthyotic' classical presentation and with connexin 26 mutations)
- Spastic paraplegia
- Myopathy
- Mental retardation

Course

There is persistent keratoderma with loss of digits around the second decade.

Laboratory findings

- Histopathology: hyperkeratosis, marked parakeratosis, hypergranulosis, acanthosis (not diagnostic)
- Radiography of phalanges

Genetics and pathogenesis

- Autosomal dominant fashion, occasionally recessive
- Mutations in gene encoding for loricrin with abnormality of a structural component of cornified

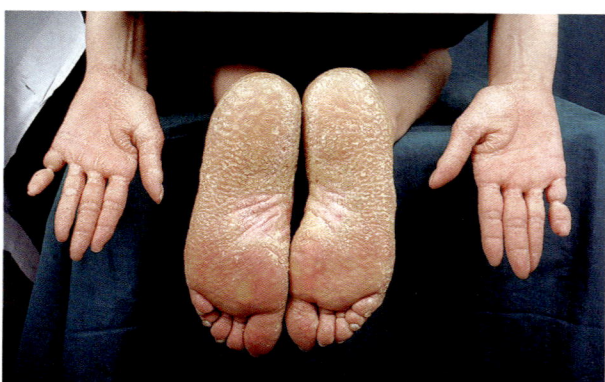

Figure 7.6

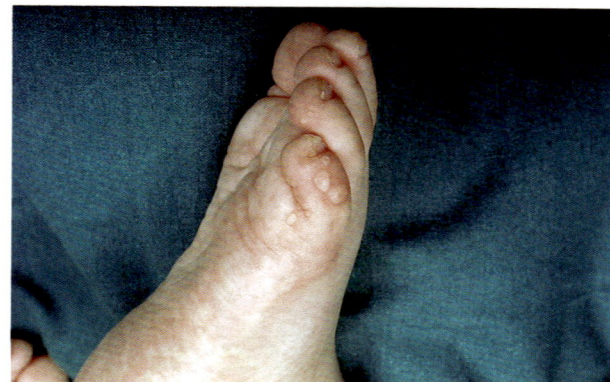

Figure 7.8

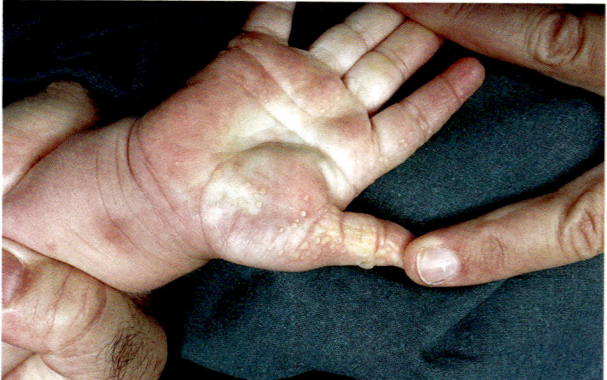

Figure 7.7

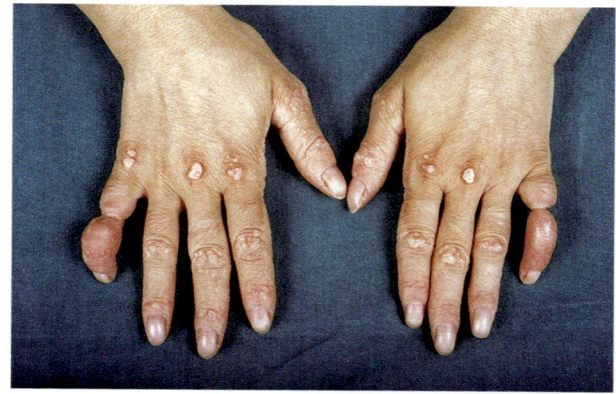

Figure 7.9

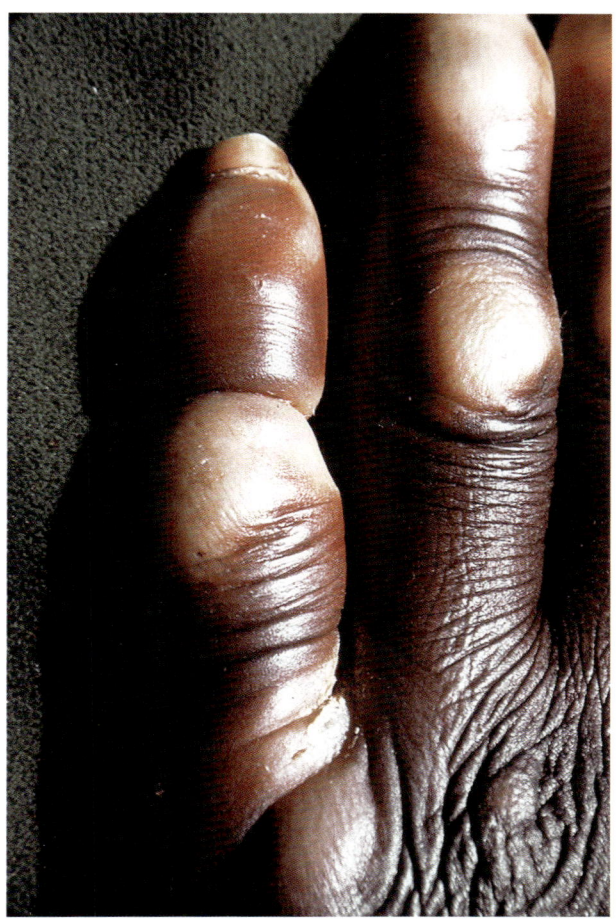

Figure 7.10

envelope and ichthyotic presentation, unrelated to deafness
* Mutations in connexin 26 (epithelial–mesenchymal interaction protein) are related to classical dominant pedigrees with severe sensorineural deafness

Differential diagnosis

* Olmsted's syndrome
* Pachyonychia congenita
* Mal de Meleda

Follow-up

* Normal life span
* Retinoids may prevent loss of digits and disability

Therapy

* Oral retinoids
* Keratolytics
* Surgical release of constriction bands

REFERENCES

Amstrong DKB, McKenna KE, Hughers AE. A novel insertional mutation in loricrin in Vohwinkel's keratoderma. J Invest Dermatol 1998; 111: 702–4

Atabay K, Yavuzer R, Latifoglu O, Ozmen S. Keratoderma hereditarium mutilans (Vohwinkel syndrome): an unsolved surgical mystery. Plast Reconstr Surg 2001; 108: 1276–80

Bakirtzis G, Choudhry R, Aasen T, et al. Targeted epidermal expression of mutant connexin 26(D66H) mimics true Vohwinkel syndrome and provides a model for the pathogenesis of dominant connexin disorders. Hum Mol Genet 2003; 12: 1737–44

Camisa C, Rossana C. Variant of keratoderma hereditaria mutilans (Vohwinkel's syndrome). Arch Dermatol 1984; 120: 1323–8

O'Driscoll J, Muston GC, McGrath JA, et al. A recurrent mutation in the loricrine gene underlies the ichthyotic variant of Vohwinkel syndrome. Clin Exp Dermatol 2002; 27: 243–6

Solis RR, Diven DG, Trizna Z. Vohwinkel's syndrome in three generations. J Am Acad Dermatol 2001; 44: 376–8

GREITHER'S DISEASE

Synonyms

- Progressive palmoplantar keratoderma
- Keratosis extremitatum

Age of onset

- Childhood

Clinical findings

Cutaneous manifestations

- Diffuse scaling palmoplantar keratoderma with an erythematous border, with slow and progressive involvement of the dorsa of the hands and feet (transgrediens pattern) (Figure 7.11)

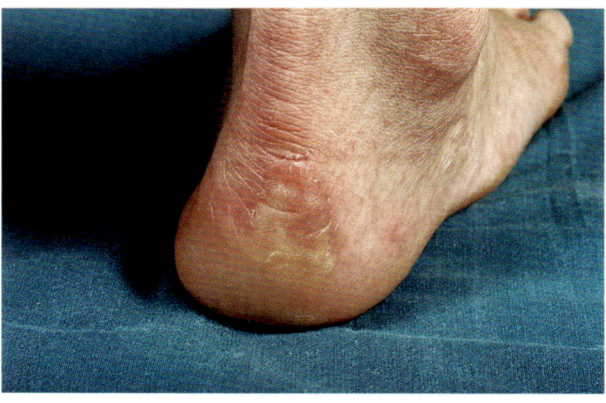

Figure 7.12

- Irregular hyperkeratotic patches on the knees, elbows and in the region of the Achilles tendon (Figure 7.12)
- Marked hyperhidrosis

Course

The disease is slowly progressive.

Laboratory investigations

Histopathologic findings include diffuse 'gothic church' hyperkeratosis without epidermolytic changes.

Genetics and pathogenesis

- Autosomal dominant inheritance
- Probable linkage to 1p36.2–34
- Possible overlapping with other PPK

Differential diagnosis

- Mal de Meleda
- Unna–Thost disease
- Vörner's epidermolytic keratoderma

Therapy

- Keratolytics
- Oral retinoids

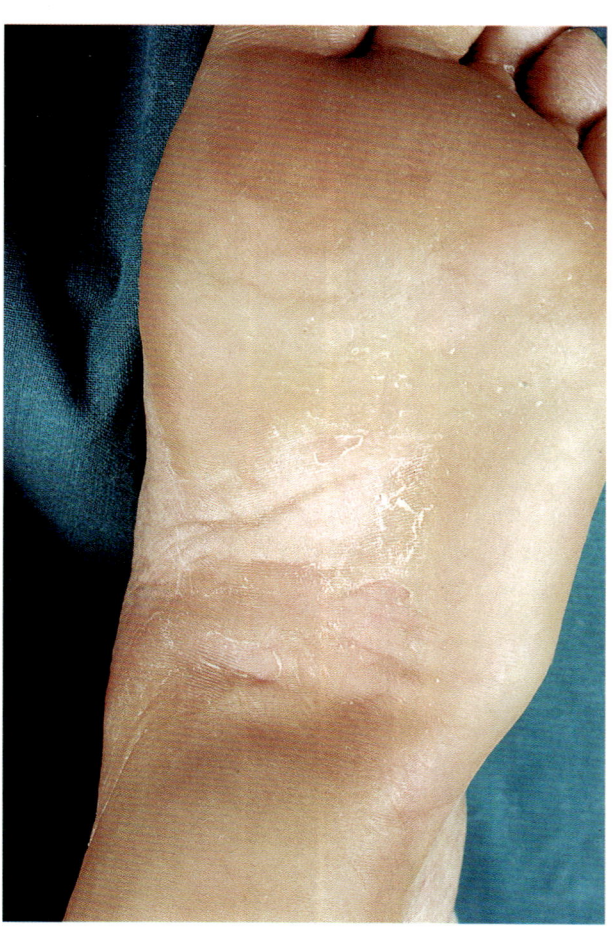

Figure 7.11

REFERENCES

Beylot-Barry M, Taieb A, Surleve-Bazeille JE, et al. Inflammatory familial palmoplantar keratoderma: Greither's disease. Dermatology 1992; 185: 210–14

Fluckiger R, Itin PH. Keratosis extremitatum (Greither's disease): clinical features, histology, ultrastructure. Dermatology 1993; 187: 309–11

Grilli R, Aguilar A, Escalonilla P, et al. Transgrediens et progrediens palmoplantar keratoderma (Greither's disease) with particular histopathologic findings. Cutis 2000; 65: 141–5

Kansky A, Arzensek J. Is palmoplantar keratoderma of Greither's type a separate nosologic entity? Dermatologica 1979; 158: 244–8

Richard G, Lin JP, Smith L, et al. Linkage studies in erythrokeratodermas: fine mapping, genetic heterogeneity and analysis of candidate genes. J Invest Dermatol 1997; 109: 666–71

Seike T, Nakanishi H, Urano Y, Arase S. Malignant melanoma developing in an area of palmoplantar keratoderma (Greither's disease). J Dermatol 1995; 22: 55–61

OLMSTED'S SYNDROME

Age of onset

- Either soon after birth or in childhood

Clinical findings

- Bilateral symmetric transgrediens palmoplantar keratoderma: the keratoderma is thick, sharply demarcated, with deep painful fissures and surrounded by an erythematous rim; ainhum-like constrictions of digits may lead to spontaneous amputation (Figures 7.13–7.15)
- Periorificial keratotic plaques (Figures 7.16–7.18)
- The plaques are symmetrical, yellow-brown in color and sharply demarcated (Figure 7.15)
- Alopecia
- Nail dystrophy (Figures 7.19 and 7.20)
- Hyperhidrosis of palms and soles
- Hyperkeratotic linear streaks
- Keratosis pilaris
- Leukokeratosis

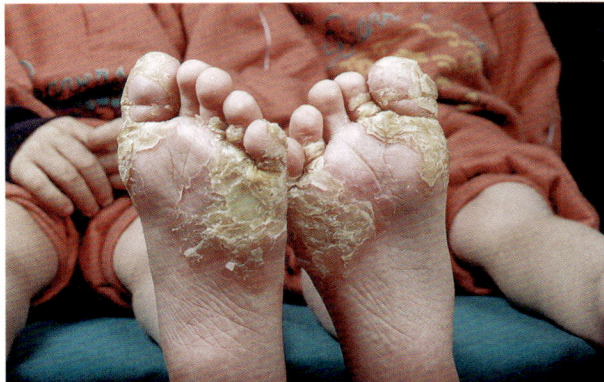

Figure 7.13

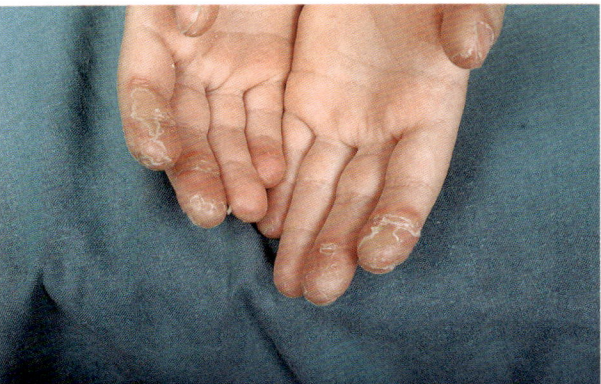

Figure 7.14

Extracutaneous findings

- Joint laxity
- Osteoporosis
- Growth retardation
- Corneal anomalies
- Immunodeficiency and lung cancer are reported

Course

The disease is slowly progressive with increasing keratoderma of the palms and soles.

Squamous cell carcinoma may appear in hyperkeratotic areas.

Laboratory findings

Histopathologic features of palmoplantar keratoderma are not diagnostic. Immunohistochemical studies have identified cytokeratin abnormalities that consist of staining involving the entire thickness of epidermis with cytokeratin AE1 (normally this cytokeratin stains only the basal layer).

Genetics and pathogenesis

The mode of inheritance is not definitely known. Transmission may be autosomal recessive, but the presence of sporadic presentation in a few cases suggests that also an autosomal dominant transmission cannot be ruled out.

The intense staining with AE1 of the entire thickness of epidermis may indicate an immature proliferative stage.

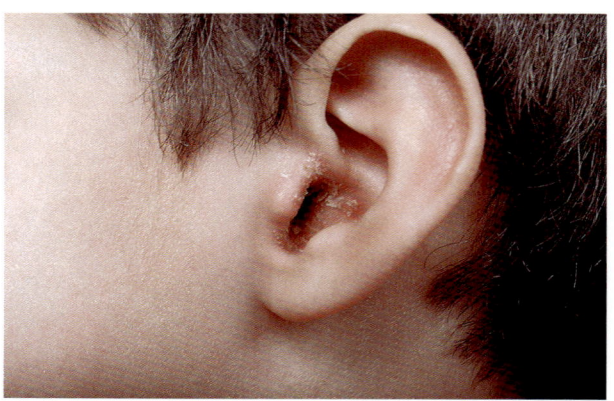

Figure 7.17

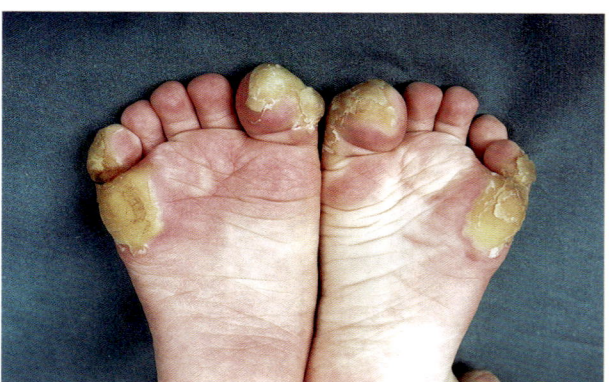

Figure 7.15

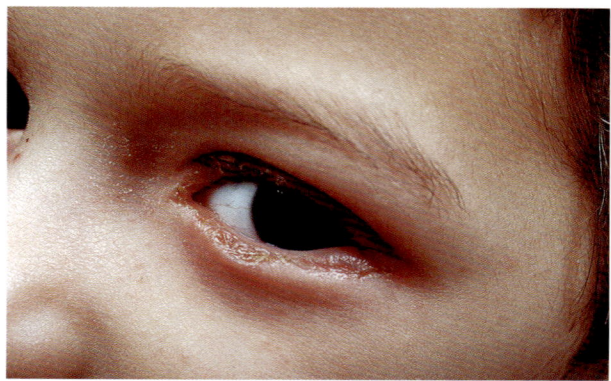

Figure 7.18

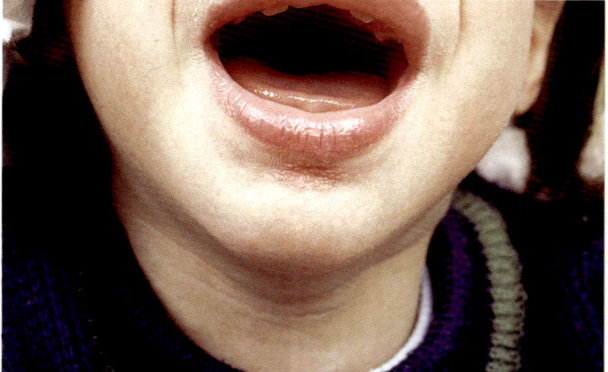

Figure 7.16

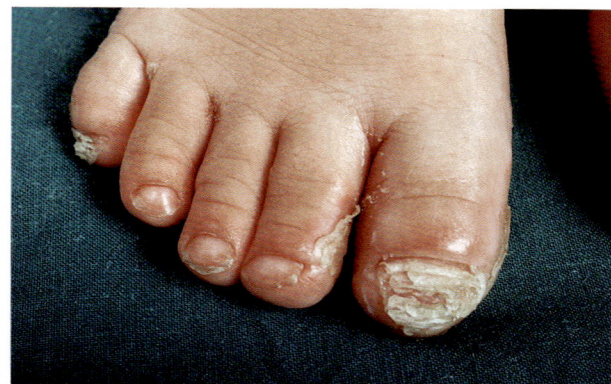

Figure 7.19

Palmoplantar keratodermas

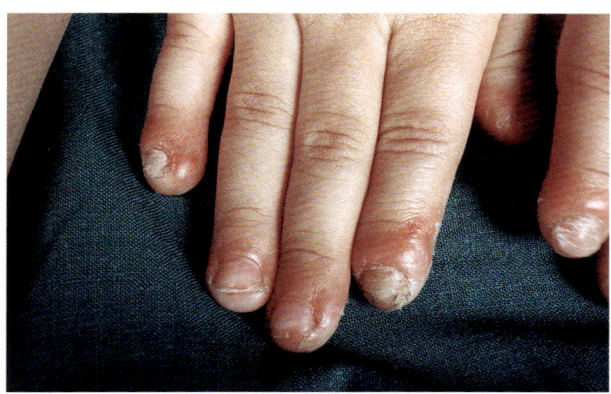

Figure 7.20

Recent studies failed to detect loricrin mutations in these patients.

Differential diagnosis

- Acrodermatitis enteropathica (periorificial lesions)
- Hidrotic ectodermal dysplasia (Clouston type)
- Pachyonychia congenita
- Mal de Meleda
- Keratoderma hereditaria mutilans (Vohwinkel)

Follow-up

The ever-increasing hyperkeratosis results in:

- Progressive contractures of fingers
- Difficulty in walking or grasping
- Cosmetic disfigurement

Treatment

It is unsatisfactory. Systemic retinoids have proved ineffective or produced moderate results. Antiseptic wet dressing, topical antibiotic ointment and emollients may be useful to give relief from pain. Attempts at autografting have been unsuccessful.

REFERENCES

Kress DW, Seraly MP, Falo L, et al. Olmsted syndrome. Case report and identification of a keratin abnormality. Arch Dermatol 1996; 132: 797–800

Larregue M, Callot V, Kanitakis J, et al. Olmsted syndrome: report of two new cases and literature review. J Dermatol 2000; 27: 557–68

Requena L, Manzarbeitia F, Moreno C, et al. Olmsted syndrome. Report of a case with study of cellular proliferation in keratoderma. Am J Dermatopathol 2001; 23: 514–20

PAPILLON–LEFEVRE SYNDROME

Synonyms

- Palmoplantar keratoderma with periodontitis
- Diffuse keratoderma with periodontopathy

Age of onset

- First 4 years of life

Clinical findings

Cutaneous manifestations

- Diffuse transgrediens palmoplantar erythrokeratoderma (main feature) (Figures 7.21 and 7.22)
- Erythematous scaly lesions over the knees, elbows, interphalangeal joints (Figure 7.23)
- Palmoplantar hyperhidrosis with fetid odor

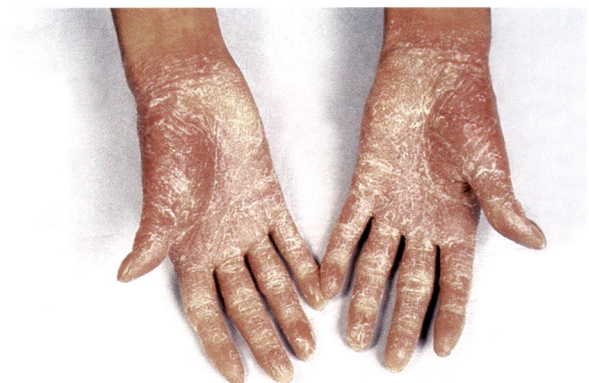

Figure 7.21

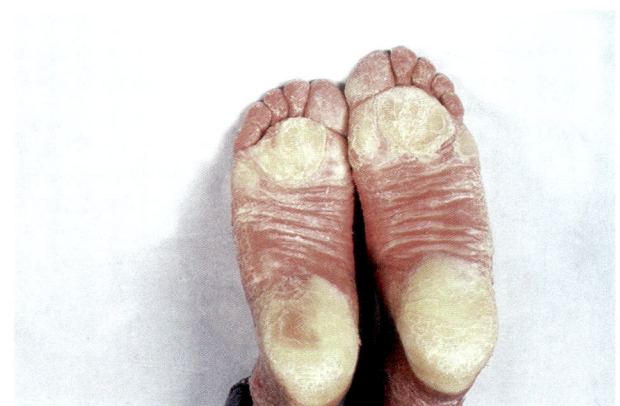

Figure 7.22

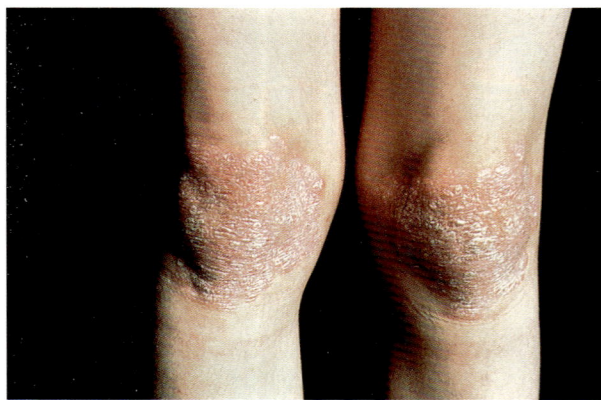

Figure 7.23

Extracutaneous manifestations

- Rapidly progressive periodontitis and severe alveolar bone destruction leading to early loss of both deciduous and permanent teeth (main feature) (Figures 7.24 and 7.25)

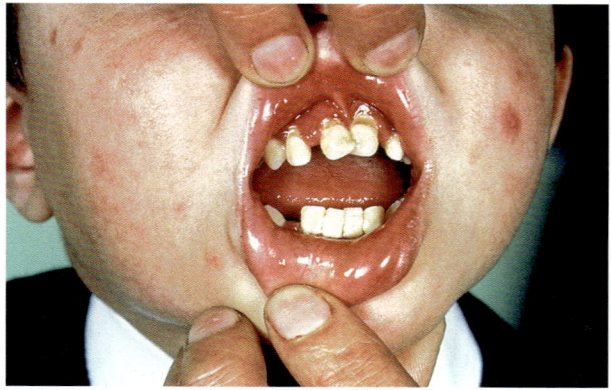

Figure 7.24

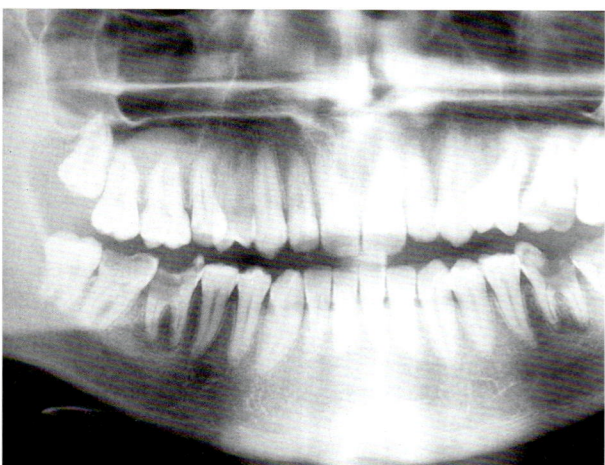

Figure 7.25

- Physical and mental retardation
- Calcifications of dura mater and falx cerebri

Course and complications

- Increased susceptibility to infections (20%)
- Persistent keratoderma with winter worsening

Laboratory findings

- Histopathological findings non specific
- Cranial radiography and orthopantomography
- Impaired leukocyte function involving chemotactic and phagocytic activity

Genetics and pathogenesis

- Autosomal recessive inheritance
- The mutated gene is called CTSC, coding for the cathepsin C protein

Differential diagnosis

- Mal de Meleda disease
- Olmsted's syndrome
- Schop–Schulz–Passarge syndrome

Therapy

Cutaneous and dental lesions may improve with oral retinoids.

REFERENCES

Angel TA, Hou S, Kornblenth J, et al. Papillon–Lefevre syndrome: a case report of four affected siblings. J Am Acad Dermatol 2002; 46: S8–S10

Gelmetti C, Nazzaro V, Cerri A. Long term preservation of permanent teeth in a patient with Papillon–Lefevre syndrome treated with etretinate. Pediatr Dermatol 1989; 6: 222–5

Lucker GPH, Van de Kerkhof PCM, Steijlen PM. The hereditary palmoplantar keratoses: an updated review and classification. Br J Dermatol 1994; 131: 1–14

HURIEZ'S SYNDROME

Synonyms

- Palmoplantar keratoderma with sclerodactyly
- Sclerotylosis

Age of onset

- At birth or in infancy

Clinical findings

- Scleroatrophy of the hands with sclerodactyly (main feature) (Figures 7.26 and 7.27)
- Mild palmoplantar keratoderma (main feature) (Figure 7.28)
- Nail changes consisting of hypoplasia, ridging, clubbing and white discoloration (main feature) (Figure 7.27)
- Palmar hypohidrosis (50%)
- Atrophic plaques on the dorsa of the hands and fingers and sclerodermatous appearance (Figure 7.28)
- Poikiloderma-like changes of the nose
- Telangiectasia on the lips

Extracutaneous findings

- Flexion contractures of the little finger
- Normal teeth

Course and complications

Lesions persist unchanged throughout life.

There is a high risk of development of squamous cell carcinomas on the affected or sun-exposed skin during the third or fourth decade of life (main feature).

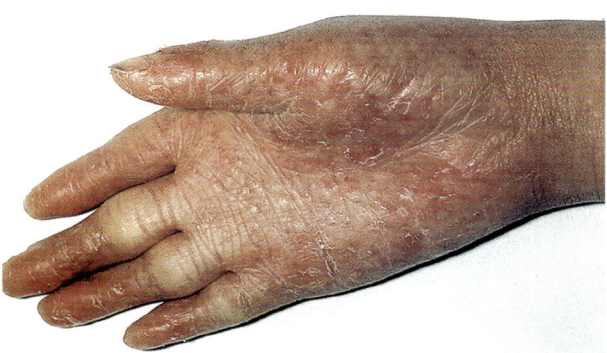

Figure 7.26

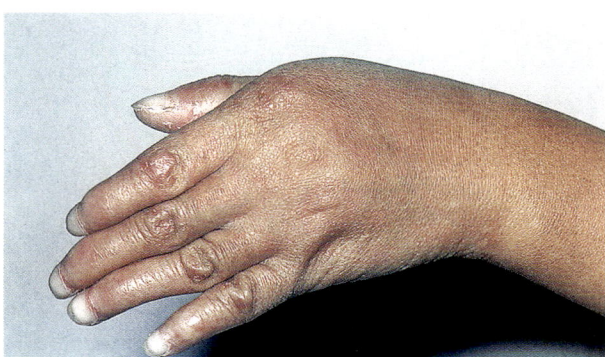

Figure 7.27

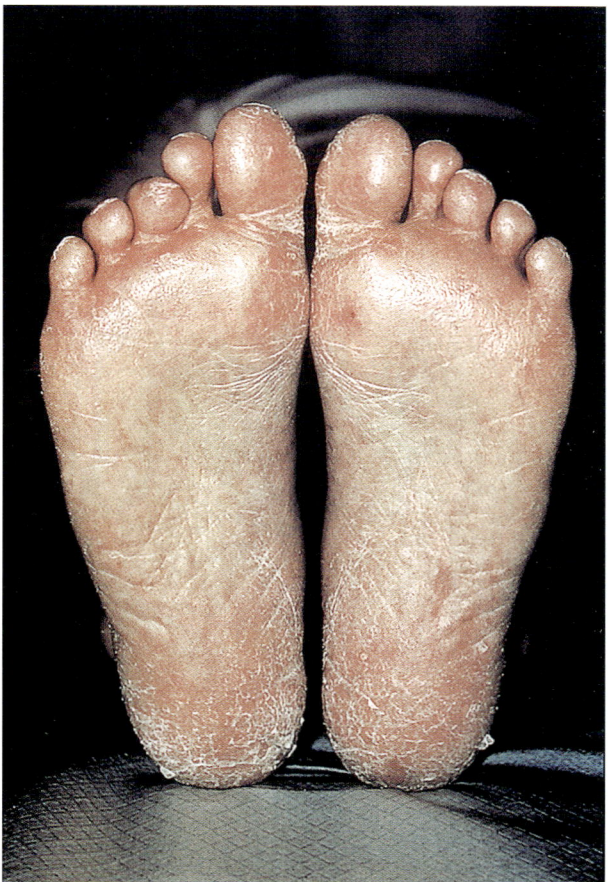

Figure 7.28

Laboratory findings

Histopathologic findings: hyperorthokeratosis and slight acanthosis; mild dermal fibrosis; and absence of Langerhans' cells in involved skin.

Genetics and pathogenesis

- Autosomal dominant inheritance
- Gene locus unknown
- Sun exposure may be a cofactor in precipitating neoplastic changes

Differential diagnosis

- Werner's syndrome
- Kindler's syndrome
- Schopf–Schulz–Passarge syndrome

Follow-up

Lifelong follow-up is necessary because there is a 13% risk of skin cancer and a 5% mortality of affected individuals.

Therapy

- Retinoids
- Early surgical excision of suspicious lesions

REFERENCES

Delaposite E, N'Guyen-Mailfer C, Janin A, et al. Keratoderma with scleroatrophy of the extremities or sclerotylosis (Huriez syndrome): a reappraisal. Br J Dermatol 1995; 133: 409–16

Hamm H, Traupe H, Broeker EB, et al. The scleroatrophic syndrome of Huriez: a cancer-prone genodermatosis. Br J Dermatol 1996; 134: 512–18

Kavanagh GM, Jardine PE, Peachy RD, et al. The scleroatrophic syndrome of Huriez. Br J Dermatol 1997; 137: 114–18

MAL DE MELEDA

Synonym

- Keratoderma palmoplantaris transgrediens

Age of onset

- From birth to the third year of life

Clinical findings

- Sharply demarcated palmoplantar keratoderma developing on erythematous base and extending to backs of the hands and feet with a 'glove and sock' distribution: transgrediens and progressive keratoderma (Figures 7.29–7.32)
- Hyperkeratotic plaques causing maceration and malodor
- Perioral erythema
- Subungual keratosis and nail abnormality (koilonychia and pachyonychia)

Extracutaneous manifestations

- Palatal abnormalities (high arched palate)
- Lingua plicata
- Syndactyly
- Knuckle pads
- Mental retardation

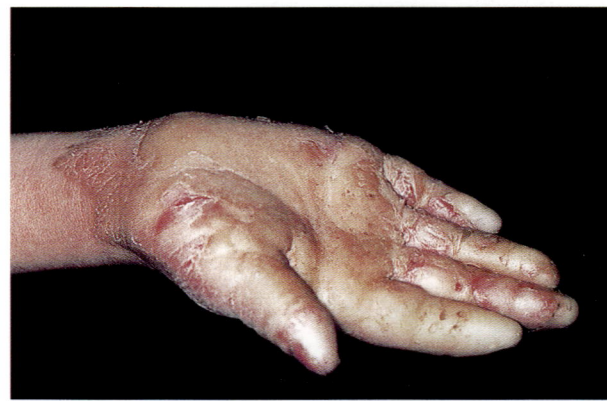

Figure 7.29

Palmoplantar keratodermas 81

Course and complications

The disease is slowly progressive with a normal life span.

- Pseudoainhum with amputation of fingers
- Secondary infections (mycotic)
- Painful fissures
- Flexion contractures of fingers

Laboratory investigations and data

- Histopathologic findings: hyperorthokeratosis, hypergranulosis, acanthosis with pseudospongiosis
- Bone radiography

Genetics and pathogenesis

- Autosomal recessive inheritance
- Caused by mutations in the ARS gene encoding the SLURP-1 protein that belongs to a superfamily of receptors and secreted proteins, which participate in signal transduction, immune cell activation and cellular adhesion. SLURP-1 shows high degree of structural similarity with some snake neurotoxins. In fact, SLURP-1 is found to be a potent modulator of human α-7 nicotinic acetylcholine receptors of the keratinocytes. SLURP-1 act as a neuromodulator which is probably relevant in the modulation of the proliferation of the keratinocytes and in preventing inflammatory cascades determined by TNF-α, thus explaining both the

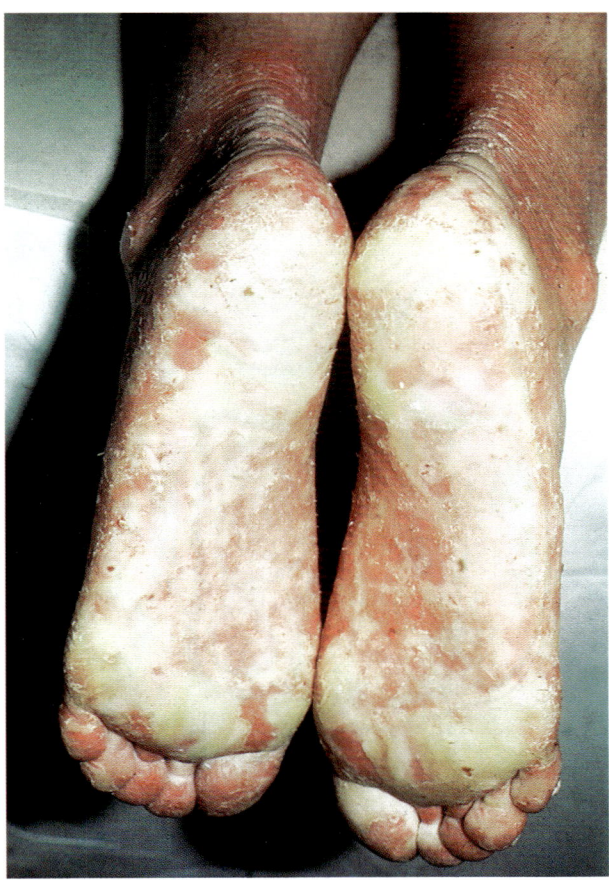

Figure 7.30

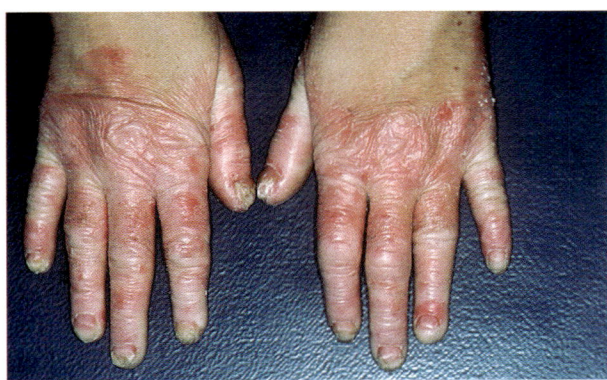

Figure 7.31

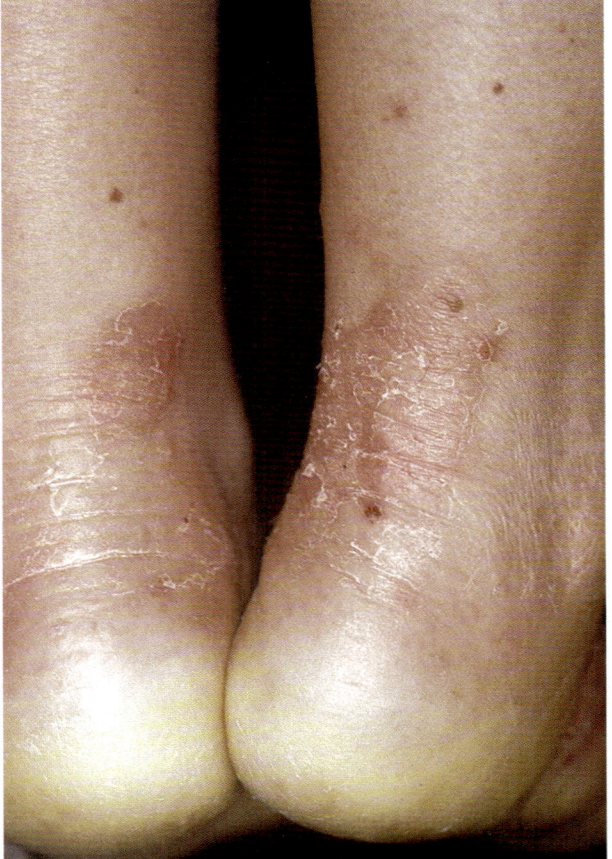

Figure 7.32

hyperproliferative and the inflammatory phenotypes of the disease

Differential diagnosis

- Vohwinkel's syndrome
- Papillon–Lefevre syndrome
- Greither's syndrome
- Olmsted's syndrome

Therapy

- Oral retinoids
- Keratolytics
- Surgery for pseudoainhum

REFERENCES

Barba Romero MA, Garcia de Lorenzo y Mateos A; Gruppo Espanol de Estudio de FOS. [Fabry's disease in Spain. Study of 24 cases] Med Clin (Barc) 2004; 123: 57–60. [Spanish]

Bonadjar B, Benmazouzia S, Prud'homme JF, et al. Clinical and genetic studies of 3 large consanguineous, Algerian families with mal de Meleda. Arch Dermatol 2000; 136: 1247–53

Chimienti F, Hogg RC, Plantard L, et al. Identification of SLURP-1 as an epidermal neuromodulator explains the clinical phenotype of Mal de Meleda. Hum Mol Genet 2003; 12: 3017–24. Epub 2003; Sep 23

Fatovic-Ferencie S. Mal de Meleda. J Invest Dermatol 2003; 121: 433

Lestringant GG, Frossard PM, Adeghate E, et al. Mal de Meleda: a report of four cases from United Arab Emirates. Pediatr Dermatol 1997; 14: 186–91

Mehta A, Ricci R, Widmer U, et al. Fabry disease defined: baseline clinical manifestations of 366 patients in the Fabry Outcome Survey. Eur J Clin Invest 2004; 34: 236–42

van Steensel MAM, van Geel M, Steijlen PH. Mal de Meleda without mutations in the ARS coding sequence. Eur J Dermatol 2002; 12: 129–32

Yerebakan O, Hu G, Yilmaz E, Celebi JT. A novel mutation in the ARS (component B) gene encoding SLURP-1 in a family with Mal de Meleda. Clin Exp Dermatol 2003; 28: 542–4

PUNCTATE PALMOPLANTAR KERATODERMA

Synonyms

- Keratosis palmaris and plantaris punctata
- Buschke–Fischer–Brauer disease

Age of onset

- Usually from the second to the fourth decade

Clinical findings

Cutaneous manifestations

- Numerous yellow to dark brown, 2–10-mm, round isolated asymptomatic keratotic papules with a central keratinic plug (Figures 7.33–7.35)
- Lesions may be represented by tiny plugs confined to palmar and digital creases, seen mostly in the black population (Figures 7.36 and 7.37)
- Occasionally nail abnormalities: longitudinal fissuring, onychogryphosis, onychomadesis
- Diffuse xerosis

Extracutaneous findings

- Gastrointestinal malignancy
- Atopy
- Spastic paralysis
- Ankylosing spondylitis

Course

This is a slowly progressive disease.

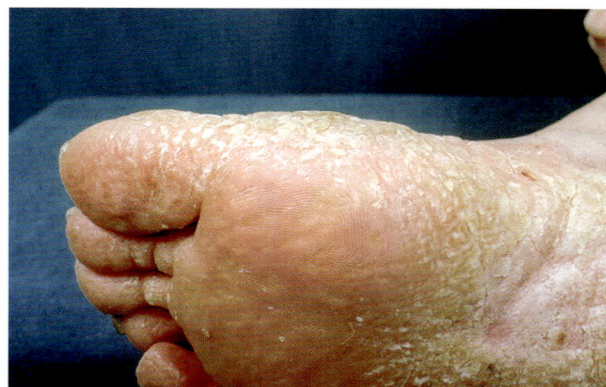

Figure 7.33

Palmoplantar keratodermas

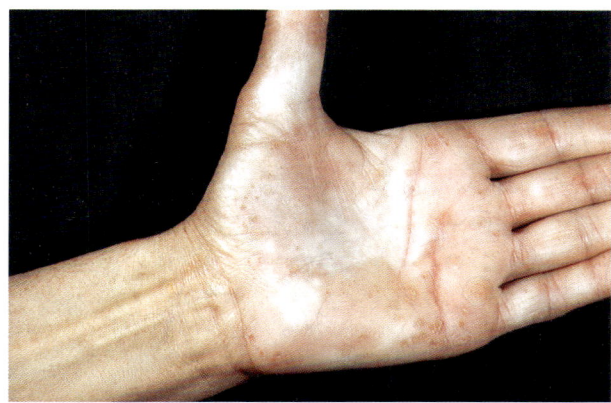

Figure 7.34

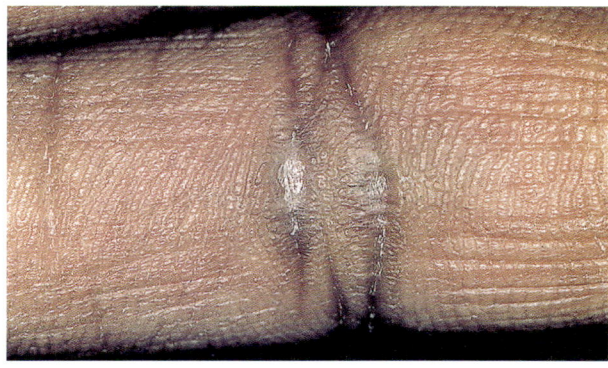

Figure 7.36

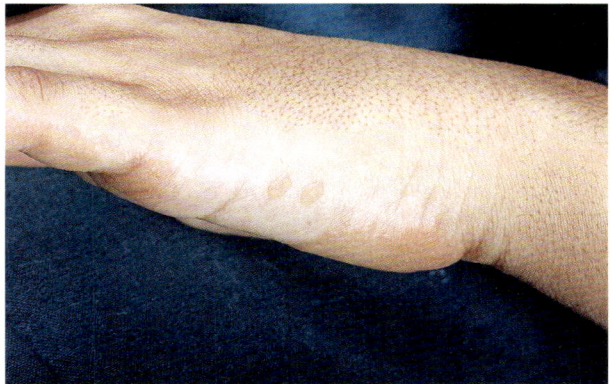

Figure 7.35

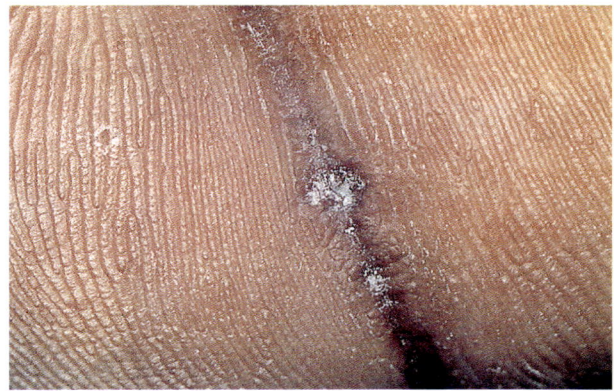

Figure 7.37

Laboratory investigations

Histopathologic findings include marked hyperkeratosis, hypergranulosis and acanthosis with a mild inflammatory dermal infiltrate around the dermal vessels.

Genetics and pathogenesis

- Autosomal dominant inheritance
- Non-linkage to keratin gene clusters
- Identification of a locus on chromosomes 8 and 15

Differential diagnosis

- Punctate porokeratosis
- Basal cell nevus syndrome
- Acrokeratosis verruciformis

Therapy

- Keratolytics
- Oral retinoids

REFERENCES

Bennion SD, Patterson JW. Keratosis punctata palmaris et plantaris and adenocarcinoma of the colon. J Am Acad Dermatol 1984; 10: 587–91

Rustad OJ, Corwin Vance J. Punctate keratoses of the palms and soles and keratotic pits of palmar creases. J Am Acad Dermatol 1990; 22: 468–76

Stevens HP, Kelsell DP, Leigh IM, et al. Punctate palmoplantar keratoderma and malignancy in a four-generation family. Br J Dermatol 1996; 134: 720–6

STRIATE KERATODERMA

Synonym

- Brunauer–Fuchs disease

Age of onset

- Puberty

Clinical findings

Cutaneous manifestations

- Linear keratotic lesions along the palmar surfaces of the fingers (Figures 7.38 and 7.39)
- Diffuse pattern (keratotic plaques) on the soles (Figure 7.40)

Course

Stable lesions are increased by mechanical trauma.

Laboratory investigations

Histopathologic findings include orthokeratotic hyperkeratosis, hypergranulosis and papillomatosis.

Genetics and pathogenesis

- Autosomal dominant inheritance
- Striated palmoplantar keratoderma type 1: mapped to the desmoglein–desmocollin locus on 18q12
- Striated palmoplantar keratoderma type 2: due to a mutation of the desmoplakin gene on chromosome 6p21 resulting in a premature termination codon
- Cadherins and keratin 1 mutations are also claimed to determine similar phenotypes

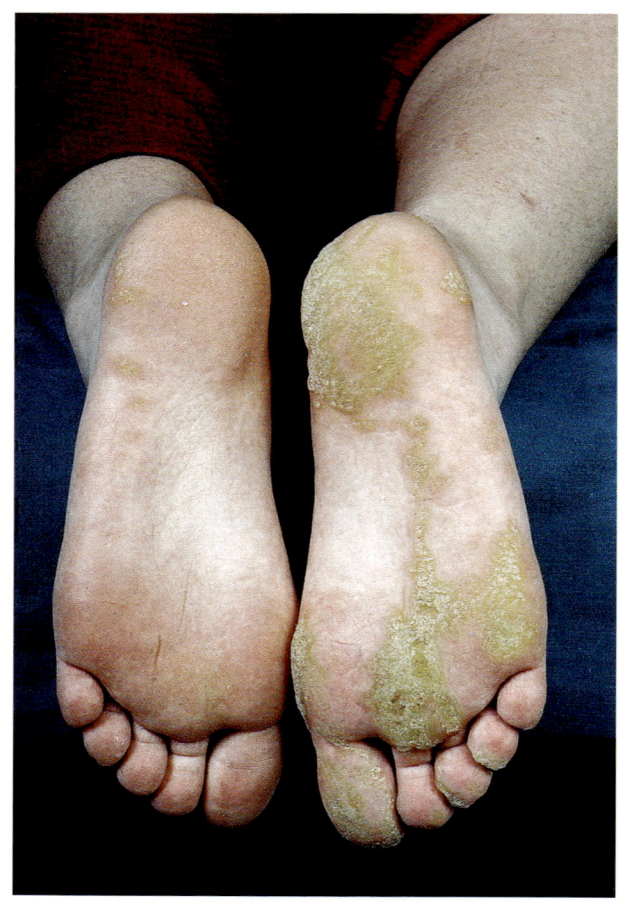

Figure 7.39

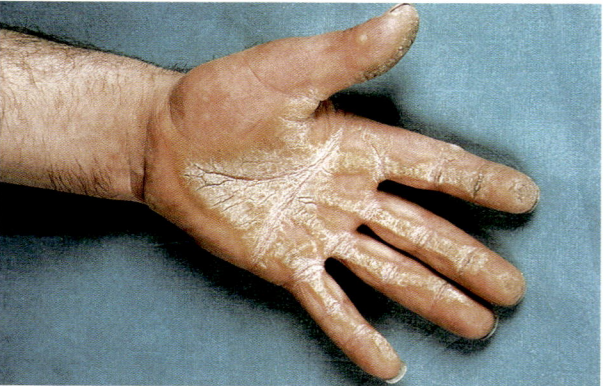

Figure 7.38

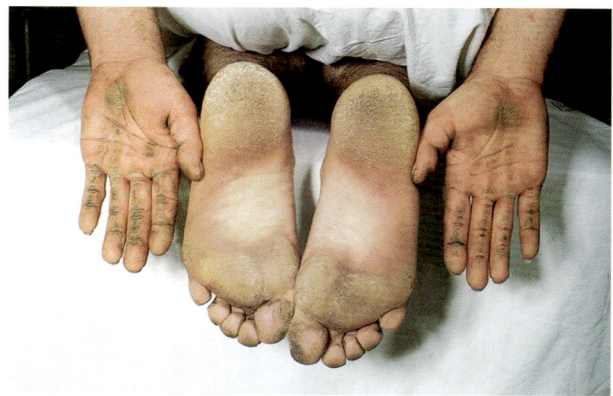

Figure 7.40

Differential diagnosis

- Other palmoplantar keratoderma

Therapy

- Keratolitics
- Oral retinoids

REFERENCES

Kotcher LB, Jih MH, White KL, et al. Striated palmoplantar keratoderma of Brunauer–Fuhs–Siemens. Int J Dermatol 2001; 40: 644–5

Ortega M, Quintane J, Camacho F. Keratosis palmoplantar striata (Brunauer–Fuhs type). Acta Dermatol Venereol 1982; 63: 273–5

Whittock NV, Ashton GHS, Dopping-Hepenstal PJC, et al. Striate palmo plantar keratoderma resulting from desmoplakin haploinsufficiency. J Invest Dermatol 1999; 113: 940–6

RICHNER–HANHART SYNDROME

Synonym

- Tyrosinemia type II

Age of onset

- From early infancy to childhood

Clinical findings

Skin and mucosal manifestations

- Circumscribed, painful hyperkeratotic plaques on the palms and soles mainly located on hypothenar or thenar eminences, fingertips (Figure 7.41) and weightbearing plantar surfaces, leading to impaired ambulation (Figure 7.42)
- Hyperkeratotic plaques on elbows and knees
- Hyperhidrosis
- Leukokeratosis of the tongue

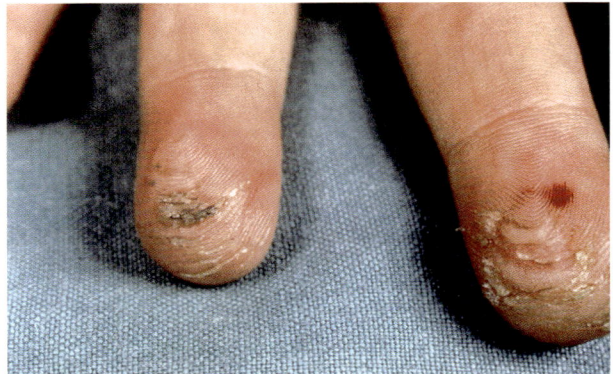

Figure 7.41

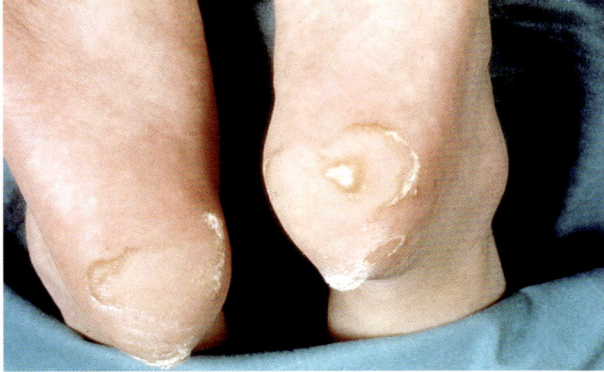

Figure 7.42

Extracutaneous manifestations

- Corneal erosions and ulcerations developing within the first months of life lead to severe keratosis and blindness (Figure 7.43)
- Mental retardation

Course

Without a special diet the disease is progressive and death occurs before adulthood.

Laboratory investigations

- Increased tyrosine levels in plasma and urine due to deficiency of hepatic tyrosine aminotransferase deficiency
- Histopathologic findings: marked orthohyperkeratosis and hypergranulosis, acantholysis (not diagnostic)
- Ultrastructural findings: intracytoplasmic tyrosine crystals

Genetics and pathogenesis

- Autosomal recessive disorder
- Disease caused by mutations of the tyrosine-aminotransferase gene that cause a deficiency of the hepatic enzyme tyrosine aminotransferase (TAT) with accumulation of tyrosine in all tissues

Differential diagnosis

- Other painful palmoplantar keratoderma
- Skin and eye manifestations absent in tyrosinemia I

Therapy

- Low-tyrosine and low-phenylamine diet as early as possible
- Systemic retinoids

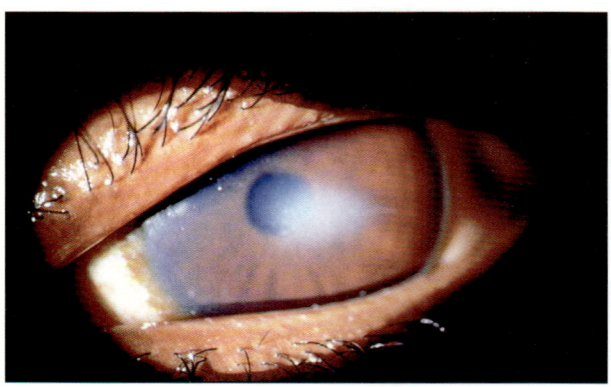

Figure 7.43

Follow-up

The dietary regimen must be continued for the patient's entire life. Early dietary intervention may prevent or limit cutaneous and ocular manifestations, but not mental retardation, and may prolong life.

REFERENCES

Huhn R, Stoermer H, Klingele B, et al. Novel and recurrent tyrosine aminotransferase gene mutations in tyrosinemia type II. Hum Genet 1998; 102: 305–13

Piccinno R, Menni S, Ermacora E, Cantoro M. [Richner–Hanhart syndrome (tyrosinemia II). G Ital Dermatol Venereol 1985; 120: 165–8

Tallab TM. Richner-Hanhart syndrome: importance of early diagnosis and early intervention. J Am Acad Dermatol 1996; 35: 857–9

PAINFUL CALLOSITIES

Synonym

- Keratosis palmoplantaris nummularis

Age of onset

- During infancy, when patient assumes erect position and starts walking

Clinical findings

Cutaneous manifestations

- Bilateral islands of hyperkeratosis mainly involving the soles at sites of maximum pressure with severe painful sensation at pressure (Figures 7.44 and 7.45)
- Similar lesions, often smaller and less painful, on the palms

Associations

- Nail anomalies: leukonychia, thickening of the toenails, koilonychia, platonychia
- Polydactyly

Course

The lesions progress slowly, with worsening of both thickness and pain.

Clinical investigations and data

- Histopathologic findings: (in nearly all patients) local epidermolytic hyperkeratosis
- Radiography of the esophagus

Genetics and pathogenesis

- Autosomal dominant inheritance

Differential diagnosis

- Clinically related to the palmoplantar lesions observed in Howel–Evans syndrome (see Chapter 24)
- Tyrosinemia type II
- Pachyonychia congenita
- Olmsted's syndrome

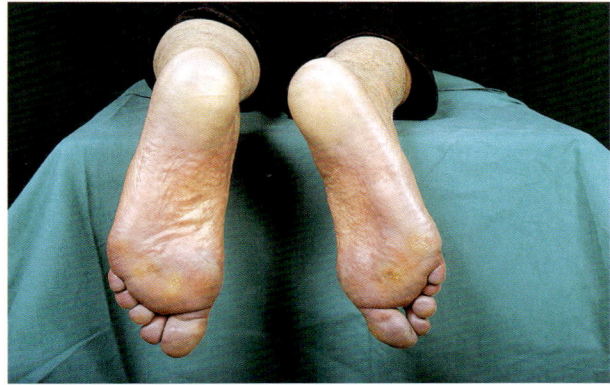

Figure 7.44

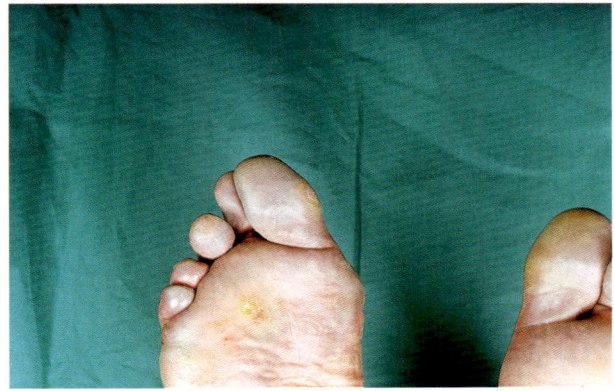

Figure 7.45

Therapy

- Resistant to many treatments
- Oral retinoids

Follow-up

The disease leads inevitably to invalidity. Esophagus monitoring is absolutely necessary.

REFERENCES

Cambiaghi S, Morel P. Hereditary painful callosities with associated features. Dermatology 1996; 193: 47–79

Risk JM, Field EA, Field JK, et al. Tylosis-oesophageal cancer mapped. Nature Genet 1994; 8: 319–21

Wachters DH, Frensdorf EL, Hausman R, et al. Keratosis palmo plantaris nummularis (hereditary painful callosities). Clinical and histopathologic aspects. J Am Acad Dermatol 1983; 2: 204–9

PACHYDERMOPERIOSTOSIS

Synonyms

- Idiopathic hypertrophic osteoarthropathy
- Touraine–Solente–Golé syndrome

Age of onset

- After puberty; male/female ratio 9:1

Clinical findings

Cutaneous manifestations

- Soft tissue hypertrophy resulting in marked thickening and furrowing of the skin of the face, eyelids (coarse facial features 60%) and scalp (cutis vertices gyrata 24%)
- Increased seborrhea (33%)
- Thickening of the skin of the hands and feet with hyperhidrosis (24%) (Figure 7.46)
- 'Watch glass' appearance of the nails (90%)

Extracutaneous manifestations

- Digital clubbing (89%) and 'spade-like' enlargement of hands and feet due to soft tissue hyperplasia and periosteal proliferation (radiologically evident in 97% of patients)
- Cylindrical thickening of legs and forearms

Associations

- Peptic ulcer
- Mental retardation
- Palmoplantar hyperkeratosis
- Papular mucinosis
- Gynecomastia
- Extramedullary hematopoiesis
- Squamous cell carcinomas

Course

The disease increases in severity for several years, then remains stable.

Laboratory investigations and data

- Radiographic examination: prominent periostosis of metatarsals, metacarpals and long bones of the limbs

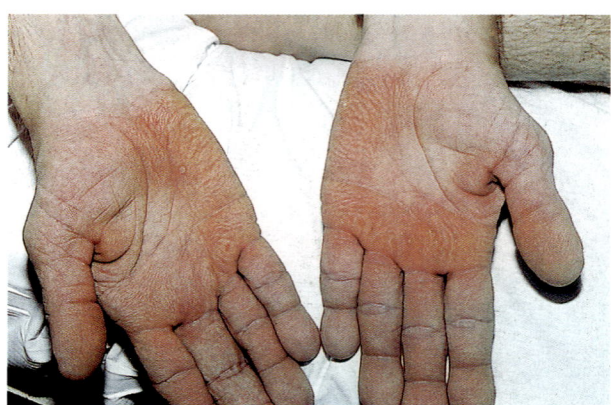

Figure 7.46

- Histopathology findings: marked thickening of the dermis with hypertrophy of collagen and increase of acid mucopolysaccharide

Genetics and pathogenesis

- Autosomal dominant inheritance
- Several serum growth factors activate the fibroblasts, endothelial cells and osteoblasts to proliferate in the soft tissue and bones

Differential diagnosis

- Acromegaly
- Lepromatous leprosy
- Secondary pachydermoperiostosis

Therapy

Surgical reductive procedures of the scalp and skin of the face and eyelids may be performed for cosmetic reasons.

REFERENCES

Lee SC, Moon HJ, Cho D, et al. Pachydermoperiostosis with cutaneous squamous cell carcinomas. Int J Dermatol 1998; 37: 687–700

Oikarinen A, Palatsi R, Kylmaniemi M, et al. Pachydermoperiostosis: analysis of the connective tissue abnormality in one family. J Am Acad Dermatol 1994; 31: 947–53

Thappe DM, Sethuraman G, Kumar CR, et al. Primary pachydermoperiostosis. A case report. J Dermatol 2000; 27: 106–9

ACROKERATOELASTOIDOSIS

Age of onset

- Childhood or adolescence

Clinical findings

Cutaneous manifestations

- Small, yellowish, firm, smooth, translucent, asymptomatic papules characteristically localized on the boundary between dorsal and palmar or plantar skin and on the dorsa of the fingers; often confluent to form plaques (Figures 7.47 and 7.48)
- Occasionally hyperhidrosis

Course

- Slow gradual increase of lesions over several years
- Rapid extension in pregnancy

Laboratory investigations and data

Histopathologic findings include epidermal hypertrophy with acanthosis and marked hyperkeratosis, and coarse fragmentation of elastic fibers in reticular dermis.

Genetics and pathogenesis

- Autosomal dominant inheritance, occasionally sporadic
- Possible linkage to chromosome 2

Differential diagnosis

- Focal acral hyperkeratosis
- Keratoelastoidosis marginalis of the hands
- Acrokeratosis verruciformis
- Degenerative collagenous plaques of the hands

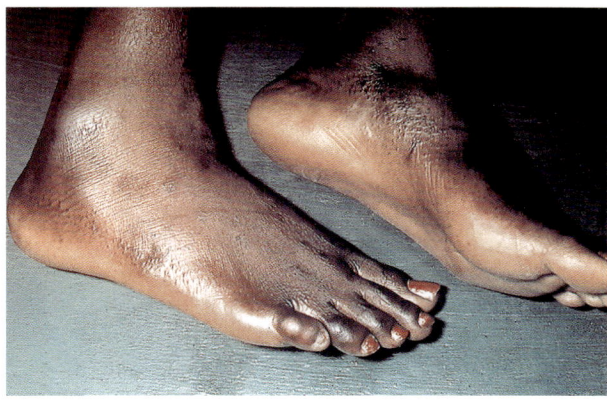

Figure 7.47

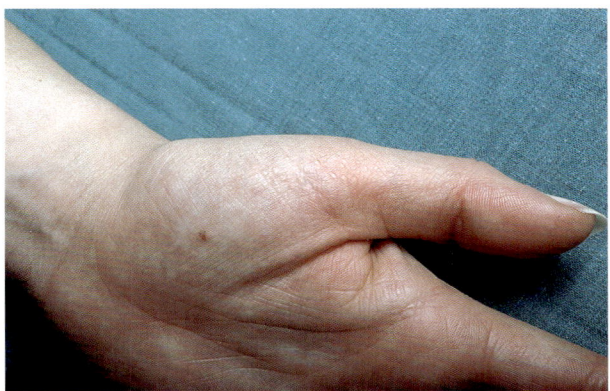

Figure 7.48

Therapy

- Keratolitics
- Oral retinoids

REFERENCES

de Boer EM, van Dijk E. Acrokeratoelastoidosis: a spectrum of diseases. Dermatologica 1985; 17: 8–11

Dyall-Smith D. Acrokeratoelastoidosis. Australas J Dermatol 1996; 37: 213–14

Greiner J, Kruger J, Palden L, et al. A linkage study of acrokeratoelastoidosis. Possible mapping to chromosome 2. Hum Genet 1983; 63: 222–7

NAXOS SYNDROME

Synonyms

- Woolly, curly and uncombable hair, palmoplantar keratoderma and right-side cardiac abnormalities syndrome

Epidemiology

Very few pedigrees have been reported since the first family on the island of Naxos, Greece.

Age of onset

- Cardiac defects at birth
- Woolly, curly hair since early childhood
- Plantar defects during childhood
- Palmar hyperkeratosis during adolescence

Clinical findings

- Thick and yellowish plantar keratoderma, especially over the pressure areas (Figures 7.49 and 7.50), and striated palmar keratoderma in others (Figure 7.51)
- Hyperkeratotic and even painful hyperkeratotic lesions over the interphalangeal joints
- Acanthosis nigricans
- Diffuse xerosis and follicular hyperkeratosis may present
- Palmoplantar hyperhidrosis
- 'Dredding' with Rastafarian curly and difficult to comb hair that is light brown, soft and matt (Figure 7.52)
- Other body hair is sparse

Extracutaneous findings

Mild to very severe heart defects are caused by right-sided fibromuscular dysplasia.

Course and complications

- Cardiac fibromuscular dysplasia may lead in some pedigrees to right-side cardiac failure
- Lifelong skin defects

Laboratory investigations

Echocardiography may reveal early right-ventricular dysfunction.

Scanning electron microscopy reveals flattening and twisting of hair shafts.

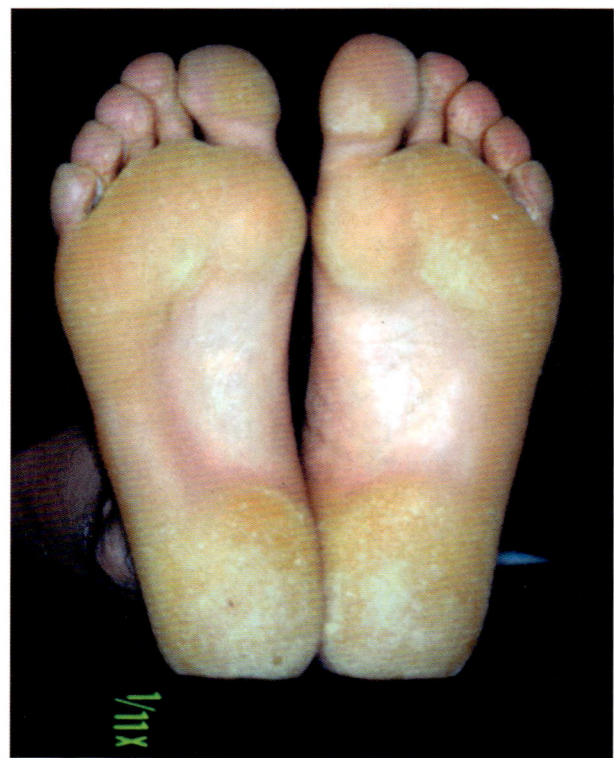

Figure 7.49

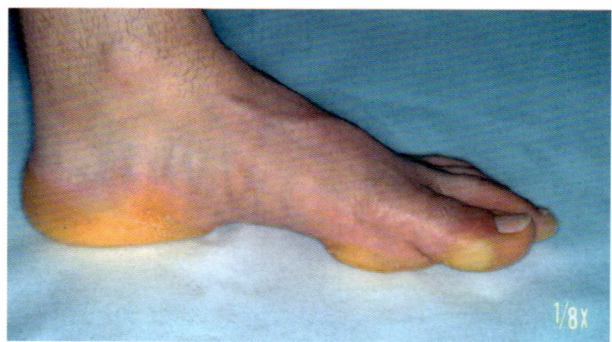

Figure 7.50

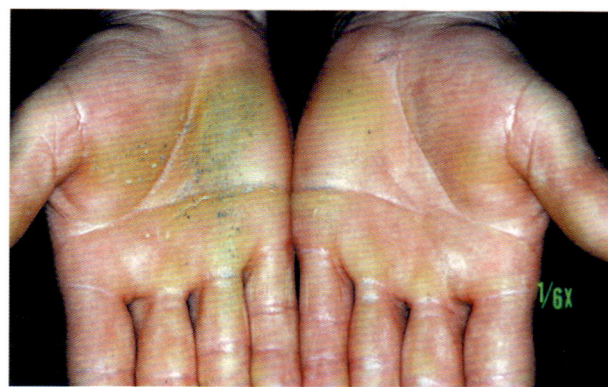

Figure 7.51

Palmoplantar keratodermas 91

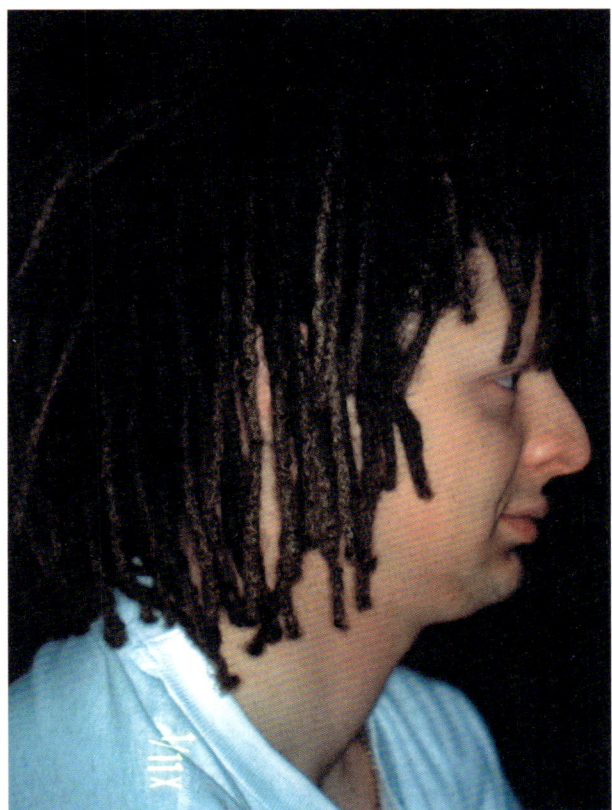

Figure 7.52

Genetics and pathogenesis

Autosomal and recessive inheritances have been demonstrated.

Mutations of the gene encoding plakoglobin, a molecule that contributes to the desmosomal structure, is demonstrated in some pedigrees. Plakoglobin is present in epidermal and neuromuscular structures as plectin, directly causing both epidermal and cardiac defects.

Follow-up and therapy

- Early echocardiography for monitoring right-sided cardiac defects
- Acitretin therapy for palmoplantar changes
- Keratolytics and emollients for hyperkeratosis and xerosis

Differential diagnosis

- Simple uncombable and woolly hair
- Other palmoplantar keratodermas

REFERENCES

McMillan JR, Shimizu H. Desmosomes: structure and function in normal and diseased epidermis. J Dermatol 2001; 28: 291–8

Protonotarios N, Tsatsopoulou A, Fontaine G. Naxos disease: keratoderma, scalp modifications, and cardiomyopathy. J Am Acad Dermatol 2001; 44: 309–11

Wichter T, Schulze-Bahr E, Eckardt L, et al. Molecular mechanisms of inherited ventricular arrhythmias. Herz 2002; 27: 712–39

CHAPTER 8

Other disorders of keratinization

POROKERATOSES

Definition

Porokeratoses are chronic keratoatrophodermas of different clinical forms histologically characterized by columns of porokeratosis termed cornoid lamellae.

Clinical forms

Porokeratosis of Mibelli (plaque porokeratosis)

- Small asymptomatic keratotic papules enlarging gradually to form plaques with a raised, wall-like border that resembles a dyke, and an atrophic depressed center (Figures 8.1 and 8.2)
- Solitary or a few lesions ranging in size from millimeters to many centimeters (giant porokeratosis) (Figure 8.3)
- Predilection for face and extremities, including the palms and soles (Figure 8.4)

Linear porokeratosis

- Linear, unilateral or diffuse coalescent keratotic papules, distributed along the Blaschko's lines, most commonly on the extremities (Figures 8.5–8.7)
- Loss of heterozygosity is relatively common, revealing exacerbation of the disease and, rarely, malignant transformation

Punctate palmoplantar porokeratosis (Mantoux)

- Multiple 1–2-mm seed-like keratotic plugs surrounded by a thin raised border (Figures 8.8 and 8.9)

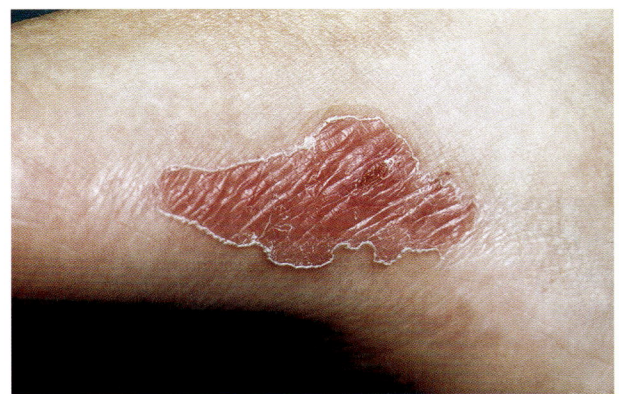

Figure 8.1

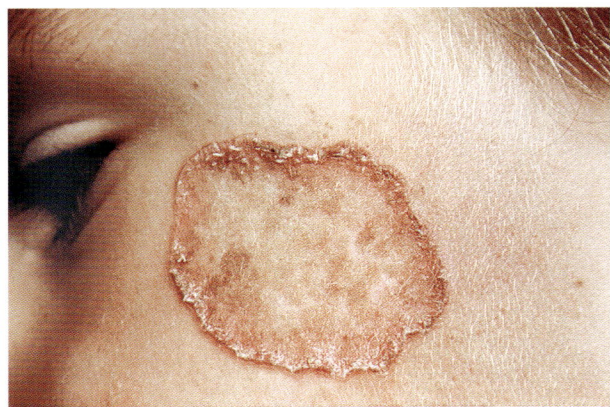

Figure 8.2

Disseminated superficial porokeratosis

- Widespread, uniform lesions not exceeding 1 cm in diameter occurring in both sun-exposed and non-sun-exposed areas (Figures 8.10 and 8.11)

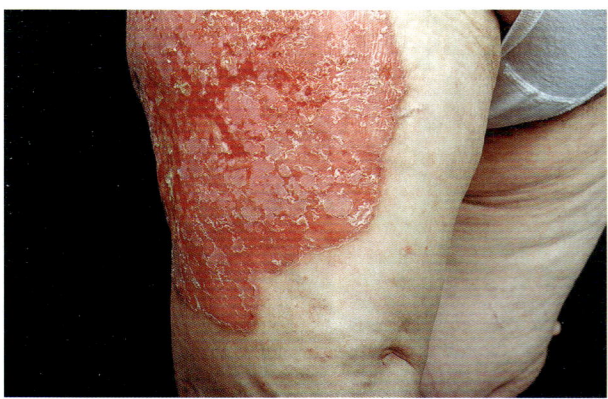

Figure 8.3

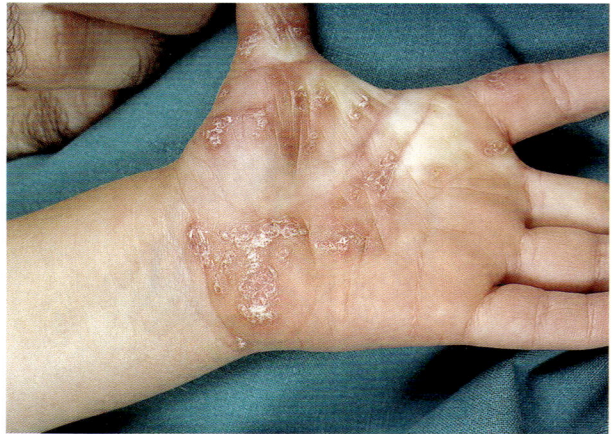

Figure 8.4

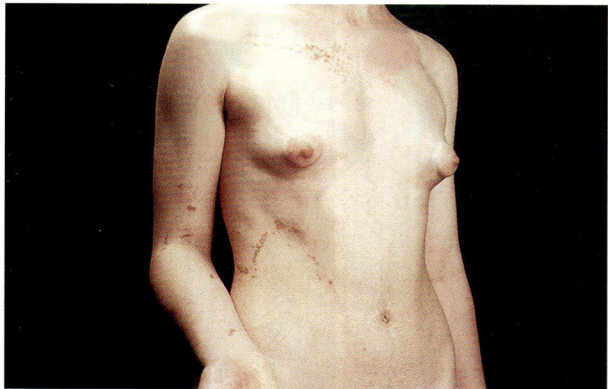

Figure 8.5

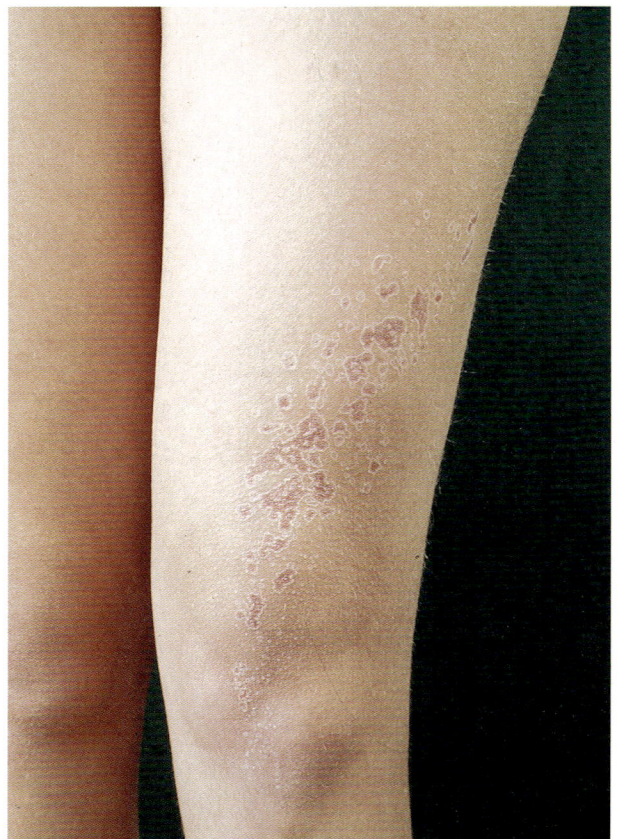

Figure 8.6

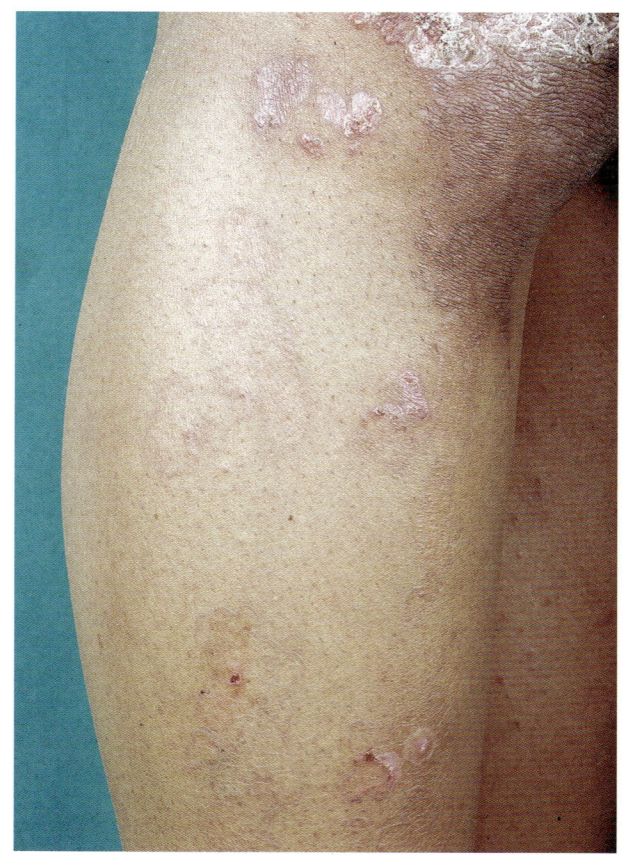

Figure 8.7

Disseminated superficial actinic porokeratosis

- Numerous pruritic papular lesions, enlarging centrifugally, confined to sun-exposed areas
- Sparing of palms, soles and mucosal surfaces
- Exacerbations during the summer (Figure 8.12)

Other disorders of keratinization

Age of onset

Onset is usually in childhood; the actinic form appears in the third or fourth decade.

Complications

About 10% of patients may develop squamous cell and basal cell carcinomas; these are most common in giant and linear forms.

- Immunosuppression (immunosuppression-induced porokeratosis) mainly revealed by transplantations (heart, kidney, bone marrow)
- Autoimmune diseases

Course

The disease is chronic and slowly progressive, with worsening after sun exposure.

Laboratory findings

Histopathologic features include the presence of cornoid lamellae, i.e. columns of parakeratosis beneath which the granular zone is thinned and, in the spinous zone, there are vacuolated and dyskeratotic cells, thinned epidermis and superficial perivascular lymphocytic infiltrate.

Genetics and pathogenesis

- Autosomal dominant diseases; many sporadic cases reported
- Mosaic forms are relatively common
- Primary defect consists of proliferation of abnormal clones of epidermal cells triggered by various factors such as actinic radiation, immunosuppression, trauma, infective agents
- Gene locus: short arm of chromosome 3 and a new locus for superficial actinic porokeratosis to chromosome 15q25.1–26.1

Differential diagnosis

- Porokeratosis of Mibelli: granuloma annularis, warts, elastosis perforans serpiginosa
- Linear porokeratosis: linear verrucous epidermal nevi, lichen striatus, linear lichen planus, linear psoriasis

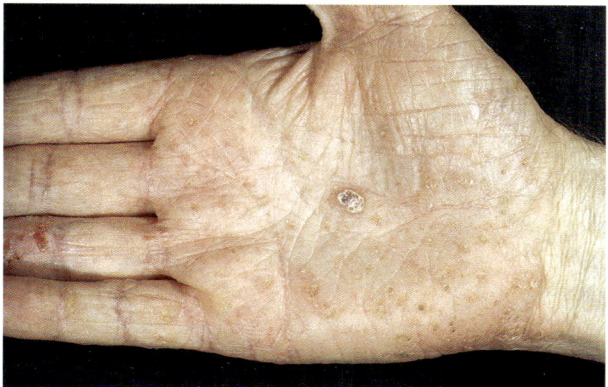

Figure 8.8

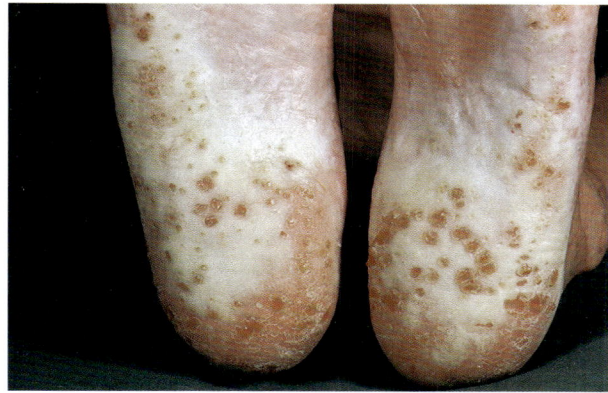

Figure 8.9

- Punctate palmoplantar porokeratosis: nevoid basal cell carcinoma syndrome, Darier's disease, pitted keratolysis, punctate palmoplantar keratoderma
- Disseminated superficial porokeratosis: pityriasis lichenoides, solar keratosis

Follow-up

- Propensity for neoplastic change requires accurate observation
- Avoid sun exposure

Therapy

This is unsatisfactory.

- Topical sunscreens, keratolytics, topical retinoids, topical steroids, 5-fluorouracil, imiquimod
- Cryotherapy, CO_2 laser, dermabrasion
- Oral retinoids

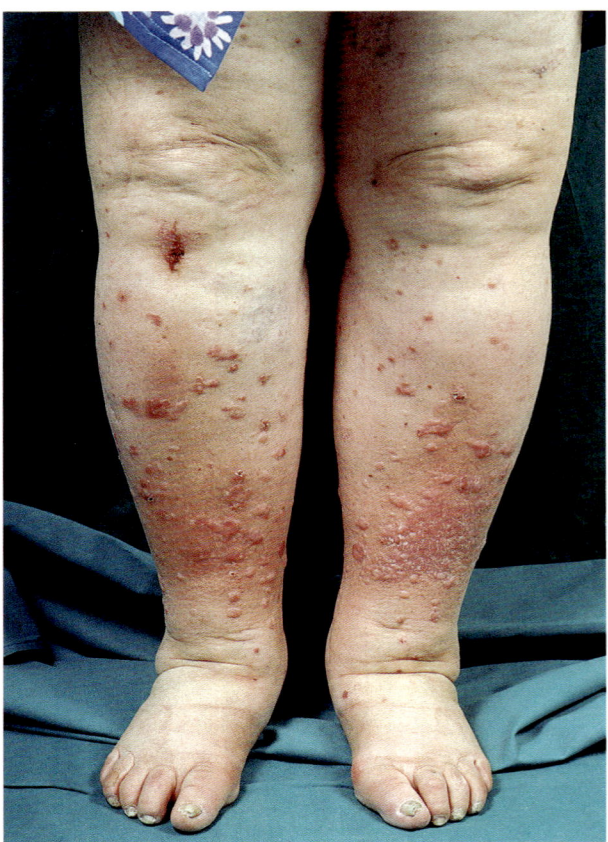

Figure 8.10

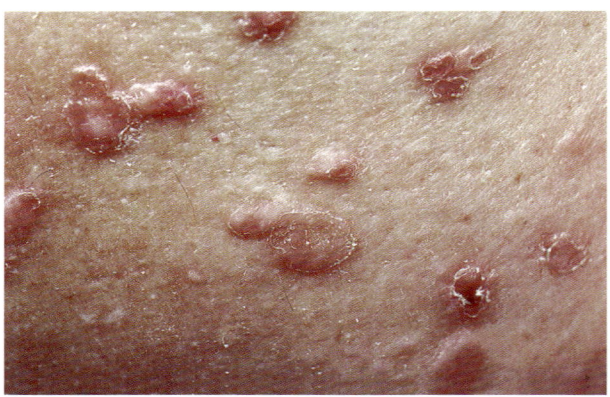

Figure 8.11

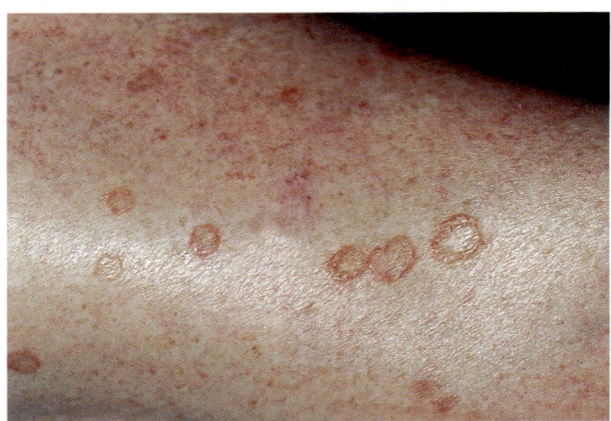

Figure 8.12

REFERENCES

Hussein MR, Wood GS. Microsatellite instability and its relevance to cutaneous tumorigenesis. J Cutan Pathol 2002; 29: 257–67

Mikhail GR, Wertheimer FW. Clinical variants of porokeratosis (Mibelli). Arch Dermatol 1968; 98: 124–31

Sasson M, Krain AD. Porokeratosis and cutaneous malignancy. Dermatol Surg 1996; 22: 339–42

Schamzoth JM, Zlotogorski A, Gilead L. Porokeratosis of Mibelli. Overview and review of the literature. Acta Dermatol Venereol 1997; 77: 207–13

Wei SC, Yang S, Li M, et al. Identification of a locus for porokeratosis palmaris et plantaris disseminata to a 6.9-cM region at chromosome 12q24.1–24.2. Br J Dermatol 2003; 149: 261–7

Xia K, Deng H, Xia JH, et al. A novel locus (DSAP2) for disseminated superficial actinic porokeratosis maps to chromosome 15q25.1–26.1. Br J Dermatol 2002; 147: 650–4

KYRLE'S DISEASE

Synonym

- Hyperkeratosis follicularis et parafollicularis in cutem penetrans

Age of onset

- From 30 to 70 years

Clinical findings

- Asymptomatic, scattered, generalized papular lesions with hyperkeratotic cone-shaped plugs (Figure 8.13)

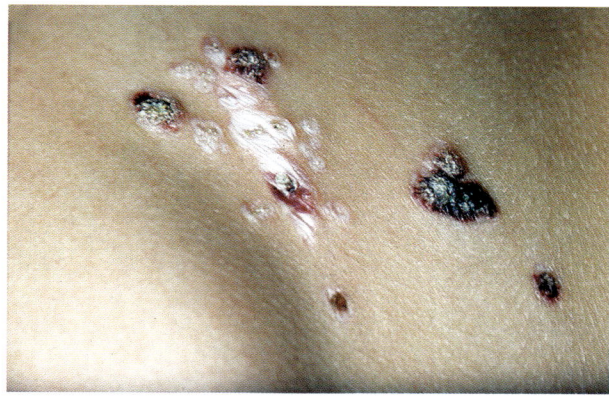

Figure 8.14

- Papules, follicular or extrafollicular (Figure 8.14)
- Possible coalescence to form verrucous plaques (mainly extensor extremities) or linear arrangements (mainly antecubital and popliteal fossae)
- Sparing of the mucous membranes and the palmar and plantar surfaces

Extracutaneous symptoms

- Diabetes mellitus
- Chronic renal failure
- Congestive cardiac failure

Course

The disease is chronic and persistent.

Laboratory investigations

Histopathologic findings:

- Keratotic plug filling an epithelial invagination
- Parakeratosis in parts of the plug
- Basophilic cellular debris within the plug
- Granulomatous reaction in the surrounding dermis

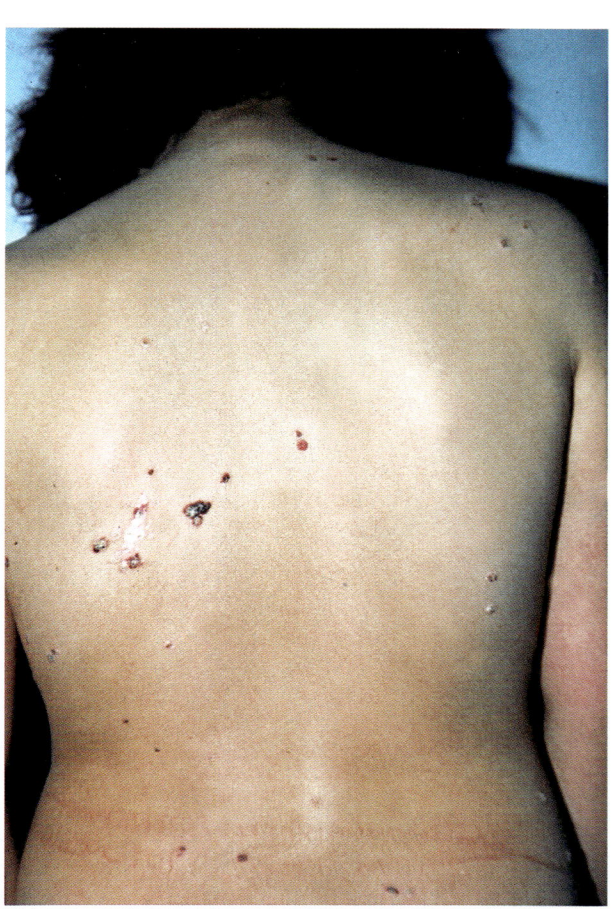

Figure 8.13

Genetics and pathogenesis

- Autosomal dominant inheritance; many sporadic cases
- Gene locus unknown
- 67-kDa elastin receptors have been detected in the epidermis eliminating altered elastic fibers (elastin–keratinocyte interaction)

Differential diagnosis

- Elastosis perforans serpiginosa
- Flegel's disease
- Reactive perforating collagenosis

Follow-up

There is a normal life span.

Therapy

- Topical keratolytic agents and retinoids
- Oral retinoids
- CO_2 laser

REFERENCES

Cunningham SR, Walsh M, Mattews MB, et al. Kyrle's disease. J Am Acad Dermatol 1987; 16: 117–123

Fujimoto N, Akagi A, Tajima S, et al. Expression of the 67 kDa elastin receptor in perforating skin disorders. Br J Dermatol 2002; 146: 74–9

Sehgal VN, Jain G, Thappe DM, et al. Perforating dermatoses: a review and report of four cases. J Dermatol 1993; 20: 329–40

CHILD SYNDROME

Synonym

- Congenital hemidysplasia, ichthyosis and limb defects

Epidemiology

This is a very rare disease. Prevalence data are unavailable. Fewer than 30 cases published.

Age of onset

- At birth or a few months after birth

Clinical findings

There is a monolateral psoriasiform erythroderma with bright erythema and seborrheic-like scales, involving half of the body, with a sharp midline border (lateralization mosaic pattern), or a bilateral presentation with lesions placed in the major folds (axillary or inguinocrural) (Figures 8.15–8.17).

Lesions are usually permanent, but rarely may disappear spontaneously, and late involvement of healthy sites is possible. On the affected side, nails are grossly dystrophic and partial alopecia may be present.

Extracutaneous findings and complications

Skeletal defects appear almost exclusively homolateral to the skin lesions, ranging from hypoplasia to aplasia of limb bones. Vertebral involvement is possible as well as defects in facial bones and upper and lower cinguli.

When cranial defects are visible, central nervous system involvement is usual, leading to mental

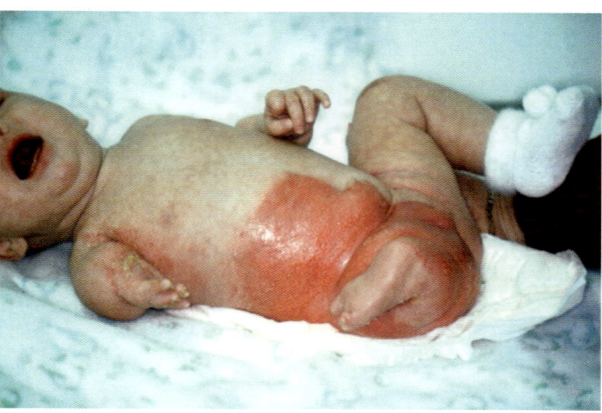

Figure 8.15

Other disorders of keratinization   99

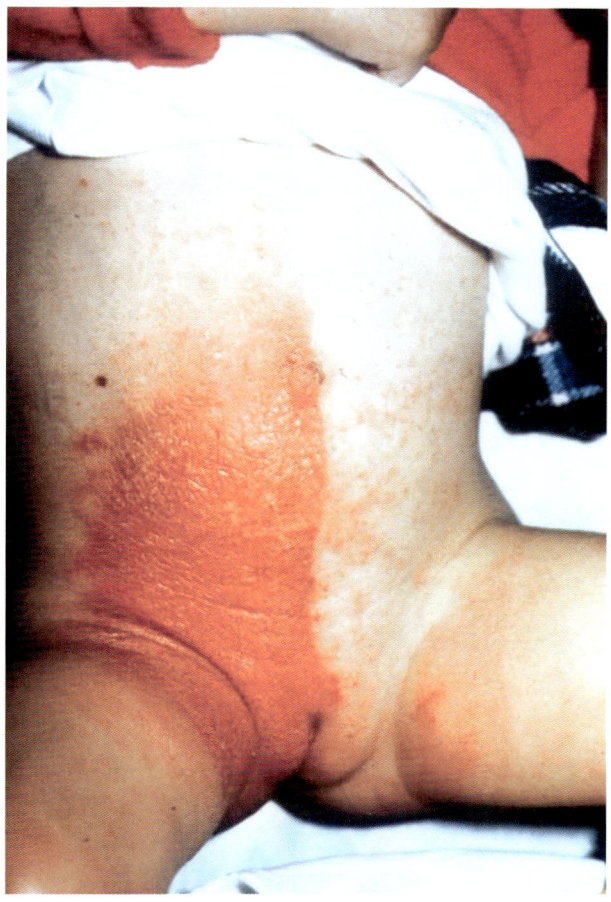

Figure 8.16

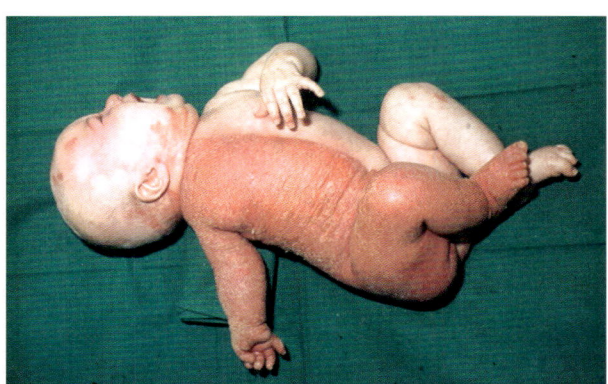

Figure 8.17

retardation. Renal and cardiac defects are relatively frequent and malformations of other entodermal-derived organs are possible.

Course

When the defects are severe and diffuse the disease may be lethal, especially for internal organ malfunctions.

Skin lesions may change during infancy and childhood.

Laboratory findings

Abnormal keratinization is found upon electron microscopy.

Genetics and pathogenesis

The disease is X-linked dominant lethal for males. Few male cases are described.

The responsible gene is called NSDHL (NadPH steroid dehydrogenase-like protein), involved in cholesterol synthesis.

The mechanism of the pattern is specific for this disease, known as 'lateralization pattern' and may reflect involvement of an ancestral gene related to modulation of the body symmetry.

Differential diagnosis

- Inflammatory linear verrucous epidermal nevus (ILVEN)
- Conradi–Hunermann–Happle disease
- Epidermal nevus syndromes
- Encephalocraniocutaneous lipomatosis
- Goltz's syndrome

Follow-up and therapy

- Assessment of limb defects and surgical correction when possible
- Study of internal organ malformations
- Emollients and keratolytics for skin lesions

REFERENCES

Bittar M, Happle R. CHILD syndrome avant la lettre. J Am Acad Dermatol 2004; 50(Suppl 2): S34–7

Koniög A, Happle R, Fink-Puches R, et al. A novel missense mutation of NSDHL in an unusual case of CHILD syndrome showing bilateral, almost symmetric involvement. J Am Acad Dermatol 2002; 46: 594–6

X-LINKED DOMINANT CHONDRODYSPLASIA PUNCTATA

Synonyms

- Conradi–Hunermann disease
- Conradi–Hunermann–Happle syndrome

Epidemiology

The disease is very rare. No further data are available.

Age of onset

- At birth

Clinical findings

- Collodion-like presentation is frequent
- Ichthyosiform linear lesions following the lines of Blaschko, composed by central adherent large scales (Figure 8.18)
- Atrophoderma vermiculatum following the lines of Blaschko, especially on arms (Figure 8.19)
- Linear alopecia and sparse hair, eyebrows and eyelashes (Figure 8.20)
- More rarely, hypo/hyperpigmented striae in a narrow-band mosaic pattern and nail dystrophies

Extracutaneous findings

- Stippled epiphyses (premature ossification) (Figure 8.21)
- Malar hypoplasia with depressed nasal bones, frontal bosses ('flat-face')
- Asymmetrical malformations of arms and legs bones with scoliosis, congenital hip dysplasia, ribs and vertebral anomalies and short stature (Figure 8.22)
- Eye abnormalities (present in over 50% of patients), striated (mosaic) cataracts, mono- and bilateral, microphthalmus, optic nerve atrophy (Figure 8.23)

Complications and course

- Ichthyotic lesions may disappear completely after adolescence
- Atrophic lesions remain steady
- Intellectual development is usually physiologic

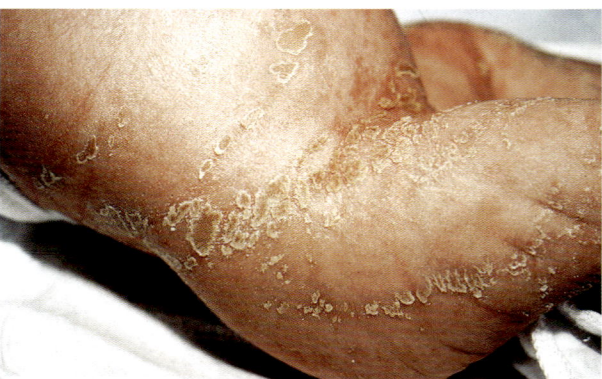

Figure 8.18

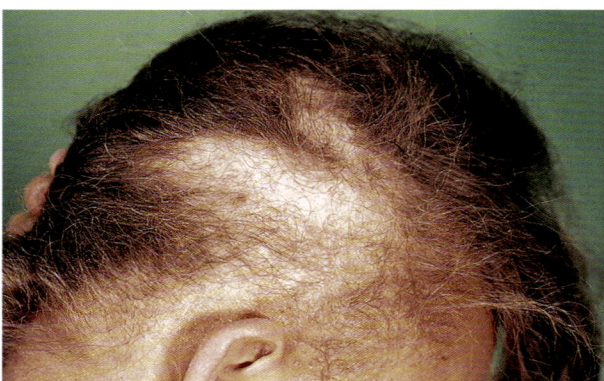

Figure 8.20

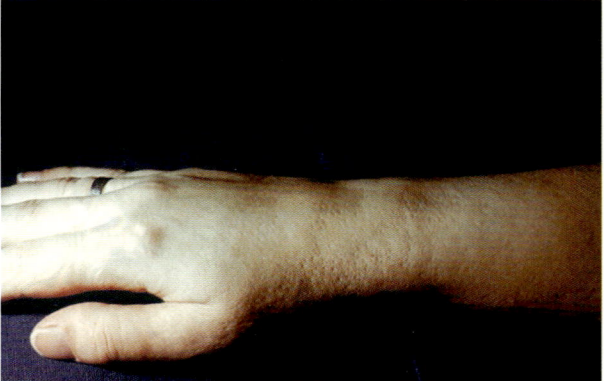

Figure 8.19

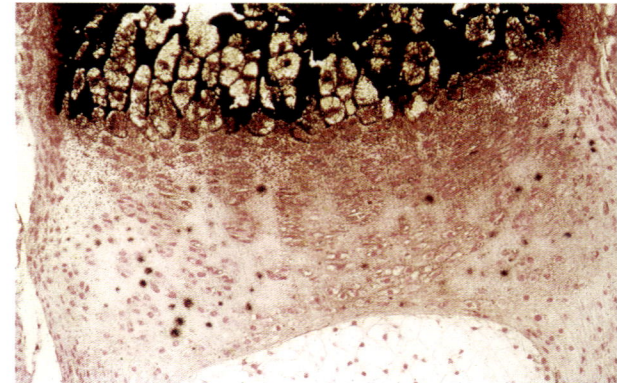

Figure 8.21

Other disorders of keratinization

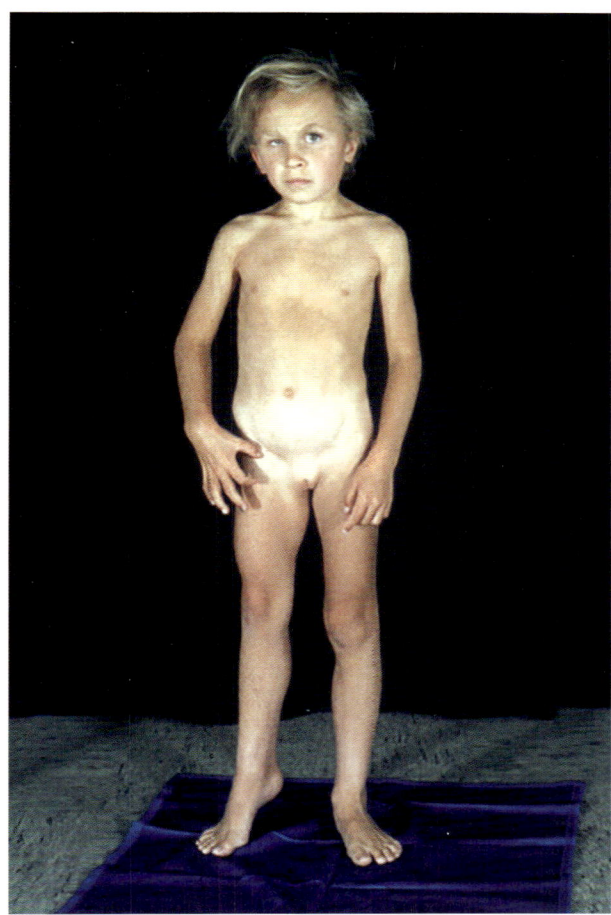

Figure 8.22

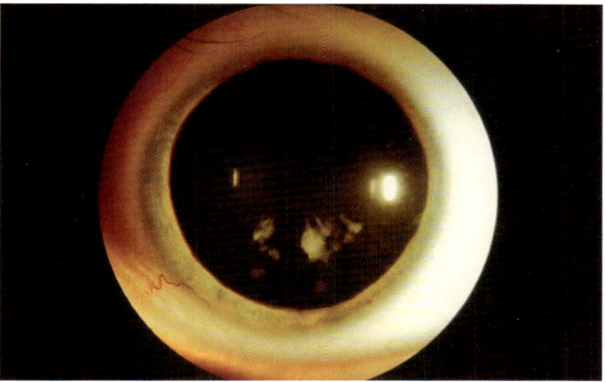

Figure 8.23

Mutations involve the Δ^8–Δ^9 sterol isomerase emopamil-binding protein (EBP) that is responsible for one of the steps of sterol biosynthesis.

Differential diagnosis

- CHILD syndrome
- Goltz's syndrome

Follow-up and therapy

- Assessment of bone defects and their correction
- Ocular defect detection and therapy
- Keratolytic agents for ichthyosis

REFERENCES

Depreter M, Espeel M, Roels F. Human peroxisomal disorders. Microsc Res Tech 2003; 61: 203–23

Herman GE, Kelley RI, Pureza V, et al. Characterization of mutations in 22 females with X-linked dominant chondrodysplasia punctata (Happle syndrome). Genet Med 2002; 4: 434–8

Milunsky JM, Maher TA, Metzenberg AB. Molecular, biochemical, and phenotypic analysis of a hemizygous male with Happle syndrome and a mutation in EBP. Am J Med Genet 2003; 116A: 249–54

Laboratory findings

- Radiography-detected stippling of epiphyses
- Peroxisomal enzyme disturbances and calcium inclusions in the dermis
- Ichthyosiform changes with aspecific stratum corneum anomalies at ultrastructural examination

Genetics and pathogenesis

The disease is transmitted with an X-linked dominant trait, usually lethal for males.

KID SYNDROME

Synonym

- Keratitis–ichthyosis–deafness syndrome

Epidemiology

This is a rare disease. No further epidemiological data are available. About 100 cases are described in the literature.

Age of onset

- At birth or shortly thereafter

Clinical findings

- Diffuse and progressive erythematous–hyperkeratotic plaques with a surface described as 'grainy' or 'leathery' (Figures 8.24 and 8.25)
- Spiny hyperkeratosis (head and extremities) (Figure 8.26)
- Palmoplantar hyperkeratosis (Figure 8.27)
- Absent or sparse hair (Figure 8.24)
- Onychodystrophy (Figures 8.25 and 8.26)
- Hypohidrosis
- Rarely, linear hyperkeratotic lesions are superimposed, explained by allelic loss
- Occurrence of squamous cell carcinomas (mucosae)

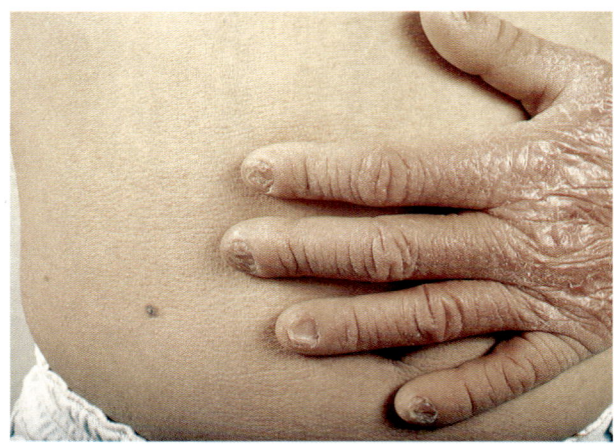

Figure 8.25

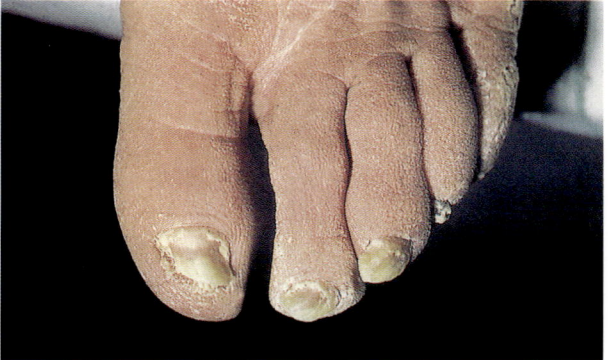

Figure 8.26

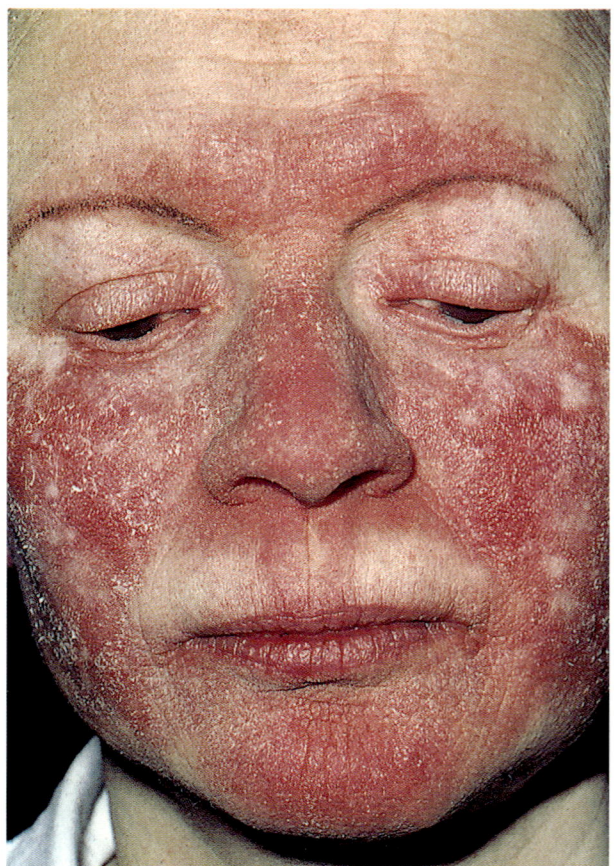

Figure 8.24

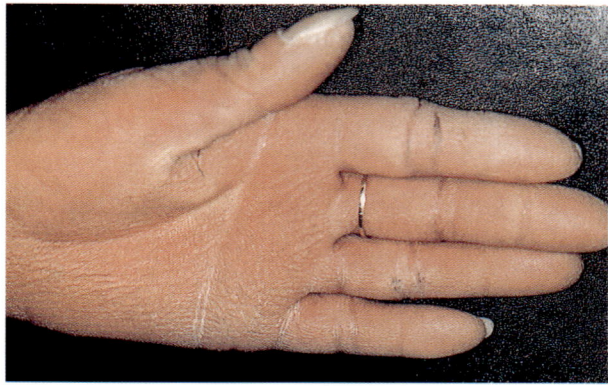

Figure 8.27

Extracutaneous findings

- Neurosensorial deafness of variable degree
- Keratoconjunctivitis, blepharitis and photophobia in over 75% of patients
- Corneal ulcerations and opacities
- Usually normal intelligence

Course and complications

Severe hearing loss may lead to impaired speech and psychomotor development.

Ocular involvement is progressive during life, leading rarely to blindness.

There is an increased risk of severe infections with pyogenes bacteria and fungi.

Laboratory findings, genetics and pathogenesis

The disease is autosomal dominant, with many sporadic cases.

Connexin 26 is the gene involved in pathogenesis of the disease. Together with other connexin-related human skin diseases, patients have palmoplantar keratoderma and deafness.

Differential diagnosis

- Epidermolytic hyperkeratosis
- Ichthyosis follicularis–alopecia–photophobia (IFAP) syndrome
- Clouston's syndrome
- The so-called 'hystrix-like ichthyosis and deafness' syndrome (HID syndrome) is just a different presentation of KID syndrome and not a separate entity

Follow-up and therapy

- Oral retinoids give controversial results
- Survey for squamous cell carcinomas in skin and mucosae
- Antibiotics and antifungal therapy for infections
- Keratolytics and emollients to relieve pruritus and xerosis
- Ophthalmological management for keratitis
- Detection and staging of neurosensory hearing loss

REFERENCES

Restano L, Cambiaghi S, Brusasco A, et al. A hyperkeratotic linear lesion in a girl with KID syndrome. A further example of early allelic loss? Eur J Dermatol 1999; 9: 143–3

van Geel M. van Steensel MA, Kuster W, et al. HID and KID syndromes are associated with the same connexin 26 mutation. Br J Dermatol 2002; 146: 938–42

Yotsumoto S, Hashiguchi T, Chen X, et al. Novel mutations in GJB2 encoding connexin-26 in Japanese patients with keratitis–ichthyosis–deafness syndrome. Br J Dermatol 2003; 148: 649–53

PITYRIASIS RUBRA PILARIS

Epidemiology

A few pedigrees have been described.

Age of onset

- Usually second–third decade

Clinical findings

- Individual erythematous-scaling lesions merging to form large patches of involved skin with characteristic islands of sparing within affected tissue (Figure 8.28), with peculiar 'dark salmon pink' color of the lesions
- Palmoplantar hyperkeratosis with progressive extension to Achilles tendon areas (Figures 8.29 and 8.30)
- As in psoriasis, extensor surfaces (Figure 8.31) are the preferred site, but erythroderma (Figure 8.32) is possible
- Aspecific nail dystrophies and scalp involvement

Extracutaneous findings

- None

Course and prognosis

Usually progressive, the disease may stabilize or relapse, with long symptom-free intervals.

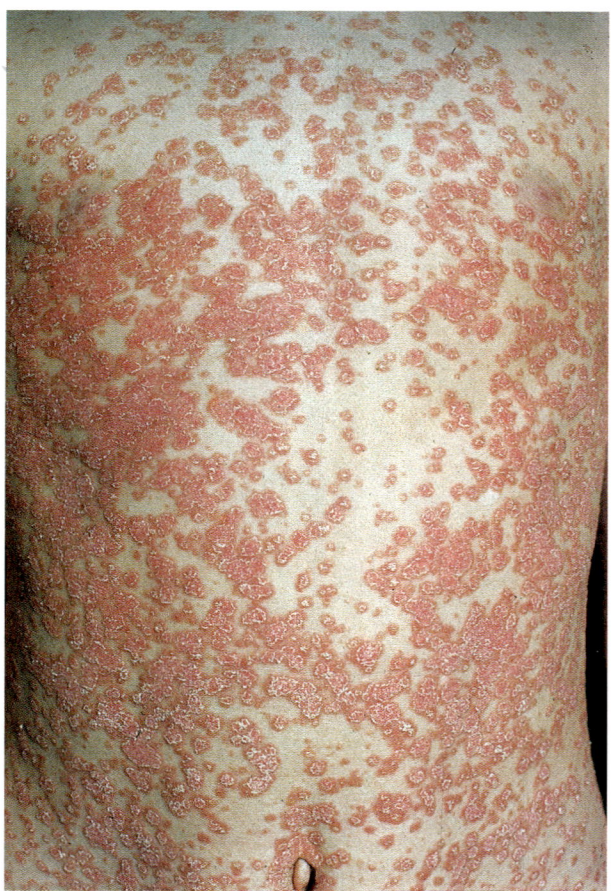

Figure 8.28

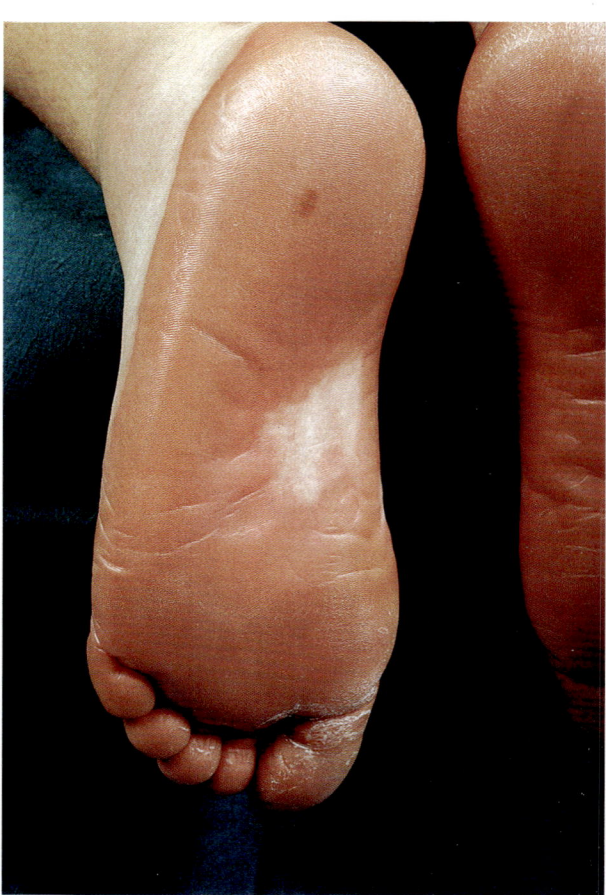

Figure 8.29

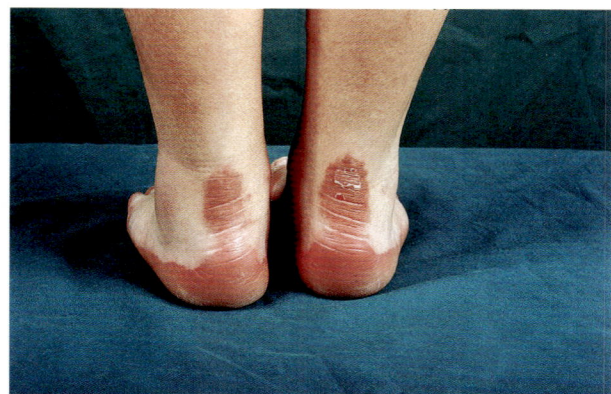

Figure 8.30

Other disorders of keratinization

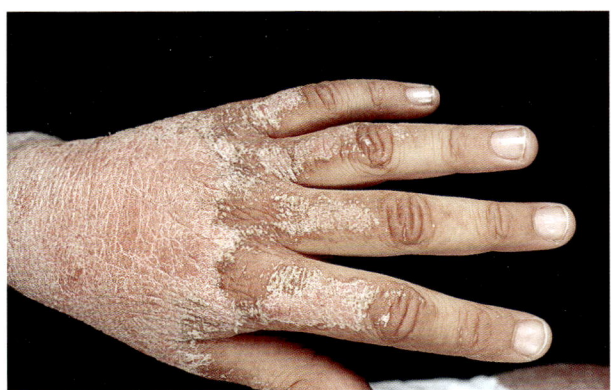

Figure 8.31

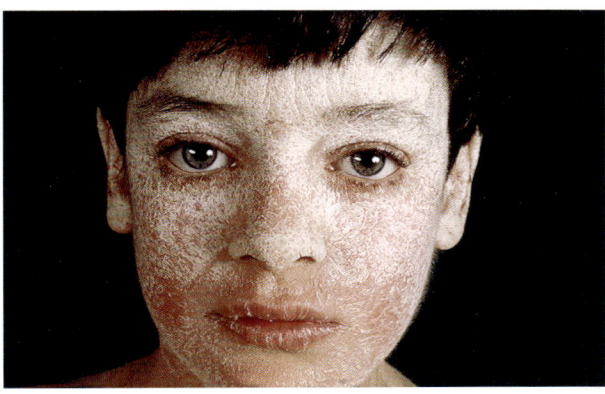

Figure 8.32

Laboratory findings

There is one report of anomalies in the expression of keratins (K6, K14, K16) and the expression of acidic non-epidermal keratins in three subjects of the same pedigree with pityriasis rubra pilaris (PRP).

Genetics and pathogenesis

- The disease is autosomal dominant
- Sporadic cases represent the vast majority
- Sporadic PRP is absolutely indistinguishable from familial PRP from the clinical point of view

Follow-up and therapy

- Keratolytics and emollients
- Calcipotriol
- Etretinate is normally prescribed in PRP with good results
- Methotrexate and azathioprine may be useful in a minority of patients

Differential diagnosis

- Psoriasis
- Seborrheic dermatitis
- Peeling skin syndrome
- Palmoplantar keratodermas

REFERENCE

Vanderhooft SL, Francis JS, Holbrook KA, et al. Familial pityriasis rubra pilaris. Arch Dermatol 1995; 131: 448–53

CHAPTER 9

Poikilodermas and aging syndromes

KINDLER'S SYNDROME

Synonyms

- Weary's syndrome
- Weary–Kindler syndrome
- Poikiloderma with bullae

Epidemiology

The disease is rare; no further prevalence data are available in the literature. We personally diagnosed eight patients in a 15-year survey.

Age of onset

- At birth or in early infancy

Clinical findings

- Acral bullae on minor trauma during childhood (Figures 9.1–9.3)
- Photosensitivity and progressive poikiloderma especially in sun-exposed areas, with atrophy (cigarette paper scars), telangiectases and macular pinpoint pigmentation (Figure 9.4)
- Proximal progressive pseudosyndactyly of cicatricial origin (pathognomonic of Kindler's syndrome) that involve characteristically the space between the metacarpophalangeal and the first interphalangeal joints (Figure 9.5)
- In adulthood a particular facies with thin nose and lips gives an appearance of scleroderma-like or xeroderma pigmentosum-like features (Figure 9.6)

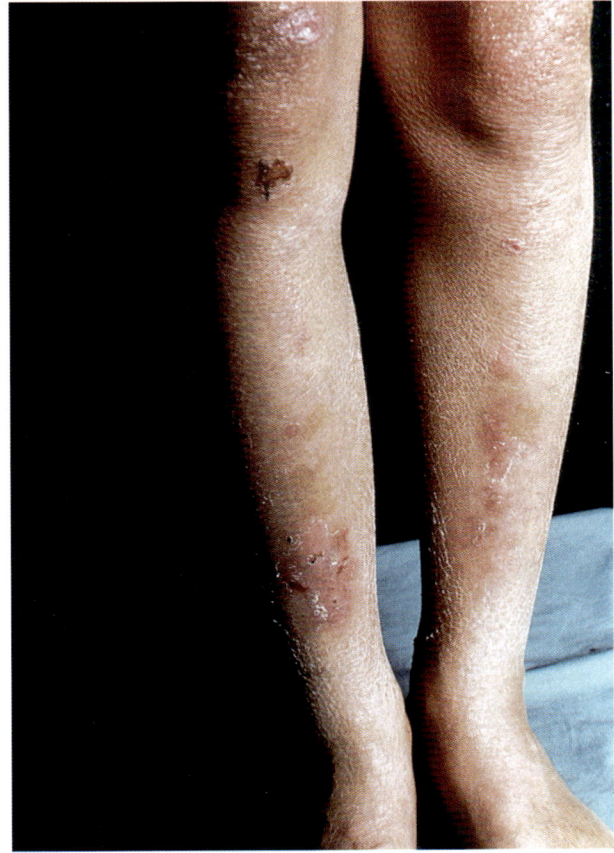

Figure 9.1

- Thickening of palms and soles
- Nail dystrophy
- Blisters may occur in oral (cheilitis) and genital mucosae

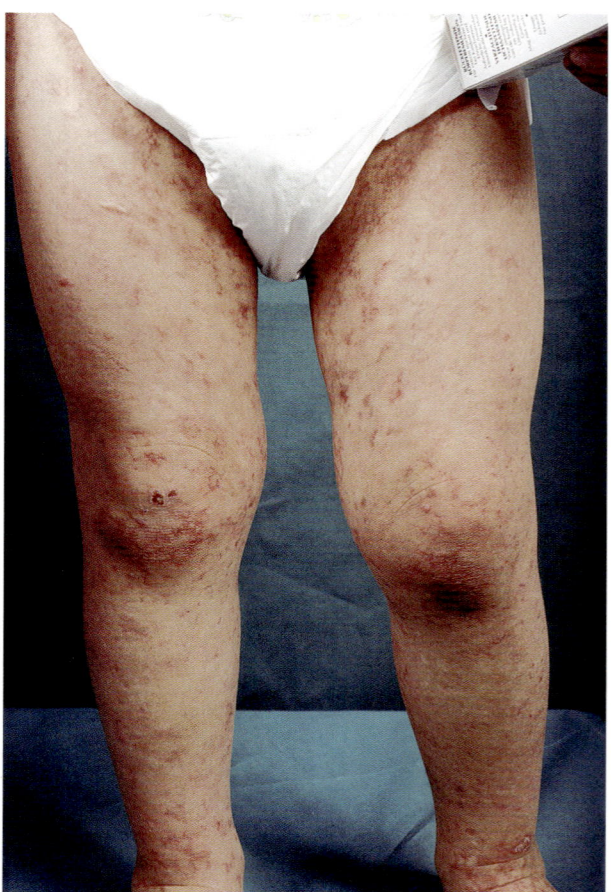

Figure 9.2

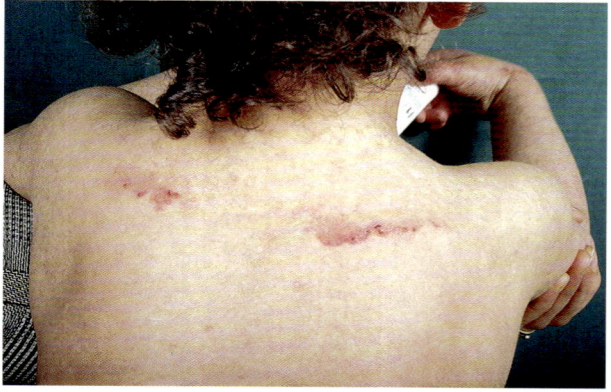

Figure 9.3

Extracutaneous findings

- Esophageal strictures in more than 60% of patients
- Cicatricial strictures may occur more rarely in conjunctivae, urethra and perianal region
- Leukokeratoses in oral mucosa with caries
- Peculiar pseudosyndactyly of the first interphalangeal spaces of hands

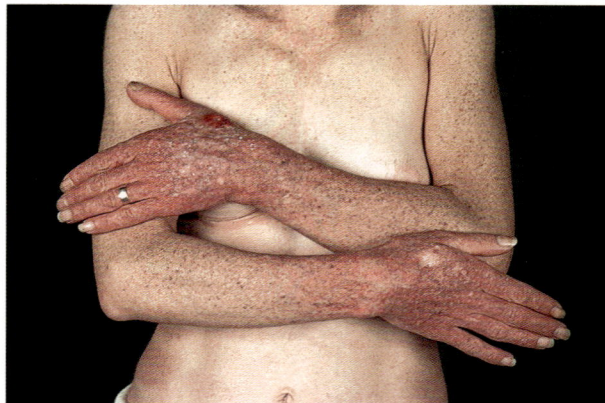

Figure 9.4

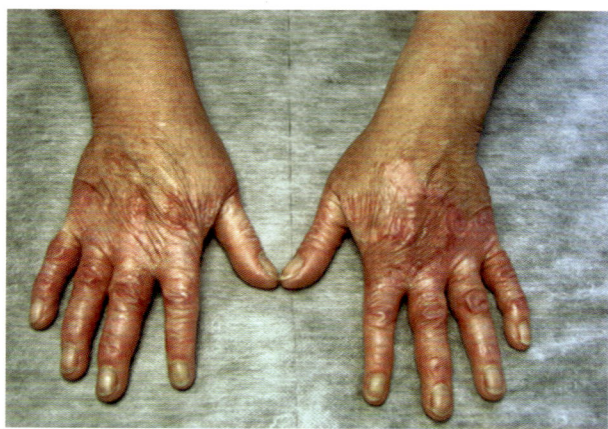

Figure 9.5

Complications and course

Blisters are frequent in infancy, and progressively decrease with age. In contrast, poikilodermatous changes are progressive and worsen with age, not only in sun-exposed areas.

Squamous cell carcinomas (dorsa of the hands, face) are a frequent complication, especially in those patients who work outdoors (Figure 9.7). Carcinomas in other regions are rare.

Esophageal strictures worsen with age in both severity and time of recurrence. Strictures in other areas are rare.

Laboratory findings

Upon electron microscopy, bullae may be intraepidermal and subepidermal, with a peculiar reduplication of the basal membrane.

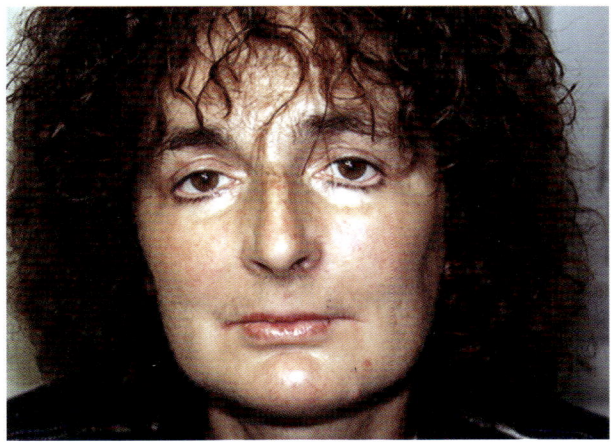

Figure 9.6

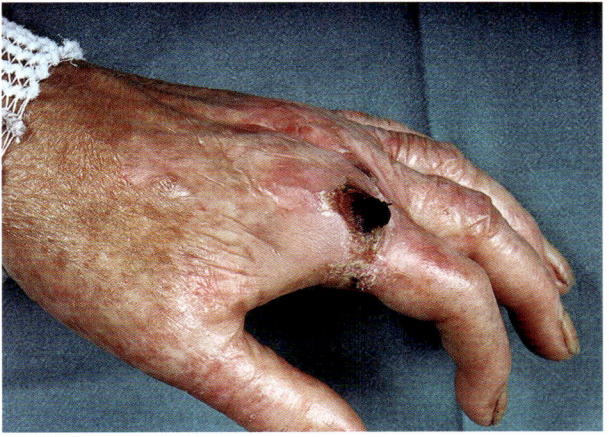

Figure 9.7

Genetics and pathogenesis

The disease is autosomal recessive. Loss of function mutations have recently been identified in the FLJ20116 gene, renamed KIND1, encoding for kindlin-1. This protein is the human homolog of the *Caenorhabditis elegans* UNC-112 protein, a membrane associated structural and signaling protein that is a link between the actin cytoskeleton and the extracellular matrix.

This phenomenon explains the formation of bullae in the early phases of the disease and the fragility of other stratified epithelia, and may be related to the poikilodermatous processes and cancer proneness. The clear ultraviolet (UV) relationship, with worsening of the disease in adulthood, represents the logical next step in research.

Differential diagnosis

- Epidermolysis bullosa
- Rothmund–Thomson syndrome
- Xeroderma pigmentosum
- Dyskeratosis congenita

Follow-up and therapy

- Photoprotection!!!
- Detection of early precancerous stages and surgery of squamous cell carcinomas in skin and mucosae
- Esophageal endoscopy and dilatations

REFERENCES

Haber RM, Hanna WM. Kindler syndrome. Clinical and ultrastructural findings. Arch Dermatol 1996; 132: 1487–90

Senturk N, Usubutun A, Sahin S, et al. Kindler syndrome: absence of definite ultrastructural feature. J Am Acad Dermatol 1999; 40: 335–7

Siegel DH, Ashton GH, Penagos HG, et al. Loss of kindlin-1, a human homolog of the *Caenorhabditis elegans* actin–extracellular-matrix linker protein UNC-112, causes Kindler syndrome. Am J Hum Genet 2003; 73: 174–87

XERODERMA PIGMENTOSUM

Synonym

- De Santis–Cacchione syndrome for XP-A

Epidemiology

The disease is rare. In a 10-year survey (mid-1970s–mid-1980s) about 1000 patients have been described in the literature.

Age of onset

- First signs of the disease may appear as soon as first UV exposure occurs
- Skin malignancies usually after the second year of life

Clinical findings

The different types of xeroderma pigmentosum (XP) (complementation groups), related to their different molecular origins, are reported in Table 9.1, but they share the following symptoms:

- Photosensitivity (severe to extreme)
- Freckling on photoexposed areas (Figure 9.8)
- Progressive premature aging with poikilodermatous changes (atrophy, lentigo, telangiectases) (Figures 9.9 and 9.10)

Solar keratoses

- Basal cell carcinomas, squamous cell carcinomas and melanoma (in decreasing order) in photo-exposed areas, lips, tongue, rarely oral and nasal mucosa (Figure 9.11)
- Disfiguring cancer on the face can cause loss of nasal pyramid, orbital structures or external ears, as occurs with repeated surgery (Figure 9.12)
- Rarely, skin angiosarcomas

Extracutaneous symptoms

- Photophobia, conjunctival cancer, blepharitis, corneal opacities and blindness
- 25% of XP patients show neurologic involvement of different degrees, with low IQ

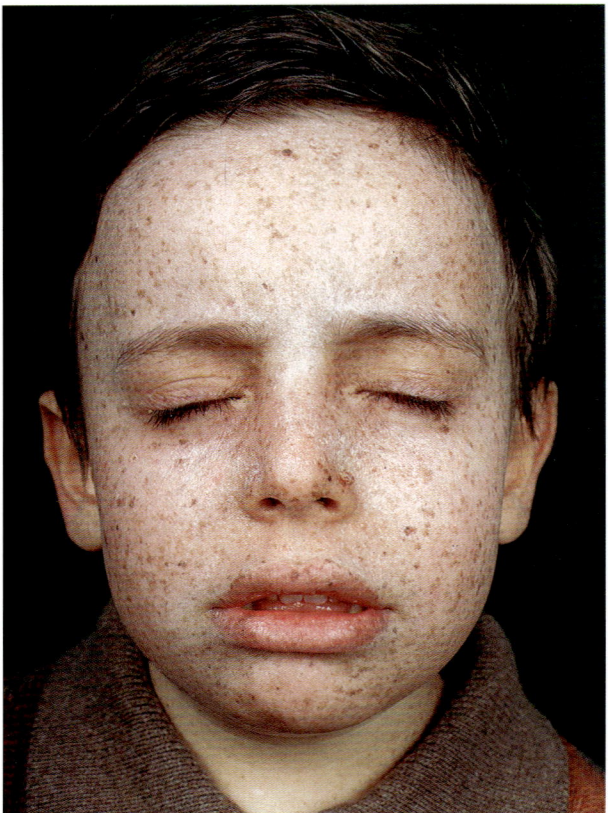

Figure 9.8

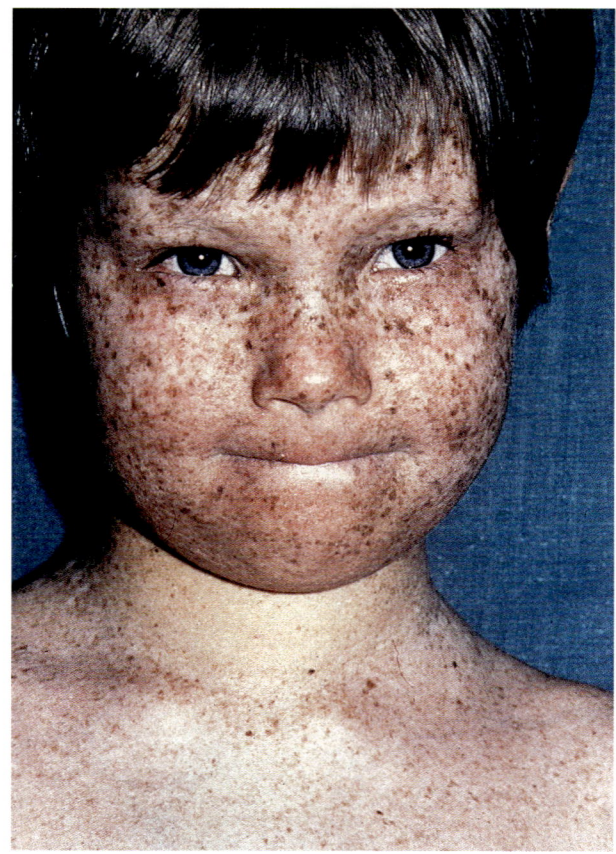

Figure 9.9

Table 9.1 Different types of xeroderma pigmentosum (XP)

Group	Enzyme encoded	Skin disease	Skin cancer
XP-A	DDB1	+++	+++
XP-B	ERCC3	++ to +++	+++
XP-C	Endonuclease	++ to +++	++ melanoma
XP-D	ERCC2	++	+
XP-E	DDB2	+	Rare
XP-F	ERCC4	++	Few or absent
XP-G	Endonuclease	+++	Few or absent
XP-V	Polymerase eta	++ to +++	Late onset ++

ERCC, excision-repair cross-complementing genes; DDB, DNA damage-binding protein; 0 = absent; + = mild; ++ = moderate; +++ = severe

- Ataxia, abnormal reflex with paresis, progressive central deafness (XP-A) (see Table 9.1)
- Microcephaly, growth retardation and abnormal sexual development in a minority of patients
- Increased risk for internal malignancies

Course and complications

- Life expectancy is greatly reduced: 90% at age 13, 80% at age 25, 70% at age 40 years
- Metastatic skin cancer occurs invariably in all patients

Genetics and pathogenesis

XP is inherited as an autosomal recessive disease.
Clinical and cellular photosensitivity is due to the inability to repair UV induced DNA damage. Two different DNA-repair processes are defective in XP, the classic nuclear excision repair, divided into two subpathways called the global genome repair (GGR) system and transcription-coupled repair (TCR) and translation synthesis (TLS).

Differential diagnosis

- Hereditary polymorphic light eruption
- Rothmund–Thomson syndrome
- Ataxia telangiectasia
- Erythropoietic protoporphyria
- Gunther's disease
- Kindler's disease

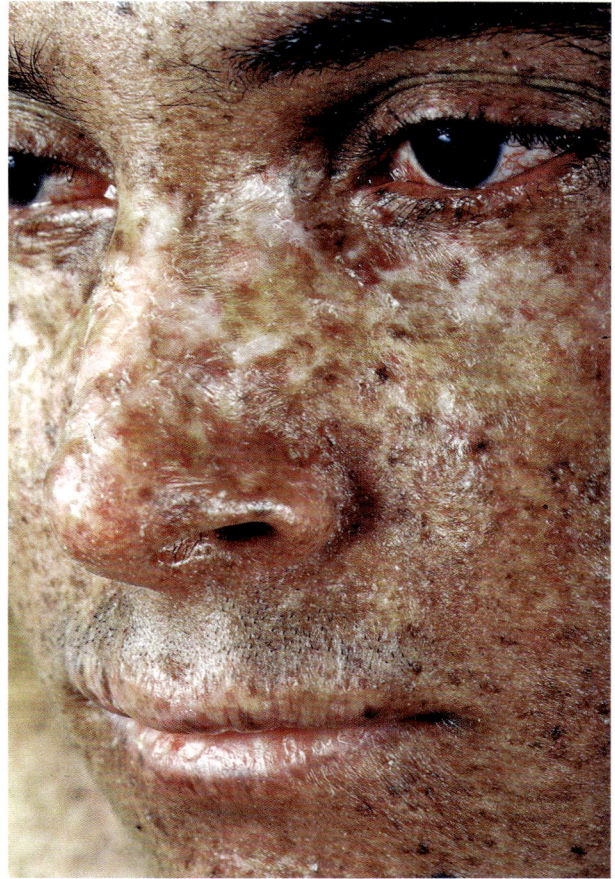

Figure 9.10

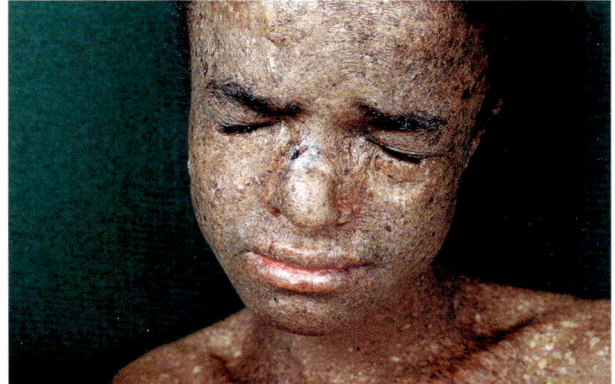

Figure 9.11

Follow-up and therapy

- Photoexposure is strictly forbidden
- Sunscreens, chemical and physical
- Adequate sunglasses, shirts, caps and gloves as well as appropriate face-masks are mandatory

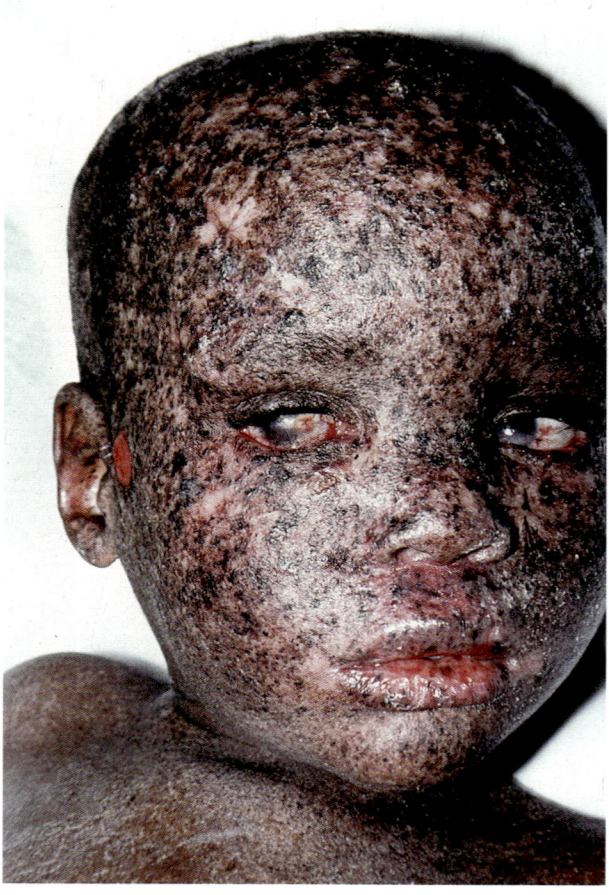

Figure 9.12

- Window screens are required at home, at school and in the car
- Psychosociological support for patients and families
- Frequent dermatological survey to prevent pre-cancerosis and skin cancers in skin and visible mucosae
- Surgical excision of pre-canceroses and skin cancers
- Plastic reconstructive surgery on the face
- Tests for internal malignancies, hematological and visceral
- Frequent ophthalmological consultations

REFERENCES

Itoh T, O'Shea C, Linn S. Impaired regulation of tumor suppressor p53 caused by mutations in the xeroderma pigmentosum DDB2 gene: mutual regulatory interactions between p48(DDB2) and p53. Mol Cell Biol 2003; 23: 7540–53

Laposa RR, Feeney L, Cleaver JE. Recapitulation of the cellular xeroderma pigmentosum-variant phenotypes using short interfering RNA for DNA polymerase H. Cancer Res 2003; 63: 3909–12

Norgauer J, Idzko M, Panther E, et al. Xeroderma pigmentosum. Eur J Dermatol 2003; 13: 4–9

ROTHMUND–THOMSON SYNDROME

Synonym

- Hereditary congenital poikiloderma

Epidermiology

This is very rare; there are no data available on the literature about incidence or prevalence.

Age of onset

- Few months to 2 years after birth

Clinical signs

Erythema and edema appear first and are located mainly in sun-exposed areas, together with photosensitivity (Figures 9.13 and 9.14).

Progression of symptoms may reveal severe telangiectases, rare blisters, hypo- and hyperpigmented macules, giving the characteristic poikilodermatous, mild atrophic pattern to UV-exposed areas.

Keratoses occur on the dorsa of the hands, and can transform into squamous cell carcinoma (25% of patients).

Hair is sparse and coarse, as well as eyebrows and eyelashes, and aspecific nail dystrophies are possible (Figure 9.13).

Extracutaneous findings

- Facies with hypotrophy of malar areas and hypertelorism
- Short stature and skeletal abnormalities (radius and hand bones)
- Early-onset cataracts, rarely leading to blindness (50%)
- Occasional hypogonadism and low fertility in a quarter of patients
- Hypodontia
- Mental retardation described

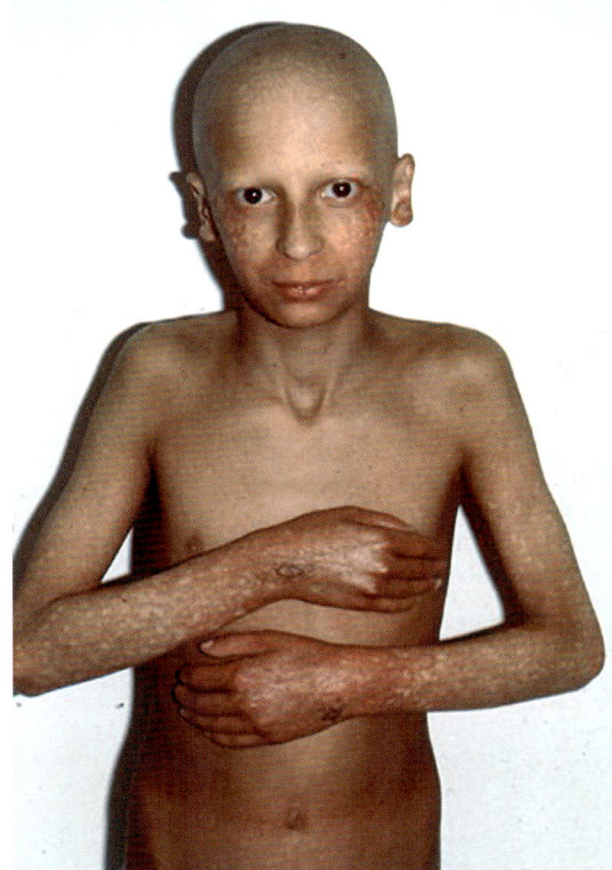

Figure 9.13

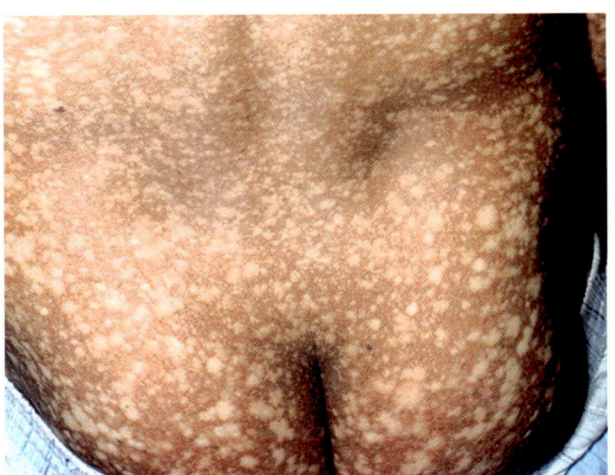

Figure 9.14

Course and prognosis

Cutaneous symptoms are progressive during infancy and until adolescence, giving a poikilodermatous appearance, especially – but not exclusively – to the face and sun-exposed areas.

Squamous cell carcinomas are frequent; in contrast, internal malignancies are rare and unrelated.

Life expectancy is reduced.

Laboratory investigations, genetics and pathogenesis

The disease is autosomal recessive and is due to mutations in the RECQ helicase gene, involved in DNA repair.

Differential diagnosis

- Xeroderma pigmentosum (early phase)
- Kindler's disease
- Ectodermal dysplasias

Follow-up and therapy

- Photoprotection!!!
- Early detection of malignancies and their correction
- Orthopedic assessment of bone anomalies

REFERENCES

Hickson ID. RecQ helicases: caretakers of the genome. Nature Rev Cancer 2003; 3: 169–78

Mohaghegh P, Hickson ID. Premature aging in RecQ helicase-deficient human syndromes. Int J Biochem Cell Biol 2002; 34: 1496–501

Wang LL, Gannavarapu A, Kozinetz CA, et al. Association between osteosarcoma and deleterious mutations in the RECQL4 gene in Rothmund–Thomson syndrome. J Natl Cancer Inst 2003; 95: 669–74

NAEGELI–FRANCESCHETTI SYNDROME

Synonyms

- Naegeli syndrome
- Naegeli–Franceschetti–Jadassohn syndrome

Epidemiology

No data are available.

Age of onset

- From early childhood to 5 years of age
- Dysplastic hyperkeratotic nails (congenital malalignment) (Figure 9.15)
- Punctate palmoplantar keratoderma with dermatoglyphic abnormalities and transient blistering
- Possible linear forms

Extracutaneous symptoms

As expected, in this rare ectodermal dysplasia enamel defects are present.

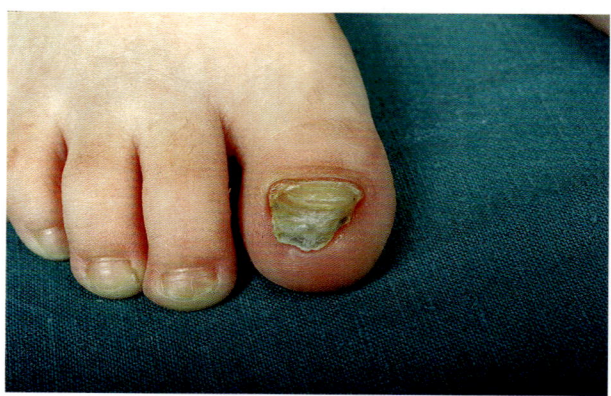

Figure 9.15

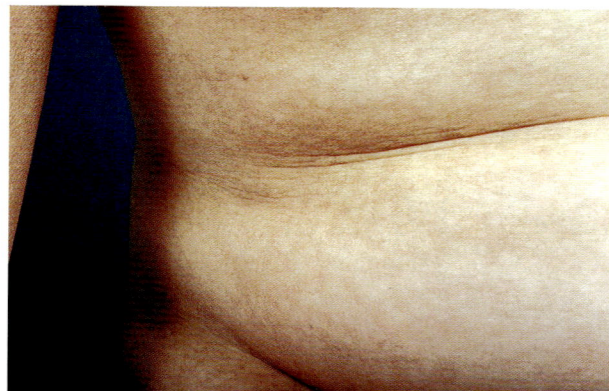

Figure 9.16

Clinical findings

- Reticulate brownish hyperpigmented macules on perioral, periocular areas, progressively extending to the neck and trunk (Figures 9.16–9.18)
- Decreased sweating and heat intolerance

Course and complications

Pigmented lesions may be less colored in adulthood.

Laboratory findings

There are none peculiar to this disease.

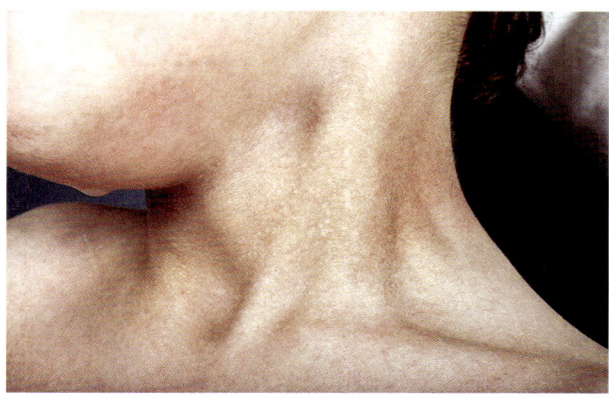

Figure 9.18

Genetics and pathogenesis

The disease is autosomal dominant, mapped to 17q11.2–q21.

Differential diagnosis

- Incontinentia pigmenti
- Kindler's disease
- Dyskeratosis congenita

Follow-up and therapy

- Protection from UV radiation
- Emollients for xerosis

REFERENCES

Itin PH, Buechner SA. Segmental forms of autosomal dominant skin disorders: the puzzle of mosaicism. Am J Med Genet 1999; 85: 351–4

Itin PH, Lautenschlager S. Genodermatosis with reticulate, patchy and mottled pigmentation of the neck – a clue to rare dermatologic disorders. Dermatology 1998; 197: 281–80

Sprecher E, Itin P, Whittock NV, et al. Refined mapping of Naegeli–Franceschetti–Jadassohn syndrome to a 6 cM interval on chromosome 17q11.2–q21 and investigation of candidate genes. J Invest Dermatol 2002; 119: 692–8

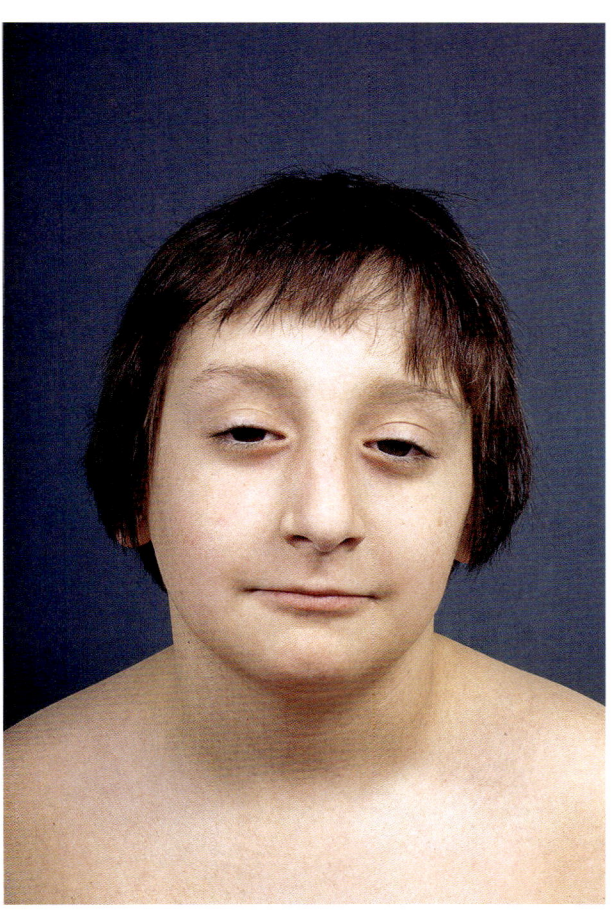

Figure 9.17

WERNER'S SYNDROME

Synonym

- Adult progeria

Epidemiology

There are no reports of epidemiological data for Werner's syndrome.

Age of onset

- Second and third decades

Clinical findings

Starting from the central years of the second decade, progressive alopecia and canities are visible. All hair is involved in this process. At the same time or shortly thereafter, sclerodermatous-like changes occur on the face, with loss of subcutaneous tissue (Figure 9.19).

There are poikilodermatous changes, including atrophy, mottled hyper- and hypopigmented macules and, less frequently, telangiectases, on the entire skin, that develop with increasing age.

Hyperkeratotic plaques and callosities are formed over elbows and knees, major joints and the palms and soles.

Ulcerations occur due to ischemic changes at trauma-prone sites.

There is mucosal atrophy in a minority of patients.

During the second or third decade typical progeroid facies is visible, leading to a variable degree of alopecia and grayish scanty hair. There are minor dystrophic nail changes and a sclerodermoid face.

Extracutaneous findings

- At puberty, growth retardation is visible; later, hypogonadism and reduced fertility
- Spindle-shaped extremities with sclerodactyly and progressive osteoporosis
- Severe atherosclerosis develops during the third decade, involving mainly cardiac valves and large vessels
- Cataracts and glaucoma
- High-pitched voice
- Early diabetes

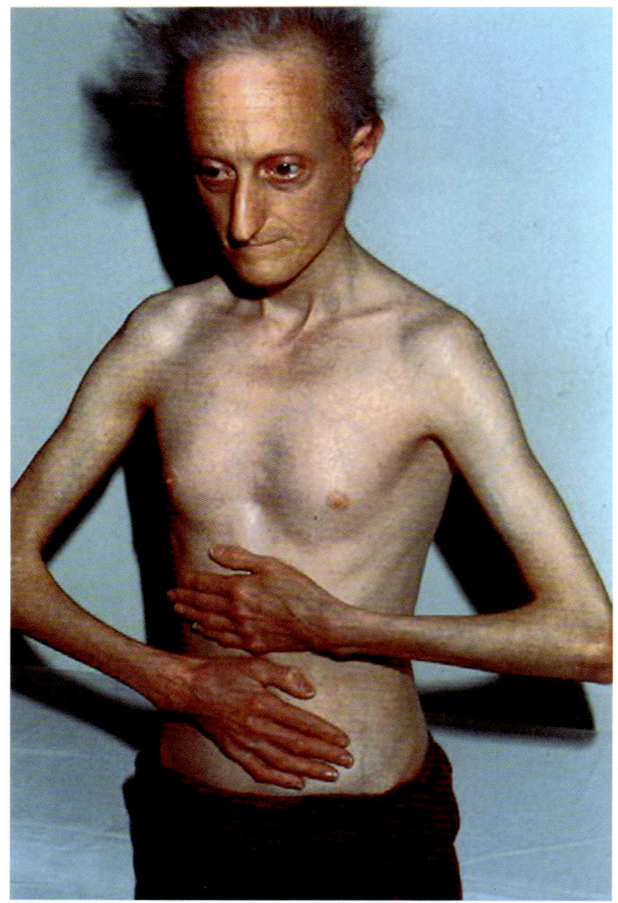

Figure 9.19

- Increased incidence of both benign tumors and malignancies (sarcomas)

Complication and course

The disease is rapidly progressive after the second decade. Heart diseases and malignancies are the major causes of death.

Laboratory findings, genetics and pathogenesis

The Werner gene codes for an exonuclease (polymerase) that is involved in the DNA repair pathway after UV damage.

Differential diagnosis

- Progeroid syndromes
- Rothmund–Thomson syndrome

REFERENCES

Kyng KJ, May A, Kolvraa S, Bohr VA. Gene expression profiling in Werner syndrome closely resembles that of normal aging. Proc Natl Acad Sci USA 2003; 100: 12259–64

Machwe A, Xiao L, Orren DK. TRF2 recruits the Werner syndrome (WRN) exonuclease for processing of telomeric DNA. Oncogene 2004; 23: 149–56

von Kobbe C, Harrigan JA, May A, et al. Central role for the Werner syndrome protein/poly(ADP-ribose) polymerase 1 complex in the poly(ADP-robosyl)ation pathway after DNA damage. Mol Cell Biol 2003; 23: 8601–13

HUTCHINSON–GILFORD SYNDROME

Synonym

- Progeria

Epidemiology

Estimated prevalence is 1 in 8 000 000 births. We have personally observed two cases in a 30-year survey.

Age of onset

- Early infancy

Clinical findings (Figures 9.20–9.23)

- Atrophic, scleroderma-like skin with progressive loss of subcutaneous fatty tissue
- Epidermis has cigarette-paper-like appearance
- Venous network becomes clearly visible, especially on the upper trunk and face (facial cyanosis)
- Hair is sparse from birth, but worsens within the first years of life to almost alopecic scalp with whitish-blond thin hair
- Poikilodermatous-like changes with prominent hyper- and hypopigmented macules from childhood
- Subcutaneous soft nodules (abdomen) have been reported in some patients
- Aspecific nail changes
- Absent or hypoplastic nipples described
- 'Bird' facies with sharp, thin nose and micrognathia with hydrocephalus-like appearance

Extracutaneous findings

- Cardiovascular anomalies (rapidly progressive atherosclerosis, early myocardial infarction and strokes, hypertension, congestive heart failure)
- Low weight and stature and general growth failure
- Coxa valga is frequent, as well as flexural contractures in major joints ('horse-rider' gait)
- Aseptic necrosis of bones reported, acro-osteolysis and osteoporosis
- Sexual secondary characteristics absent
- Delayed and abnormal dentitions
- High-pitched voice

Complications and course

- Life expectancy is at the end of the second decade due to major cardiovascular events

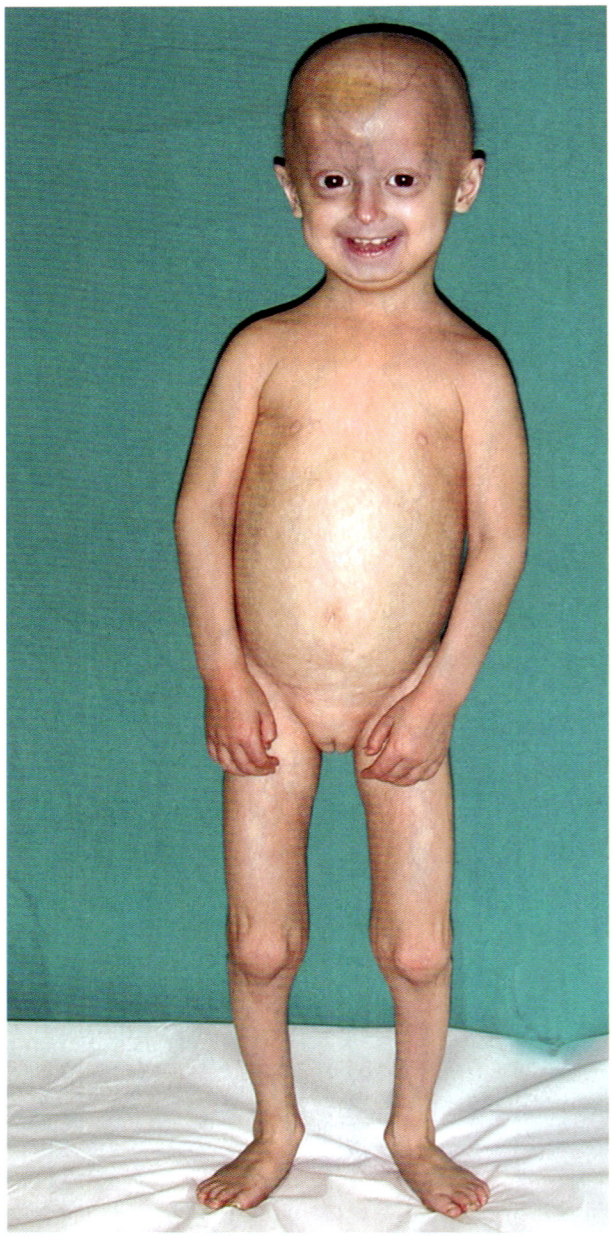

Figure 9.20

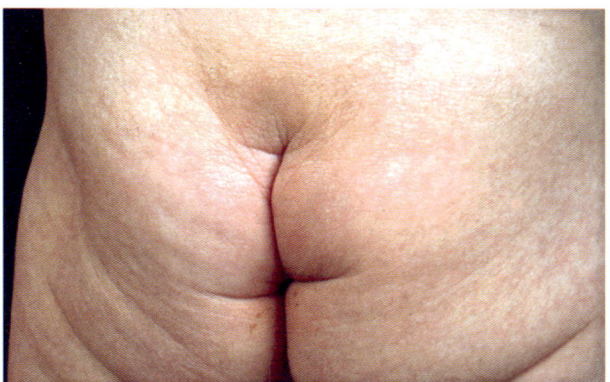

Figure 9.21

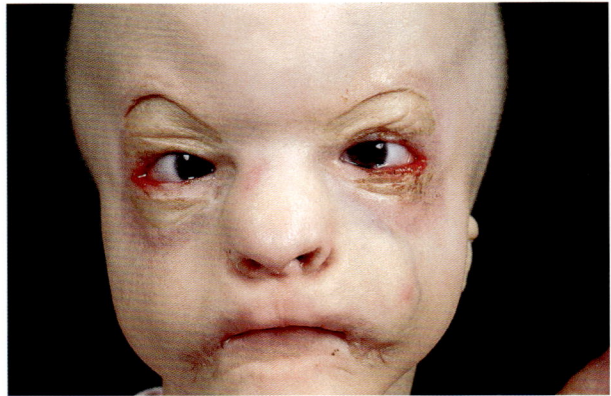

Figure 9.22

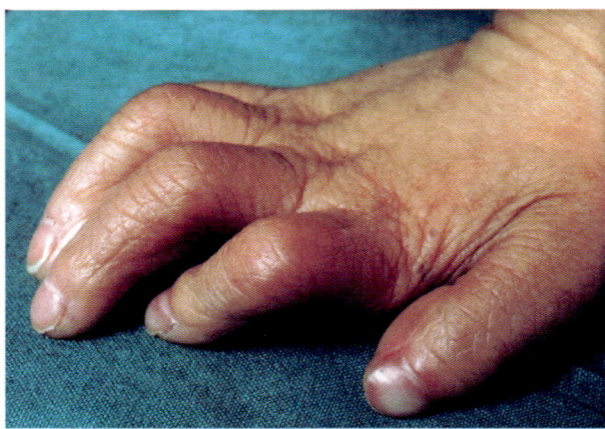

Figure 9.23

- Myocardial infarction within the first decade is frequent
- Rapidly progressive poikilodermatous skin and hair changes
- Normal development of intelligence

Laboratory findings

Optical and electron microscopy examinations show aspecific atrophic changes.

Genetics and pathogenesis

The disease is autosomal recessive. The causative gene is LMNA, coding for lamins A and C. These structures are important components of the nuclear membrane (envelope) and are responsible for premature cellular death.

Differential diagnosis

- Rothmund–Thomson syndrome
- Cockayne's syndrome
- Werner's syndrome and other progerias

Follow-up and therapy

- Cardiovascular support is mandatory

REFERENCES

Cao H, Hegele RA/LMNA is mutated in Hutchinson–Gilford progeria (MIM 176670) but not in Wiedemann–Rautenstrauch progeroid syndrome (MIM 264090). J Hum Genet 2003; 48: 271–4

Eriksson M, Brown WT, Gordon LB, et al. Recurrent de novo point mutations in lamin A cause Hutchinson–Gilford progeria syndrome. Nature (London) 2003; 423: 293–8

Fong LG, Ng JK, Meta M, et al. Heterozygosity for Lmna deficiency eliminates the progeria-like phenotypes in Zmpste24-deficient mice. Proc Natl Acad Sci USA 2004 28; 101: 18111–16. Epub 2004 Dec 17

Hegele RA. Drawing the line in progeria syndromes. Lancet 2003; 362: 416–7

Pollex RL, Hegele RA. Hutchinson–Gilford progeria syndrome Clin Genet 2004; 66: 375–81

Prufert K, Vogel A, Krohne G. The lamin CxxM motif promotes nuclear membrane growth. J Cell Sci 2004; 117: 6105–16. Epub 2004 Nov 16

Strelkov SV, Schumacher J, Burkhard P, et al. Crystal structure of the human lamin A coil 2B dimer: implications for the head-to-tail association of nuclear lamins. J Mol Biol 2004 29; 343: 1067–80

Vantyghem MC, Pigny P, Maurage CA, et al. Patients with familial partial lipodystrophy of the Dunnigan type due to a LMNA R482W mutation show muscular and cardiac abnormalities. J Clin Endocrinol Metab 2004; 89: 5337–46

KITAMURA–DOWLING–DEGOS DISEASE

Synonyms

Kitamura's disease, or reticulate acropigmentation, and Dowling–Degos disease were considered separate entities, until recent reports demonstrated a definite clinical overlap. In contrast, malignant atrophic papulosis of Degos is a different disease.

- (Familial) reticular pigmented anomaly of flexures

Epidemiology

The disease is rare. There are no reports on prevalence in the literature, but some pedigree has been reported in the French literature.

Age of onset

- Second to fourth decades of life

Clinical findings

- Isolated or confluent asymptomatic macules giving a reticulate appearance on major folds (Figure 9.24) (Dowling–Degos disease) or on the dorsa of the hands and feet (Kitamura disease) (Figure 9.25)
- Mild atrophy may be visible
- Palpable lesions are less frequent
- Perioral punctate atrophoderma is described

Extracutaneous findings

There is mental retardation in some cases.

Course and complications

- The disease is progressive with age; lesions may become confluent and darker
- Tendency to acne and hidradenitis (Haber's syndrome)
- Rarely, neoplastic transformation

Laboratory findings

At the ultrastructural examination there is an increased number of normal melanosomes in the keratinocytes.

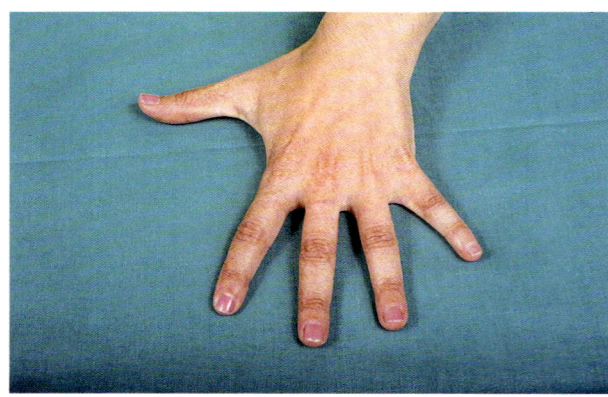

Figure 9.24

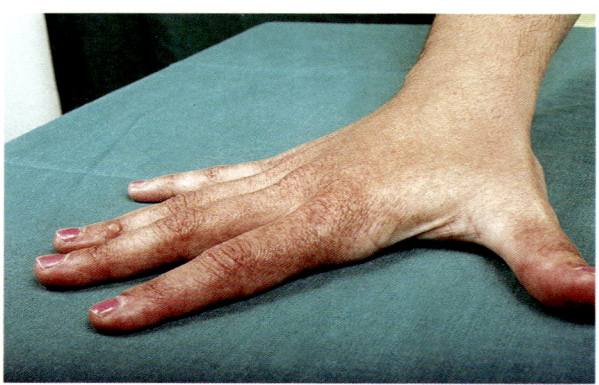

Figure 9.25

Genetics and pathogenesis

- Mostly sporadic, but several pedigrees with autosomal dominant inheritance exist
- The involved gene remains to be investigated

Follow-up and therapy

- UV protection

Differential diagnosis

- Lentiginoses, syndromic and non-syndromic
- Naegeli–Franceschetti syndrome
- Acanthosis nigricans
- Carney's complex

REFERENCE

Al Hawsawi K, Al Aboud K, Alfadley A, Al Aboud D. Reticulate acropigmentation of Kitamura–Dowling Degos disease overlap: a case report. Int J Dermatol 2002; 41: 518–20

COCKAYNE'S SYNDROME

Epidemiology

- The disease is rare: 180 patients have been described in the literature

Age of onset

Is very variable. Normally CS children appear normal at birth, developing symptoms during childhood (CS type I). Nevertheless a few patients may be affected from birth (CS type II) and another group may have late or very late onset of typical symptoms (CS type III).

Clinical findings

- Thinning of the skin and hair
- Photosensitivity
- Premature aging appearance
- Loss of subcutaneous adipose tissue

Extracutaneous symptoms

- Microcephaly with sunken eyes, beaked nose and prominent ears (Figures 9.26 and 9.27)
- Short stature ('cachectic dwarfism')
- Progressive spastic quadraparesis with stooped posture and joint contractures
- Mental retardation (demyelinization, brain calcifications, severe neuronal loss)
- Cataracts
- Overcrowded mouth with severe caries
- Hearing loss
- Osteoporosis

Course and prognosis

- The disease is inexorable and progressive with a greatly reduced life-expectancy in 80% of those affected

Laboratory findings

- MRI may be useful for detecting early phases of demyelinization and/or brain calcification

Genetics and pathogenesis

CS may be due to two different genes: CKN1 (CSA) and ERCC6 (CSB), but additionally, there are three

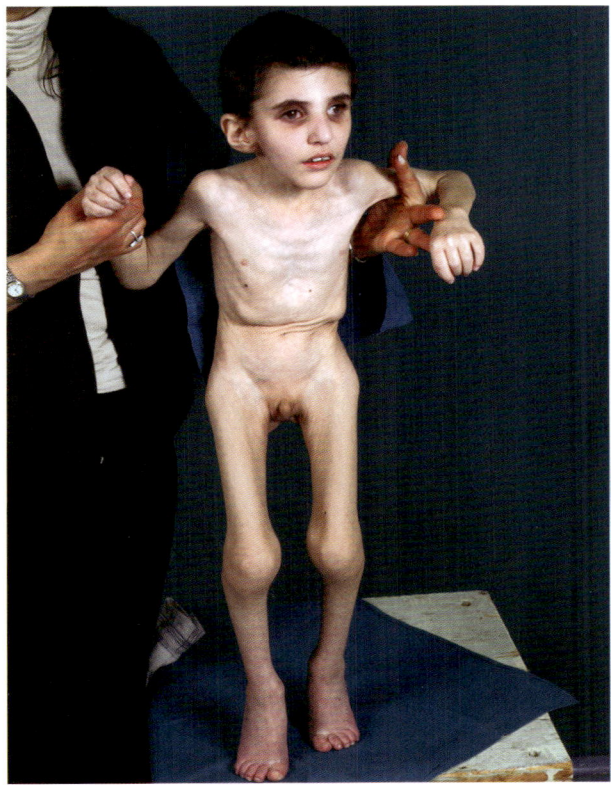

Figure 9.26

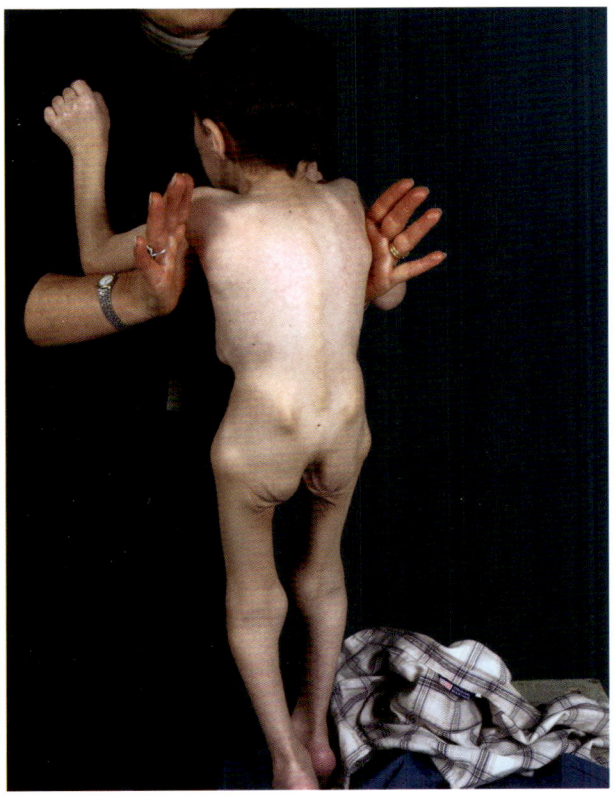

Figure 9.27

different xeroderma pigmentosum genes that can cause CS-like phenotypes.

All the genes involved in the pathogenesis of CS are related to the nucleotide excision repair mechanism that is responsible for DNA-repair caused by UV radiation.

The two involved genes may be related to other processes: lack of DNA-repair caused by oxidative damage in active genes, methylation and demethylation processes, excessive cell death by apoptosis induced by blocked transcription. The non cancer-proneness of CS patients remains to be elucidated.

CSB gene is also related to other diseases:

- The De Santis-Cacchione syndrome (a variant of XP)
- The cerebro-oculo-facial-skeletal syndrome
- The 'ultraviolet-sensitivity syndrome', characterized by a high degree of photosensitivity with abnormal skin pigmentation but not cancer proneness with normal growth and development

Follow-up and therapy

- There is no treatment for the disease
- Neurological assessment is mandatory
- Orthopedic devices are suggested for joint contractures
- Physiotherapy is suggested in milder cases

Differential diagnosis

- Other progeroid syndromes

REFERENCE

Spivak G. The many faces of Cockayne syndrome. Proc Natl Acad Sci USA 2004; 101: 15273–4

CHAPTER 10

Hair diseases

Alopecias

MARIE–UNNA HYPOTRICHOSIS

Synonym

- Marie–Unna-type hereditary hypotrichosis simplex of the scalp

Age of onset

- At birth or during first years of life

Clinical findings

- Affected individuals may be born with normal to coarse hair
- During early infancy the scalp hairs become more coarse, wiry and twisted. Eyebrows, eyelashes and body hair are sparse to absent (Figure 10.1)
- At puberty scalp hair is progressively lost, mainly from the vertex and scalp margins
- During adolescence a scarring alopecia of varying extent develops in a pattern suggestive of androgenetic alopecia (Figure 10.2). Anomalies remain confined to the hair. Teeth, nails, physical and mental development are normal

Extracutaneous findings

- Juvenile macular degeneration

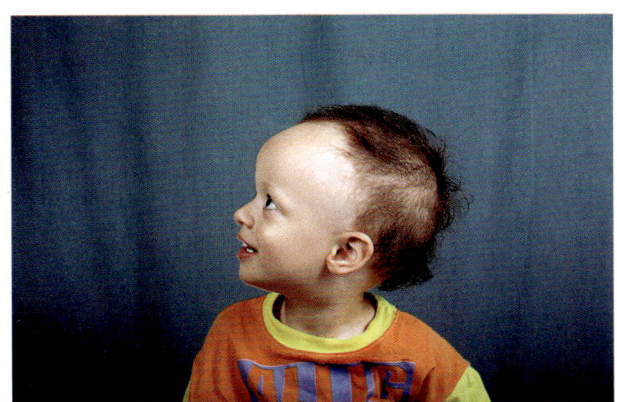

Figure 10.1

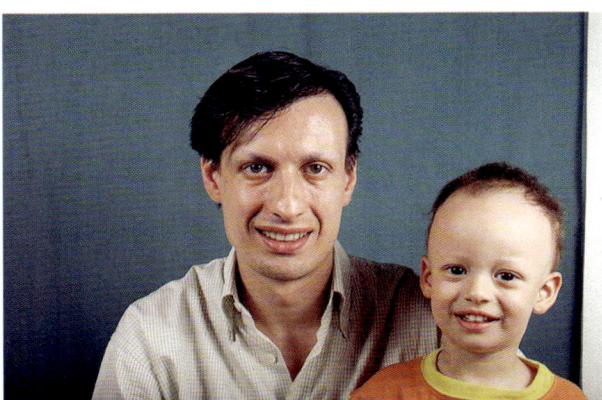

Figure 10.2

Laboratory findings

- Individual hair shafts are deeply pigmented, increased in diameter and twisted. The combination of longitudinal growing and twisting of the shaft at irregular intervals is unique
- There is a reduction in the number of follicles per unit area, with little fibrosis

Genetics and pathogenesis

- Autosomal dominant disorder
- Pathogenesis is unknown

Differential diagnosis

- Ectodermal dysplasias
- Menkes' syndrome
- Hypotrichosis *simplex* of the scalp

Follow-up

The condition becomes stable and is persistent. It is more evident in males.

REFERENCES

Marren P, Wilson C, Dawber RPR, et al. Hereditary hypotrichosis (Marie–Unna type) and juvenile macular degeneration (Stargardt's maculopathy). Clin Exp Dermatol 1992; 17: 189–91

Papadavid E, Dover R, Mallon E, et al. Marie–Unna hypotrichosis: an autosomal dominant hair disorder. J Eur Acad Dermatol Venereol 1996; 7: 279–83

Roberts JL, Whiting DA, Henry D, et al. Marie–Unna congenital hypotrichosis: clinical description, histopathology, scanning electron microscopy of a previously unreported large pedigree. J Invest Dermatol Symp Proc 1999; 4; 261–7

HYPOTRICHOSIS SIMPLEX OF THE SCALP

Age of onset

- During the first decade

Clinical findings

- Marked hypotrichosis of the scalp, resulting in nearly complete alopecia by the beginning of the third decade (Figure 10.3)
- Scalp hair is sparse, short and lighter than normal; terminal hair without signs of inflammation or scarring of the skin
- Eyelashes, eyebrows, axillary and pubic hair are not affected and are normal
- Males and females are affected equally
- No associated anomalies
- Normal intelligence

Course

The disease is slowly progressive.

Laboratory investigations and data

- Microscopic examination of hair shaft: no morphological alterations
- Trichogram: decrease in the percentage of follicles at developed anagen and a progression of the follicles from intermediate anagen towards catagen
- Histologic findings: hair follicle miniaturization

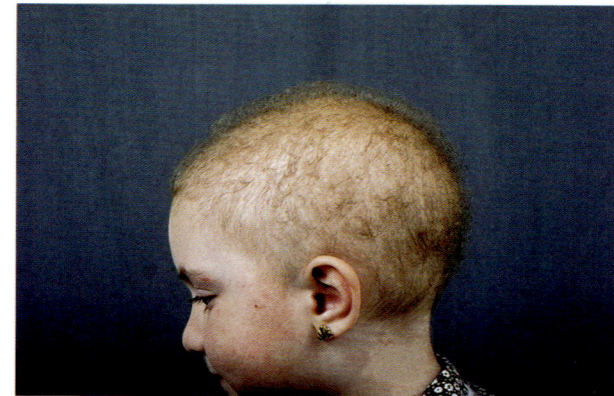

Figure 10.3

Genetics and pathogenesis

- Autosomal dominant inheritance
- Gene locus unknown

Differential diagnosis

- Marie–Unna hypotrichosis
- Ectodermal dysplasias

Treatment

No therapy is available.

REFERENCES

Rodriguez Diaz E, Fernandez Blasco G, Martin Pascual A, et al. Hereditary hypotrichosis simplex of the scalp. Dermatology 1995; 191: 139–41

Rodriguez Vazquez M, Rodriguez RR, Tapia AG, et al. Hereditary hypotrichosis simplex of the scalp. Pediatr Dermatol 2002; 19: 148–50

Toribio J, Quinones PA. Hereditary hypotrichosis simplex of the scalp. Br J Dermatol 1974; 91: 687–9

ICHTHYOSIS FOLLICULARIS WITH ATRICHIA AND PHOTOPHOBIA

Synonym

- IFAP syndrome

Age of onset

- At birth

Clinical findings

Cutaneous manifestations

- Extensive, non-inflammatory follicular hyperkeratosis (ichthyosis follicularis): dry harsh skin with follicular fine scaliness on the scalp, extensor surfaces of the limbs and hands (Figures 10.4 and 10.5)
- Ulerythema ophryogenes (Figure 10.6)

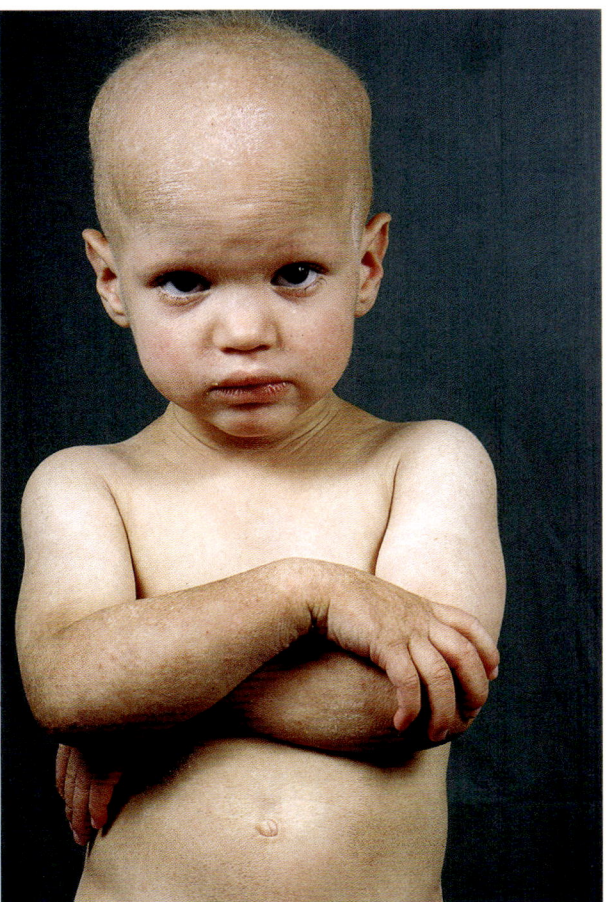

Figure 10.4

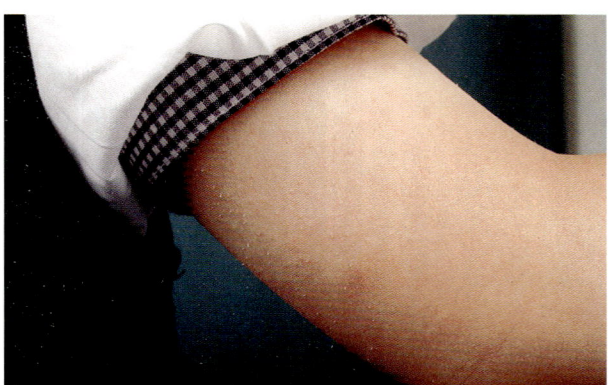

Figure 10.5

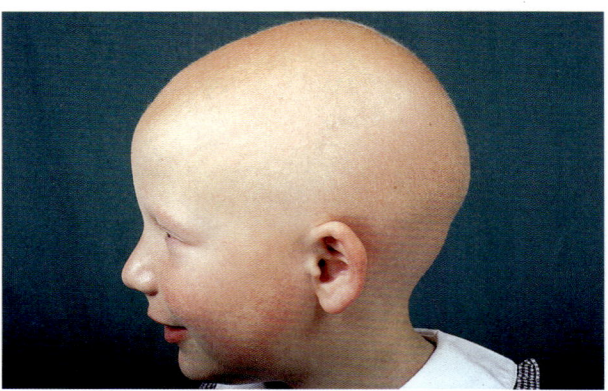

Figure 10.7

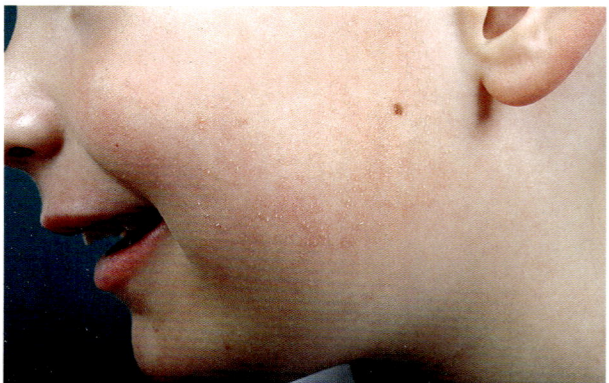

Figure 10.6

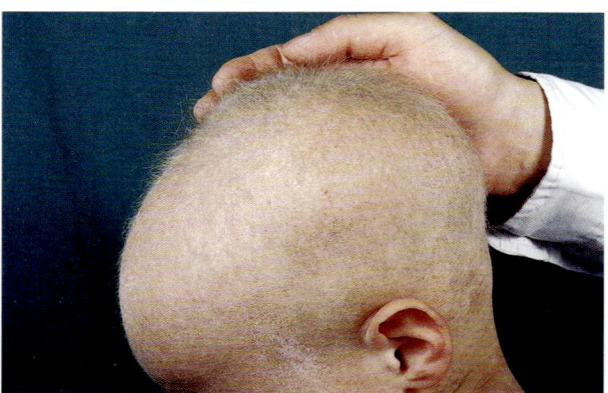

Figure 10.8

- Widespread non-scarring alopecia (Figures 10.7 and 10.8)
- Hypohidrosis in some pedigree
- Atrophoderma vermiculatum-like lesions (segmental presentation in carriers)
- Atopic eczema is frequently a feature in childhood

Extracutaneous manifestations

- Severe photophobia with progressive improvement
- Epilepsy
- Mental retardation is reported
- Skeletal abnormalities
- Megacolon

Course and complications

- Skin abnormalities are lifelong
- Photophobia improve with age
- Tendency to infections

Laboratory investigations and data

- Histopathologic finding: keratin plugs occupying dilated hair follicles
- Hair shaft aspecific abnormalities an scanning electron microscopy (Figure 10.9)

Genetics and pathogenesis

- X-linked recessive inheritance; recessive inheritance
- Female patients generally less severely affected than male

Differential diagnosis

- Keratosis follicularis spinulosa decalvans
- Other diseases with atrophoderma vermiculatum
- Monilethrix
- KID syndrome (keratitis–ichthyosis–deafness)
- Atrichia with papular lesions
- Hypotrichosis simplex of the scalp

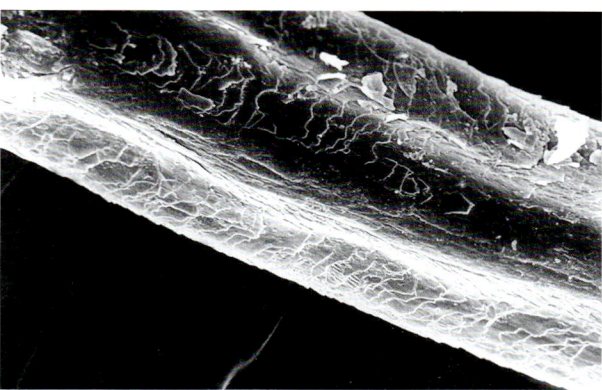

Figure 10.9

Follow-up and therapy

- Ophthalmological examination and sun-protective glasses
- Neurological evaluation to detect epilepsy and psychomotor delays
- Local emollients for xerosis
- Dietary prescriptions for food intolerance
- Prosthetic devices

REFERENCES

Cambiaghi S, Barbareschi M, Tadini G. Ichthyosis follicularis with atrichia and photophobia (IFAP) syndrome in two unrelated female patients. J Am Acad Dermatol 1992; 46: S156–8

Keyvani K, Paulus W, Traupe H, et al. Ichthyosis follicularis, alopecia and photophobia (IFAP) syndrome: clinical and neuropathological observations in a 33 year old man. Am J Med Genet 1998; 78: 371–7

Konig A, Happle R. Linear lesions reflecting lyonization in women heterozygous for IFAP syndrome (ichthyosis follicularis with atrichia and photophobia). Am J Med Genet 1999; 85: 365–8

ALOPECIA AREATA

Age of onset

- Any age

Clinical findings

- Asymptomatic hair loss from round or oval, sharply circumscribed, smooth, discrete areas (alopecia areata); from the entire scalp (totalis), and from the entire body (universalis) (Figure 10.10)
- 'Exclamation point' hair
- Dystrophic nail changes

Association

- Autoimmune disease, e.g. vitiligo, pernicious anemia, Hashimoto's thyroiditis

Course

- Unpredictable and exceedingly variable
- Recurrences are frequent

Laboratory findings

Histopathologic findings include infiltrates of lymphocytes around bulbs of hair follicles in anagen.

Genetics and pathogenesis

- Familial incidence is between 10 and 20%
- Postulated autosomal dominant condition with limited penetrance (Figure 10.10)

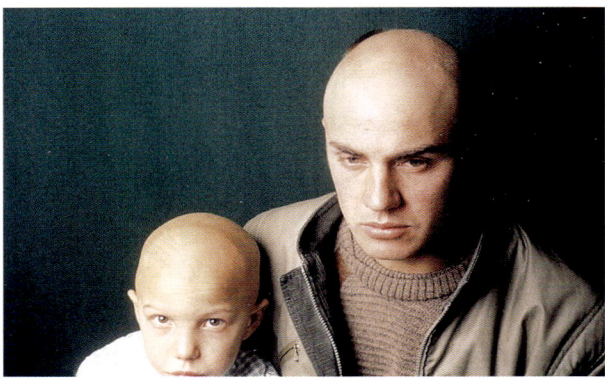

Figure 10.10

- Alopecia areata is an organ-specific autoimmune disease directed against the hair follicle occurring in individuals with a genetic predisposition and exposed to different environmental triggers

Differential diagnosis

- Other genetic disorders causing hair loss or balding

Therapy

- Topical corticosteroid
- Sensitization with squaric acid dibutyl ester
- Minoxidil
- Phototherapy
- Prosthetic devices

REFERENCES

Duvic M, Nelson A, de Andrade M. The genetics of alopecia areata. Clin Dermatol 2001; 19: 135–9

Mcdonagh AJG, Messenger AG. Alopecia areata. Clin Dermatol 2001; 19: 141–7

Valsecchi R, Vicari O, Frigeni A, et al. Familial alopecia areata. Genetic susceptibility or coincidence? Acta Dermatol Venereol 1985; 65: 175–7

ULERYTHEMA OPHRYOGENES

Synonyms

- Keratosis pilaris atrophicans faciei
- Keratosis pilaris rubra atrophicans faciei
- Folliculitis rubra

Age of onset

- Infancy

Clinical findings

- Erythematous keratotic follicular papules typically involving the lateral third of eyebrows (Figure 10.11)
- Subsequent extension to the cheeks, forehead, ears and scalp
- With resulting scarring, atrophy and alopecia

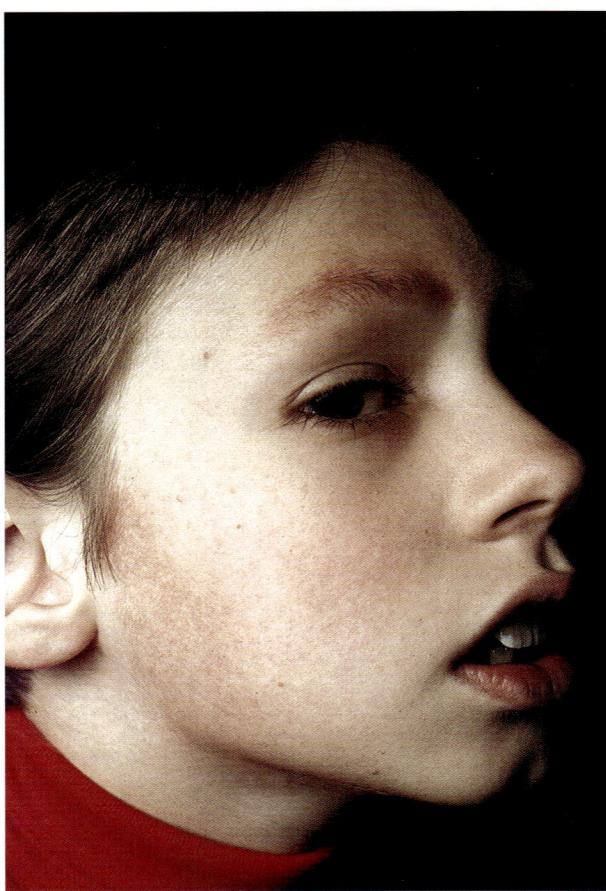

Figure 10.11

- Keratosis pilaris of the lateral aspects of the arms and thighs
- Atopy
- Woolly hair

Extracutaneous findings

- Mental retardation is rarely reported in the literature

Course

The disease is progressive, with permanent follicular destruction.

Laboratory findings

Histopathologic findings include dilated hair follicles plugged by keratin masses, and perifollicular inflammatory infiltration.

Genetics and pathogenesis

- Autosomal dominant transmission (Figure 10.12)
- Association with chromosome 18p deletion defect

Differential diagnosis

- Atrophoderma vermiculatum
- Follicular keratosis

Therapy

- Topical tretinoin
- Pulsed dye laser to remove erythematous–violaceous lesions

REFERENCES

Florez A, Fernandez-Rolando V, Toribio J. Ulerythema ophryogenes in Cornelia de Lange syndrome. Pediatr Dermatol 2002; 19: 42–5

Gomez Centeiro P, Roson E, Poteiro C, et al. Rubinstein–Taybi syndrome and ulerythema ophryogenes in a 9 year old boy. Pediatr Dermatol 1999; 16: 134–6

Zouboulis CC, Stratakis CA, Rinck G, et al. Ulerythema ophryogenes and keratosis pilaris in a child with monosomy 18p. Pediatr Dermatol 1994; 11: 172–5

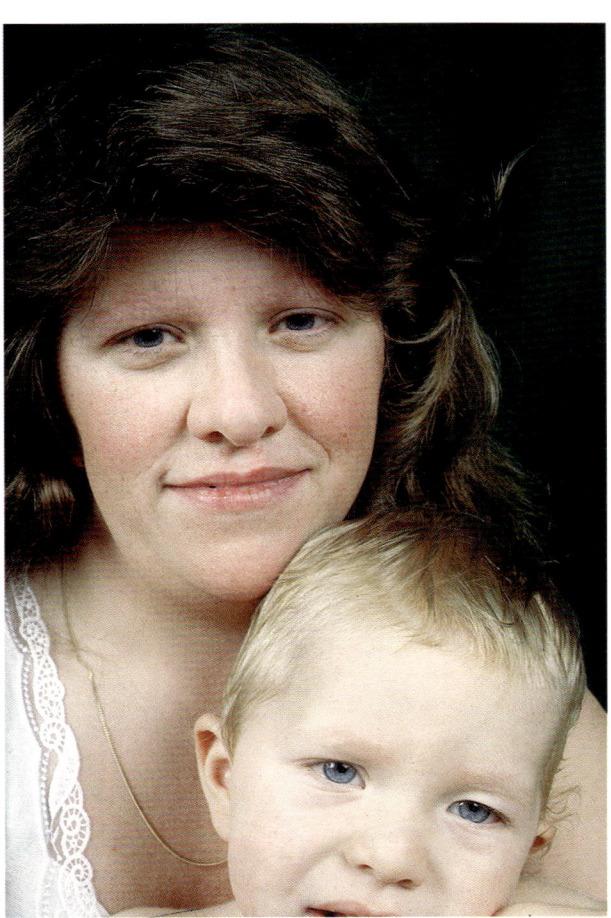

Figure 10.12

TRIANGULAR ALOPECIA

Synonym

- Congenital temporal triangular alopecia

Epidemiology

The disorder is not so rare. There are a few reported familial pedigrees.

Age of onset

- Within 6 years of life

Clinical findings

There is a triangular temporal area of partial alopecia with vellus and intermediate hair (Figure 10.13).

Extracutaneous findings
Non-reported

Course and prognosis

- Lifelong

Laboratory findings

There are none specific.

Genetics and pathogenesis

This is an autosomal dominant disease (Figure 10.14). The disease may underlie an abnormal distribution of hair follicles during the late phase of haembriogenesis.

Follow-up and therapy

- There is no effective therapy

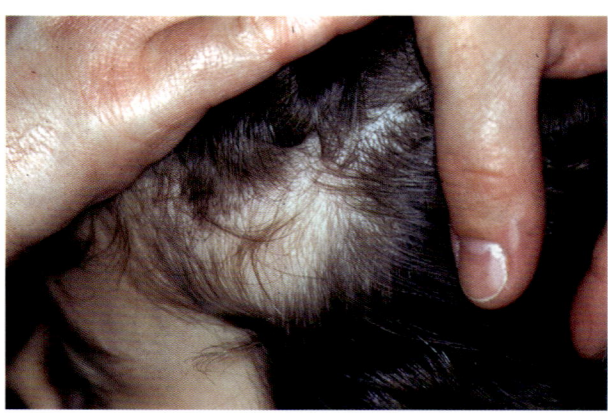

Figure 10.13

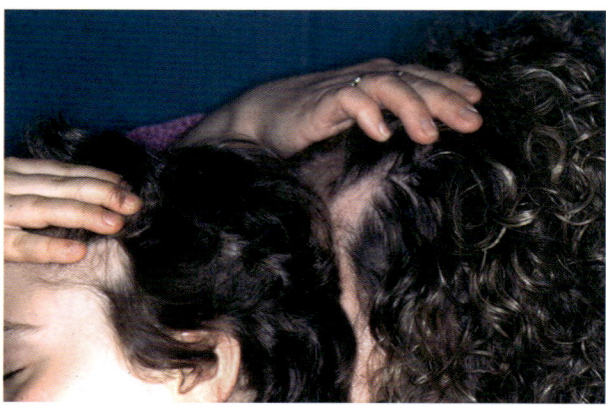

Figure 10.14

Differential diagnosis

- Seborrheic alopecia

REFERENCES

Elmer KB, George RM. Congenital triangular alopecia: a case report and review. Cutis 2002; 69: 255–6

Happle R. Congenital triangular alopecia may be categorized as a paradominant trait. Eur J Dermatol 2003; 13: 346–7

Hirsutism

HYPERTRICHOSIS CONGENITA

Synonyms

- Hypertrichosis universalis
- Generalized hypertrichosis
- Hypertrichosis lanuginosa

Epidemiology

About 100 cases have been described.

Age of onset

- Usually at birth

Clinical findings

- Generalized hypertrichosis lanuginosa, sparing palms, soles and mucosae (Figures 10.15–10.17)
- Hair is curly and color depends on the racial background
- Distribution of body hair may create areas of minor involvement (Figures 10.16 and 10.17)
- Clinical presentation may be different within the same family

Extracutaneous findings

A miscellanea of abnormalities has been described in these patients:

- Mental retardation
- Cataracts
- Dentition anomalies
- Skeletal abnormalities

Course and prognosis

Hypertrichosis may change during life.

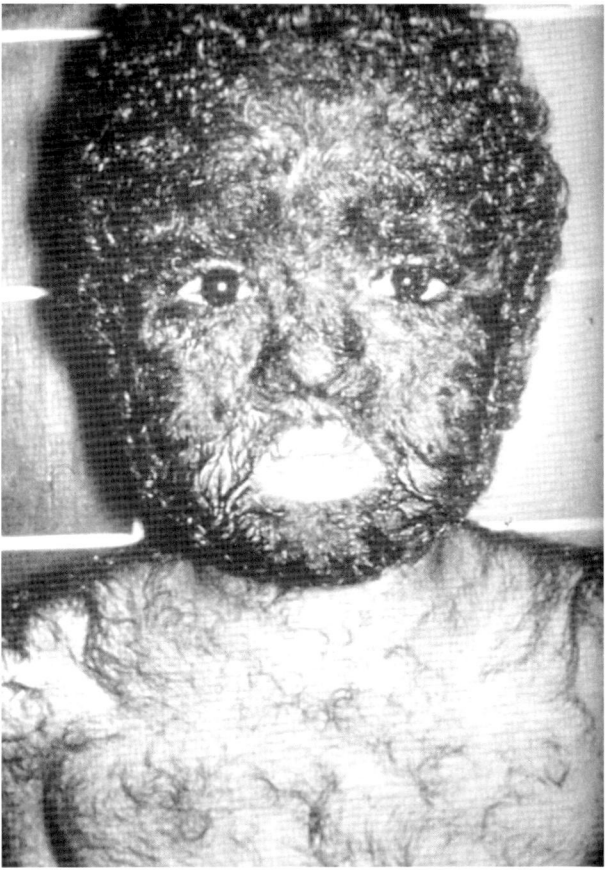

Figure 10.15

Laboratory findings

Increased numbers of hairs are found on histopathologic examination.

Genetics and pathogenesis

- X-linked inheritance
- Female carriers show hypertrichosis distributed in a checkerboard pattern

132 Atlas of Genodermatoses

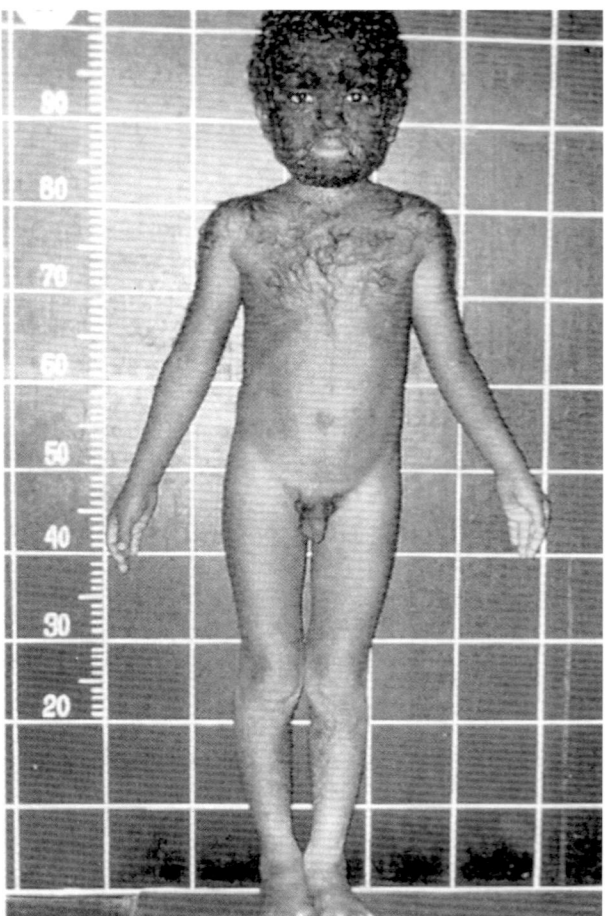

Figure 10.16

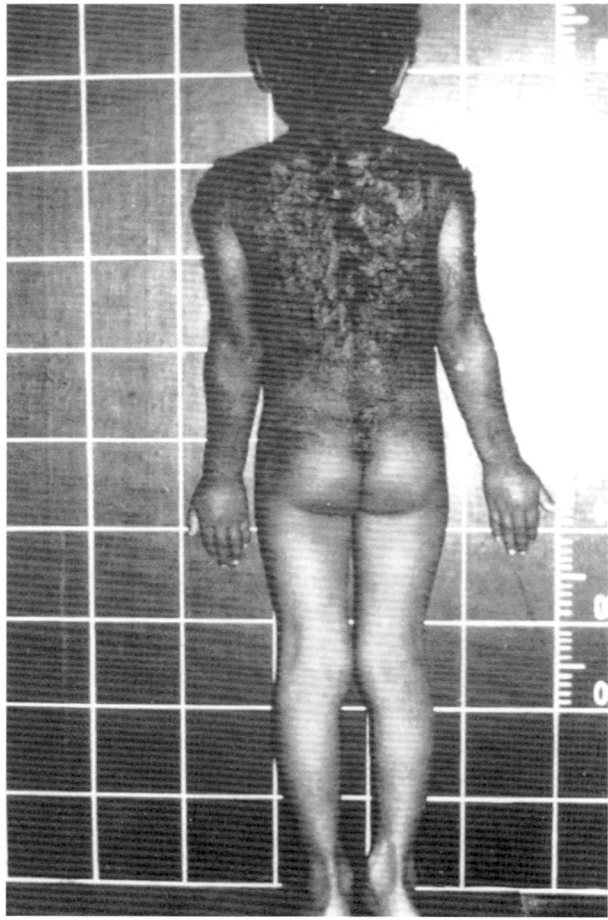

Figure 10.17

Follow-up and therapy

- Search for associated anomalies
- Psychological consultation
- Laser for epilation

Differential diagnosis

- Barber–Say syndrome
- Ambras syndrome
- Hirsutism (hormone-dependent)

REFERENCES

Tadin-Strapps M, Salas-Alanis JC, Moreno L, et al. Congenital universal hypertrichosis with deafness and dental anomalies inherited as an X-linked trait. Clin Genet 2003; 63: 418–22

Trueb RM. Causes and management of hypertrichosis. Am J Clin Dermatol 2002; 3: 617–27

Wendelin DS, Pope DN, Mallory SB. Hypertrichosis. J Am Acad Dermatol 2003; 48: 161–79

LOCALIZED HYPERTRICHOSIS

Synonyms

- Hairy elbows
- Hairy neck
- Hypertrichosis cubiti

Epidemiology

The condition is uncommon.

Clinical findings

In 'hairy elbows' fine and long hairs are visible within the first years of life on the extensor surface of the arms (Figure 10.18).

Patches of hypertrichosis may be visible on lumbar and sacral areas (Figures 10.19), without any underlying hamartomas or skeletal abnormalities; also posterior cervical and sternal areas may host patches of isolated long and fine hair.

Lesions are usually single but may be rarely multifocal.

Extracutaneous findings

Localized hypertrichosis (neck, lumbar region) may be isolated or associated with underlying abnormalities (skeletal, nervous system).

Hairy elbows are associated in one publication with short stature.

Course and prognosis

A certain degree of amelioration of symptoms is described for the hairy elbows condition.

Laboratory findings

There are none specific.

Genetics and pathogenesis

The disease is sporadic and probably autosomal dominant.

In hairy elbows there may be an abnormal distribution during haembryogenesis and/or a different maturation of hair follicles due to hormonal stimuli.

In other areas the localized hypertrichosis may be considered as a hamartomatous lesion.

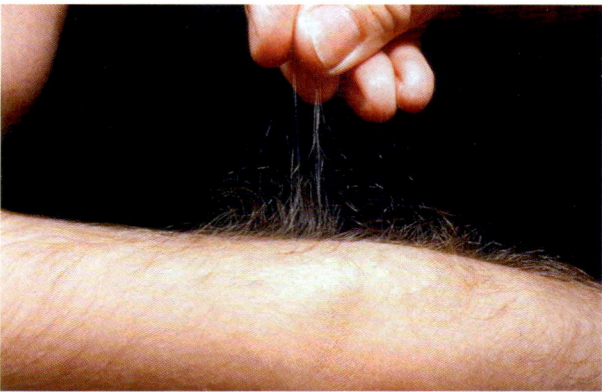

Figure 10.18

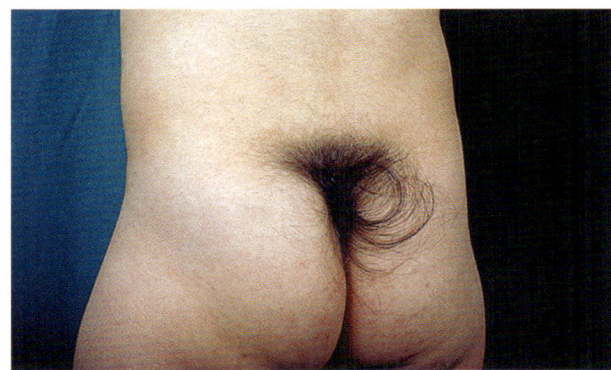

Figure 10.19

Follow-up and therapy

- Search for associated abnormalities
- Laser epilation

Differential diagnosis

- Neurofibromatosis type 1 (plexiform tumors with hypertrichosis)
- Becker's nevus

REFERENCES

Garcia-Hernandez MJ, Ortega-Resinas M, Camacho FM. Primary multifocal localized hypertrichosis. Eur J Dermatol 2001; 11: 35–7

Vashi RA, Mancini AJ, Paller AS. Primary generalized and localized hypertrichosis in children. Arch Dermatol 2001; 137: 877–84

Visser R, Beemer FA, Veenhoven RH, De Nef JJ. Hypertrichosis cubiti: two new cases and a review of the literature. Genet Couns 2002; 13: 397–403

Hair shaft abnormalities

MONILETHRIX

Synonym

- Beaded hair

Age of onset

- First few months of life after shedding of lanugo hair

Clinical findings

Cutaneous manifestations

- Very short, dry, fragile, sparse, lusterless, brittle and beaded hair (Figures 10.20 and 10.21)
- Alopecia of the occipital region slowly extending over the entire scalp and occurring also occasionally on eyelashes, eyebrows and general body hair
- Keratosis pilaris presenting as red follicular papules is in most cases associated with abnormal hairs, mainly on the nape and occipital areas (Figures 10.21 and 10.22)
- Nails may be brittle

Extracutaneous manifestations

- Teeth abnormalities
- Cataracts
- Syndactyly
- Oligophrenia

Course

This is variable. Lesions are persistent in many cases. Spontaneous improvement may occur with age, puberty or pregnancy.

Laboratory investigations and data

- Light microscopy of hair shaft: presence of knots and narrowing along the hair shaft similar to a pearl necklace. Elliptical knots show a regular periodicity (0.7–1 mm) (Figure 10.23)
- Electron microscopy of hair shaft: narrowing hair are amedullated with cortical and cuticular alterations, with regular periodicity knots (Figure 10.24)

Genetics and pathogenesis

- Autosomal dominant inheritance
- Mutations in human hair keratin genes KRTHB6 and 1 are responsible for the disease

Differential diagnosis

This is straightforward and based on clinical, optical microscopic and scanning microscopic features.

Therapy

There is no effective treatment; oral retinoids induce only marginal benefit.

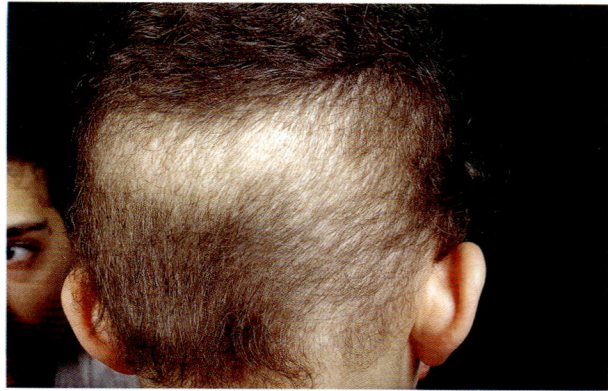

Figure 10.20

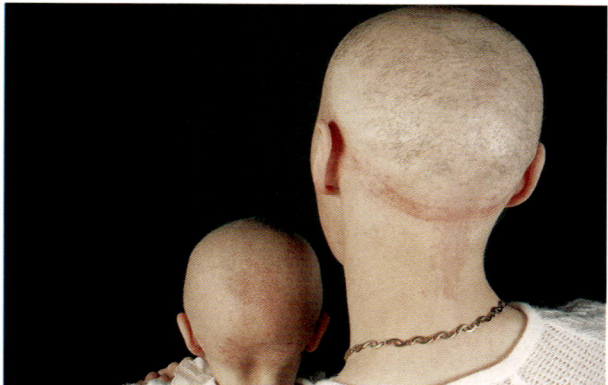

Figure 10.21

Hair diseases

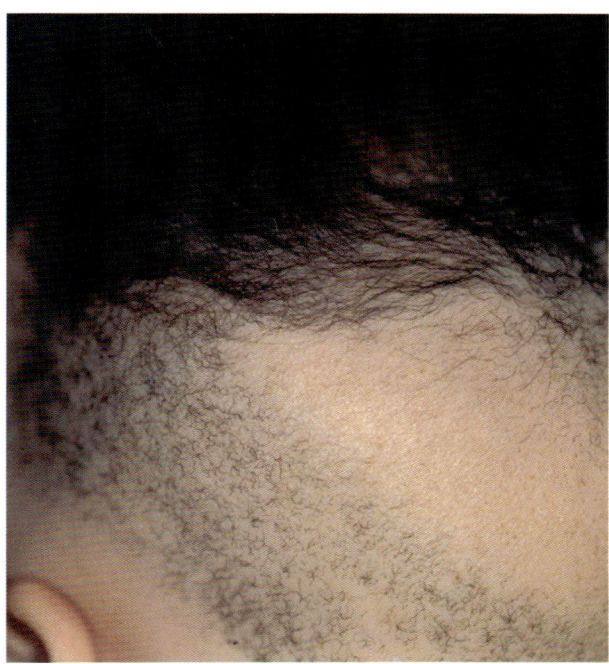

Figure 10.22

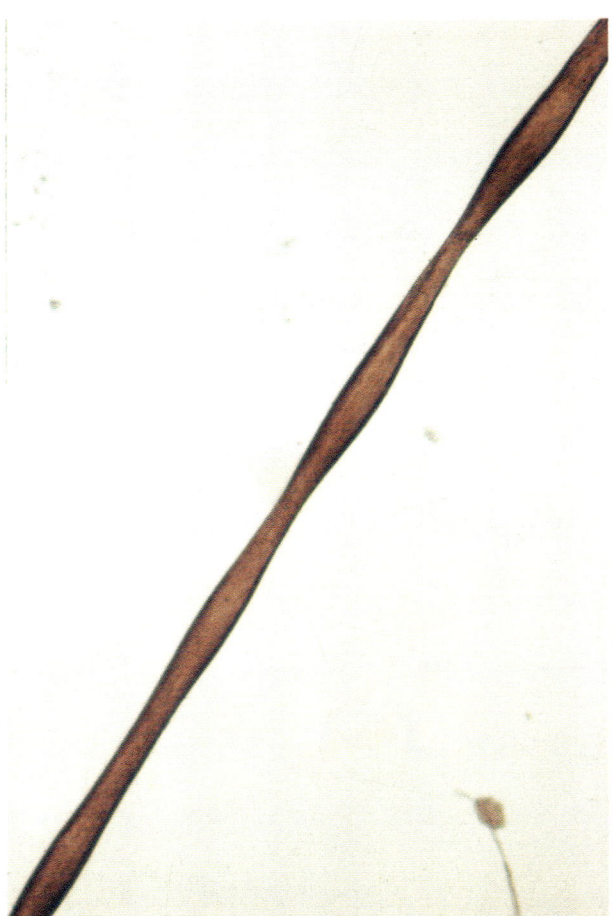

Figure 10.23

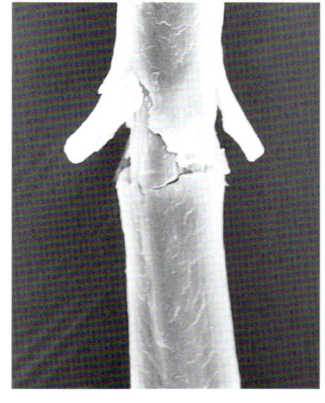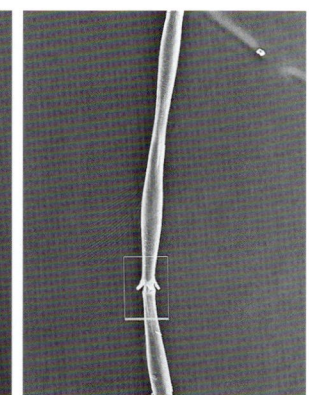

Figure 10.24

REFERENCES

Dawber RPR. An update of hair shaft disorder. Dermatol Clin 1996; 14: 753–72

De Berker DAR, Ferguson DJP, Dawber RPR. Monilethrix: a clinicopathological illustration of a cortical defect. Br J Dermatol 1993; 128: 327–31

Horev L, Djabali K, Green J, et al. De novo mutations in monilethrix. Exp Dermatol 2003; 12: 882–5

Horev L, Glaser B, Metzker A, et al. Monilethrix: mutational hotspot in the helix termination motif of the human hair basic keratin 6. Hum Hered 2000; 50: 325–30

Khandpur S, Bairwa NK, Reddy BS, Bamezai R. A study of phenotypic correlation with the genotypic status of HTM regions of KRTHB6 and KRTHB1 genes in monilethrix families of Indian origin. Ann Genet 2004; 47: 77–84

Stevens HP, Kelsell DP, Bryant SP, et al. Linkage of monilethrix to the trichocyte and epithelial keratin gene cluster on 12q11–q13. J Invest Dermatol 1996; 106: 795–7

PILI ANNULATI

Synonym

- Ringed hair

Age of onset

- During infancy

Clinical findings

- Scalp hair with a banded appearance, with alternating segments of dark and light color (Figures 10.25 and 10.26)
- Diffuse defect or limited to certain areas
- Occasional involvement of axillary hair
- Variable degree of hair shaft fragility
- Slow growth of hair

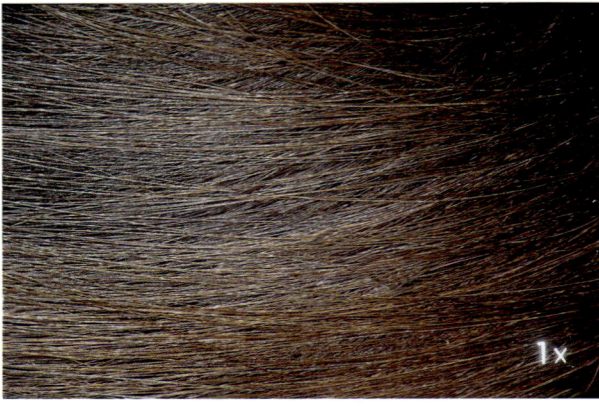

Figure 10.26

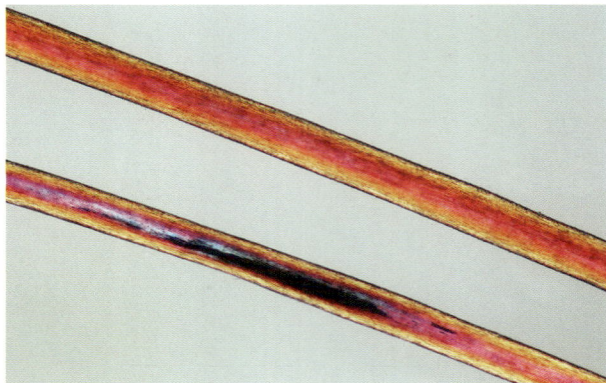

Figure 10.27

Course

The disease is lifelong.

Laboratory investigations and data

- Polarized light microscopy of hair shaft: light bands are morphologically normal and dark bands are abnormal (Figure 10.27)
- Transmission electron microscopy of hair shaft: abnormal bands reveal cavities in the cortex (Figure 10.28)
- Scanning electron microscopy of hair shaft: structural alterations of the cuticle where the underlying cortical areas are air-filled (Figure 10.29)
- Normal caliber of the hair shaft

Genetics and pathogenesis

Normally sporadic cases at the consultation, but there is some reported autosomal dominant pedigree.

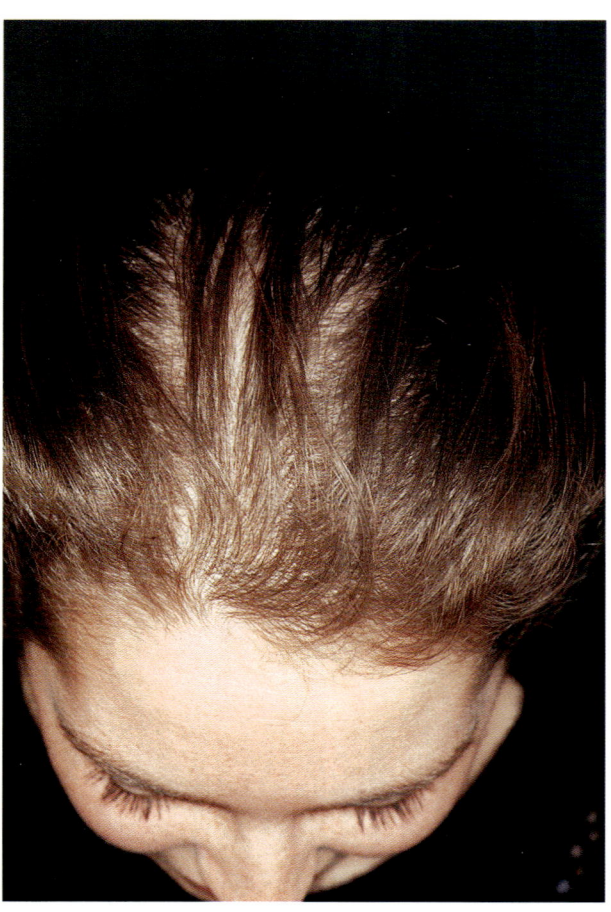

Figure 10.25

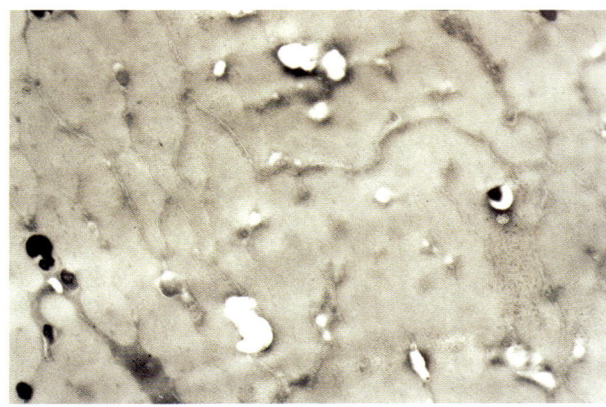

Figure 10.28

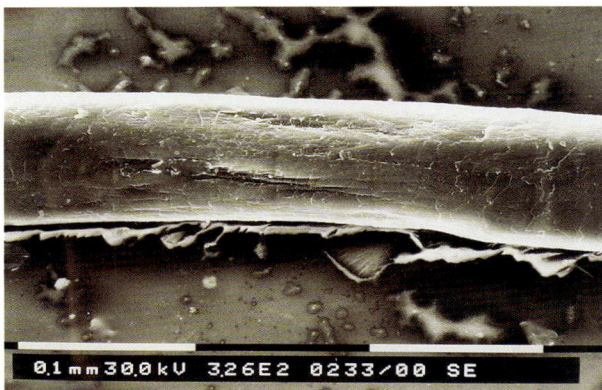

Figure 10.29

Differential diagnosis

- Pseudopili annulati
- Bubble hair
- Pseudopili torti

Therapy

No treatment is available.

REFERENCES

Dini G, Casigliani R, Rividi L, et al. Pili annulati: optical and scanning electron microscopic studies. Int J Dermatol 1988; 27: 256–7

Price VH, Thomas RS, Jones FT. Pili annulati: optical and electron microscopy studies. Arch Dermatol 1968; 98: 640–7

Wade MS, Sinclair RD. Disorders of hair in infants and children other than alopecia. Clin Dermatol 2002; 20: 16–28

PILI TORTI

Synonym

- Twisted hair

Age of onset

- During the first 3 years of life
- After puberty (rare postpubertal form)

Clinical findings

- Dry, brittle, straight, short hair with a spangled appearance in reflected light (Figures 10.30 and 10.31)
- Wide variation in the fragility of the hair with circumscribed or diffuse areas of alopecia
- Inconstant involvement of eyebrows and other body hair
- Occasionally keratosis pilaris
- The postpubertal form presents as patchy alopecia; the hair is black and mental retardation may be present

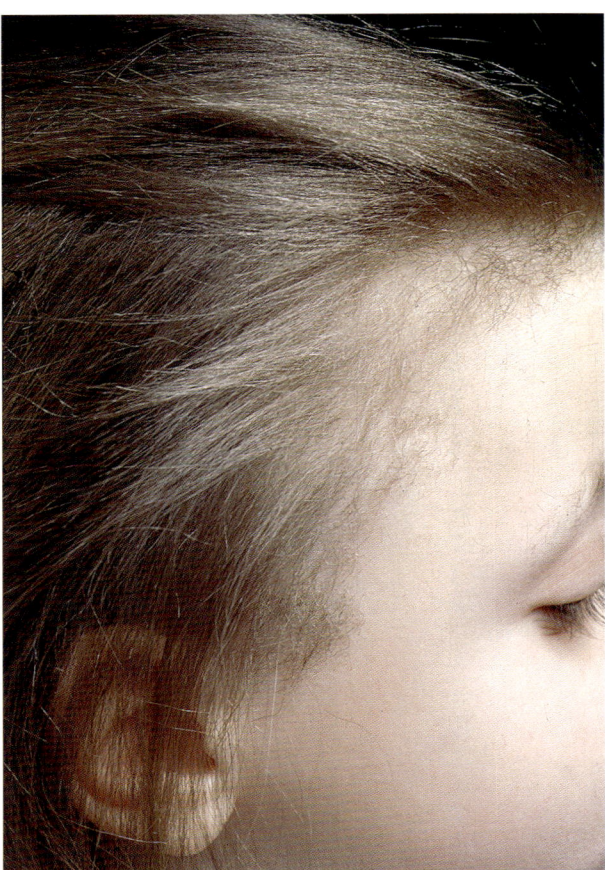

Figure 10.30

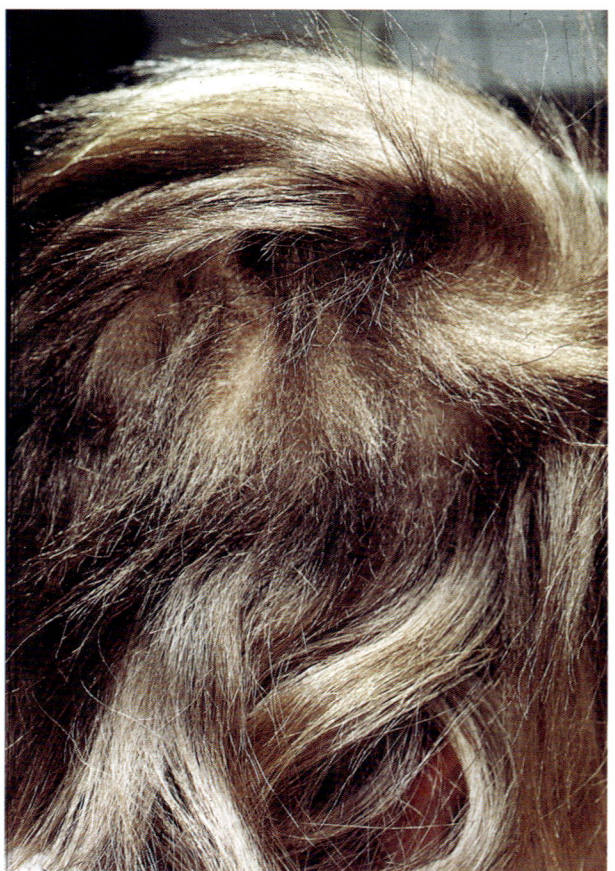

Figure 10.31

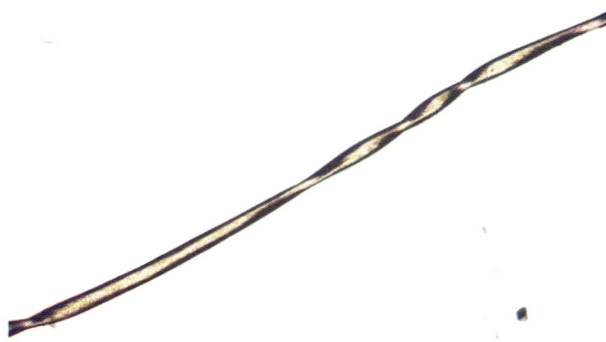

Figure 10.32

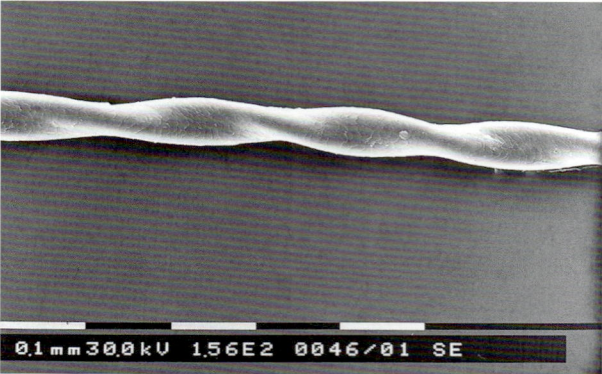

Figure 10.33

Syndromes of which pili torti is a feature

- Menkes' syndrome
- Björnstad's syndrome
- Crandall's syndrome
- Trichothiodystrophy
- Pseudomonilethrix
- Hypohidrotic ectodermal dysplasia

Course

The hair remains abnormal until puberty, when it darkens, becomes less fragile and grows to an acceptable length.

Laboratory investigations and data

- Microscopic examination of hair shaft: flattened and twisted through 180° at irregular intervals along the shaft (Figure 10.32)
- Upon scanning electron microscopy abnormal spiraloid pattern of the hair follicle is clearly visible (Figure 10.33)

Genetics and pathogenesis

There is autosomal dominant inheritance.

Differential diagnosis

See 'Syndromes of which pili torti is a feature', above.

Therapy

- No effective treatment
- Avoid physical and chemical trauma

REFERENCES

Camacho Martinez F, Ferrando J. Hair shaft dysplasias. Int J Dermatol 1988; 27: 71–80

Wade MS, Sinclair RD. Disorders of hair in infants and children other than alopecia. Dermatol Clin 2002; 20: 16–28

WOOLLY HAIR

Age of onset

- At birth or during infancy

Clinical findings (Figures 10.34–10.36)

- Unruly scalp hair that curls in a spiral but does not form locks and shows a slow twist on its long axis
- Hair is extremely thin, brittle, light colored, tightly curled, very fragile
- Eyebrows and body hair may be affected

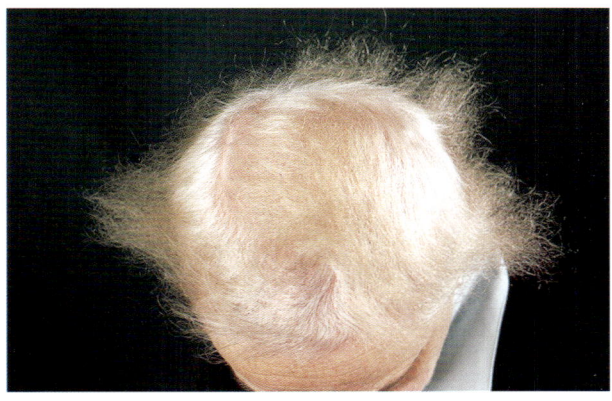

Figure 10.35

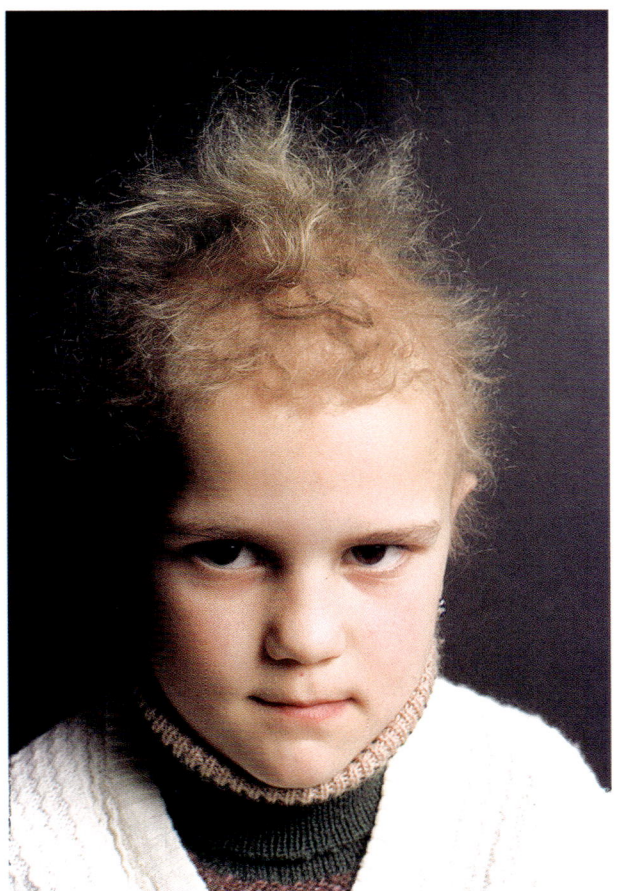

Figure 10.34

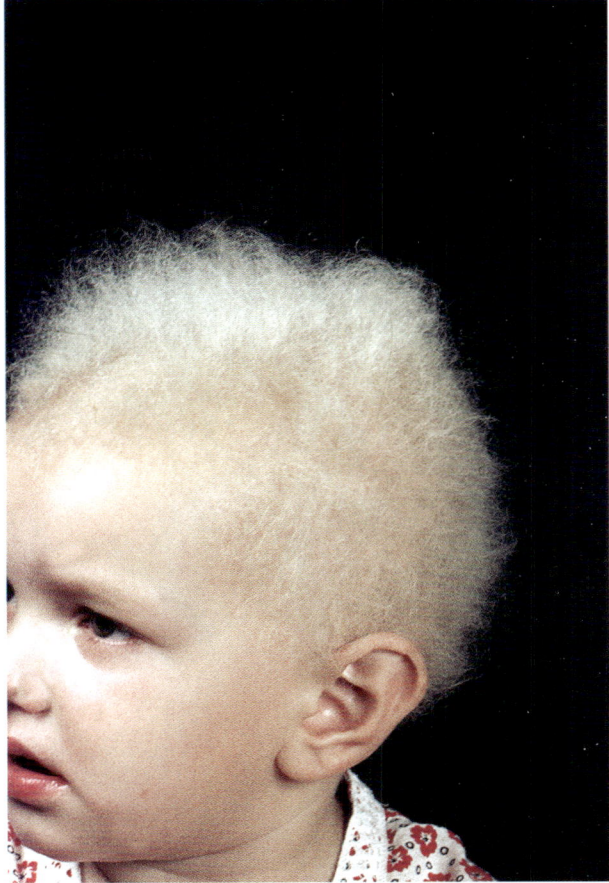

Figure 10.36

Extracutaneous findings

- Ocular defects
- Deafness
- Keratosis pilaris atrophicans

Course

- Usually lifelong

Genetics and pathogenesis

- Autosomal dominant and recessive inheritances are reported in the literature

Laboratory investigations

- Microscopic examination of hair shaft:
  - important cuticular damage
- Histopathologic findings: curved follicle within the dermis

Differential diagnosis

- Woolly hair nevus
- Other diseases with structural hair shaft defects

Follow-up and therapy

There is no treatment available.

REFERENCES

Camacho Martinez F, Ferrando J. Hair shaft dysplasias. Int J Dermatol 1988; 27: 71–80

Hutchinson PE, Cairns RJ, Wells RS. Woolly hair, clinical and general aspects. Trans St John's Hosp Dermatol Soc 1974; 60: 160–77

Taylor AEM. Hereditary woolly hair with ocular involvement. Br J Dermatol 1990; 123: 523–5

ELEJALDE'S SYNDROME

Synonym

- Neuroectodermal melanolysosomal disease

Epidemiology

The disease is very rare.

Age of onset

- At birth

Clinical findings

- Generalized hypopigmentation (Figure 10.37, showing a Mexican girl)
- Silvery hair

Extracutaneous symptoms

- Severe mental and motor retardation
- Seizures

Course and complications

Psychomotor retardation is progressive and may become very severe.

Laboratory findings

Hair shaft pigment inclusions are found an ultrastructural examination.

Genetics and pathogenesis

It is an autosomal recessive disease caused by a mutation in the gene MYO5 A (see Griscelli's syndrome) that causes impairment of intracellular vesicular trafficking in melanocytes and central nervous system cells.

Follow-up and therapy

Neurologic consultation is required for psychomotor delay.

Hair diseases

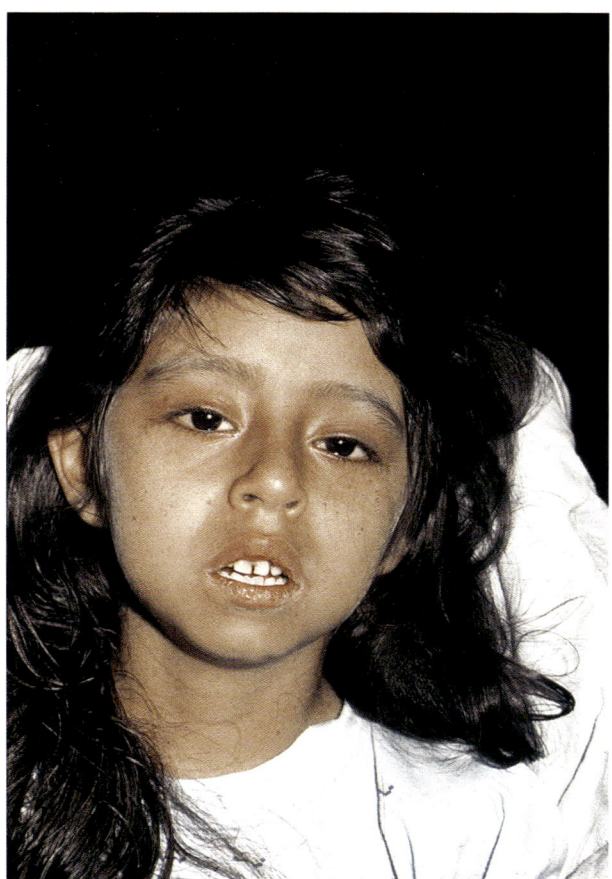

Figure 10.37

Differential diagnosis

- Griscelli's syndrome
- Chediak–Higashi syndrome
- Hermansky–Pudlak syndrome

REFERENCES

Bahadoran P, Ortonne JP, Ballotti R, de Saint-Basile G. Comment on Elejalde syndrome and relationship with Griscelli syndrome. Am J Med Genet A 2003 1; 116: 408–9

Cahali JB, Fernandez SA, Oliveira ZN, et al. Elejalde syndrome: report of a case and review of the literature. Pediatr Dermatol 2004; 21: 479–82. Review

Scheinfeld NS. Syndromic albinism: a review of genetics and phenotypes. Dermatol Online J 2003; 9: 5. Review

GRISCELLI'S SYNDROME

Synonym

- Partial albinism with immunodeficiency

Epidemiology

The disease is very rare. There are no data available in the literature on incidence or prevalence.

Age of onset

Hair anomalies are visible soon after birth, immunodeficiency in early childhood.

Clinical findings

- Diffuse hypopigmented areas
- Silvery hair, eyebrows and eyelashes (Figure 10.38)

Extracutaneous symptoms

- Immunodeficiency with both immunoglobulin (A and G) and cellular immunity
- NK (natural killer) cell abnormalities
- Hypotonia and motor retardation due to demyelinization and atrophy of central nervous system
- Lymphadenopathy, hepatosplenomegaly, anemia, neutropenia and thrombocytopenia
- Hemophagocytic syndrome with platelet storage pool deficiency
- Prolonged bleeding times

Course and complications

Immunodeficiency can cause frequent pyogenic infections of the skin and elsewhere, and could cause neurologic abnormalities.

Laboratory findings

Clumping of pigment in the hair shaft is found an ultrastructural examination.

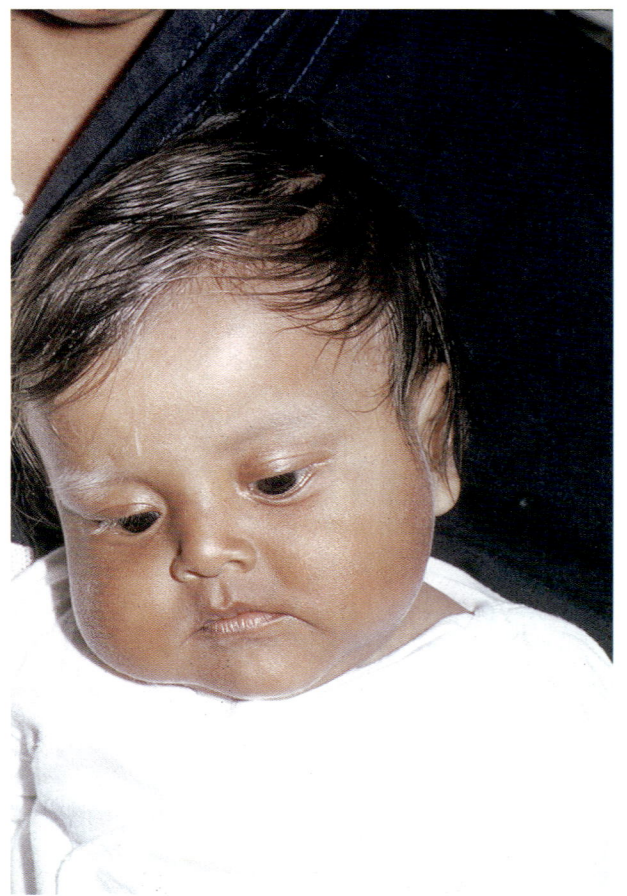

Figure 10.38

Genetics and pathogenesis

This is an autosomal recessive disease.

Mutations in the Rab27a gene, which encodes guanosine triphosphatase (GTPase) and appears critical for the secretion of specialized granules both in melanocytes and immune cells, and the MYO5 A gene, which encodes an actin-dependent molecular motor, can cause Griscelli's syndrome.

Rab27a and MYO5 A gene products interact with each other in the intracellular vesicular trafficking compartment. Mutated cells (melanocytes, platelets and immune cells) that act via complex vesicular pathways (melanosomes and melanin distribution to keratinocytes and lysosomal vesicle trafficking of cytotoxic T lymphocytes and formation of platelet-dense granules) cannot complete their functions, and directly cause silvery hair and depigmentation, immunodeficiency and prolonged bleeding time.

Follow-up and therapy

- Immune functions and bleeding abnormalities must be strictly monitored, as well as neurological abnormalities
- Antibiotics for pyogenic infections
- Successful bone marrow transplantations have been reported

Differential diagnosis

- Elejalde's syndrome (now considered to be synonymous with Griscelli's syndrome)
- Albinisms
- Chediak–Higashi syndrome
- Hermansky–Pudlak syndrome

REFERENCES

Neeft M, Wieffer M, de Jong AS, et al. Munc13-4 is an effector of Rab27a and controls secretion of lysosomes in haematopoietic cells. Mol Biol Cell 2005; 16: 731–41

Sheela SR, Latha M, Injody SJ. Griscelli syndrome: Rab 27a mutation. Indian Pediatr 2004; 41: 944–7

Tomita Y, Suzuki T. Genetics of pigmentary disorders. Am J Med Genet 2004; 131C: 75–81

UNCOMBABLE HAIR SYNDROME

Synonyms

- Pili triangulari et canaliculi
- 'Cheveux incoiffables'
- Spun-glass hair

Age of onset

- From infancy to childhood

Clinical findings

- Dry, coarse, fuzzy, reddish blond shiny hairs that stand straight out from the scalp, arranged in different directions and impossible to comb (Figures 10.39 and 10.40)
- These hairs are usually normal in length, quantity and tensile strength and not fragile
- Eyelashes and eyebrows are unaffected
- Localized forms have been described
- Atopy

Course

- Slow growth percentiles
- The condition may improve with age

Laboratory investigations

- Scanning electron microscopy: individual hair shaft shows a longitudinal groove and in cross-section is triangular, hence pili canaliculi et trianguli (~ 80% of hairs of affected patients)
- Histopathologic findings: irregularity in shape of the inner root sheath with premature maturation

Genetics and pathogenesis

This is an autosomal dominant disease with incomplete penetrance, but there are many sporadic cases.

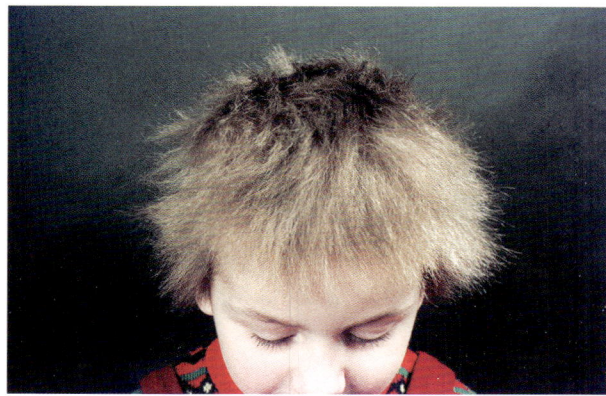

Figure 10.39

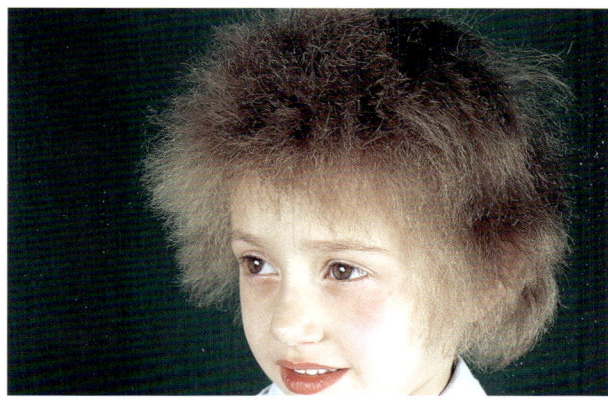

Figure 10.40

Differential diagnosis

- Woolly hair
- Ectodermal dysplasias

Therapy

There are no effective treatments, but oral biotin may induce improvements.

REFERENCES

Mallon E, Dawber DPR, De Berker D, et al. Cheveux incoiffables – diagnostic, clinical and hair microscopic findings, and pathogenic studies. Br J Dermatol 1994; 131: 608–14

Matis WL, Baden H, Green R, et al. Uncombable hair syndrome. Pediatr Dermatol 1987; 4: 215–19

MENKES' KINKY HAIR SYNDROME

Synonyms

- Kinky hair syndrome
- Menkes' disease
- Steely hair syndrome

Age of onset

- First few months of life

Clinical findings

Cutaneous manifestations

- Scalp hair and eyebrows, normal at birth, at approximately 3 months of age become kinky, sparse, light-colored, lusterless and fragile. They feel like steel wool (Figure 10.41)
- Skin laxity is most prominent in the region of the posterior neck and leg folds
- Pudgy face with 'Cupid's bow' upper lip
- Areas of skin depigmentation

Extracutaneous manifestations

- Progressive neurodegenerative processes starting at about 2 months: seizures, developmental regression, hypothermia, lethargy, hypertonia
- Musculoskeletal abnormalities: failure to thrive, wormian bones of the skull and spurring of long bone metaphyses, high arched palate, micrognathia
- Cardiovascular abnormalities: increased tortuosity of arteries, intracranial hemorrhages
- Genitourinary abnormalities: hydronephrosis, hydroureter, bladder diverticula

Course and complications

There is susceptibility to infections.
The disease is rapidly fatal (death at third or fourth year of life).

Laboratory investigations and data

- Light and scanning electronmicroscopy of hair shaft: pili torti demonstrate a flattened appearance with multiple twists of 180° around the long axis, trichorrhexis nodosa, trichoptilosis
- The free sulfhydryl content of hair is nine-fold increased
- Low plasma and ceruloplasmin levels
- Prenatal diagnosis based on increased incorporation of copper by cultured amniotic fluid cells

Genetics and pathogenesis

- X-linked recessive disorder; all patients are male; some clinical and laboratory findings observed in heterozygous females (Lyon's hypothesis of random X inactivation)
- Gene for Menkes' syndrome designated ATP7A and located on chromosome Xq12–q13, responsible for control of the function of copper-requiring enzymes
- Defect in the action of lysyloxidase is responsible for hair abnormality and alterations of elastic lamina of arteries
- Defect in tyrosinase activity is responsible for decreased melanin synthesis and hypopigmentation
- Defects in cytochrome c oxidase, superoxide dismutase and dopamine B hydroxylase are responsible for thermoregulatory instability, neurologic symptoms and developmental decline

Differential diagnosis

- Occipital horn syndrome is allelic to Menkes' disease (mutations in the ATP7A gene)
- Björnstad's syndrome
- Arginosuccinic aciduria

Follow-up and therapy

- None

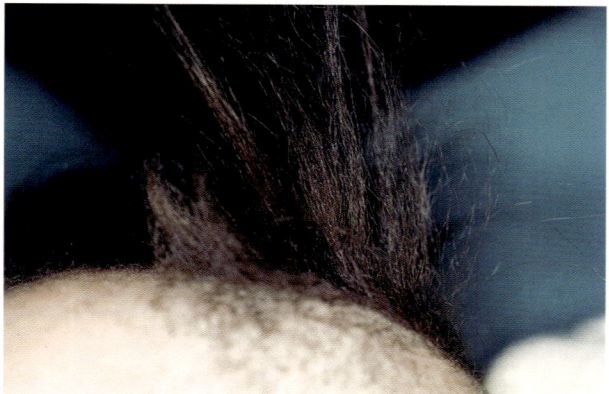

Figure 10.41

REFERENCES

Borm B, Moller LB, Hausser I, et al. Variable clinical expression of an identical mutation in the ATP7A gene for Menkes disease/occipital horn syndrome in three affected males in a single family. J Pediatr 2004; 145: 119–21

Dawber RPR. An update of hair shaft disorders. Dermatol Clin 1996; 14: 753–72

Greenough M, Pase L, Voskoboinik I, Petris MJ, et al. Signals regulating trafficking of Menkes (MNK; ATP7A) copper-translocating P-type ATPase in polarized MDCK cells. Am J Physiol Cell Physiol 2004; 287: C1463–71. Epub 2004 Jul 21

Hart DB. Menkes' syndrome: an updated review. J Am Acad Dermatol 1983; 9: 145–52

Stratigos AJ, Baden HP. Unraveling the molecular mechanism of hair and nail genodermatosis. Arch Dermatol 2001; 137: 1465–71

Tumer Z, Horn N, Tonnesen T, et al. Gene symbol: ATP7A. Disease: Menkes disease. Hum Genet 2004; 114: 606

Wojewodzka U, Gajewska A, Gajkowska B, et al. Impaired somatostatin accumulation within the median eminence in mice with mosaic mutation. Neuro Endocrinol Lett 2004; 25: 78–82

TRICHORHINOPHALANGEAL SYNDROME

Synonyms

- TRPS type I: Giedion–Gurish syndrome
- TRPS type II: Langier–Giedion syndrome
- TRPS type III: Sugio–Kajii syndrome

Age of onset

- At birth

Clinical findings

Cutaneous manifestations

- Fine, sparse, slowly growing scalp hair; eyebrows with growth abnormalities (Figure 10.42)
- Dystrophic, hypoplastic, brittle, slow growing nails; occasionally koilonychia and leukonychia (Figure 10.43)

Extracutaneous manifestations

- Pear-shaped nose tented alae, long extended filtrum, thin upper lip: characteristic facies (Figure 10.42)
- Brachyphalangia with deviation of fingers and toes and with shortened phalanges and metacarpals (Figure 10.43)

Clinical variants

These clinical variants are cited for didactic reasons, being determined merely by different mutations in the responsible gene.

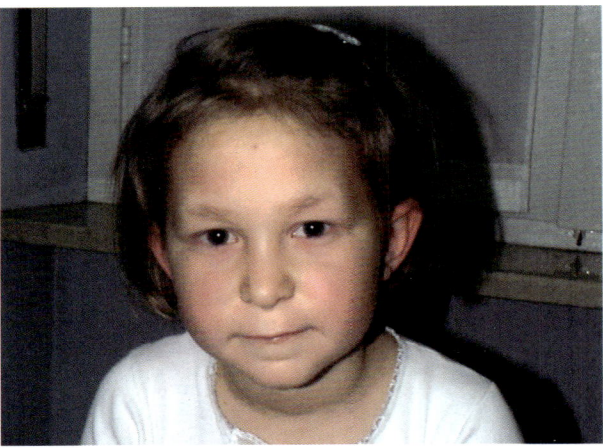

Figure 10.42

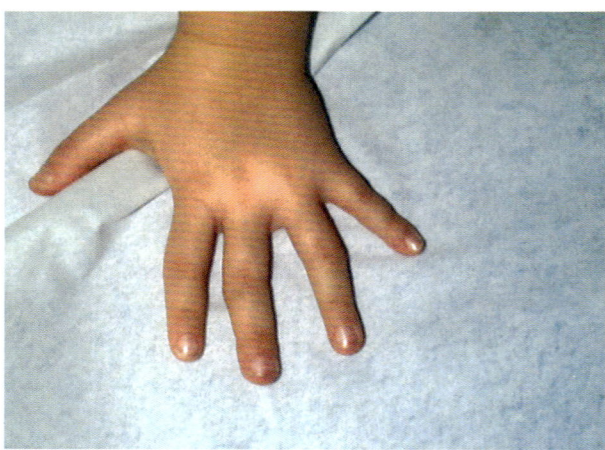

Figure 10.43

- TRPS type I: short stature
- TRPS type II: presence of multiple cartilaginous exostoses, redundant and loose skin, microcephaly and mental retardation
- TRPS type III: marked short stature, severe brachydactyly, pronounced cone-shaped epiphyses

Course

The disease is lifelong.

Laboratory investigations

Radiography of bones shows cone-shaped epiphyses of the hands and feet.

Genetics and pathogenesis

Linked to mutations on TRPS1 gene, a putative localization signal nuclear protein.

Follow-up and therapy

- Multidisciplinary approach
- No treatment is available

REFERENCES

Böni R, Böni RH, Tsambaos D, et al. Trichorhinophalangeal syndrome. Dermatology 1995; 190: 152–5

Carrington PR, Chen H, Altick JA. Trichorhinophalangeal syndrome, type I. J Am Acad Dermatol Venereol 1994; 31: 331–6

McCloud DJ, Solomon LM. The trichorhinophalangeal syndrome. Br J Dermatol 1977; 96: 403–7

ATRICHIA WITH PAPULAR LESIONS

Epidemiology

The disease is rare: about 50 pedigrees have been described.

Age of onset

- Within the first year of life

Clinical findings

- Progressive alopecia leading to complete absence of scalp, axilla and body hair (Figure 10.44)
- Eyebrows and eyelashes may be hypotrophic or absent
- Small hyperkeratotic papules scattered on the upper part of the body, but especially on the face (Figure 10.45)
- Normal sweating and nails

Course and prognosis

The disease is rapidly progressive.

Laboratory investigations

Scalp biopsy shows the absence of mature hair follicles.

Genetics and pathogenesis

The disease is autosomal recessive and is due to mutations in the hairless gene, a transcription factor protein expressed in the maturation of hair follicles in humans and animals.

Follow-up and therapy

- Cosmetic evaluation
- Cosmetic devices
- Psychological support

Differential diagnosis

- Familial area celsi (alopecia areata)
- Decalvans folliculitis
- Ectodermal dysplasias (Clouston's syndrome)

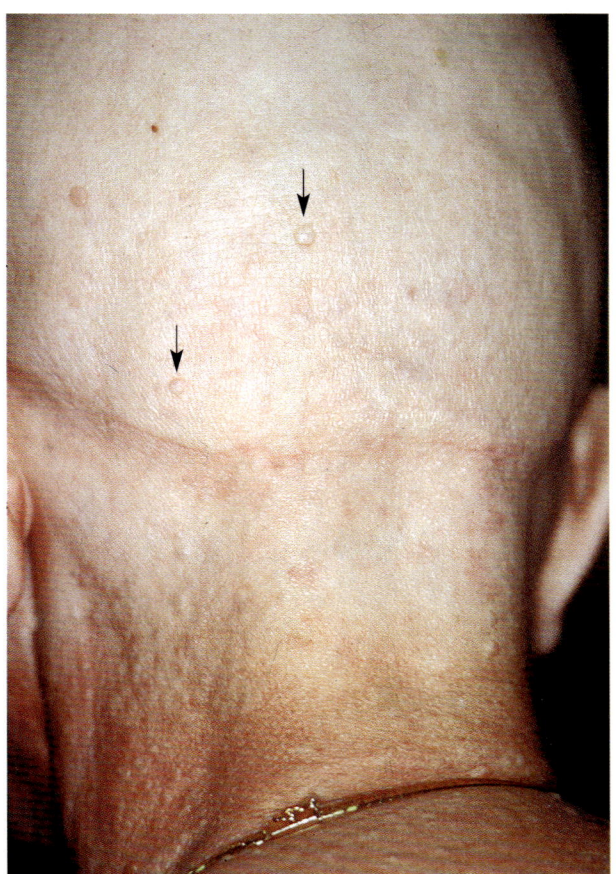

Figure 10.44

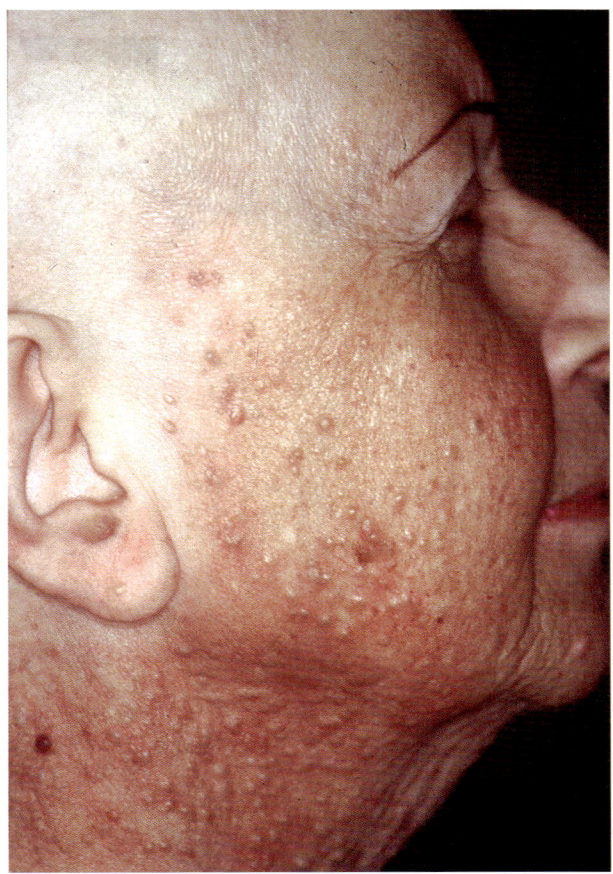

Figure 10.45

REFERENCES

Paller AS, Varigos G, Metzker A, et al. Compound heterozygous mutations in the hairless gene in atrichia with papular lesions. J Invest Dermatol 2003; 121: 430–2

Paradisi M, Chuang GS, Angelo C, et al. Atrichia with popular lesions resulting from a novel homozygous missense mutation in the hairless gene. Clin Exp Dermatol 2003; 28: 535–8

Zlotogorski A, Hochberg Z, Mirmirani P, et al. Clinical and pathologic correlations in genetically distinct forms of atrichia. Arch Dermatol 2003; 139: 1591–6

LOOSE ANAGEN SYNDROME

Synonym

- Short anagen syndrome

Age of onset

- Early childhood (2–5 years of age), more often in girls

Clinical findings

- Diffuse or patchy alopecia with painless loss of clumps of hair by accidental or deliberate pulling of scalp hair
- The hairs are blond, dry, lusterless (Figure 10.46), loosely anchored and easily removed
- The occipital hair is matted and feels sticky
- There is no increase in fragility of the hair

Associations

- Hypohidrotic ectodermal dysplasia
- Ocular coloboma

Course

The condition often recedes with age.

Laboratory investigations and data

A trichogram reveals that all anagen hairs are without root sheaths; the proximal ends of the hairs may have a curled appearance.

Genetics and pathogenesis

- Autosomal dominant inheritance; many sporadic cases
- Gene locus unknown
- Pathogenesis related to the expression of adhesion molecules

Differential diagnosis

- Alopecia areata
- Trichotillomania
- Uncombable hair syndrome

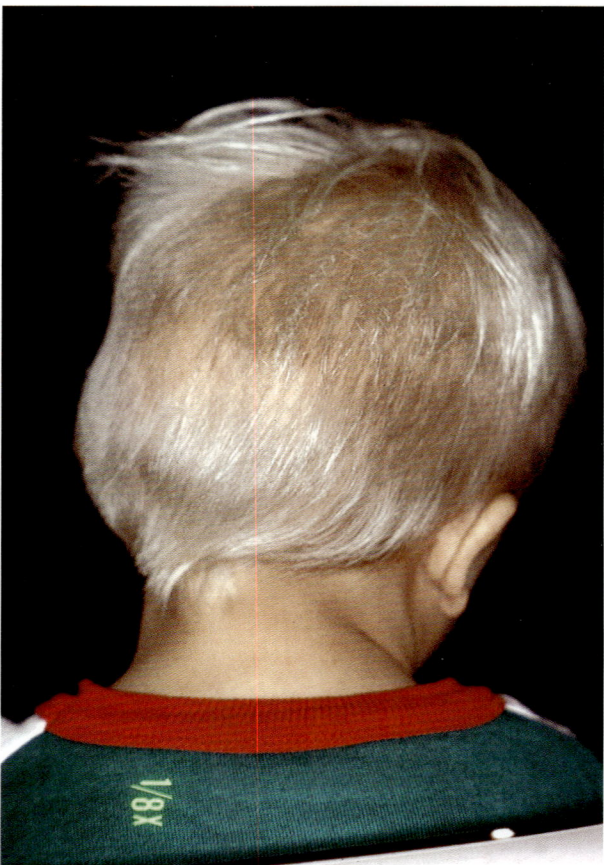

Figure 10.46

Follow-up and therapy

The severity of hair loss varies considerably among affected members of a family, the children being more severely affected.

There is no effective therapy.

REFERENCES

Baden HP, Kvedar JC, Magro CM. Loose anagen hair as a cause of hereditary hair loss in children. Arch Dermatol 1992; 128: 1349–53

Price VH, Gummer CL. Loose anagen syndrome. J Am Acad Dermatol 1989; 20: 249–56

Tosti A, Peluso AM, Misciali C, et al. Loose anagen hair. Arch Dermatol 1997; 133: 1089–93

KERATOSIS FOLLICULARIS SPINULOSA DECALVANS

Synonym

- Keratosis pilaris decalvans

Age of onset

- Infancy or early childhood

Clinical findings

Cutaneous manifestations

- Widespread filiform follicular hyperkeratosis evolving with follicular atrophy (main feature)
- Scarring alopecia of scalp, eyebrows and eyelashes (Figure 10.47)
- Occasionally calcaneal hyperkeratosis

Extracutaneous manifestations

- Ophthalmological disturbances are reported in some pedigrees

Course

The disease is usually lifelong and progressive.

Laboratory findings and data

Histopathologic findings include follicular plugging with perifollicular fibrosis and normal sebaceous glands.

Genetics and pathogenesis

- X-linked inheritance
- Gene locus mapped to chromosome Xp21, 2p22.2, related to a gene called SSAT (spermidin–spermin $N(1)$-acetyltransferase. Mutations cause putrescin accumulation that may cause the related phenotype
- Female carriers frequently show signs of the condition

Differential diagnosis

- IFAP syndrome (ichthyosis follicularis with atrichia and photophobia)
- KID syndrome (keratitis–ichythyosis–deafness)

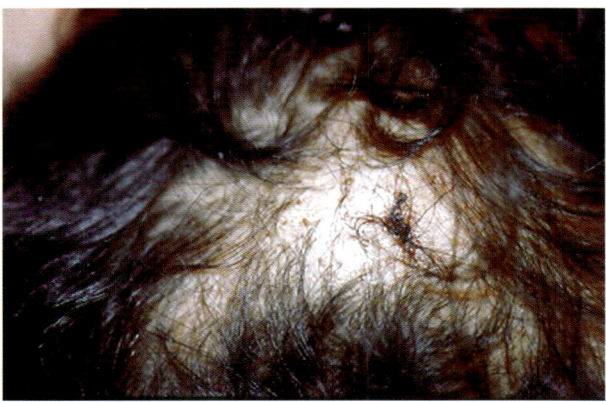

Figure 10.47

Therapy

Oral retinoids may induce improvement of the inflammatory alopecia and scarring.

REFERENCES

Alfadley A, Al Hawsawi K, Hainau B, Al Aboud K. Two brothers with keratosis follicularis spinulosa decalvans. J Am Acad Dermatol 2002; 47(5 Suppl): S275–8. Review

Gimelli G, Giglio S, Zuffardi O, et al. Gene dosage of the spermidine/spermine $N(1)$-acetyltransferase (SSAT) gene with putrescine accumulation in a patient with a Xp21.1p22.12 duplication and keratosis follicularis spinulosa decalvans (KFSD). Hum Genet 2002; 111: 235–41. Epub 2002 Aug 01

Herd RM, Benton EC. Keratosis follicularis spinulosa decalvans: report of a new pedigree. Br J Dermatol 1996; 134: 138–42

Rand R, Baden HP. Keratosis follicularis spinulosa decalvans. Report of two cases and literature review. Arch Dermatol 1983; 199: 22–6

Van Osch LDM, Oranje AP, Kenkens FM, et al. Keratosis follicularis spinulosa decalvans: a family study of seven male cases and six female carriers. J Med Genet 1992; 29: 36–40

CHAPTER 11

Nail disorders

PACHYONYCHIA CONGENITA

Synonyms

- Jadassohn–Lewandowsky syndrome
- Pachyonychia ichthyosiformis
- Keratosis multiformis idiopathica

Age of onset

- Birth; first months of life

Clinical findings

Skin and mucosal lesions

- Symmetrical, progressive thickening of all fingernails and toenails (main clinical feature: 97–100%): the distal two-thirds of the nails are yellow-brown, thick and dystrophic, distal subungual keratinous material elevates and transversally arches the nail plate (pincer nails) (Figures 11.1–11.3)
- Diffuse or focal symmetrical hyperkeratosis of palms and soles (62%) (Figure 11.4)
- Painful blisters on palms and soles (36%)
- Follicular keratosis and verrucous lesions on the extensor surfaces of the arms and legs and on the buttocks (36%) (Figures 11.5 and 11.6)
- Palmoplantar hyperhidrosis (20%)
- Leukokeratosis of the mouth (60%): white striae or plaques involving buccal mucosa, tongue and lips (Figures 11.7 and 11.8)
- Leukokeratosis of the larynx (6%) causing hoarseness
- Angular cheilosis (10%)
- Neonatal teeth (15%)
- Hair anomalies (9%): thin, dry, kinky, sparse

Extracutaneous lesions

- Corneal dyskeratosis (7%), cataracts (6%)
- Mental retardation (4%)
- Leukokeratosis of tympanic membrane causing deafness

Complications

- Candidal paronychial superinfections
- Chronic oral candidiasis
- Steatocystoma multiplex (5%)
- Hidradenitis suppurativa

'Historical' clinical classification (Feinstein *et al.*, 1988)

- Pachyonychia congenita type I: hypertrophy of nails, palmoplantar hyperkeratosis, follicular keratosis and oral leukokeratosis
- Pachyonychia congenita type II: clinical findings of type I plus blisters of palms and soles, hyperhidrosis, neonatal teeth, steatocystoma multiplex

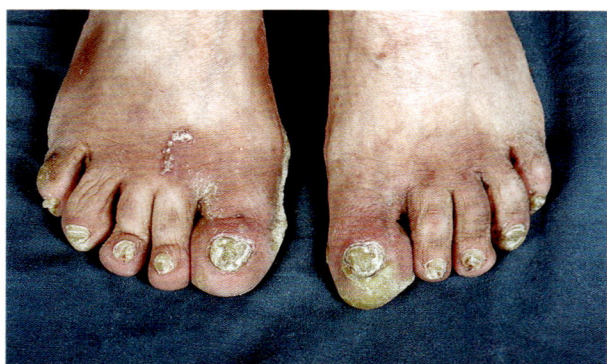

Figure 11.1

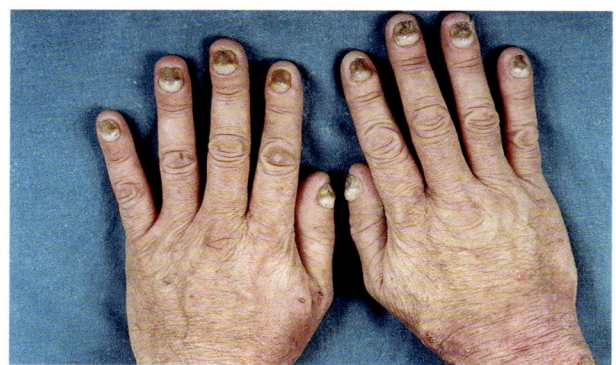

Figure 11.2

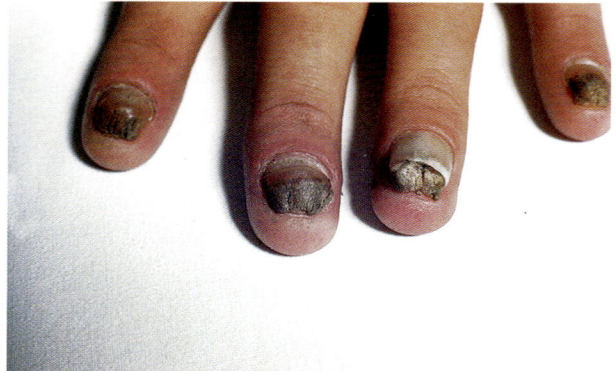

Figure 11.3

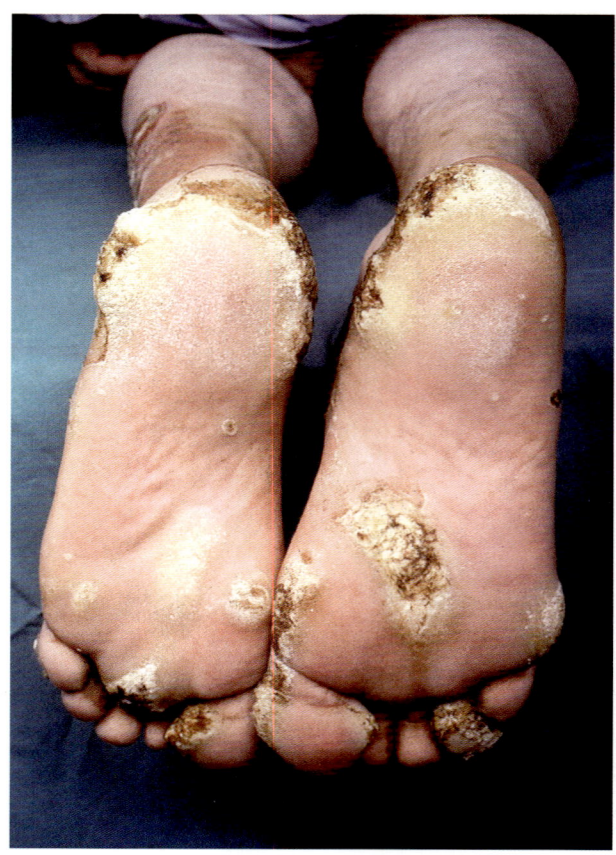

Figure 11.4

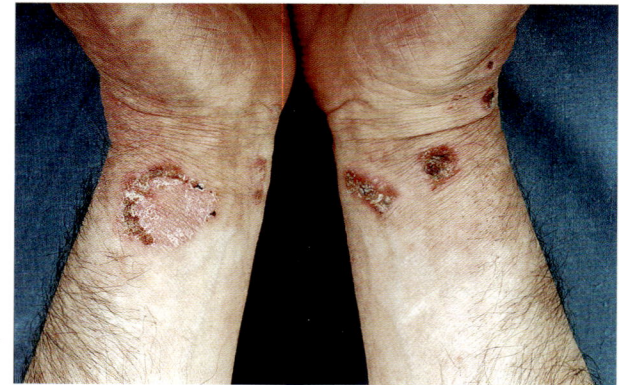

Figure 11.5

- Pachyonychia congenita type III: clinical findings of types I and II plus angular cheilosis, corneal dyskeratosis, cataracts
- Pachyonychia congenita type IV: clinical findings of types I, II and III plus laryngeal lesions, hoarseness, mental retardation, hair anomalies

Course

- Usually by 6 months of life the characteristic clinical manifestations have developed in 83%
- Lesions persist throughout life
- Growth and development usually normal

Nail disorders 153

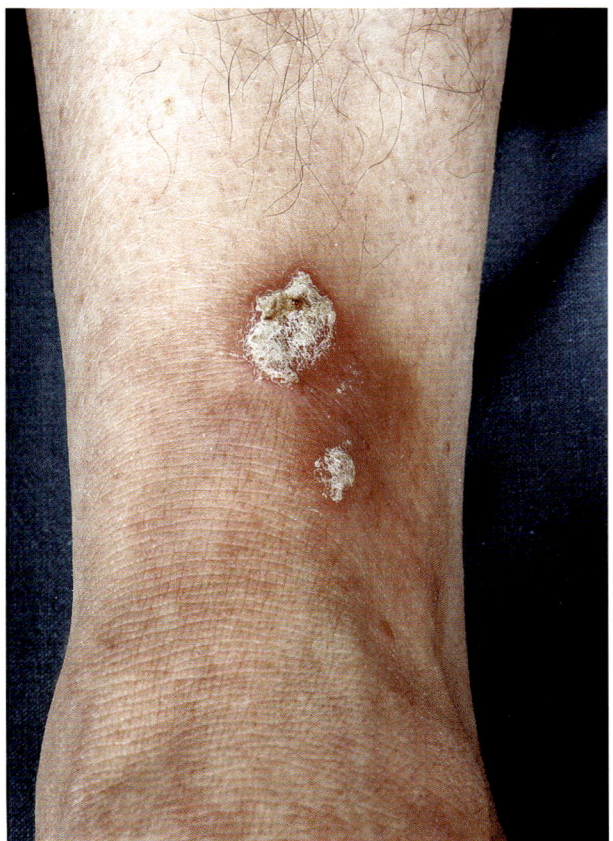

Figure 11.6

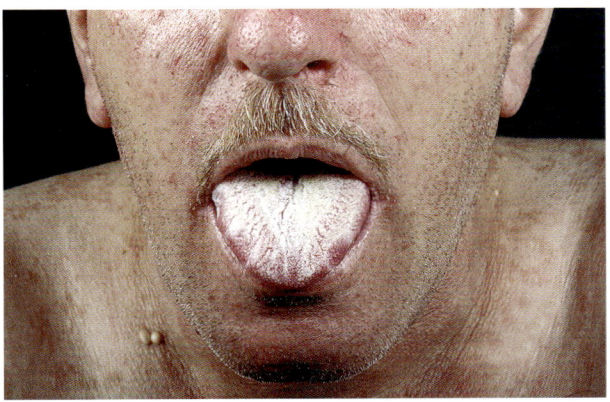

Figure 11.7

Laboratory findings

- Histopathologic features: marked hyperkeratosis of the nail bed

Genetics and pathogenesis

- Autosomal dominant disease; possibly autosomal recessive

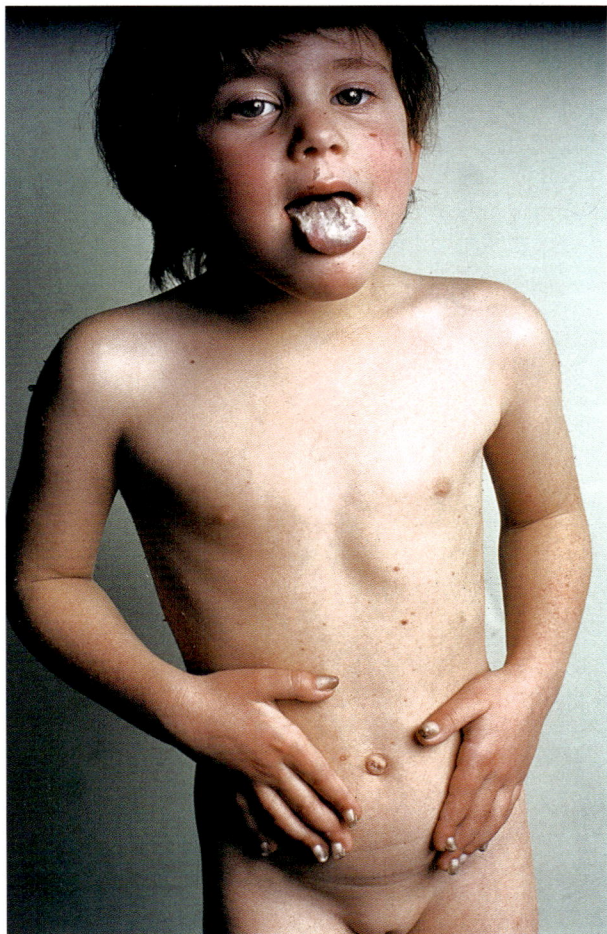

Figure 11.8

- Mutations in the genes encoding keratin 6,16,17 and desmoglein I

Differential diagnosis

- Other focal palmoplantar keratodermas
- Dyskeratosis congenita
- Psoriasis
- Congenital onychogryphosis
- Pityriasis rubra pilaris

Follow-up

- Oral leukokeratosis does not have a propensity for neoplastic changes
- Frequent difficulty in walking and using hands

Therapy

Treatment is palliative and frequently disappointing.

- Nail lesions: surgical treatments (radical excision and curettage)
- Skin lesions: lubricants, keratolytic agents, antiseptic dressings, special shoes
- Mucosal lesions: surgical or CO_2 laser excision; removal of natal and neonatal teeth
- Use of systemic retinoids may improve lesions

REFERENCES

Bowden PE, Haley JL, Kansky A, et al. Mutation of a type II keratin gene (K6a) in pachyonychia congenita. Nature Genet 1995; 10: 363–5

Dahl PR, Dand MS, Su WPD. Jadassohn–Lewandowsky syndrome (pachyonychia congenita). Semin Dermatol 1995; 14; 129–34

Feinstein A, Friedman J, Schewach-Millet M. Pachyonychia congenital. J Am Acad Dermatol 1988; 19: 705–11

Lin MT, Levy ML, Bowden PE, et al. Identification of sporadic mutations in the helix initiation motif of keratin 6 in two pachyonychia congenita patients: further evidence for a mutational hot spot. Exp Dermatol 1999; 8: 115–9

McLean WH, Rugg EL, Lunny DP, et al. Keratin 16 and keratin 17 mutations cause pachyonychia congenita. Nature Genet 1995; 9: 273–8

Sobecki R, Jaroszewicz C, Czechowicz-Janicka K. [A case of Jodassohn–Lewandowsky syndrome] Klin Oczna 1996; 98: 385–6. Polish

Su WPD, Chin SI, Hammond DE, et al. Pachyonychia congenita: a clinical study of 12 cases and review of the literature. Pediatr Dermatol 1990; 7: 33–8

NAIL–PATELLA–ELBOW SYNDROME

Synonyms

- Nail–patella syndrome
- Osteo-onychodysplasia

Age of onset

- At birth

Clinical findings

Cutaneous manifestations

- Fingernails involved in a symmetrical fashion (98%) with anonychia, hyponychia, koilonychia, onychorrhexis (Figure 11.9)
- Characteristic triangular or 'V'-shaped lunula
- Fingernail abnormalities are most severe on the ulnar side of the thumb, decreasing to the little finger
- Toenails rarely involved
- Palmoplantar hyperhidrosis

Extracutaneous manifestations

Bone involvement:

- Hypoplasia of capitulum and radial heel (90%)
- Patella aplasia with recurrent or permanent luxation (90%) (Figures 11.10 and 11.11)
- Bilateral posterior iliac horns (30%)
- Scapular hypoplasia
- Scoliosis
- Genu valgum
- Hyperextensible joints of digits

Renal involvement:

- Renal dysplasia (40%)
- Urethral duplication (25%)
- Glomerulonephritis
- Renal failure

Ocular involvement:

- Heterochromia of the iris, with hyperpigmentation of the papillary margin: Lester's iris (45%)
- Microcornea
- Glaucoma

Nail disorders 155

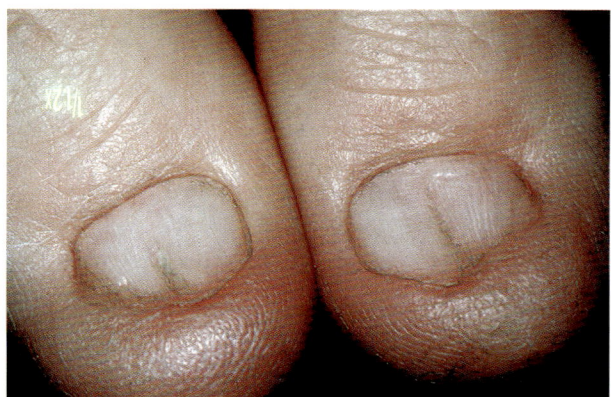

Figure 11.9

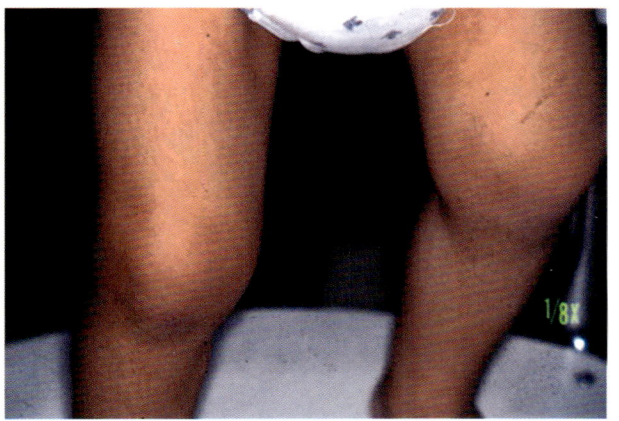

Figure 11.10

Course

The disease is lifelong.

Laboratory investigations

There are none specific.

Genetics and pathogenesis

- Autosomal dominant inheritance
- The disease is caused by mutations in the LIM homeodomain encoding LMX1B gene. The LMX1B transcription factor plays a role in defining the

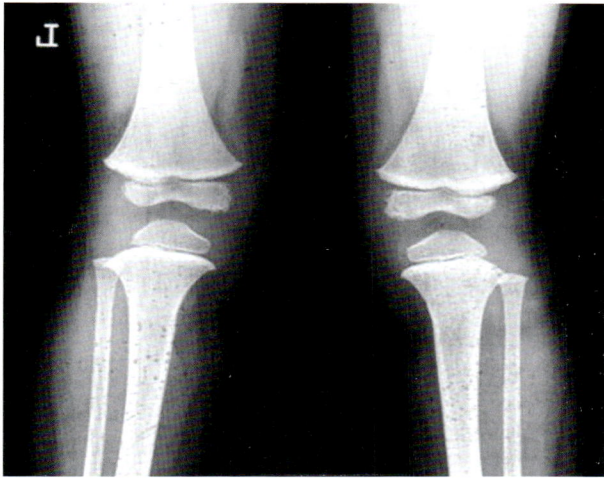

Figure 11.11

development of dorsal-specific structures during limb development
- Association with Buschke–Ollendorff syndrome (see also Chapter 17)

Differential diagnosis

- Hypo-anonychia congenita

Follow-up and therapy

- Examination of bones
- Renal and ocular evaluation
- Management of bone problems by orthopedists
- Management of kidney failure by nephrologists

REFERENCES

Chen H, Lun Y, Ovehinnikov D, et al. Limb and kidney defects in Lmx1b mutant mice suggest an involvement of LMX1B in human nail patella syndrome. Nature Genet 1998; 19: 51–5

Drouin CA, Grenon H. The association of Buschke-Ollendorff syndrome and nail patella syndrome. J Am Acad Dermatol 2002; 46: 621–5

McIntosh I, Clough MV, Shäffer AA, et al. Fine mapping of nail–patella syndrome locus at 9q34. Am J Hum Genet 1997; 60: 133–42

TWENTY-NAIL DYSTROPHY

Age of onset

- At birth

Clinical findings

Nails show thinning, thickening, pitting, ridging, koilonychia, opalescence and loss of luster (Figures 11.12 and 11.13).

Association

- Dental deformities

Course

This is a lifelong disease.

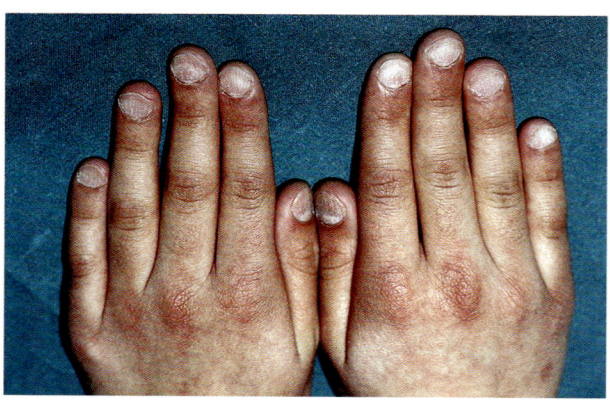

Figure 11.12

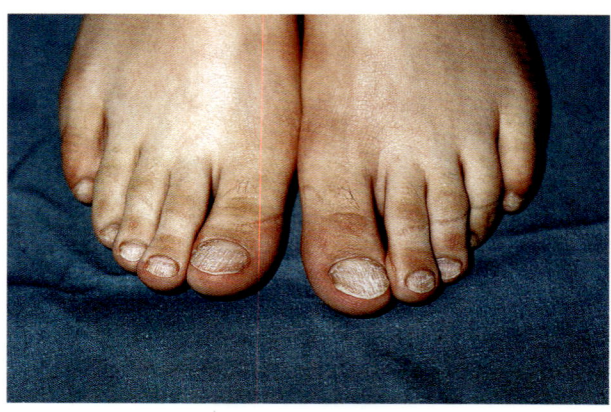

Figure 11.13

Genetics and pathogenesis

There is autosomal dominant inheritance.

Differential diagnosis

- Acquired twenty-nail dystrophy
- Pachyonychia congenita
- Nail–patella syndrome

REFERENCES

Arias AM, Yung CW, Rendler S, et al. Familial severe twenty-nail dystrophy. J Am Acad Dermatol 1982; 7: 349–52

Menni S, Piccinno R, Sala F, et al. Twenty nail dystrophy of childhood; two cases in one family. Clin Exp Dermatol 1984; 9: 604–7

Pavone L, Volti S, Guarnieri B, et al. Hereditary twenty nail dystrophy in a Sicilian family. J Med Genet 1982; 19: 337–40

MALALIGNMENT OF THE GREAT TOENAILS

Epidemiology

- This is a very rare disorder.

Age of onset

- At birth

Clinical findings

- Monolateral or bilateral deviation of the toenail plate (Figure 11.14)
- Nails may be thickened and dystrophic (Figure 11.15)

Course and prognosis

- Spontaneous improvement is reported
- Ingrown nails or onychogryphosis

Laboratory findings

There are none specific.

Genetics and pathogenesis

The disease is autosomal dominant.

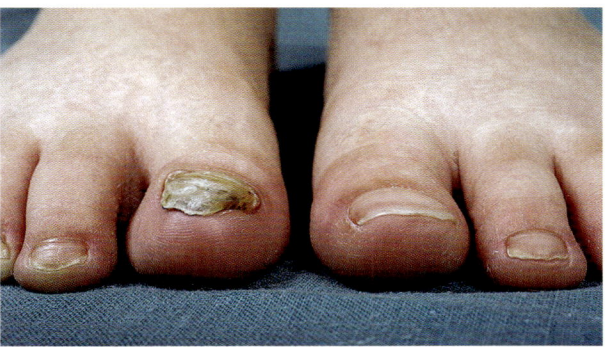

Figure 11.14

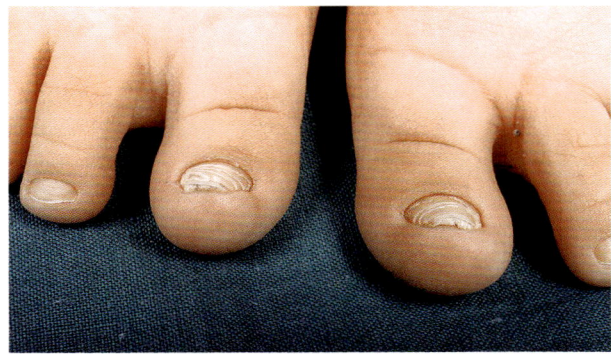

Figure 11.15

Follow-up and therapy

- Surgical treatment for ingrown nails
- Cosmetic treatment (artificial nail implantation)

Differential diagnosis

- Naegeli–Franceschetti syndrome

LEUKONYCHIA

Age of onset

- From birth to childhood

Clinical findings

- Nails may be completely white (leukonychia totalis) or incompletely white (leukonychia partialis, striata or punctata) (Figure 11.16)
- The color may be white, milky or porcelain

Associations

- Pili torti
- Sebaceous cysts
- Koilonychia
- Palmoplantar keratoderma
- Knuckle pads
- Dental changes
- Keratosis pilaris
- Hypoparathyroidism
- Cataracts
- LEOPARD syndrome (lentigines, electrocardiographic abnormalities, ocular hypertelorism, pulmonary stenosis, abnormalities of genitalia, retardation of growth, sensorineural deafness)
- Renal calculi
- Personal observation of a single patient with total leukonychia, vitiligo and hearing loss due to a mutation in the connexin 26 gene

Course

This disease is lifelong.

Laboratory investigations and data

Nail plate biopsy shows parakeratosis and immature keratinocytes.

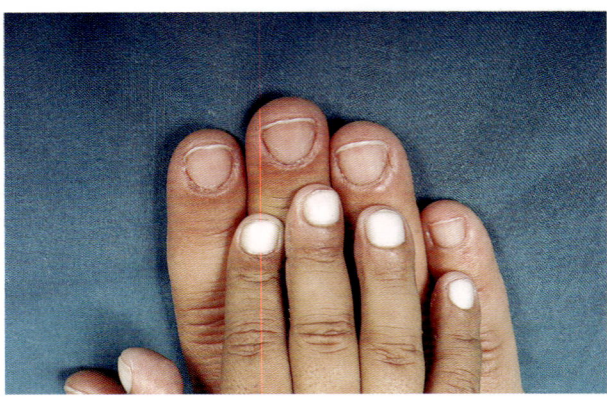

Figure 11.16

Genetics and pathogenesis

- Autosomal dominant inheritance
- Leukonychia is probably due to an abnormal keratinization of the nail plate: large immature keratohyaline granules reflect light, resulting in a white nail that prevents visualization of the underlying pink vascular bed

Therapy

- Cosmetics

REFERENCES

Grossman M, Scher RK. Leukonychia: review and classification. Int J Dermatol 1990; 29: 535–41

Stevens KR, Leis PF, Peter S, et al. Congenital leukonychia. J Am Acad Dermatol 1998; 39: 509–12

Stewart L, Young E, Lim HW. Idiopathic leukonychia totalis and partialis. J Am Acad Dermatol 1985; 13: 157–8

PTERYGIUM INVERSUM OF NAILS

Synonym

- Familial subungual pterygium of nails

Age of onset

- At birth

Clinical findings

- The distal part of the nail bed remains adherent to the ventral surface of the nail plate, eliminating the distal groove (Figures 11.17 and 11.18)
- Fingers of both hands affected symmetrically
- Occasional paroxysms of digital pain

Course

The disease is lifelong.

Genetics and pathogenesis

- Autosomal dominant and autosomal recessive inheritance
- The suggested cause is a disproportional extension of the nail bed epithelium with dislocation of the hyponychium

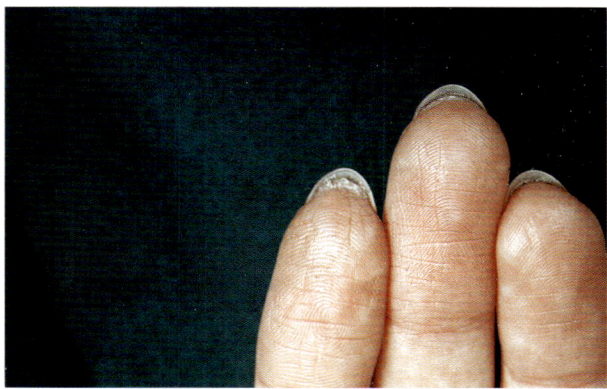

Figure 11.17

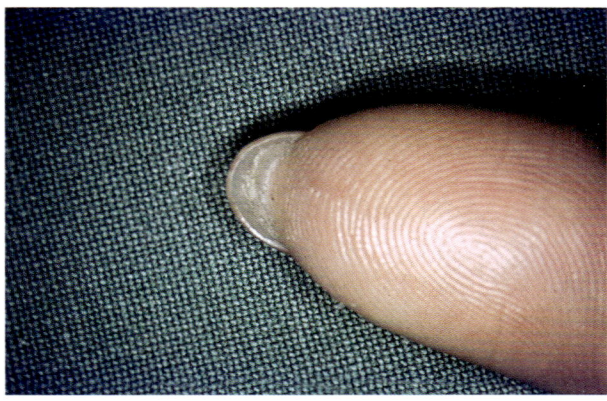

Figure 11.18

REFERENCES

Caputo R, Prandi G. Pterygium inversum unguis. Arch Dermatol 1973; 108: 817–18

Christophers E. Familiare subungueal pterygium. Hautarzt 1975; 26: 543–4

Dugois P, Amblard P, Martel C, et al. Pterygium inversum unguis familial. Bull Soc Franc Dermatol Syph 1975; 82: 283–84

ISO-KIKUCHI SYNDROME

Synonym

- Congenital onychodysplasia of the index finger(s)

Epidemiology

- More than 200 cases reported in the literature

Age of onset

- At birth

Clinical findings

- Hypoplastic nail and hypoplasia of the index finger are the hallmarks of the disease (Figure 11.19)
- Defects of different degrees may involve other fingers and/or nails and toes
- The full spectrum of onychodysplasias may be present: irregular lunula, malalignment, micronychia, polyonichia and anonychia

Extracutaneous findings

- Brachydactyly and short hands
- Bilateral inguinal hernia

Course and prognosis

Progressive delineation of nail, finger (toe) defects

Laboratory findings

- X-rays of hands or feet may reveal phalanx and metatarsal bone defects
- Arteriography reveals stenosis in the radial artery or palmar digital artery (Figure 11.20)

Genetics and pathogenesis

- Autosomal dominant with many sporadic cases
- The disease is caused by different degrees of stenosis of the radial artery or digital palmar (plantar) arteries
- The delineation of the syndrome may disclose a more complex malformative disease

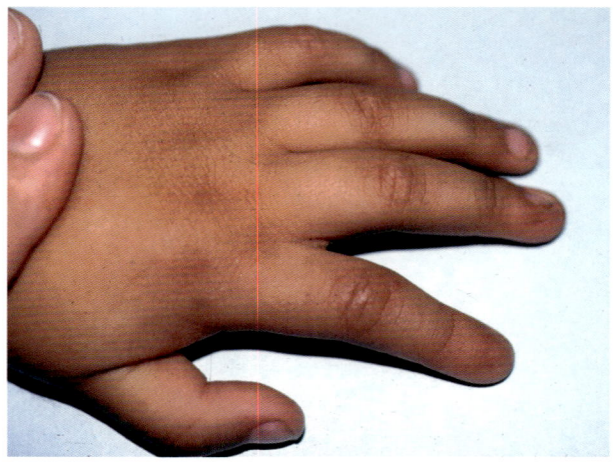

Figure 11.19

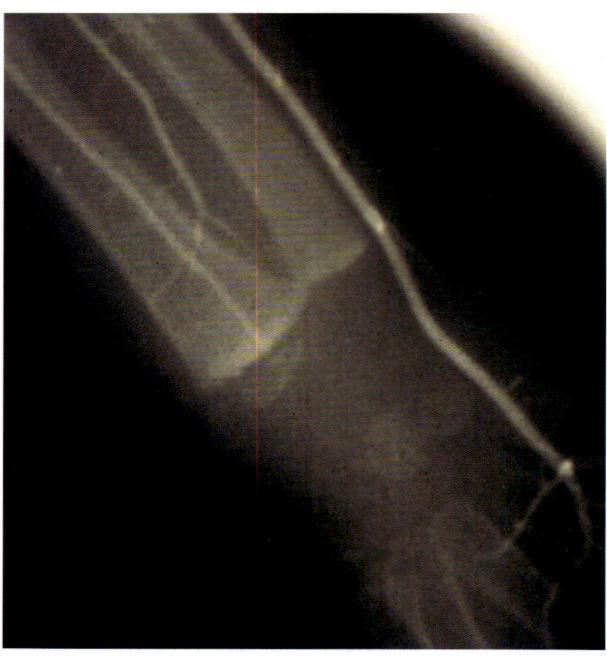

Figure 11.20

Follow-up and therapy

- Cosmetic surgery

Differential diagnosis

- Other isolated or complex onychodysplasias

REFERENCE

Franceschini P, Licata D, Guala A, et al. Peculiar facial appearance and generalized brachydactyly in a patient with congenital onychodysplasia of the index fingers (Iso-Kikuchi syndrome). Am J Med Genet 2001; 98: 330–5 [Review]

CHAPTER 12

Sebocystomatosis

Synonyms

- Steatocystoma multiplex
- Eruptive vellus hair cysts
- Multiple pilosebaceous cyst syndrome
- Hereditary epidermal polycystic disease

Age of onset

- Adolescence

Clinical findings

Cutaneous manifestations

- Asymptomatic, multiple (up to hundreds) dome-shaped smooth papulonodular lesions, skin colored or variably pigmented (yellow, blue, red brown) varying in diameter from 1 to 20 mm
- The cysts commonly involve the face, scalp, arms, trunk and thighs (Figures 12.1–12.5)

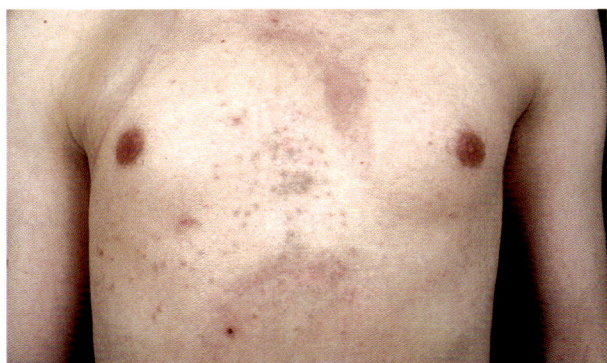

Figure 12.1

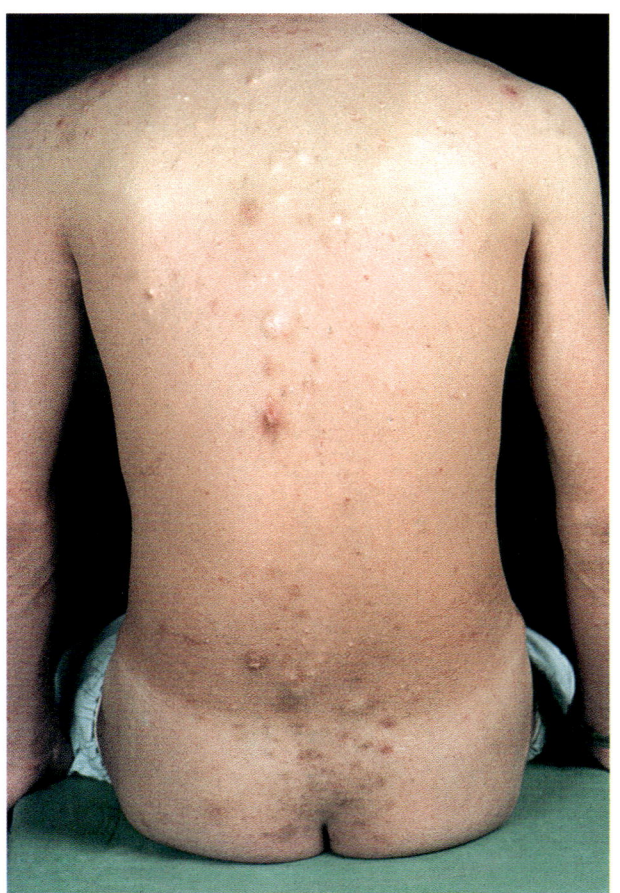

Figure 12.2

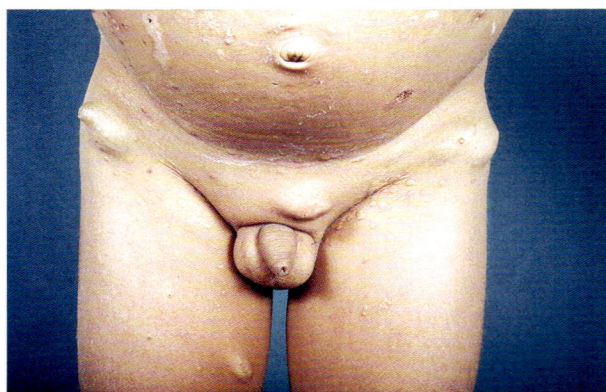

Figure 12.3

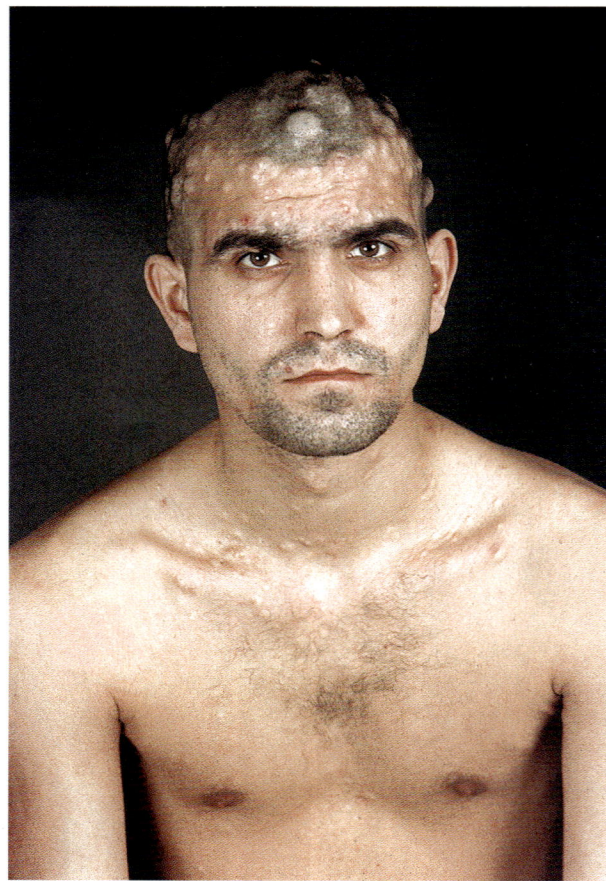

Figure 12.4

- The cysts contain an oily, clear or opaque, milky or yellowish, odorless fluid or cheesy solid material
- Occasionally lesions may be localized

Associations

- Pachyonychia congenita
- Hidradenitis suppurativa
- Koilonychia

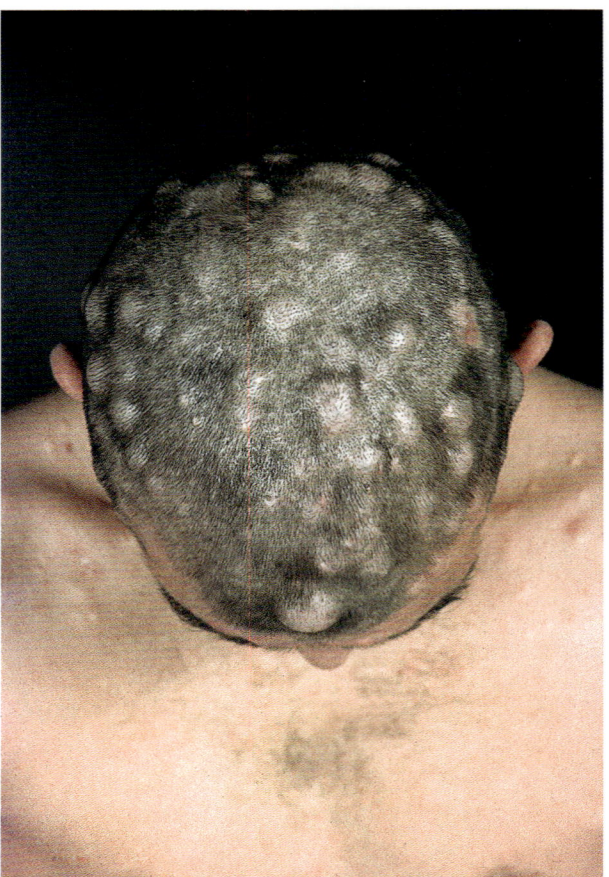

Figure 12.5

Complications

- Infections

Course

After eruption the lesions become stationary; occasional spontaneous resolution occurs through transepidermal elimination.

Laboratory investigations

Histopathologic findings:

- Eruptive vellus hair cysts: cystic proliferation lined by squamous epithelium with an evident granular layer and containing keratinous material and vellus hairs
- Steatocystoma multiplex: cystic proliferation characterized by stratified squamous epithelium without a granular layer and associated with large sebaceous glands located within the cyst wall

Genetics and pathogenesis

- Autosomal dominant diseases
- Gene locus unknown
- Multiple pilosebaceous cysts seems to be a nevoid malformation of the pilosebaceous duct junction zone. The resulting cystic tumors may develop with a predominantly follicular differentiation as in eruptive vellus hair cysts, or with differentiation and imitation of the sebaceous duct as in steatocystoma multiplex

Differential diagnosis

- Adnexal tumors
- Epidermoid cysts
- Trichilemmal cysts
- Perforating dermatoses
- Milia
- Acne cysts

Therapy

- Incisions of the cysts
- Oral retinoids
- YAG (yttrium–aluminum–garnet) and CO_2 lasers

REFERENCES

Cho S, Chang SE, Choi JH, et al. Clinical and histologic features of 64 cases of steatocystoma multiplex. J Dermatol 2002; 29: 152–6

Kiene P, Hauschild A, Christophers E. Eruptive hair cysts and steatocystoma multiplex. Variants of one entity? Br J Dermatol 1996; 134; 365–7

Patrizi A, Neri I, Guerrini V, et al. Persistent milia, steatocystoma multiplex and eruptive vellus hair cysts: variable expression of multiple pilosebaceous cysts within an affected family. Dermatology 1998; 196: 392–6

CHAPTER 13

Oral mucosa

WHITE SPONGE NEVUS

Synonyms

- Familial white folded dysplasia of the mucous membranes
- Nevus of Cannon

Age of onset

- From birth (rarely) to the third decade of life

Clinical findings

- Asymptomatic, diffuse soft, white, spongy, hyperkeratotic plaques on oral mucous membranes with a velvety or rugose surface
- Sites of predilection: buccal mucosa, labial mucosa, gingiva (Figures 13.1 and 13.2) and floor of the mouth; tongue; nasal, esophageal, genital and anal mucosae rarely affected

Extracutaneous findings

Ocular coloboma has been reported in the literature.

Course and prognosis

The disease is lifelong, without potential for malignancy.

Laboratory findings and data

Histopathologic findings include hyperkeratosis and acanthosis with cellular vacuolization in the

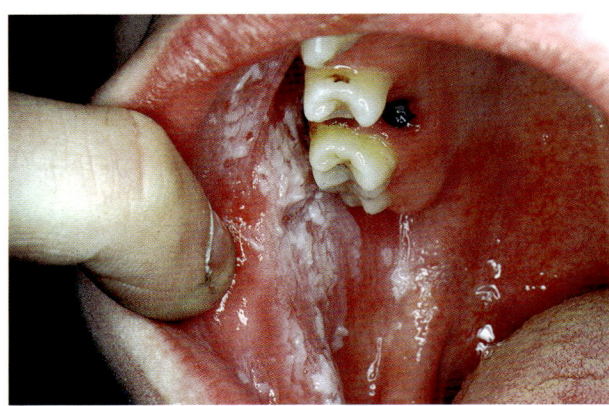

Figure 13.1

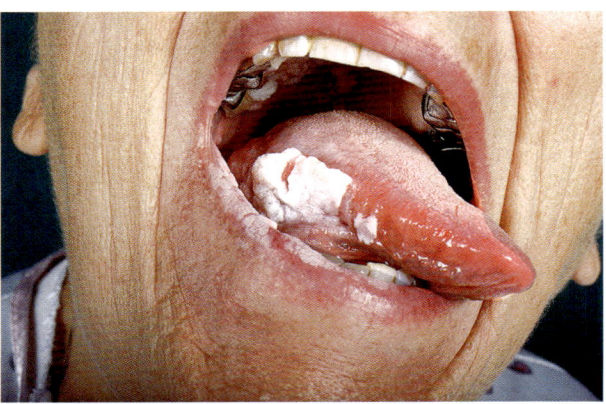

Figure 13.2

granular and squamous layers due to intracellular edema without nuclear atypia.

Genetics and pathogenesis

- Autosomal dominant inheritance
- Mutations in keratin 4 (K4) and keratin 13 (K13) genes
- Consequence of an alteration in the distribution of tonofilaments in epithelial cells

Differential diagnosis

- Pachyonychia congenita
- Darier's disease
- Benign intraepithelial dyskeratosis
- Dyskeratosis congenita
- Acquired white oral lesions
- Leukoplakia and lichen planus
- Human papilloma virus-related lesions

Follow-up and therapy

- Local tretinoin
- CO_2 laser
- Rarely, surgery is indicated

REFERENCES

Hernandez-Martin A, Fernandez-Lopez E, de Unamuno P, et al. Diffuse whitening of the oral mucosa in a child. Pediatr Dermatol 1997; 14: 316–20

Jorgenson RJ, Levin LS. White sponge nevus. Arch Dermatol 1981; 117: 73–6

Terrinoni A, Candi E, Oddi S, et al. A glutamine insertion in the 1° alpha helical domain of keratin 4 gene in a familial case of white sponge nevus. J Invest Dermatol 2000; 114: 388–91

DYSKERATOSIS CONGENITA

Synonym

- Zinsser–Cole–Engman syndrome

Age of onset

- Generally before puberty

Epidemiology

The disease is rare. No further data are available.

Clinical findings

- Lacy reticulated telangiectatic hyperpigmentation (poikilodermatous appearance) with interposed zones of hypopigmentation (100%) on face, neck, trunk, upper thighs (Figures 13.3 and 13.4)
- Atrophy and cyanosis of the dorsal aspects of the hands and feet (93%) (Figure 13.5)

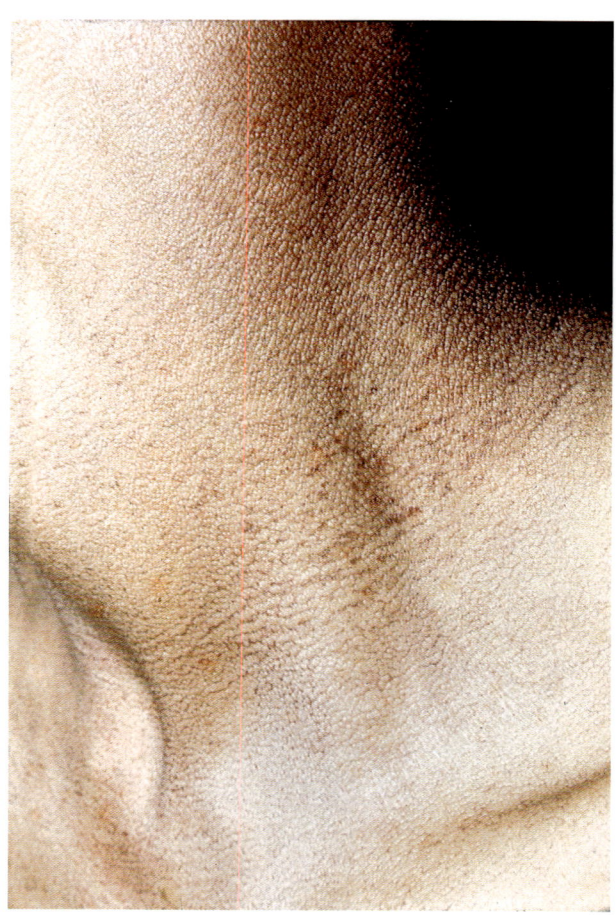

Figure 13.3

- Hyperkeratosis and hyperhidrosis of palms and soles (72%) (Figure 13.6)
- Bullae are visible especially during childhood and adolescence or in sun-exposed areas (78%)
- Nail dystrophy (98%): longitudinal ridges, thinning (Figure 13.5)

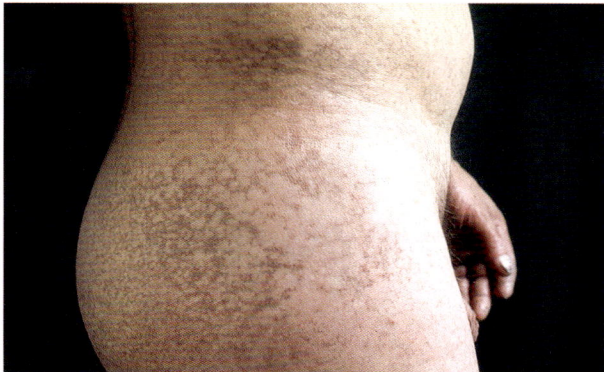

Figure 13.4

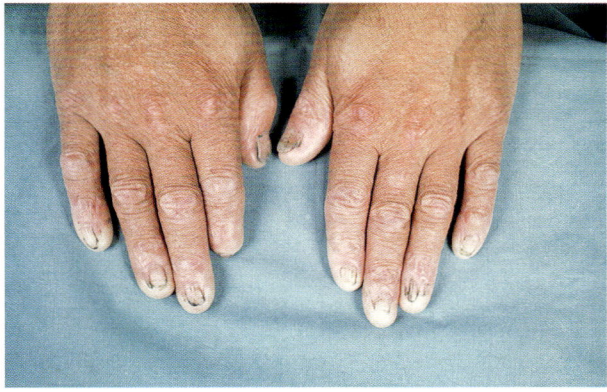

Figure 13.5

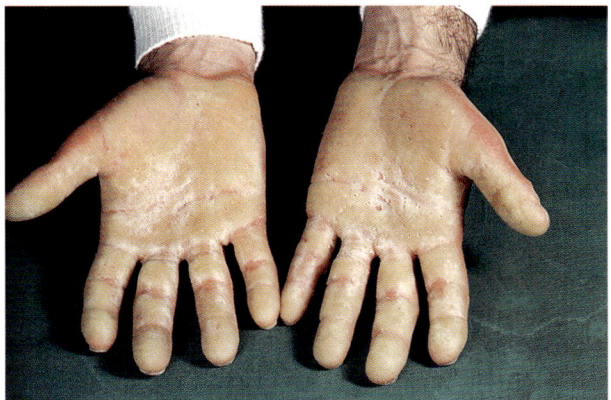

Figure 13.6

- Thin, lusterless sparse hair (51%)
- Leukokeratosis of oral mucosa (87%) (Figures 13.7 and 13.8) and less frequently of pharynx, anorectal and urogenital mucosae

Extracutaneous manifestations

- Epiphora, i.e. persistent overflow of tears due to obstruction of lachrymal ducts (78%): blepharitis, conjunctivitis
- Early dental loss (63%) or extensive caries
- Aplastic anemia (50%) with bleeding problems and purpura
- Esophageal diverticuli with dysphagia (59%)
- Retardation of growth (50%)
- Hypogonadism (40%)
- Mental retardation (42%)
- Macular amyloidosis

Course and complications

There is a poor prognosis. Death is the rule, often in the third decade

- Malignant neoplasms, most often squamous cell carcinomas of mucosal surfaces
- Infection by opportunistic agents
- Irreversible condition with high mortality owing to failure of bone marrow, hematologic malignancies (mainly in the second or third decade)

Laboratory investigations

- Blood count
- Bone marrow biopsy
- Accurate study of cellular immunity
- X-ray of bones
- Histopathological findings:
  - skin: thinned epidermis, vacuolar alterations, sparse perivascular lymphocytic infiltrate
  - mucous membranes: atypical keratinocytes with thickened ortho- and parakeratotic epithelium

Genetics and pathogenesis

Mutations in the gene called DKC1 encoding a modulator of the telomerase RNA and for ribosomal RNA processing (X-linked form) and in the gene called hTERC (RNA telomerase) (autosomal dominant form) are strictly related to the symptoms (premature aging, anemia and bone marrow malignancies and neoplastic proneness) of dyskeratosis congenita.

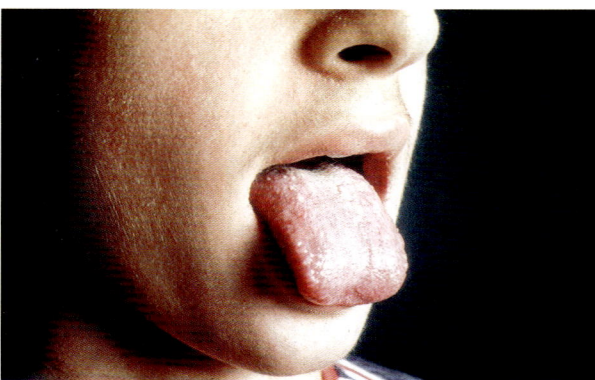

Figure 13.7

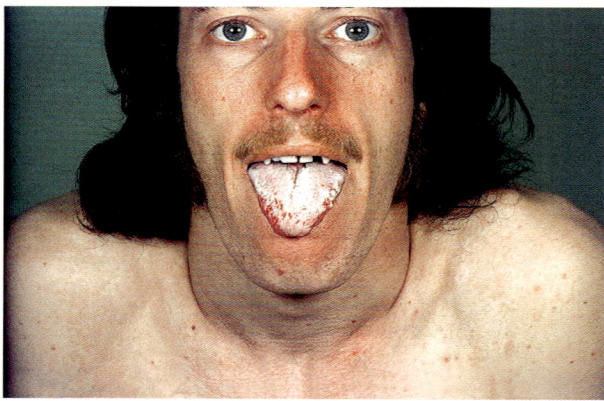

Figure 13.8

Follow-up and therapy

- Close observation to detect early signs of bone marrow failure and malignant neoplasm
- Bone marrow transplantation
- Oral retinoids
- Transfusions

Differential diagnosis

- Fanconi's anemia
- Kindler syndrome
- Rothmund–Thomson syndrome
- White sponge nevus

REFERENCES

Bessler M, Wilson DB, Mason PJ. Dyskeratosis congenita and telomerase. Curr Opin Pediatr 2004; 16: 23–8. Review

Ding YG, Zhu TS, Jiang W, et al. Identification of a novel mutation and a de novo mutation in DKC1 in two Chinese pedigrees with dyskeratosis congenita. J Invest Dermatol 2004; 123: 470–3

Dokal I, Vulliamy T. Dyskeratosis congenita: its link to telomerase and aplastic anaemia. Blood Rev 2003; 17: 217–25. Review

Marrone A, Mason PJ. Dyskeratosis congenita. Cell Moll Life Sci 2003; 60: 507–17

Marrone A, Stevens D, Vulliamy T, et al. Heterozygous telomerase RNA mutations found in dyskeratosis congenita and aplastic anemia reduce telomerase activity via haploinsufficiency. Blood 2004 15; 104: 3936–42. Epub 2004 Aug 19. PMID: 15319288 [PubMed – in process]

Mochizuki Y, He J, Kulkarni S, et al. Mouse dyskerin mutations affect accumulation of telomerase RNA and small nucleolar RNA, telomerase activity, and ribosomal RNA processing. Proc Natl Acad Sci USA 2004 20; 101: 10756–61. Epub 2004 Jul 07

Yamaguchi H, Baerlocher GM, Lansdorp PM, et al. Mutations of the human telomerase RNA gene (TERC) in aplastic anemia and myelodysplastic syndrome. Blood 2003; 102: 916–18

ORAL–FACIAL–DIGITAL SYNDROME TYPE I

Synonym

- Orofaciodigital syndrome type I

Epidemiology

There are more than 200 cases reported in the literature. The other types of oral–facial–digital syndrome may be unified as a single disease with a different phenotype.

Age of onset

- At birth

Clinical findings

- Cleft, lobulated or bifid tongue with possible ankyloglossia (Figure 13.9)
- Multiple accessory frenulae
- Lip nodules and pseudoclefting (Figure 13.9)
- Multiple milia of face and hands that heal spontaneously leaving cribrous areas (Figures 13.9 and 13.10)
- Thin and fragile hair leading to alopecia (Figure 13.11)

Extracutaneous symptoms

- Complete or partial cleft palate and lip
- Defective or supernumerary teeth
- Facies with frontal bossing, hypertelorism and 'dystopia canthorum', micrognathia and malar hypoplasia (Figure 13.10)
- 'True' syndactyly and brachydactyly of hands (feet are less involved) are characteristic, less frequently clino- and camptodactyly (Figure 13.12)
- Central nervous system defects, including corpus callosum agenesis and cortical atrophy
- Mild to severe mental deficit is frequent
- Polycystic kidney disease

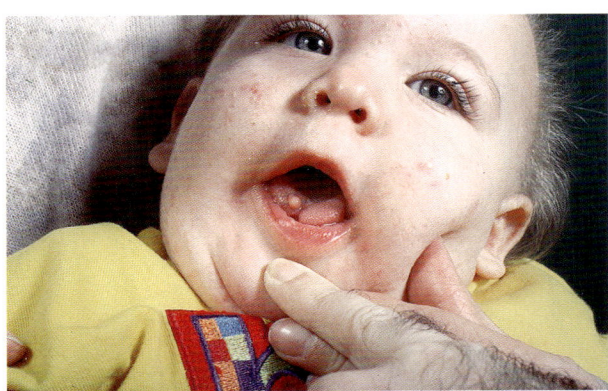

Figure 13.9

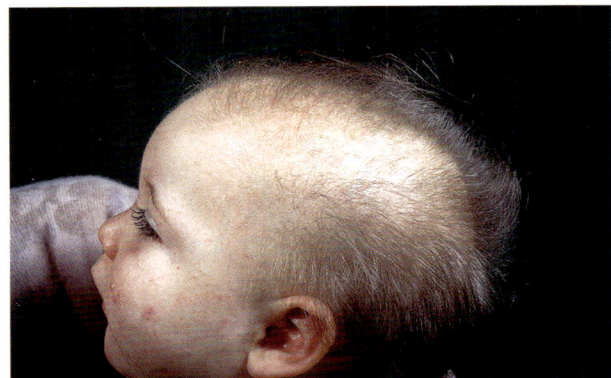

Figure 13.11

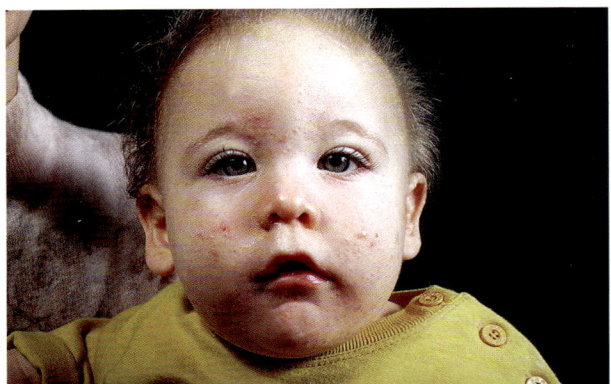

Figure 13.10

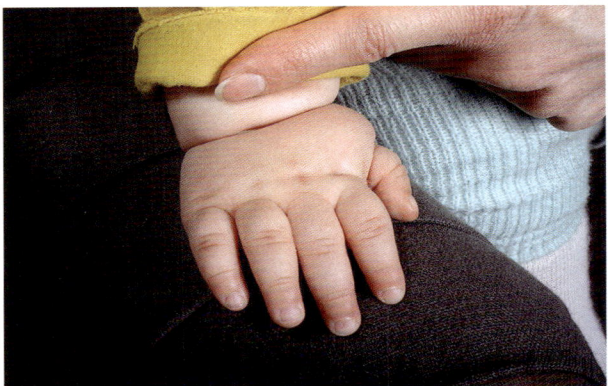

Figure 13.12

Complications and course

Development of mental deficiency is progressive.

Laboratory findings

Nodular tongue lesions are mixed hamartomas.

Genetics and pathogenesis

The disease is transmitted with an X-linked dominant trait with male lethality; nonetheless, a few surviving males are described, as occur in incontinentia pigmenti and Goltz's syndrome.

The OFD1 gene is expressed in mesenchymal cells and the metanephron during embryogenesis.

Differential diagnosis

- Other syndromes sharing multiple oral and lip defects
- Trichorhinophalangeal syndrome

Follow-up and therapy

Oral surgery is recommended to improve speech.

REFERENCES

Emes RD, Ponting CP. A new sequence motif linking lissencephaly, Treacher–Collins and oral-facial-digital type 1 syndromes, mictotubule dynamics and cell migration. Hum Mol Genet 2001; 10: 2813–20

King NM, Sanares AM. Oral-facial-digital syndrome, type I: a case report. J Clin Pediatr Dent 2002; 26: 211–15

Romio L, Wright V, Price K, et al. OFD1, the gene mutated in oral-facial-digital syndrome type 1, is expressed in the metanephros and in human embryonic renal mesechymal cells. J Am Soc Nephrol 2003; 14: 680–9

CHAPTER 14

Neurocutaneous syndromes

NEUROFIBROMATOSIS TYPE 1

Synonym

- Von Recklinghausen's disease

Epidemiology

Neurofibromatosis type 1 (NF1) is one of the most frequent genetic diseases involving the skin. The estimated prevalence is 1 : 500 to 1 : 3000.

Age of onset

- Lesions of NF1 (as well as those of tuberous sclerosis) have specific age of onset: at birth for café-au-lait spots, during childhood for freckling, and in late childhood and puberty for neurofibromas and plexiform tumors

Clinical findings

- Café-au-lait spots: light-brown macules present at birth and slowly growing with age, distributed randomly with sharp borders and round–oval shape (Figures 14.1–14.4)
- Freckling: small lentiginous-like lesions distributed preferentially on large folds (Figures 14.4 and 14.5)
- Neurofibromas: nodules ranging from 2–3 mm to 1–2 cm in dimension, flesh colored, subcutaneous and slightly protruding, randomly distributed or focused along the course of peripheral nerves (Figures 14.6–14.8)
- Plexiform tumors: large subcutaneous soft tumors (Figures 14.9 and 14.10), with a particular 'full bag'

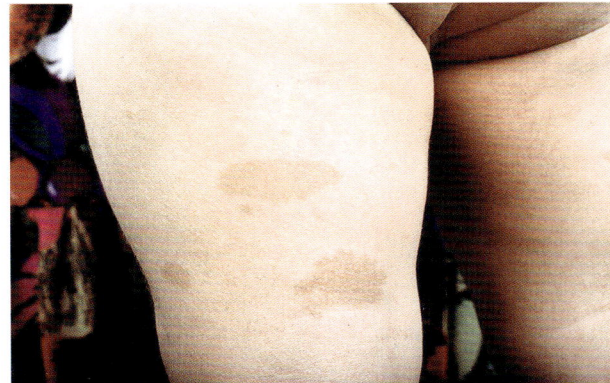

Figure 14.1

texture, located elsewhere on the skin and potentially reaching huge dimensions, becoming the so-called 'tumeurs royales' (Figures 14.11–14.13)
- Less frequently hypopigmented ovalar spots similar to those occurring in tuberous sclerosis are noted, as well as angiomatous-like lesions (Figures 14.14 and 14.15)
- Rarely, alopecic lesions are visible on the vertex (Figure 14.16)
- Mucosal lesions are very rare
- Darker colored skin compared with healthy family subjects
- A soft skin touch, similar to that occurring in Ehlers–Danlos subjects, is detectable in over 70% of patients
- Itching
- A higher incidence of juvenile xanthogranulomas (Figure 14.17)
- Segmental presentation for both café-au-lait spots and neurofibromas is possible (Figure 25.28)

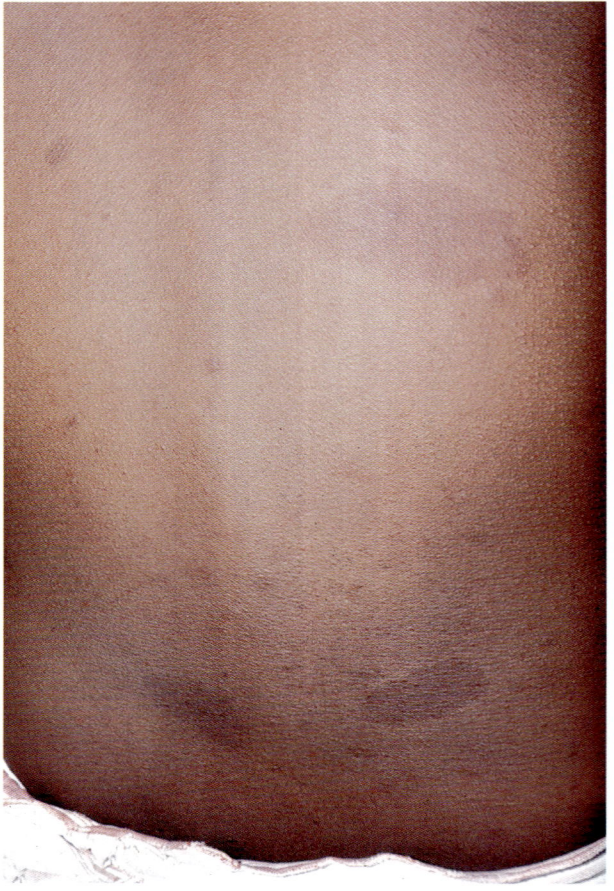

Figure 14.2

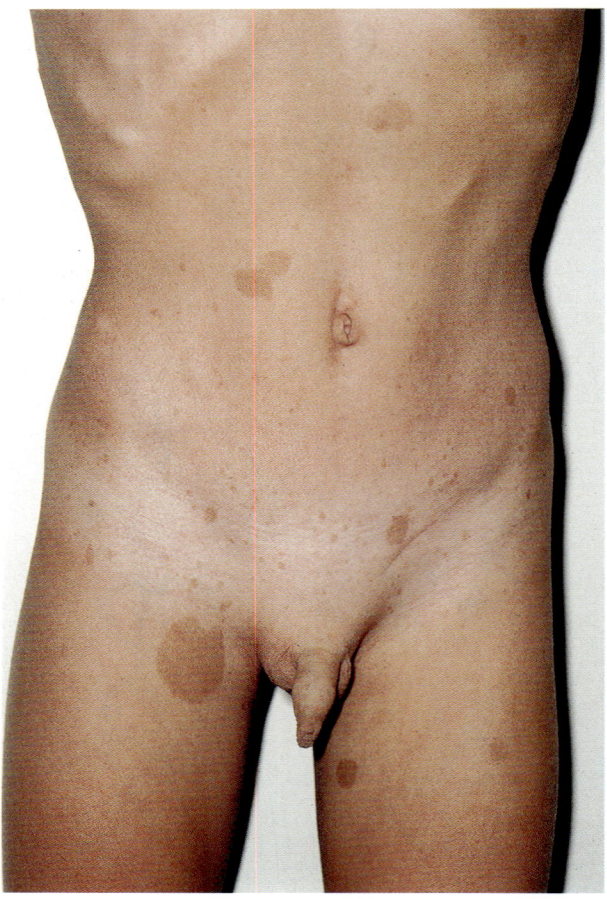

Figure 14.4

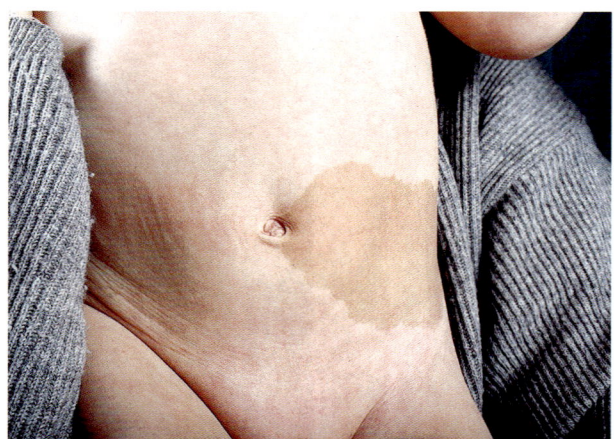

Figure 14.3

- Cutaneous lesions vary widely from subject to subject and even among members of the same family

Extracutaneous symptoms

- Lisch nodules, small multiple papules on iris, pathognomonic of NF1
- Macrocephaly with hypertelorism (Figure 14.18)
- Fibrous dysplasia of the sphenoid, highly characteristic of the disease and usually monolateral
- Scoliosis, lordosis (Figure 14.19) and pseudoarthrosis of joints and dysplastic lesions of the bones
- Optic nerve and chiasmal gliomas, peculiar to NF1
- Rarely, other tumors of the nervous tissue may be detected, such as malignant peripheral nerve sheath tumors but, in general, malignant transformation of tumors is rare
- Early-onset hypertension
- Pulmonary stenosis (this association is known as **Watson syndrome**)
- Classic mental retardation is overemphasized but rarely present and frequently confused with the typical poor performance at school of these patients
- Low attention, dyslexia, scarce propensity to scholar discipline may be severe during the first years of maternal or elementary school, but this gap may be solved during late childhood and pre-puberty
- Soft tissue tumors (retroperitoneal or pelvic)
- Rarely, leukemias in patients with xanthogranulomas

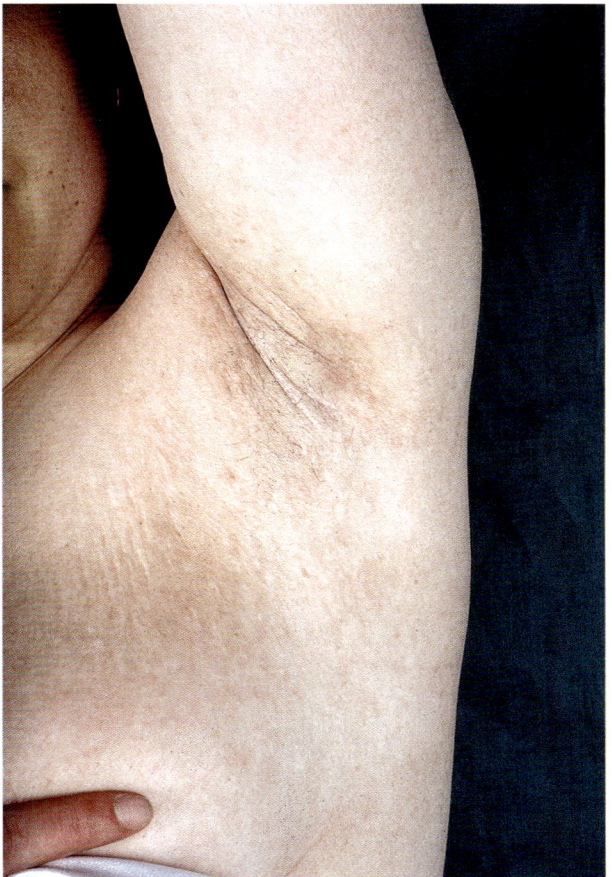

Figure 14.5

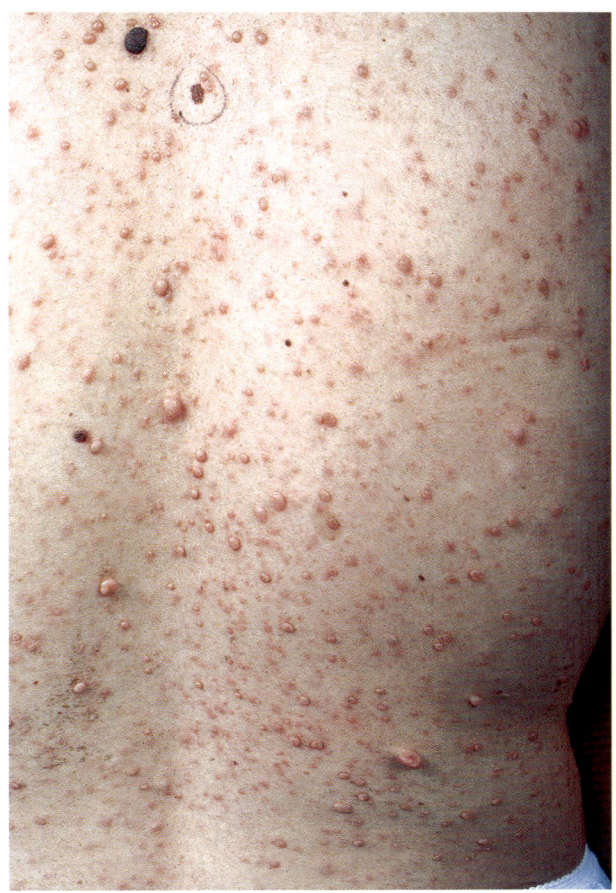

Figure 14.7

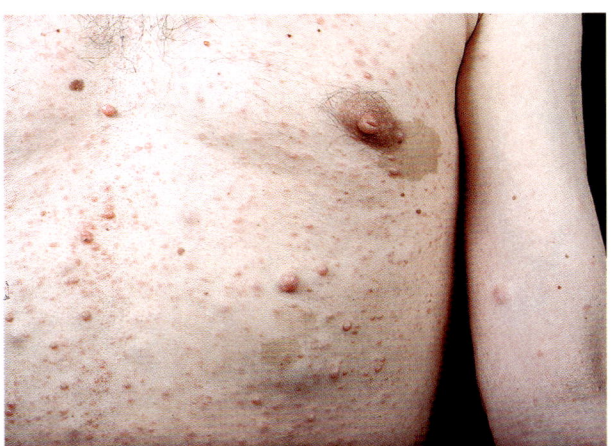

Figure 14.6

Finally, we experienced in our consultations four subtypes of clinical presentation that may reflect a specific genetic pattern:

- Classic NF1 with café-au-lait spots, neurofibromas and plexiform tumors, with associated CNS symptoms (40% of patients)
- Café-au-lait spots alone, without any other cutaneous or extracutaneous sign (Figure 14.19) (40%)
- Almost 'complete' or generalized lentiginosis with intermingled café-au-lait spots with 'buttonhole' (soft-tumors, easily compressible lesions) (5%) (Figure 14.20)
- Generalized neurofibromas, usually of small dimension (100–200 lesions), with plexiform tumors, 'tumeurs royales' and usually very few or absent café-au-lait spots with CNS-associated symptoms (15%) (Figure 14.7)

Course and prognosis

The course of the disease is strictly dependent on the extracutaneous involvement.

Genetics and pathogenesis

- Transmitted as an autosomal dominant trait
- The gene has been mapped on chromosome 17 and called 'neurofibromin'

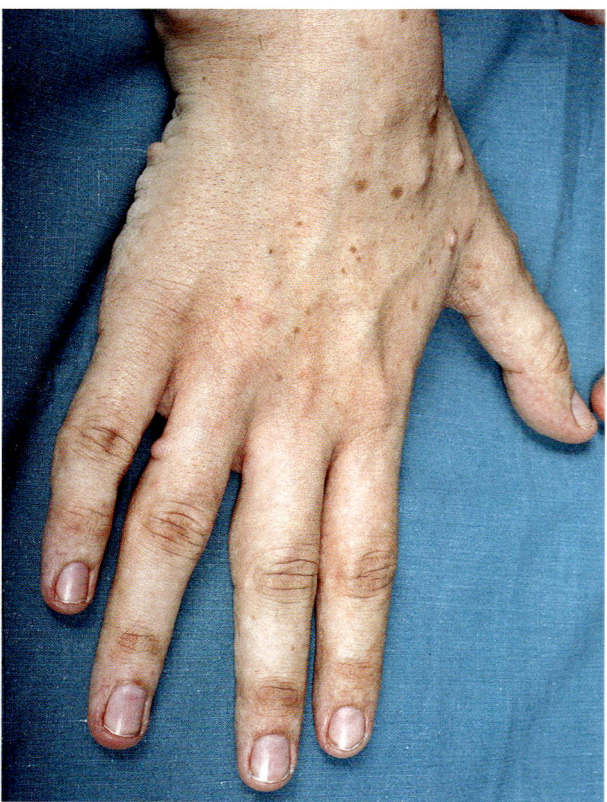

Figure 14.8

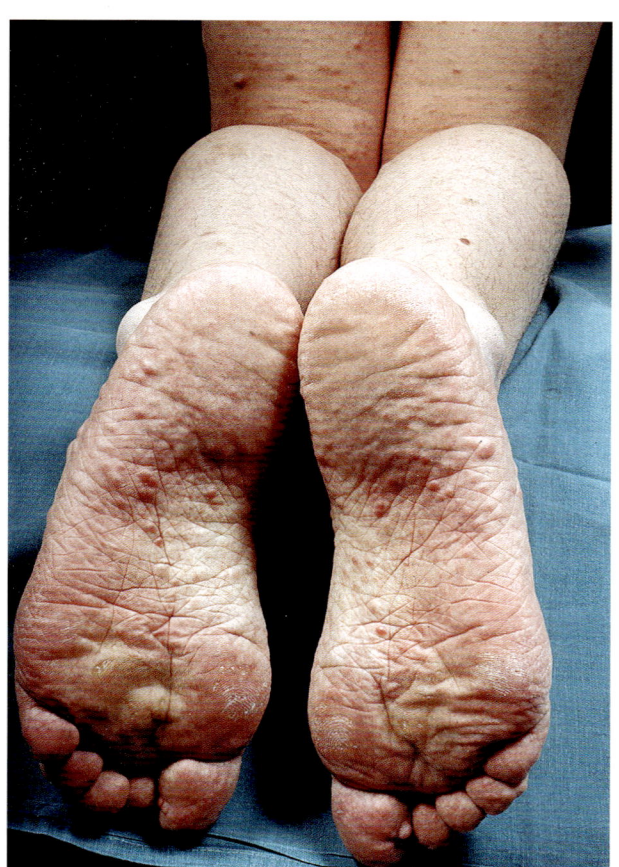

Figure 14.9

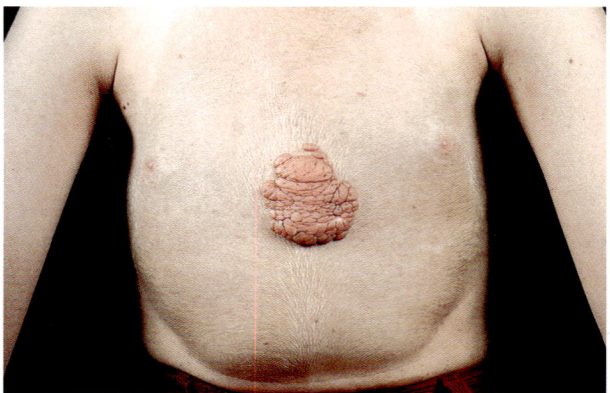

Figure 14.10

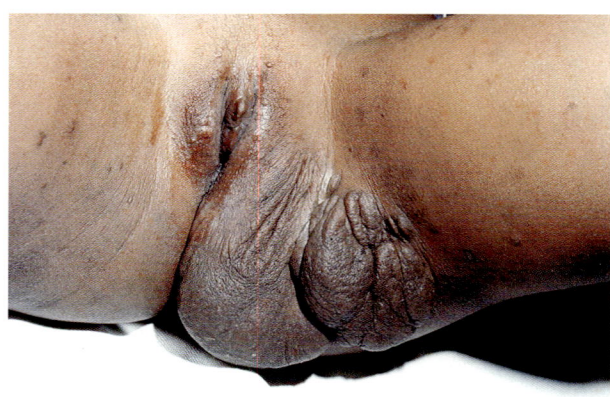

Figure 14.11

- This gene is very large, encodes a member of the GTPase-activating protein (GAP) family and is known to modulate the activity of the *ras* oncogene
- The mutated protein can lead to an impaired cell-cycle control and to abnormal proliferation and differentiation of melanocytes (café-au-lait spots and freckling), Schwann cells (neurofibromas and plexiform tumors) and keratinocytes (modulation of other cell types)
- Molecular search for the mutation is not routinely available and is successful only in half of patients. Prenatal diagnosis is frequently inaccurate
- In the majority of cases a second, postzygotic, mutation is needed to obtain the phenotype of NF1 in patients with 'tumeurs royales' (Figures 14.10–14.12), ('doubling of severity' of a pre-existing dominantly inherited disease)
- Microdeletions in NF1 gene have been recently linked to multiple neurofibromas phenotype

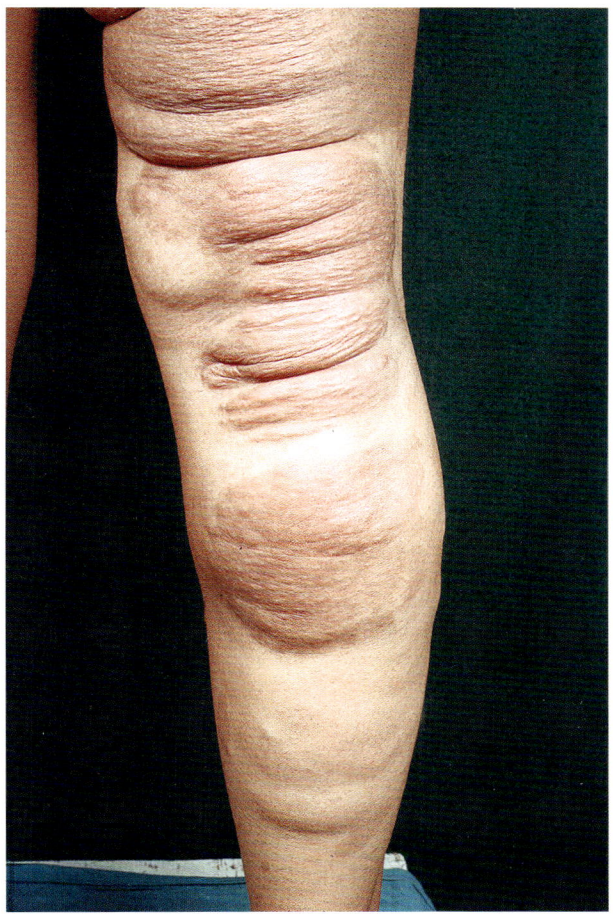

Figure 14.12

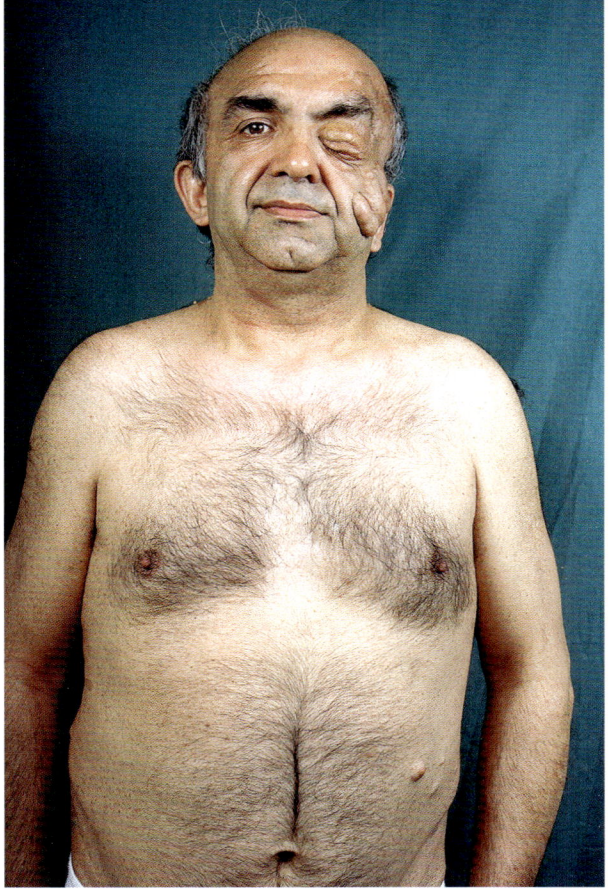

Figure 14.13

Differential diagnosis

Diseases with café-au-lait spots (CLS):

- McCune–Albright syndrome (CLS, polyostotic fibrous dysplasia, hormonal dysfunctions)
- LEOPARD syndrome (CLS diffuse lentiginosis, electrocardiogram abnormalities, pulmonary stenosis, abnormalities of genitalia deafness, growth retardation and ocular hypertelorism)
- Ataxia–telangiectasia (CLS, ataxia and telangiectasis, facial)
- Watson's syndrome (CLS, pulmonary artery stenosis and mental retardation); this is thought to be an allelic form of NF1
- Ringed chromosome disease (CLS and complex malformations)
- Tuberous sclerosis complex
- Turner's syndrome (CLS, pterygium colli, low stature and XO genotype)
- Gorlin syndrome (multiple basal cell tumors, palmoplantar pits, odontogenous cysts, medulloblastomas)

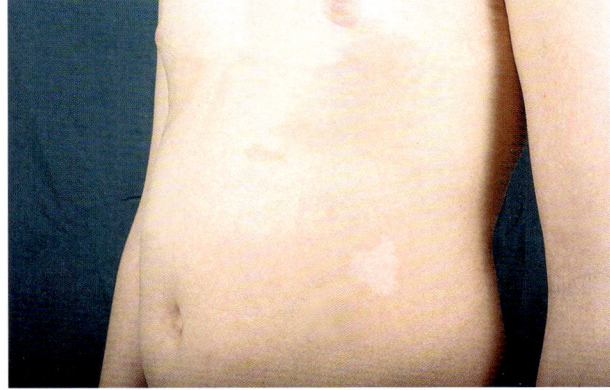

Figure 14.14

- Bloom's syndrome (CLS, erythematous–telangiectatic and poikilodermatous photoexposed skin, photosensitivity, neoplasias)
- Diffuse mastocytosis
- And other, rarest, such as Silver–Russell syndrome, Jaffé's syndrome and Gaucher's syndrome

176 Atlas of Genodermatoses

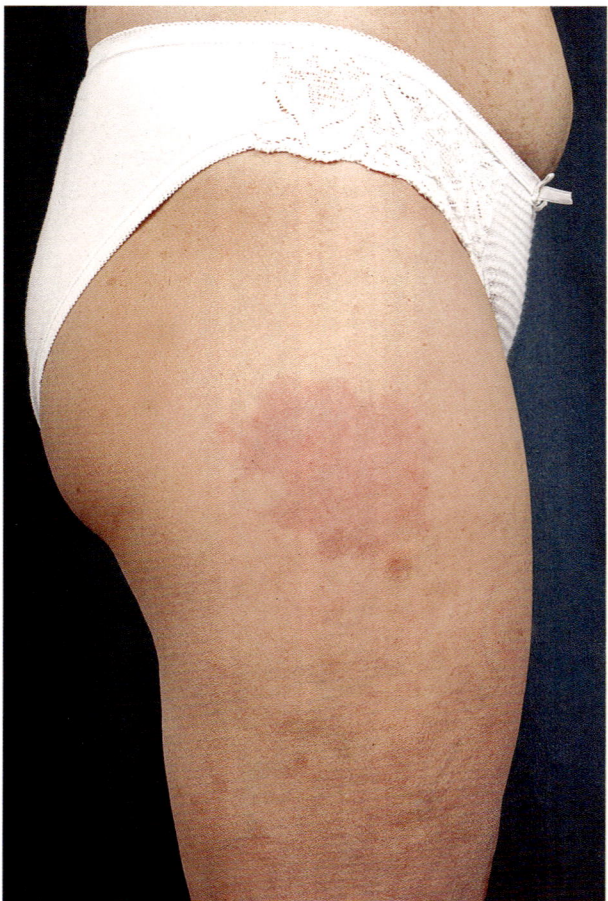

Figure 14.15

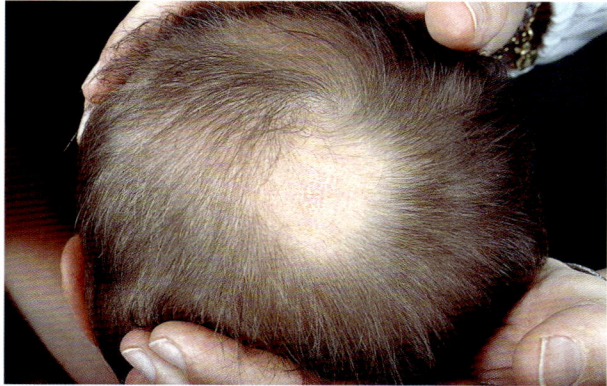

Figure 14.16

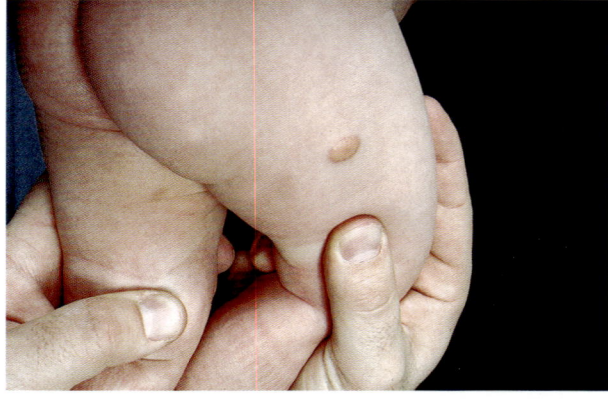

Figure 14.17

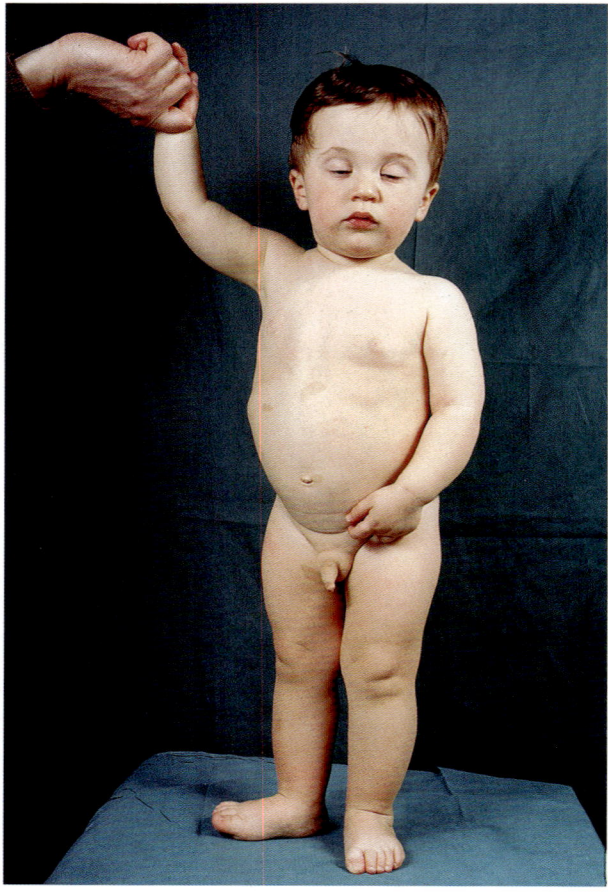

Figure 14.18

Diseases with nodules and soft subcutaneous tumors

- Proteus syndrome
- Encephalocraniocutaneous lipomatosis
- Familial lipomatoses
- Klippel–Trénaunay syndrome
- Bannayan's syndrome
- Maffucci syndrome

Follow-up

- Cutaneous assessment for potentially malignant disease and for borderline cases
- Echotomography to detect visceral lesions or cardiac abnormalities
- Magnetic resonance imaging (MRI) and computed tomography (CT) scan for cerebral or visceral localization

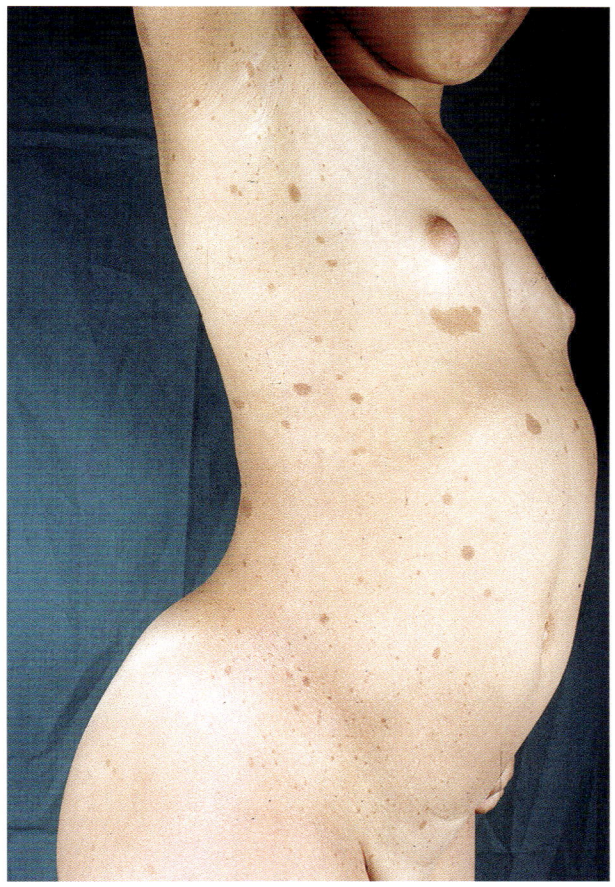

Figure 14.19

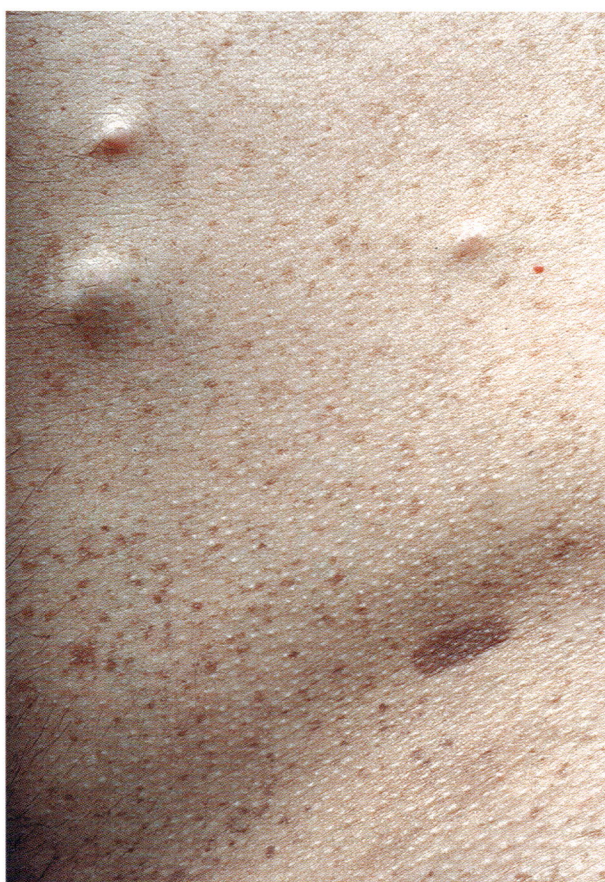

Figure 14.20

- Ophthalmological consultation for Lisch nodules for patients and relatives and detection of chiasmal lesions
- Blood pressure measurement

Therapy

- Surgery is mandatory when hamartomas are painful or for esthetic reasons
- Neurosurgery is rarely recommended for chiasmal or intracranial tumors or for neurofibromas along the peripheral nerve sheath
- Orthopedic support for scoliosis and different osseous abnormalities
- Psychotherapy is advised to detect the degree of mental retardation and for support at school
- Antihypertensive drugs are used to optimize blood pressure
- Antihistaminic drugs for pruritus in case of severe symptoms

REFERENCES

Agesen TH, Florenes VA, Molenaar WM, et al. Expression patterns of cell cycle components in sporadic and neurofibromatosis type 1-related malignant peripheral nerve sheath tumors. J Neuropathol Exp Neurol 2005; 64: 74–81

De Schepper S, Boucneau J, Lambert J, et al. Pigment cell-related manifestations in neurofibromatosis type 1: an overview. Pigment Cell Res 2005; 18: 13–24

Korf BR. The phakomatoses. Clin Dermatol 2005; 23: 78–84 [Review]

Spiegel M, Oexle K, Horn D, et al. Childhood overgrowth in patients with common NF1 microdeletions. Eur J Hum Genet 2005; 13: 883–8

NEUROFIBROMATOSIS TYPE 2

Epidemiology

The disease is rare, with an estimated prevalence of 1 : 20 000–40 000.

Age of onset

- At birth for cutaneous lesions, during childhood or adolescence for extracutaneous symptoms

- Central nervous system (CNS) tumors
- Schwannomas along peripheral nerves
- Mental retardation has been reported

Course and prognosis

The neurinomas of the acoustic nerve may be asymptomatic or create severe impairment of auditory function.

Malignant transformation of CNS tumors is possible.

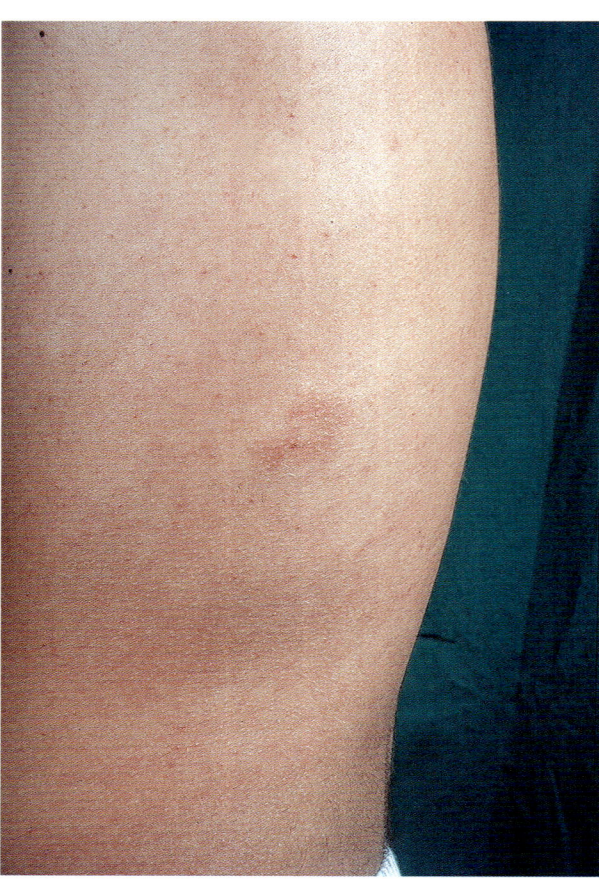

Figure 14.21

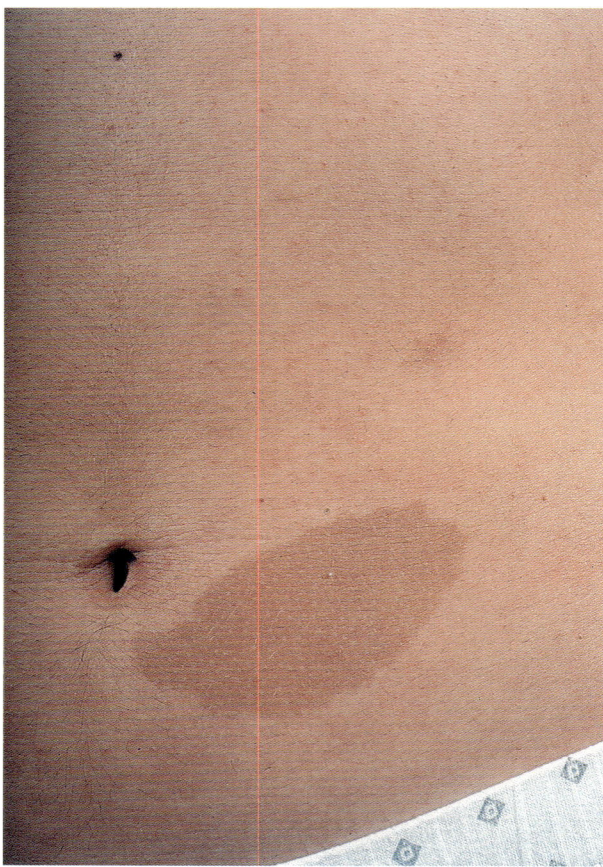

Figure 14.22

Clinical findings

- Café-au-lait spots in 10% of patients (Figure 14.21)
- Small, soft subcutaneous, hamartomatous red-bluish lesions (Figure 14.22)

Extracutaneous findings

- Neurinomas of the acoustic nerve (100% of patients), usually monolateral

Laboratory findings

CT scans and MRI show clearly the intracranial neurinomas and other CNS neoplasias.

Genetics and pathogenesis

- Autosomal dominant inheritance
- Due to mutations of an oncogene suppressor gene encoding 'merlin' that is probably a further

modulator of the cell cycle expressed in neuroectodermally derived cells

Follow-up and therapy

- Acoustic evoked potential in the study of intracranial neurinomas
- Rarely, surgical approach for the latter

Differential diagnosis

- NF1
- Multiple isolated schwannomas (schwannomatosis)

REFERENCES

Chen R, Diamond AS, Vaheesan KR, et al. Retroperitoneal neurofibrosarcoma in a patient with neurofibromatosis 2: A case report and review of the literature. Pediatr Pathol Mol Med 2003; 22: 375–81

Kim H, Kwak NJ, Lee JK, et al. Merlin neutralizes the inhibitory effect of Mdm2 on p53. J Biol Chem 2004; 279: 7812–18

Surace EI, Haipek CA, Gutmann DH. Effect of merlin phosphorylation on neurofibromatosis 2 (NF2) gene function. Oncogene 2004; 23: 580–7

NOONAN'S SYNDROME

Age of onset

- At birth

Clinical findings

Cutaneous manifestations

- Lymphedema of dorsa of hands and feet
- Coarse, curly scalp hair with a low posterior hairline (Figure 14.23)
- Scanty pubic, axillary and beard hair
- Short, wide dystrophic nails
- Increase in the number of pigmented nevi
- Ulerythema ophryogenes
- Elastic skin
- Increased keloid formation

Extracutaneous manifestations

- Typical facies including hypertelorism, downward sloping of the palpebral fissures, low-set ears with a thick helix, depressed nasal bridge, high arched palate, micrognathia, broad or webbed neck (Figure 14.24)
- Short stature with pectus excavatum or carinatum
- Congenital heart defects (pulmonary valvular stenosis)
- Mental retardation
- Cryptorchidism, hypogonadism

Course

This is a lifelong disease.

Laboratory investigations and data

- Radiography of bones and lungs
- Electrocardiography (ECG), electroencephalography (EEG)

Genetics and pathogenesis

There is autosomal dominant inheritance, but also many sporadic cases.

This syndrome is related to mutations in PTPN11 ('non-receptor protein tyrosine phosphatase SHP-2') gene.

Differential diagnosis

- Turner's syndrome

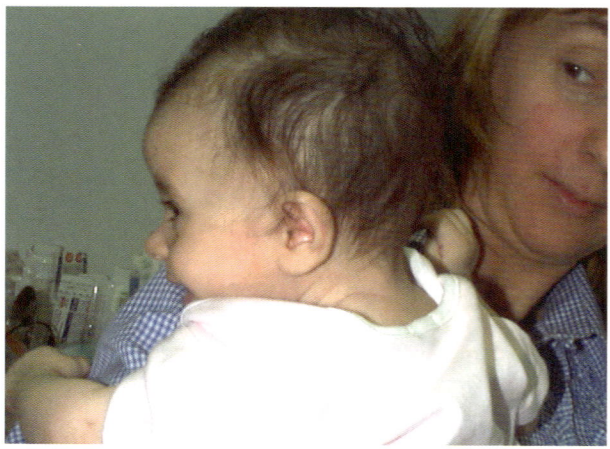

Figure 14.23

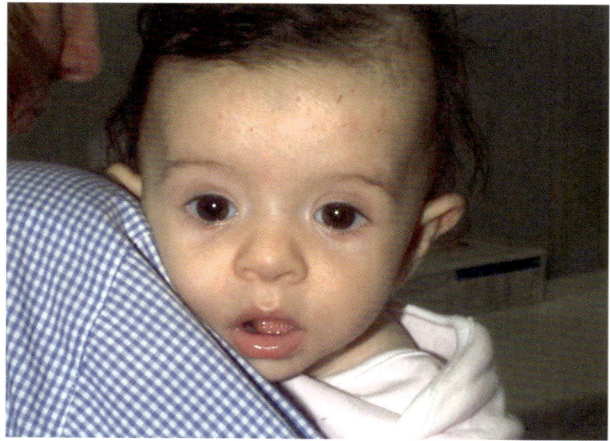

Figure 14.24

Follow-up and therapy

- Multidisciplinary approach
- Prognosis determined by cardiac complications

REFERENCES

Grob JJ, Laure M, Berge G, et al. Les signes cutanées du syndrome de Noonan. Ann Dermatol Venereol 1988; 115: 303–10

Tartaglia M, Cordeddu V, Chang H, et al. Paternal germline origin and sex-ratio distortion in transmission of PTPN11 mutations in Noonan syndrome. Am J Hum Genet 2004; 75: 492–7. Epub 2004; Jul 09

Yoshida R, Hasegawa T, Hasegawa Y, et al. Protein-tyrosine phosphatase, nonreceptor type 11 mutation analysis and clinical assessment in 45 patients with Noonan syndrome. J Clin Endocrinol Metab 2004; 89: 3359–64

TUBEROUS SCLEROSIS COMPLEX

This is described as a complex of cutaneous and extracutaneous symptoms due to the formation of hamartomas.

The prevalence of the disease is 1 : 6000–7000 births, with no racial or sex predilection.

Age of onset

- Hypopigmented macules: (congenital) birth to 3–4 years
- Shagreen patches: up to 3–4 years
- Angiofibromata of the face: 4 years to puberty
- Angiomyolipomas: up to 7–8 years
- Koenen tumors: from puberty

Clinical findings

Skin and mucosae are involved in about 70% of cases.

Hypopigmented macules (HM) are the first visible sign of tuberous sclerosis complex (TSC) and usually precede epilepsy.

- They are oval or leaf shaped, multiple (3–6 on average), visible on any part of the body and normally 1–3 cm in length along the major axis (Figures 14.25–14.28)
- Rarely HM are present on the scalp and are easily visible because of white surrounding hair (Figure 14.29)
- 80% of TSC patients have these whitish macules
- In some cases a picture of irregular diffuse, marble-like hypopigmentation is visible (Figure 14.30)
- Café-au-lait macules are present in a minority of patients (Figure 14.31)
- HM are highly diagnostic in the examination of subjects with early episodes of epilepsy and in families at risk for TSC (Wood's lamp examination)

Angiofibromas of the face (often erroneously described as sebaceous adenomas) are a pathognomonic sign of TSC and are present in more than half of patients.

- Small papules ranging from 1 to 10 mm, pink or frankly red-purple on the cheeks and nose, and less frequently on other areas of the face or neck, in a very variable number from a few papules to hundreds, and rarely can merge to form large plaques (Figures 14.32–14.35)
- Rarely they can be visible in the oral mucosa (Figure 14.36)

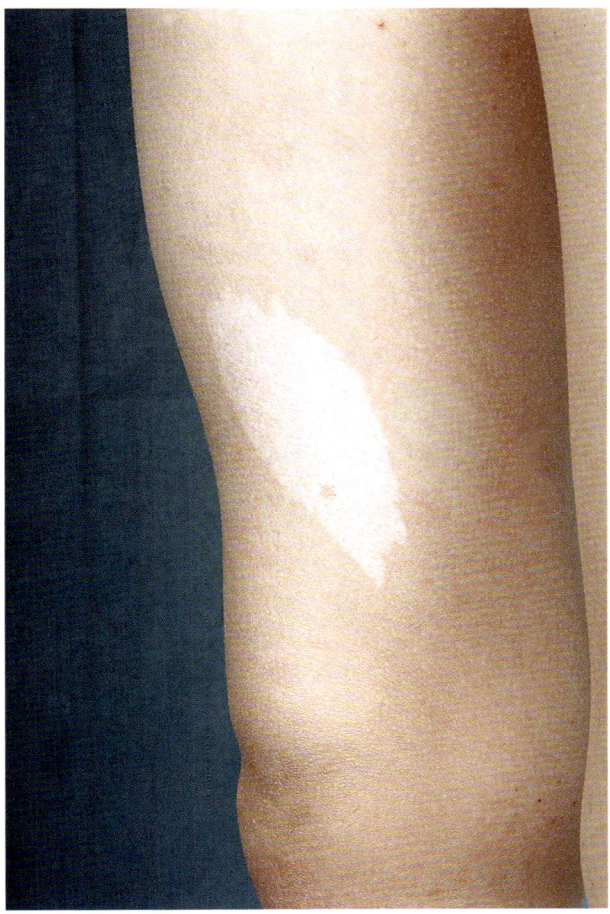

Figure 14.25

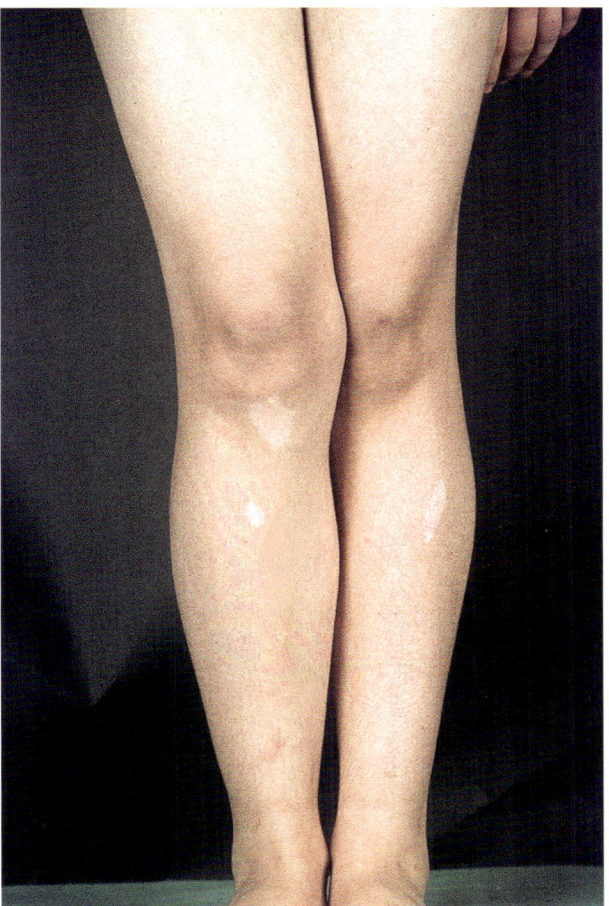

Figure 14.26

- Histologically they show hyperplastic small blood vessels, hyperplastic collagen bundles and normal sebaceous glands
- Differential diagnosis includes acne, trichoepitheliomas and syringomas and xanthomatous lesions
- Segmental (mosaic) forms are possible (Figure 14.37)

Shagreen patches are small hamartomas in plaques of irregular shape and dimension with a pigskin surface, pinkish or light brown colored.

- They can be found elsewhere on the body but are very characteristic of the face and the frontal region, where they are highly diagnostic of TSC (Figures 14.38 and 14.39)

Angiomyolipomas

- They usually have a cobblestone surface appearance and are localized particularly on the trunk and lumbar areas, where they can reach 10–15 cm or more in dimension (Figures 14.40 and 14.41)

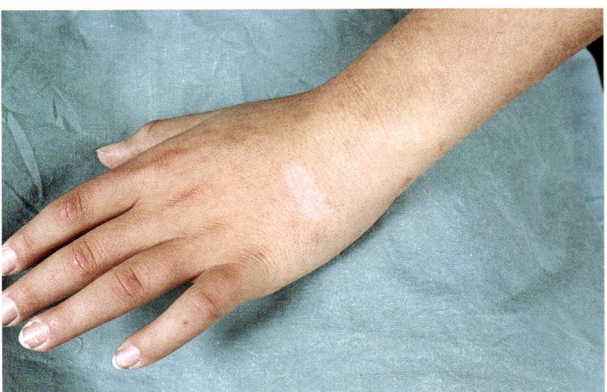

Figure 14.27

- Histologically they are mixed hamartomatous lesions

Koenen tumors or periungual fibromas are firm, rice-grain-like nodules, irregular in shape and dimension and number, that arise from the periungual folds on toes and fingers (Figures 14.42–14.44)

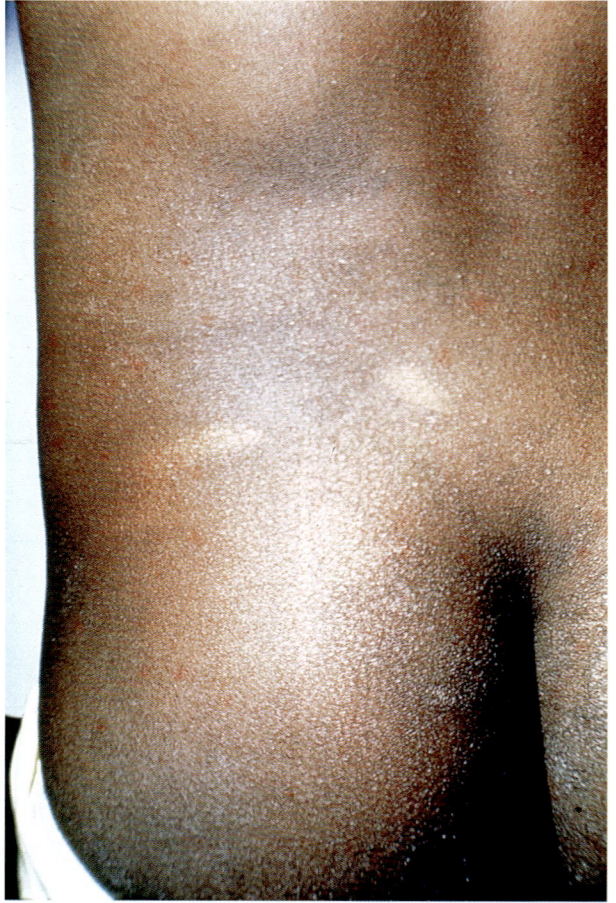

Figure 14.28

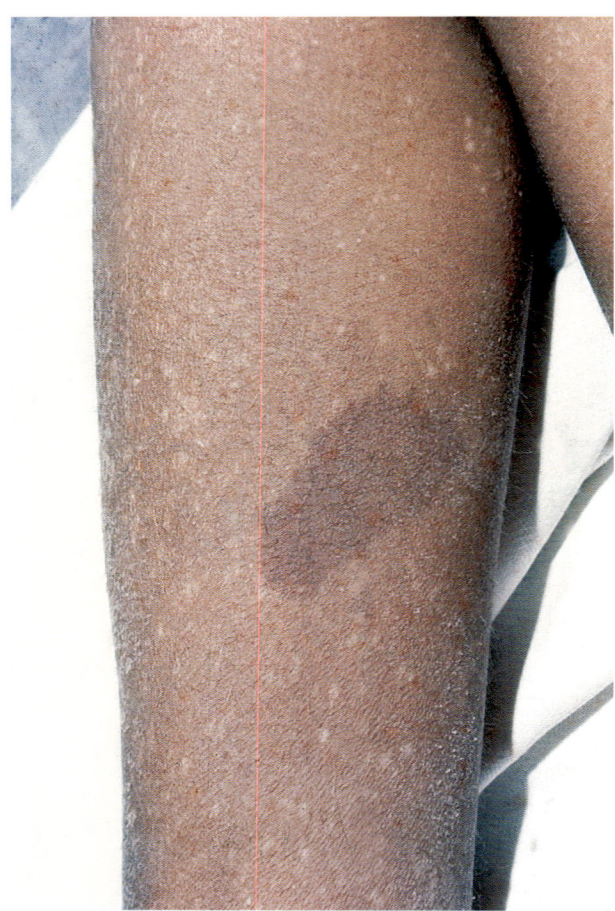

Figure 14.30

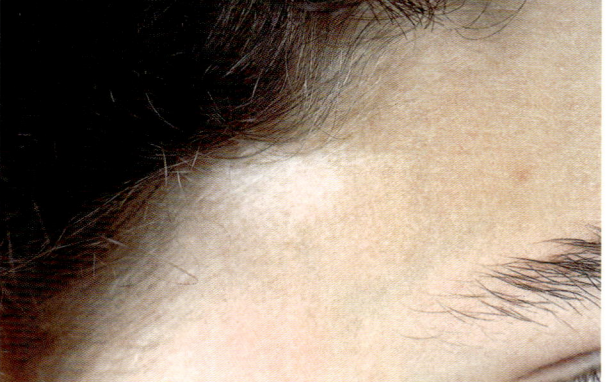

Figure 14.29

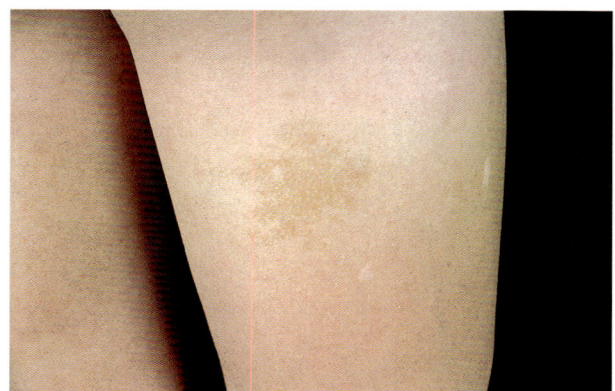

Figure 14.31

- They range from 2 to 20 mm, are usually multiple, and have variable scaling on the surface. Periungual fibromas are usually painless but disabling
- Other cutaneous symptoms are café-au-lait spots (Figures 14.30 and 14.31) and cervical skin tags. More rarely, angiomatous lesions can be detected

- In the oral mucosa (30% of patients) gingival hyperproliferative lesions can be found, papular or in plaques (Figure 14.45), less frequently visible on the tongue or in the palate
- Dental pitting is referred to in the literature
- In rare cases hamartomas are present in the upper digestive or respiratory tracts

Neurocutaneous syndromes

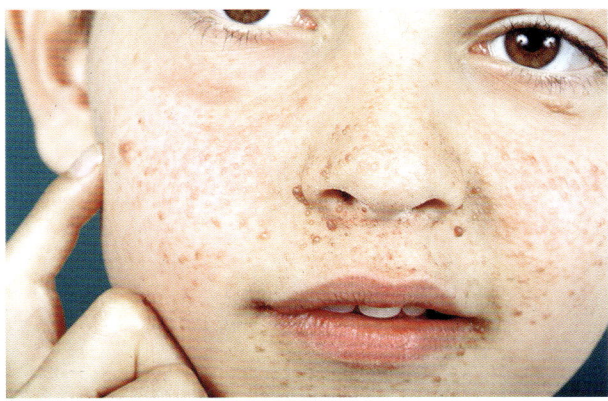

Figure 14.32

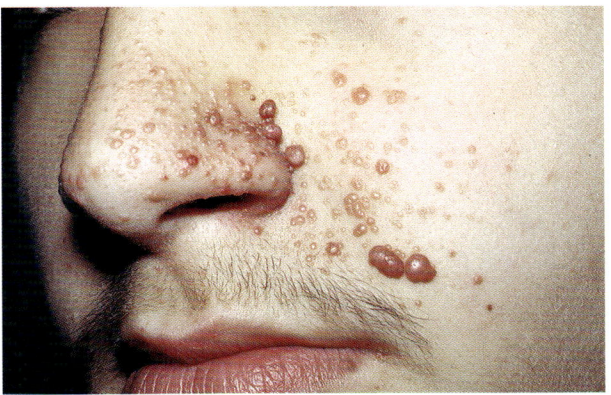

Figure 14.33

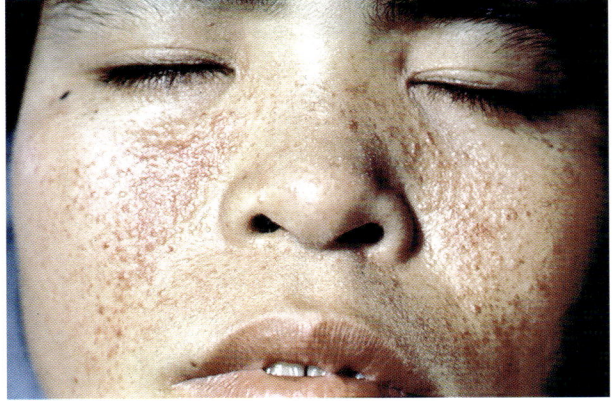

Figure 14.34

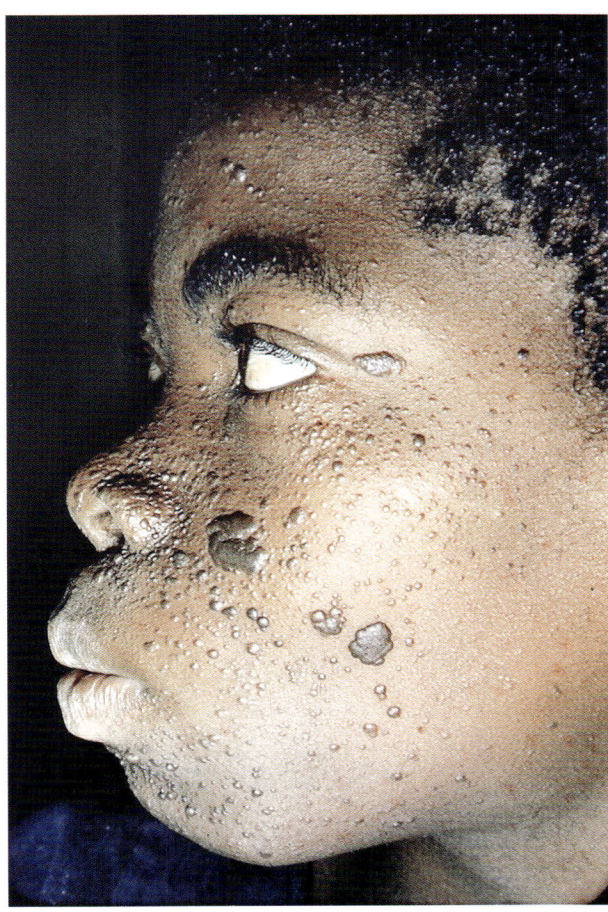

Figure 14.35

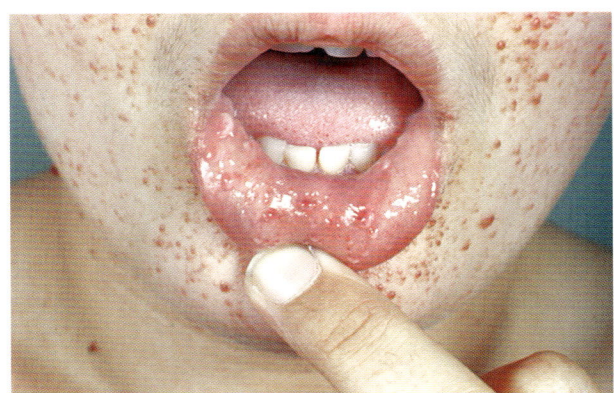

Figure 14.36

Extracutaneous findings

Central nervous system

- Epilepsy is the most common sign of TSC (90%) and represents the first symptom of the disease, given that more than two-thirds of patients with epilepsy show this symptom before the second year of life
- Epilepsy is of the infantile spasms type or West's ipsarrhythmia, but later different kinds of seizure are diagnosed (focal or generalized epilepsy)
- Mental retardation (60–70% of patients) is linked almost always with seizures and is of very variable severity
- In some patients anomalies of behavior are present, and less frequently schizophrenia and

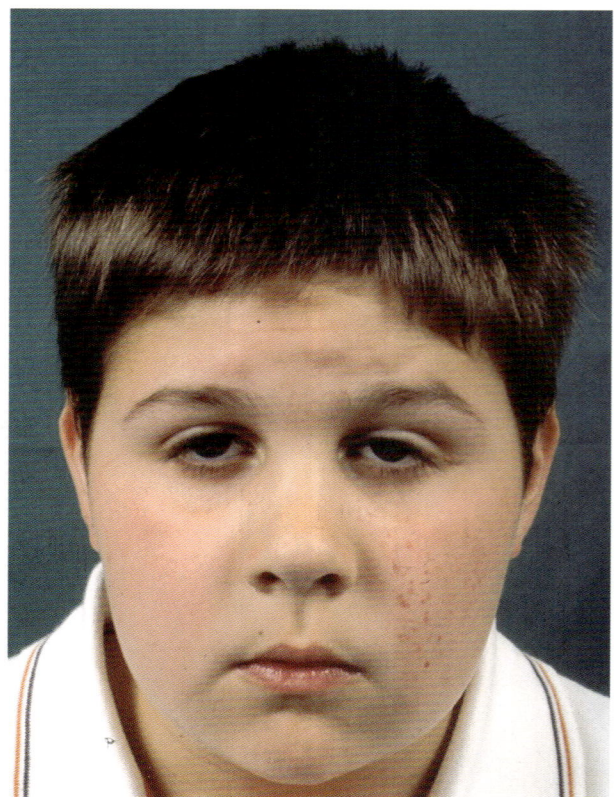

Figure 14.37

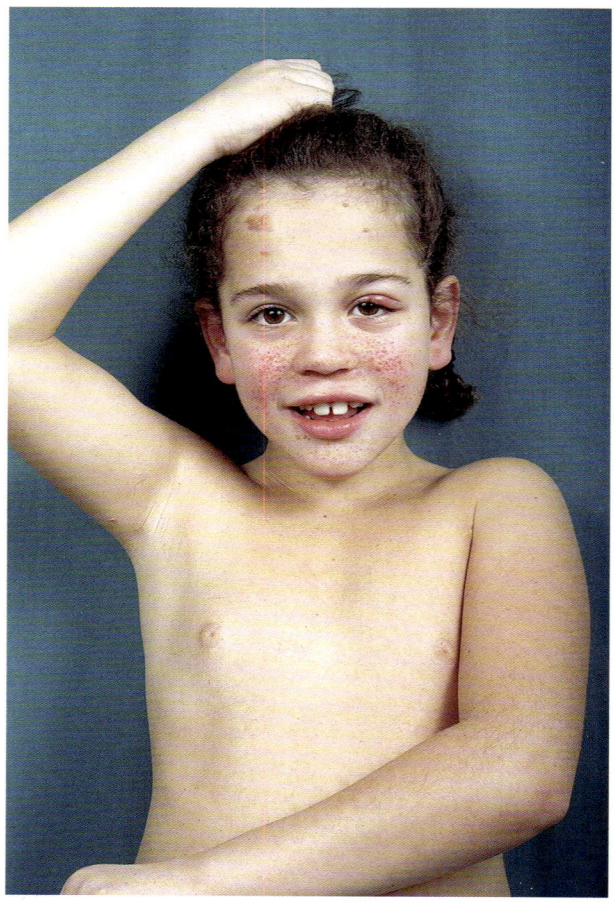

Figure 14.39

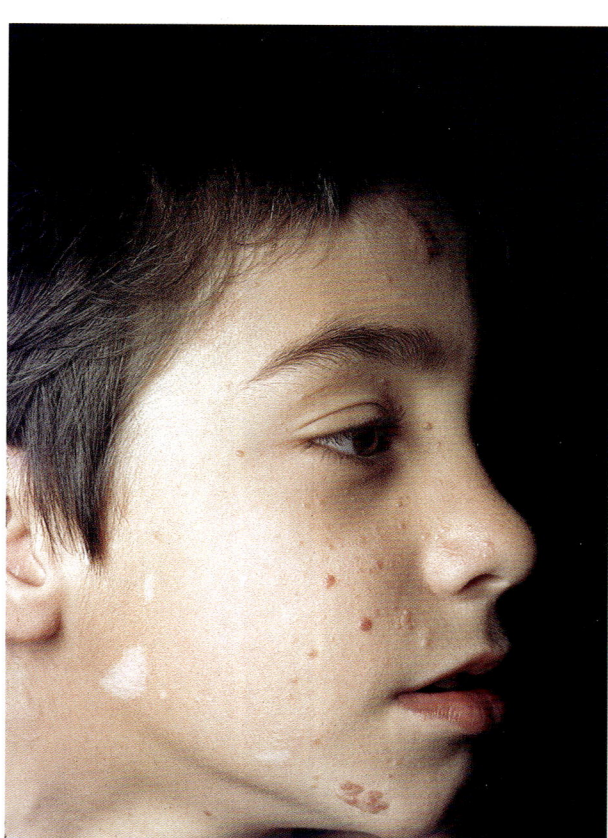

Figure 14.38

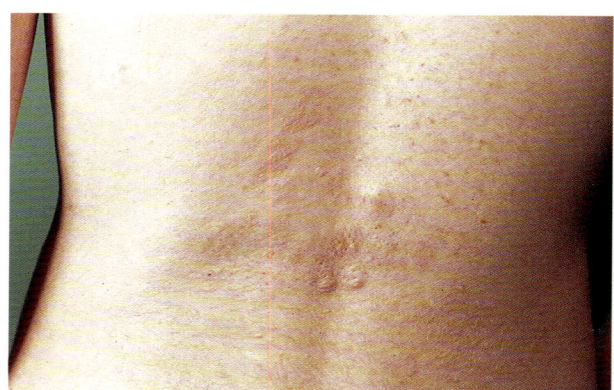

Figure 14.40

autism are diagnosed. The severity of the CNS symptoms is strictly due to the presence of cerebral hamartomas, the 'tuberi', to their localization, number and size

- Tuberi are usually cortical but are detected at the subependymal level around the foramen of Munro and the nucleus caudatus, rarely causing

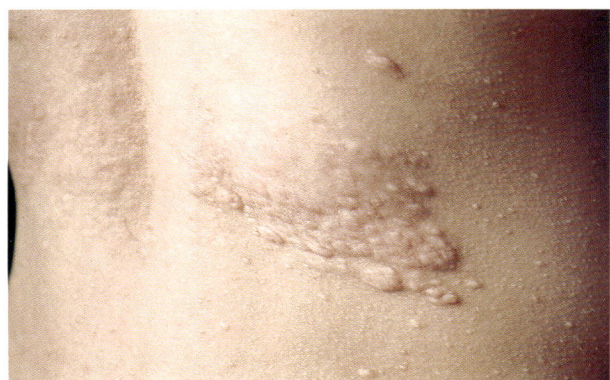

Figure 14.41

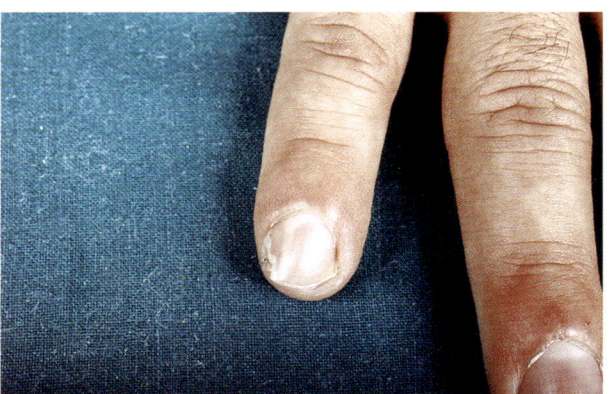

Figure 14.44

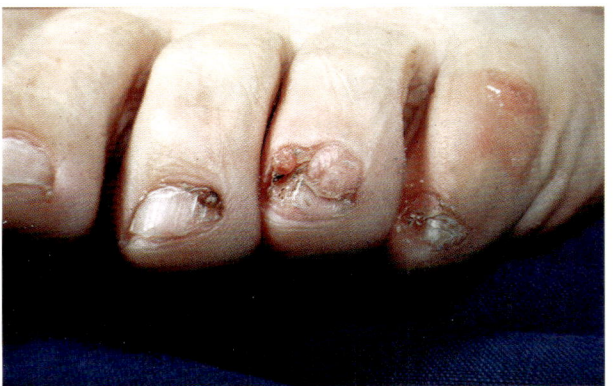

Figure 14.42

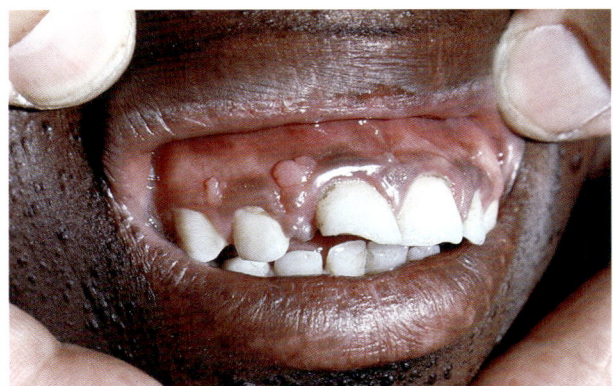

Figure 14.45

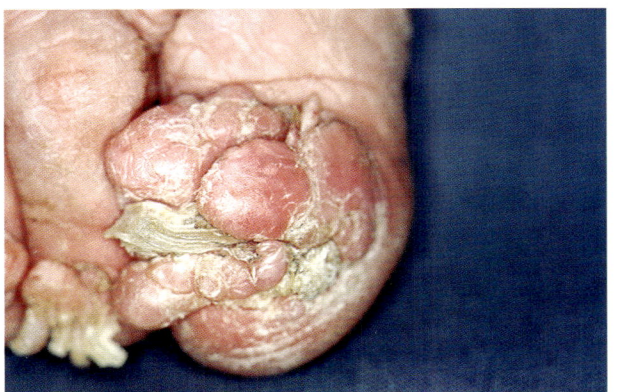

Figure 14.43

- Cardiac rhabdomyomas are present during pregnancy, when they are diagnosed by ultrasonography
- 80% of patients suffering from rhabdomyomas at birth are affected by TSC
- Usually rhabdomyomas are asymptomatic and resolve spontaneously within 2–3 years
- Wolff–Parkinson–White arrhythmias are possible
- More than 70% of patients affected by TSC develop renal angiolipomas that are usually multiple and bilateral and can reach large dimensions
- Polycystic kidney is associated with TSC in about 10% and in this case chronic renal failure is possible
- In some female subjects pulmonary lymphangiomatosis is present as a sign of segmental TSC

hydrocephalus. Malignant tumors (subependymal giant-cell astrocytoma) associated with TSC are reported

Other clinical signs

- Ophthalmologically, the so-called 'phakomas' are visible as small yellow-grayish nodules on the retina, asymptomatic; very rarely macular depigmentation is detectable on the iris

Diagnostic protocol

- Clinical examination for cutaneous signs with Wood's lamp
- Neurological examination and EEG for epilepsy
- Psychological and psychiatric examination for behavioral disturbances
- MRI and CT for the detection of 'tuberi' and striae that are highly diagnostic for TSC, and represent the

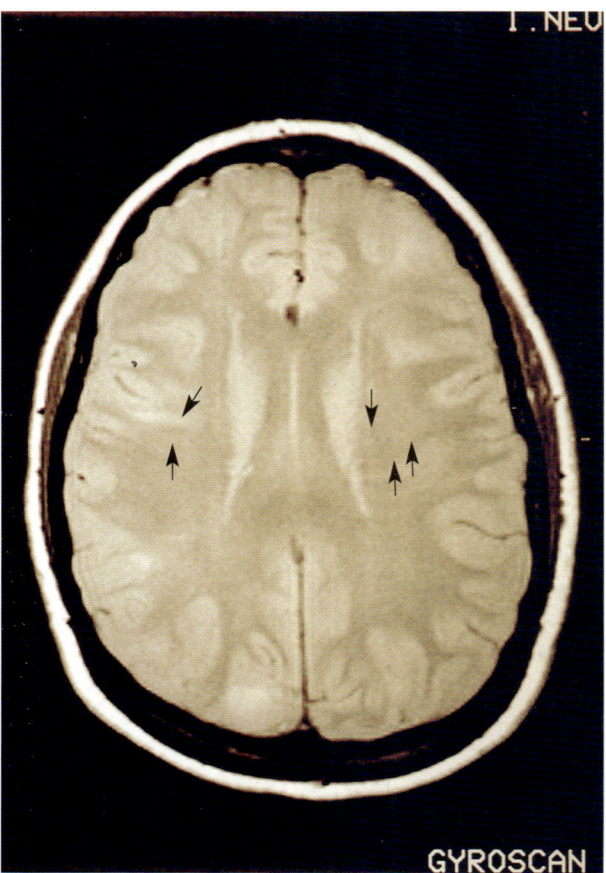

Figure 14.46

putative cerebral Blaschko's lines that the affected stem cells follow, tracing their pathway, starting from the ependyma to reach the cortex. Obviously, as they occur in epidermis (see also Figure 25.3), these embryological pathways are always the same and are reproducible in each patient, as demonstrated by the examination of RMI of different STC patients (Figure 14.46, arrows)
- Echocardiography for rhabdomyomas
- Echotomography for renal and hepatic localizations
- Ophthalmological examination
- Molecular biology for the detection of mutations on STC1 and STC2 genes (blood and tissues)

Genetics and pathogenesis

In one-third of patients an autosomal dominant inheritance is demonstrable for the pedigree.

About two-thirds are so-called 'sporadic cases' due to 'spontaneous mutations' that could be a result of gonadal (germinal) mutations in the parents of a somatic mutation. In this case the affected patients are true 'mosaic', and this possibly explains the finding of 'mosaic TSC' affecting only one area of skin (Figure 14.37).

For TSC to be fully developed, a second mutation ('two-step' disease) is needed other than the first inherited, in the second allele (allelic loss). The severity and diffusion of the disease depends on the precocity of the second mutation (early embryonic mutation = very severe disease, late mutation = milder phenotype). This phenomenon explains the wide phenotypic variability in TSC patients, even in the same pedigree.

Two genes have been detected and related to TSC, TSC1 (9q34) that encodes a nuclear protein called 'hamartin', and TSC2 (16p13.3) that encodes a Golgi apparatus protein called 'tuberin'. Both molecules have a role in the regulation of proliferation and differentiation, and their mutation leads to hyperproliferation (hamartomas). Mutations of TSC1 and TSC2 account for at least 60% of TSC patients, and 'low-level mosaicism' can explain the negativity in the other 40%, given that molecular tests are performed on blood cells and not in other cell lines or tissues.

TSC1 accounts for 80% of mutations, and TSC2 for 20%.

TSC2 seems to be related to epilepsy.

Follow-up and therapy

This is similar to the above 'diagnostic protocol', and includes:

- Clinical examination for cutaneous signs with Wood's lamp
- Neurological examination and EEG for epilepsy
- Psychological and psychiatric examination for behavioral disturbances
- MRI and CT for the detection of 'tuberi', their localization, size and number
- Echocardiography for rhabdomyomas
- Echotomography for renal and hepatic localizations
- Ophthalmological examination
- Surgical and laser therapy (combined CO_2 and dye laser) for angiofibromas of the face
- Pharmacological therapy for epilepsy (vigabatrim)
- Rarely, cardiosurgery for rhabdomyomas or β-blockers for arrhythmias
- Psychological approach for school and social problems

Differential diagnosis

- Neurofibromatoses (angiolipomas)
- Hypomelanotic nevi (segmental hypomelanotic lesions)
- Fabry's disease (angiofibromas)
- Acne vulgaris

REFERENCES

Ali M, Girimaji SC, Markandaya M, et al. Mutation and polymorphism analysis of TSC1 and TSC2 genes in Indian patients with tuberous sclerosis complex. Acta Neurol Scand 2005; 111: 54–63

Conrad GR, Sinha P. FDG PET imaging of subependymal gray matter heterotopia. Clin Nucl Med 2005; 30: 35–6

Crooks DM, Pacheco-Rodriguez G, DeCastro RM, et al. Molecular and genetic analysis of disseminated neoplastic cells in lymphangioleiomyomatosis. Proc Natl Acad Sci USA 2004; 101: 17462–7. Epub 2004; Dec 06

Govindarajan B, Brat D, Csete M, et al. Transgenic expression of dominant negative tuberin through a strong constitutive promoter results in a tissue-specific tuberous sclerosis phenotype in the skin and brain. J Biol Chem 2004; 2

Mak BC, Yeung RS. The tuberous sclerosis complex genes in tumor development. Cancer Invest 2004; 22: 588–603

CARDIOFACIO-CUTANEOUS SYNDROME

Synonym

- CFC syndrome

Epidemiology

More than 100 cases have been described, with many having different conditions (Noonan's syndrome).

Age of onset

- At birth

Clinical findings

- Usually mild, patchy ichthyosiform condition on arms and legs to severe generalized ichthyosis and palmoplantar hyperkeratosis (Figure 14.47)
- Keratosis pilaris (scalp) (Figure 14.48)
- Occasionally pigmentation disorders
- Sparse, friable and curly hair (Figure 14.48)
- Sparse or absent eyebrows

Extracutaneous symptoms

- Turricephalic vault with high forehead
- Bitemporal constriction

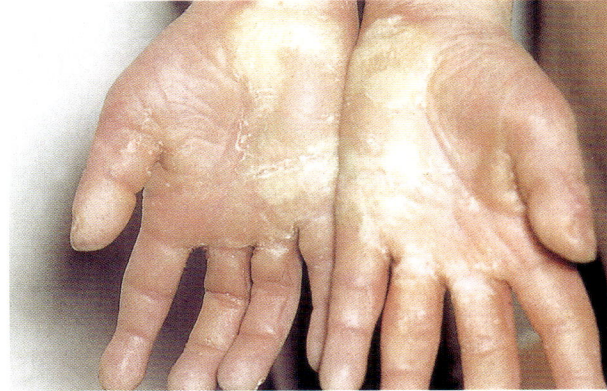

Figure 14.47

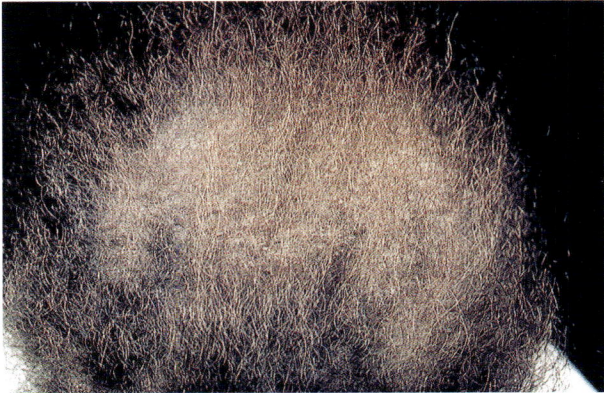

Figure 14.48

- Hypoplastic supraorbitary ridges
- Low nasal bridge, large alae
- Upturned nose
- Protruding upper lip
- Short neck
- Ptosis, strabismus and nystagmus are common
- Growth retardation is usual (>75%)
- Macrocephaly
- Mental retardation with speech impairment and epilepsy
- Pulmonary stenosis (50%) and atrial and ventricular septal defects

Laboratory findings

There are none specific.

Genetics and pathogenesis

CFC is sporadic; true familial cases are not demonstrated and probably have Noonan's syndrome.

The gene responsible for CFC is mapped to locus 12q21.2.

Exclusion of PTPN11 mutations in CFC syndrome.

Follow-up and therapy

- Early detection of cardiac defect and surgery when appropriate
- Neurologic consultation and rehabilitation for mental retardation
- Emollients for dry skin

Differential diagnosis

- Noonan's syndrome
- NF1/Watson's syndrome

REFERENCES

Kavamura MI, Pomponi MG, Zollino M, et al. PTPN11 mutations are not responsible for the cardiofaciocutaneous (CFC) syndrome. Eur J Hum Genet 2003; 11: 64–8

Musante L, Kehl HG, Majewski F, et al. Spectrum of mutations in PTPN11 and genotype-phenotype correlation in 96 patients with Noonan syndrome and five patients with cardio-facio-cutaneous syndrome. Eur J Hum Genet 2003; 11: 201–6. Erratum in: Eur J Hum Genet 2003; 11: 551

Neri G, Kavamura MI, Zollino M, et al. CFC syndrome. Am J Med Genet A 2003; 116: 410

Tartaglia M, Cotter PD, Zampino G, et al. Exclusion of PTPN11 mutations in Costello syndrome: further evidence for distinct genetic etiologies for Noonan, cardio-facio-cutaneous and Costello syndromes. Clin Genet 2003; 63: 423–6

PHAKOMATOSIS PIGMENTOKERATOTICA

Synonym

- Epidermal–melanocytic twin nevus syndrome

Epidemiology

Since our first description in the early 1990s, at least 20 other cases have been described or communicated.

Clinical findings

This recently recognized disease is characterized by the contemporaneous presence of an epidermal–sebaceous nevus (ESN) and a speckled lentiginous nevus (SLN) (Figures 14.49–14.52) (or more rarely a melanocytic nevus (Figure 14.53)) associated with body hemihypotrophy (Figures 14.54–14.56) and neurological abnormalities such as dysesthesia and hyperhydrosis (Figures 14.57).

The two nevoid lesions are distributed along the lines of Blaschko (ESN) and as a checkerboard pattern (SLN), following the rules of 'twin-spot' lesions. They

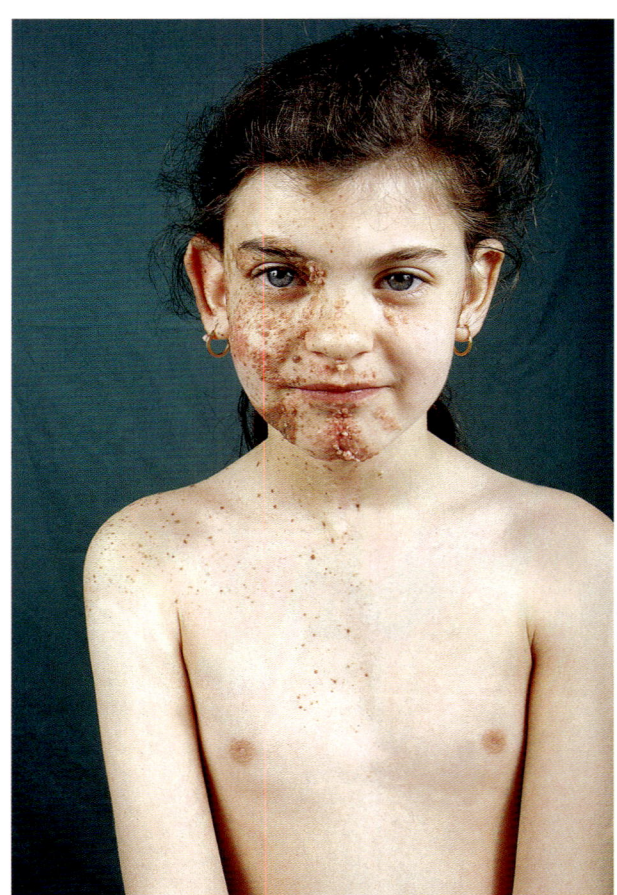

Figure 14.49

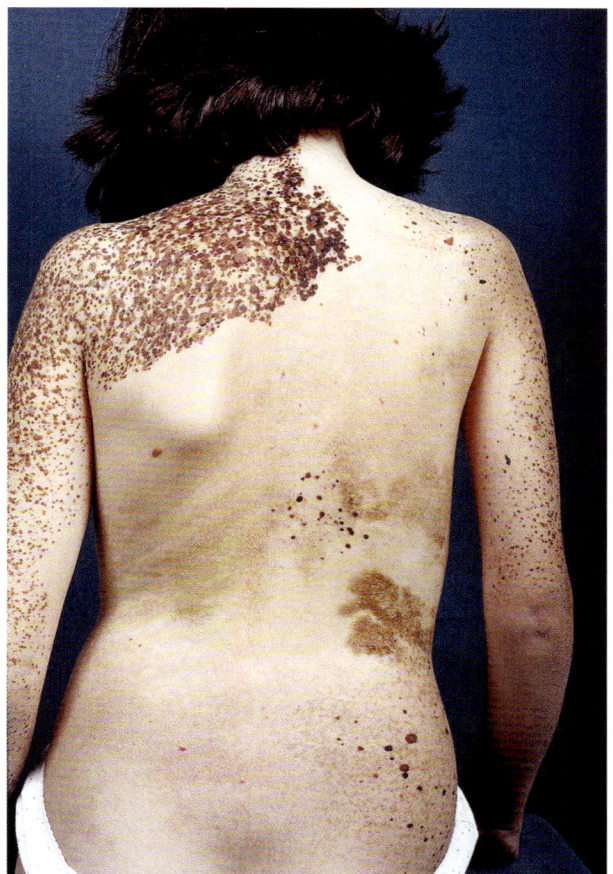

Figure 14.50

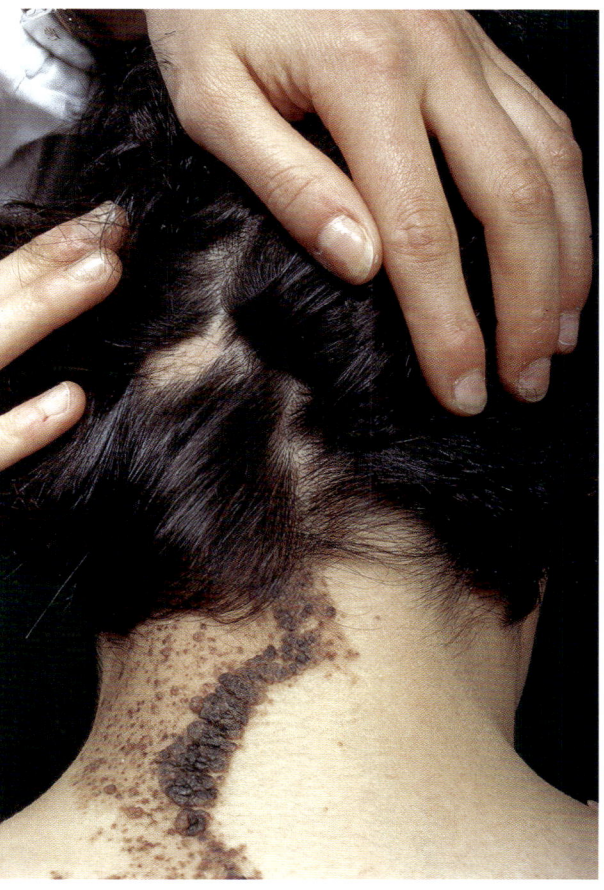

Figure 14.51

may occur in any part of the body, and may be homo- or contralateral.

Extracutaneous symptoms

The hemiatrophy is strictly related to the presence of the nevi, as are the neurological abnormalities. The former can be visible as a minor asymmetry of the face, or may be related to the whole body with true hemiatrophy (Figures 14.54–14.56) with reactive scoliosis (Figure 14.58) and shortening of the arms and/or legs (Figure 14.55). The latter are present as peculiar tactile disturbances (the patient feels a disturbing sensation even when touched during the consultation) or as hyperhydrosis, i.e. superimposed to the SLN (Figure 14.57). In a few patients, various degrees of mental retardation have been reported, as well as ocular anomalies (colobomas).

Course and prognosis

Nevi grow progressively with age. In SLN there is an increased risk of melanoma.

Dysesthesias persist steadily with age.

Hemiatrophy may cause major orthopedic conditions, such as severe scoliosis or impairment of walking.

Laboratory findings

To date, neither ESN nor SLN has its genetic counterpart.

The involved autonomous peripheral fibers have abnormal speed of progression of the nervous signals, as demonstrated by the evoked potentials measured in comparison with those associated with healthy sites.

Genetics and pathogenesis

This complex is the result of a very precocious postzygotic mutation involving the whole ectodermal sheet and is a further example of the 'twin-spots' theory (see Chapter 25, 'Cutaneous mosaicism'). The hemiatrophy is due to possible involvement of an ancestral gene responsible for the symmetry and metamerical division of the body.

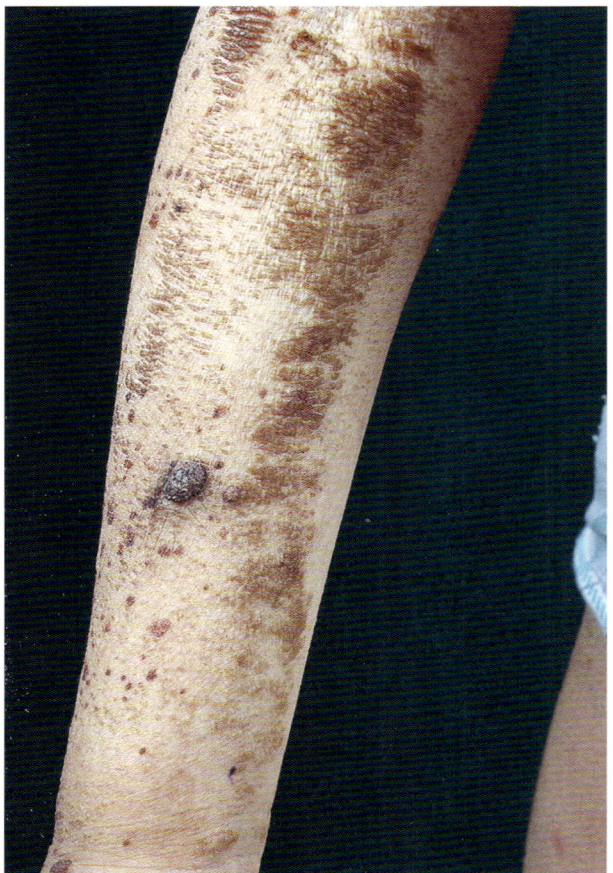

Figure 14.52

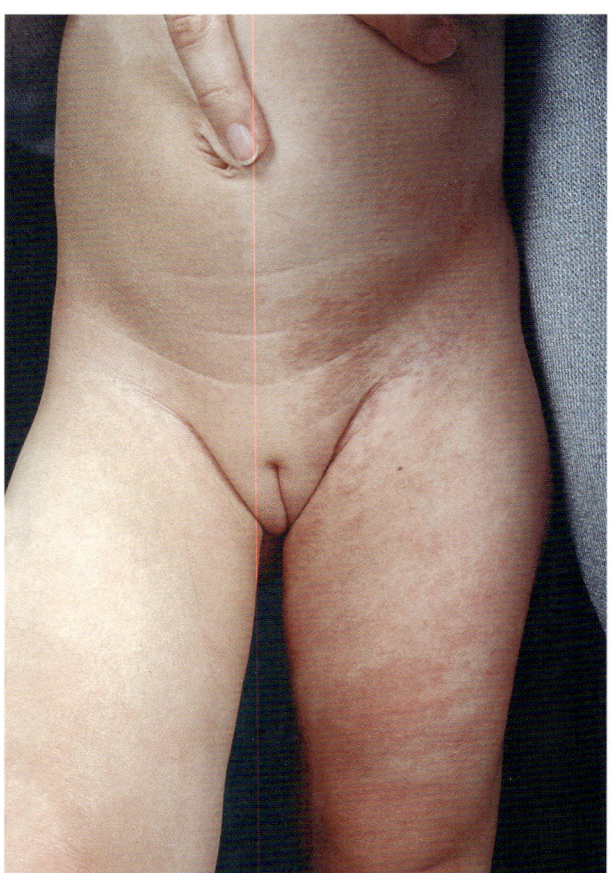

Figure 14.53

Follow-up and therapy

The SLN must be monitored for potential malignant transformation. A multidisciplinary approach is recommended for the evaluation of orthopedic anomalies such as scoliosis and asymmetry of the arms and legs. CT and MRI are used to detect eventual central nervous system anomalies when the disease is located on the face and head. Dysesthesias may be painful or greatly uncomfortable for patients, and modulatory neuropharmacological therapy is advised as well as psychological support.

A surgical approach is recommended to remove potentially evolving lesions, both melanocytic and epidermal nevi. Laser therapy may be helpful to remove large lesions for esthetic reasons. Orthopedic devices and physical therapy are suggested for scoliosis and asymmetries.

Differential diagnosis

- Epidermal–sebaceous nevus syndrome
- Proteus syndrome
- Phakomatosis pigmentovascularis

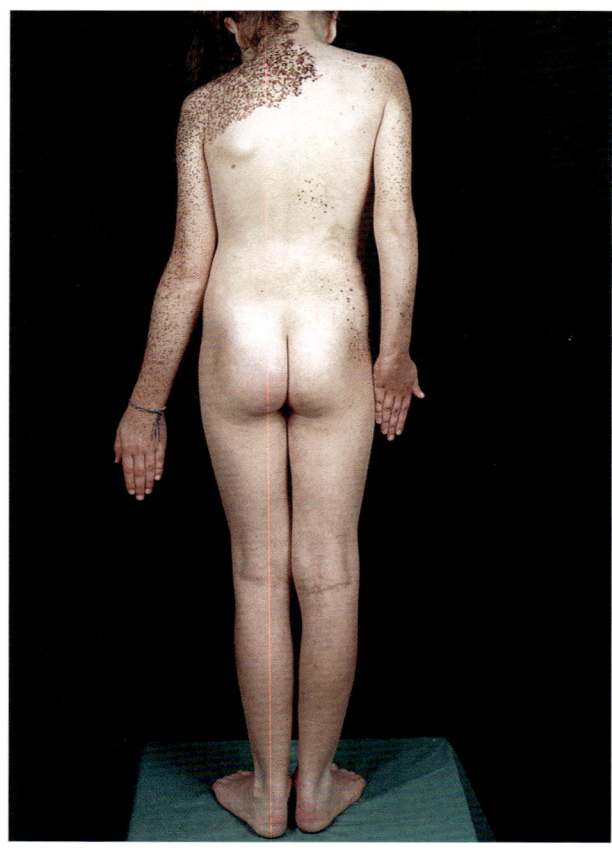

Figure 14.54

Neurocutaneous syndromes

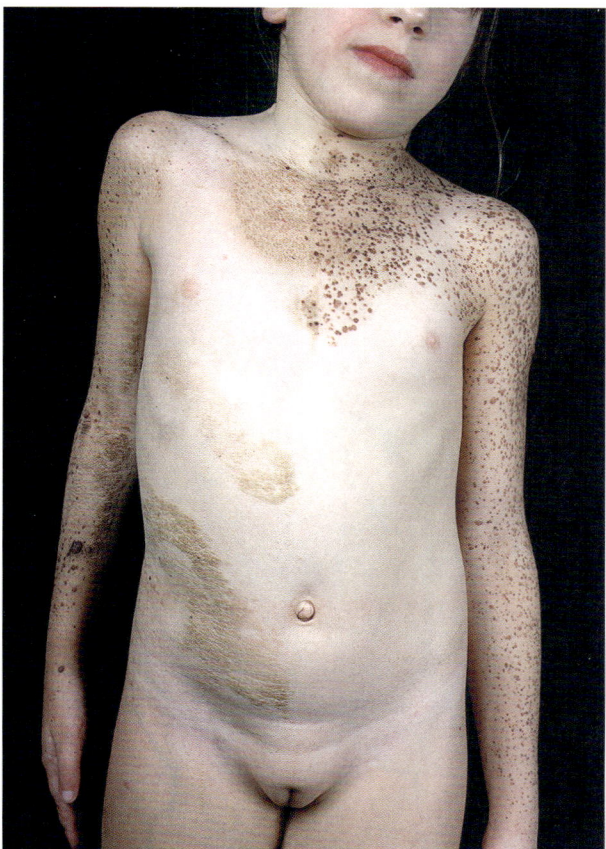

Figure 14.55

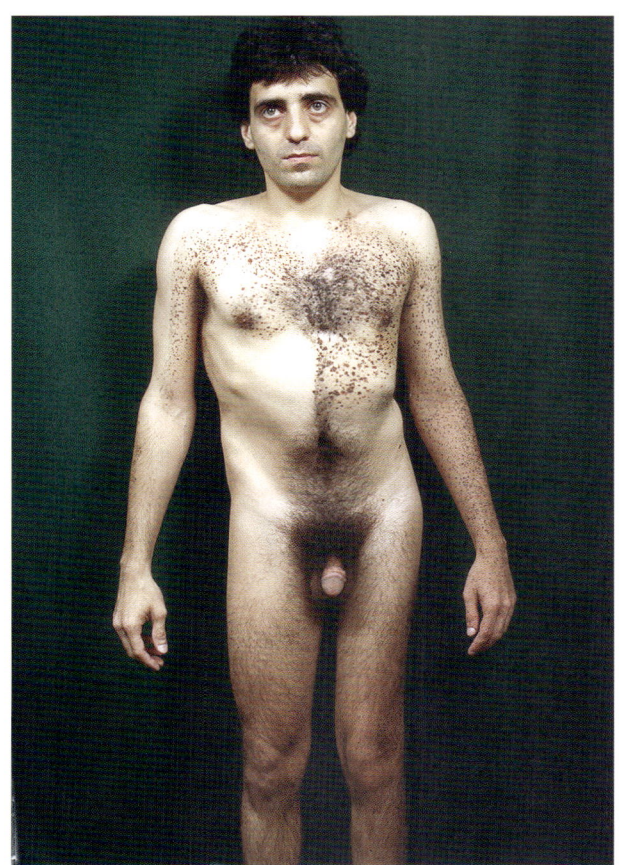

Figure 14.56

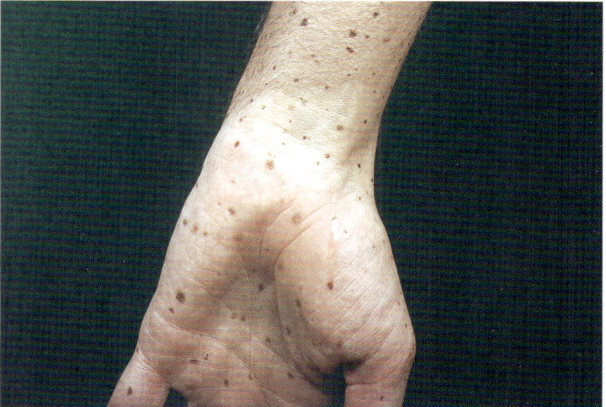

Figure 14.57

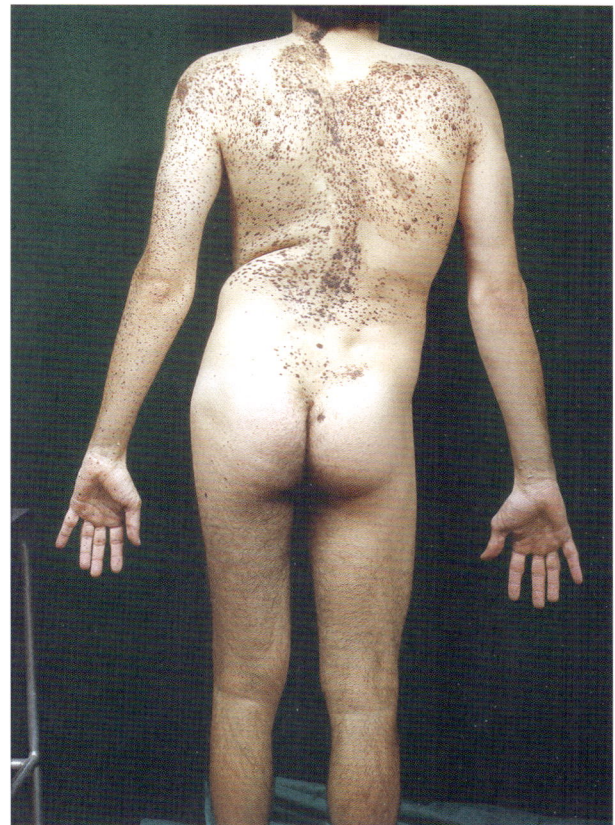

Figure 14.58

REFERENCES

Boente MC, Pizzi de Parra N, Larralde de Luna M, et al. Phacomatosis pigmentokeratotica: another epidermal nevus syndrome and a distinctive type of twin spotting. Eur J Dermatol 2000; 10: 190–4

Happle R, Hoffmann R, Restano L, et al. Phacomatosis pigmentokeratotica: a melanocyctic–epidermal twin nevus syndrome. Am J Med Genet 1996; 65: 363–5

Tadini G, Restano L, Gonzales-Perez R, et al. Phacomatosis pigmentokeratotica: report of new cases and further delineation of the syndrome. Arch Dermatol 1998; 134: 333–7

EPIDERMAL NEVI AND EPIDERMAL NEVUS SYNDROMES

Introduction

(See also Chapter 25 'Cutaneous mosaicism'.)

Epidermal nevi (EN) arise from postzygotic mutations in ectoderm-derived cell lines (except melanocytes), namely keratinocytes and cells forming adnexa. EN may be present alone without any associated abnormality, or be a part of a syndrome.

Epidermal nevus syndrome (ENS) is defined by a complex of different diseases sharing common features of a nevus of epidermal origin (from keratinocytes or adnexa) arranged in a mosaic distribution, and the involvement of extracutaneous structures such as the CNS and bones.

A tentative effort to list these syndromes is as follows.

ENS with a single origin nevus and extracutaneous involvement

- The former epidermal–sebaceous nevus syndrome (Schimmelpenning syndrome)
- Nevus comedonicus syndrome
- Angora hair nevus syndrome
- Gobello's nevus syndrome

ENS associated with mosaicism of different origin

- Phakomatosis pigmentokeratotica (see section above in this chapter)
- Proteus syndrome (see section below in this chapter)
- Becker's nevus syndrome
- EN with vitamin D-resistant rickets
- EN with angiodysplasia and aneurysms

Epidermal–sebaceous nevus (ESN) and ESN syndrome (Schimmelpenning syndrome)

- Areas of yellow-pinkish color, frequently arranged as a single patch or distributed in a linear multiple fashion, usually located on the scalp, face and neck but visible at any site on the body
- Histologically the nevus may be purely epidermal or containing organoid sebaceous and even apocrine differentiation that, in our opinion, is due simply to the localization of the nevus
- You may find almost pure sebaceous nevi in the areas of face (Figure 14.59), neck (Figure 14.60), scalp (Figure 14.61), or in other areas rich in sebaceous glands, such as the sternal region or intrascapular region
- In contrast, almost pure epidermal nevus (without any organoid–adnexal differentiation) is more probably found in areas such as the arms, legs, trunk and abdomen (Figures 14.62 and 14.63)
- Less frequently mixed apocrine–sebaceous nevus has been reported arising from cervical areas (Figure 14.64) or axillae
- Associated anomalies are:
  - CNS involvement with psychomotor retardation and epilepsy

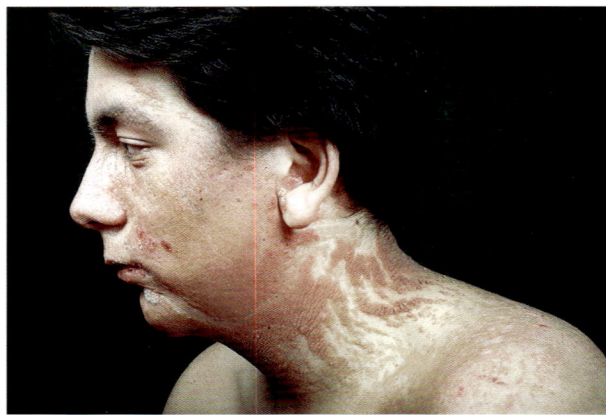

Figure 14.59

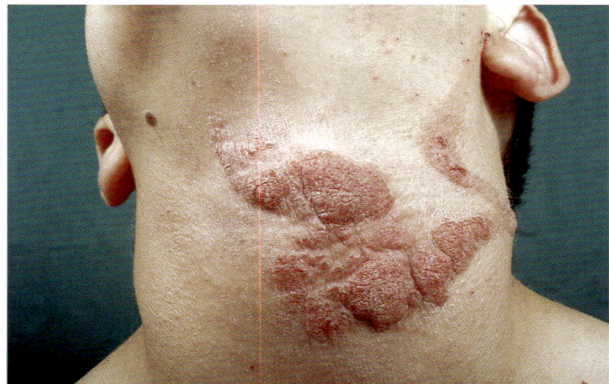

Figure 14.60

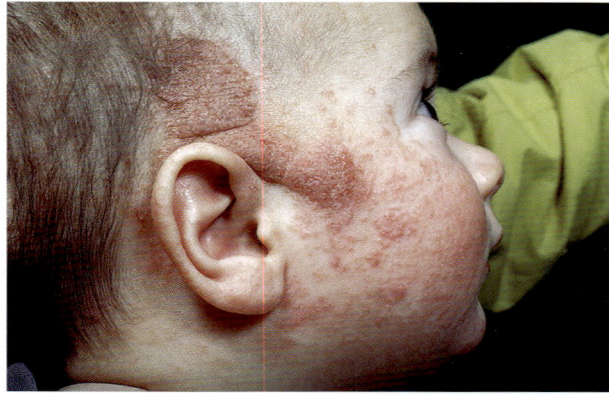

Figure 14.61

- colobomas and lipodermoid cysts
- osseous asymmetry and malformations topographically related to the above-lying nevus

- This complex is a classic example of an autosomal dominant lethal trait being non-lethal in the mosaic form

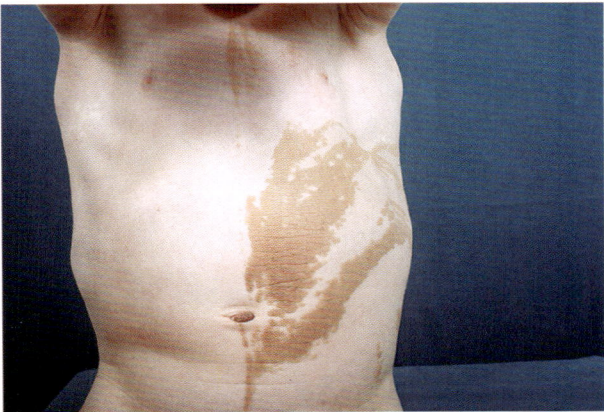

Figure 14.62

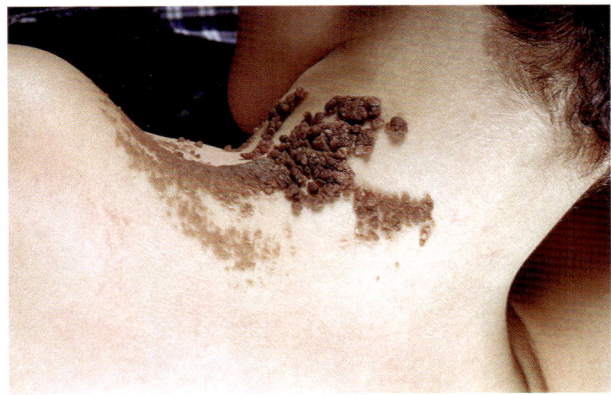

Figure 14.64

Nevus comedonicus (NC) and NC syndrome

- Comedones, sebaceous cysts and atrophic pointed scars (atrophoderma-like lesions) arranged in a mosaic pattern (Figures 14.65–14.66), more frequently visible on the face
- Associated anomalies are:

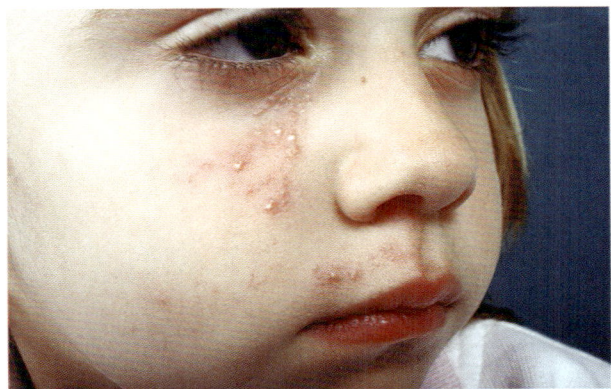

Figure 14.65

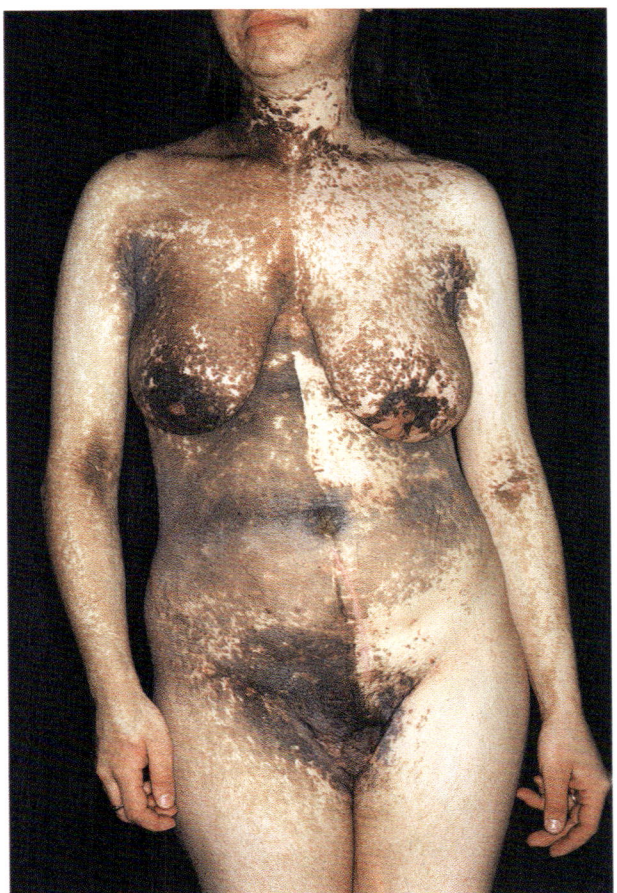

Figure 14.63

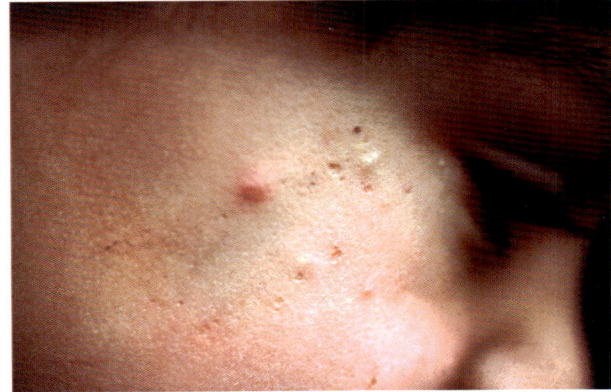

Figure 14.66

- Homolateral cataract
- Skeletal abnormalities
- Mental retardation

- NC is a disease that is non-lethal in the mosaic form
- A recently described entity called **porokeratotic eccrine ostial and dermal duct nevus** shares clinical similarities with nevus comedonicus (Figure 14.67), but on histological examination shows large superficial corneal lamellae, similar to those occurring in porokeratosis, and hamartomatous feature of eccrine glands. No systemic signs have been so far associated with this nevus

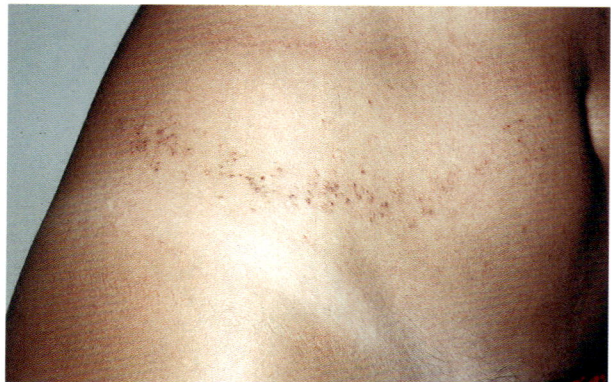

Figure 14.67

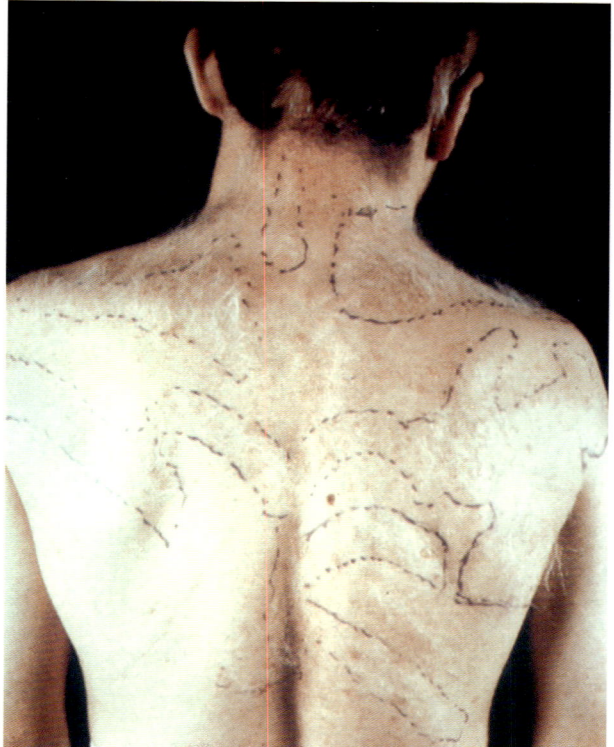

Figure 14.68

Angora hair nevus syndrome

- There is just a single report from Schauder in the literature
- The clinical picture is represented by bilateral diffuse broad bands covered by white, long and fine hair (Figure 14.68)
- Associated anomalies are:
  - bone defects such as short stature, hemihypotrophy and malformation of the skull and face
  - CNS involvement with brain malformation (porencephaly and asymmetry of the hemispheres) leading to seizures and mental retardation

Becker's nevus (BN) and BN syndrome

- Characterized by a well-known triad of an epidermal, pigmented and hairy nevus with irregular borders
- Because of its hormonal dependence, Becker's nevus is visible from puberty, usually located on the superior girdle, arms and trunk, rarely on other body sites
- The nevus is associated with an ipsilateral hypoplasia of subcutaneous tissues, including breasts (Figure 14.69), and related osseous malformations of the thorax and also the long bones
- BN is relatively frequent but, in contrast, severe associated abnormalities are rare
- BN may be transmitted to offspring with a paradominant trait

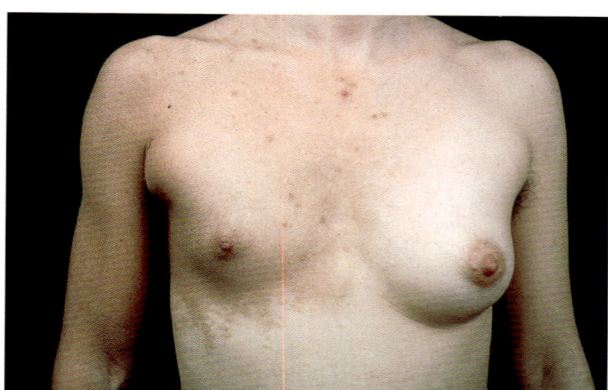

Figure 14.69

Neurocutaneous syndromes

Gobello's nevus syndrome

- Gobello described recently a single case of an epidermal nevus composed of a systematized linear epidermal (non-acantholytic, non-sebaceous) nevus characterized by follicular hyperkeratosis and an increased amount of superimposed hair (Figure 14.70)

- Associated anomalies are:
  - Brachydactyly, clinodactyly and onychodystrophy (Figure 14.71)
  - Body asymmetry due to osseous defects (Figure 14.72)
  - Onychodystrophy

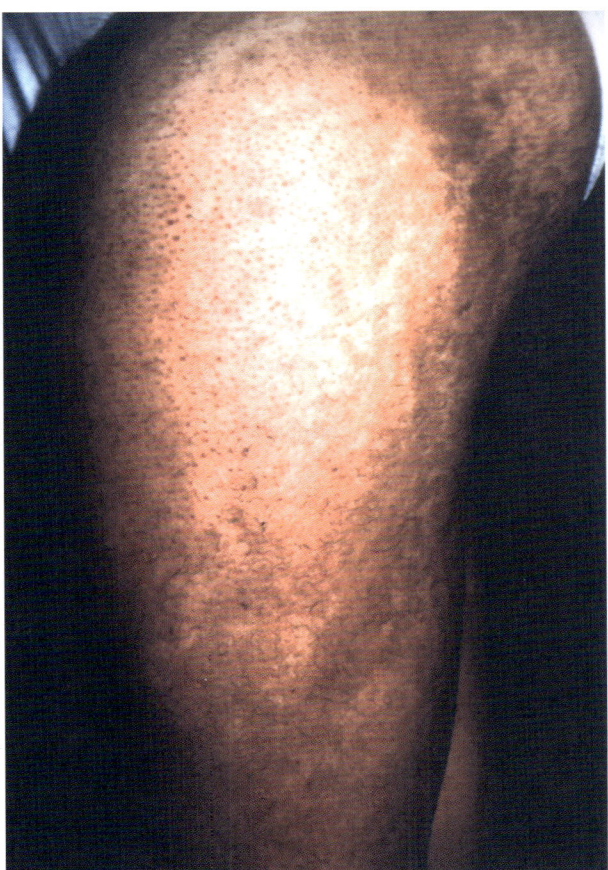

Figure 14.70

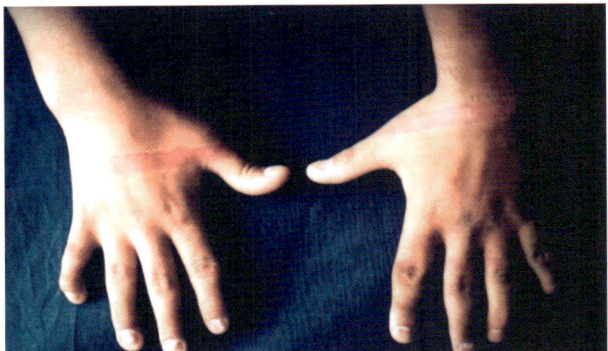

Figure 14.71

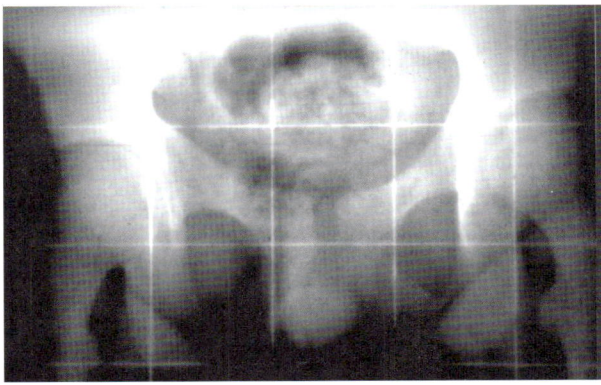

Figure 14.72

EN with vitamin D-resistant rickets

- Organoid nevus (multiple streaks), associated with:
  - Hypophosphatemia
  - Vascular cutaneous and visceral tumors
  - In a personal observation, speckled lentiginous nevus, severe osseous abnormalities, mental retardation, strabismus, lipodermoid cysts and xanthogranulomas (Figures 14.73 and 14.74)

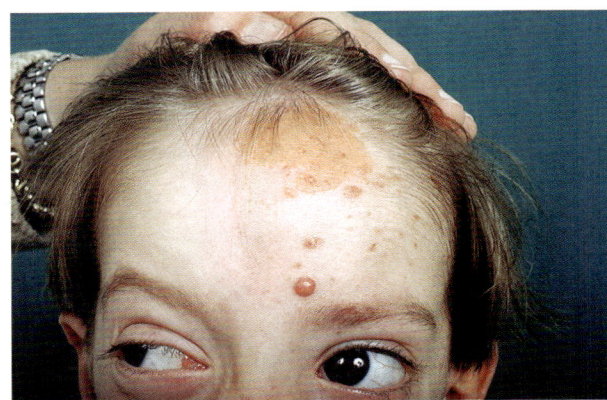

Figure 14.73

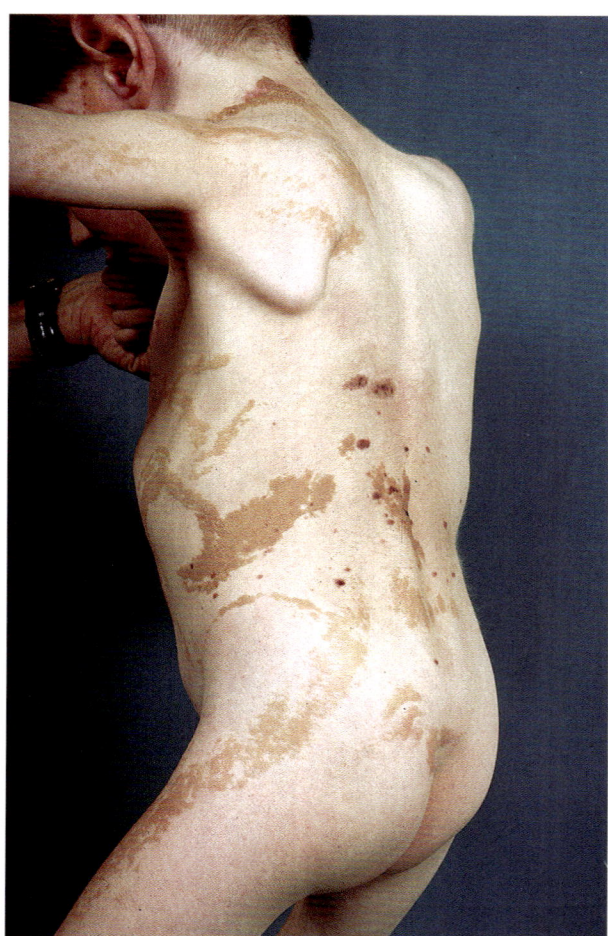

Figure 14.74

REFERENCES

Happle R, Gustav Schimmelpenning and the syndrome bearing his name. Dermatology 2004; 209: 84–7

O'Shaughnessy RF, Christiano AM. Inherited disorders of the skin in human and mouse: from development to differentiation. Int J Dev Biol 2004; 48: 171–9. Review

Randerson-Moor JA, Gaut R, Turner F, et al. The relationship between the epidermal growth factor (EGF) 5′UTR variant A61G and melanoma/nevus susceptibility. J Invest Dermatol 2004; 123: 755–9

Sugarman JL. Epidermal nevus syndromes. Semin Cutan Med Surg 2004; 23: 145–57. Review

WAXY KERATOSIS OF CHILDHOOD

Epidemiology

Five cases have been described.

Age of onset

- A few lesions may be visible at birth

Clinical findings

- Hyperkeratotic 'waxy' yellowish, flesh-colored or light brown papules (Figure 14.75), preferentially on the trunk (Figures 14.76 and 14.77) and flexures (Figure 14.78), with few lesions on arms and legs
- Papules are not follicular and scales may be easily detachable, without pruritus, pain or bleeding
- One of the five patients described in the literature had a segmental mosaic distribution

Extracutaneous findings

- Epilepsy and mental retardation (two of four patients with generalized symptoms)
- Delayed puberty
- Dolichocephaly, low-placed ears, elongated face, hypoplastic mandible (Figure 14.79)

Course and prognosis

Papules may be few and tiny at birth, gradually increasing in size and number with age.

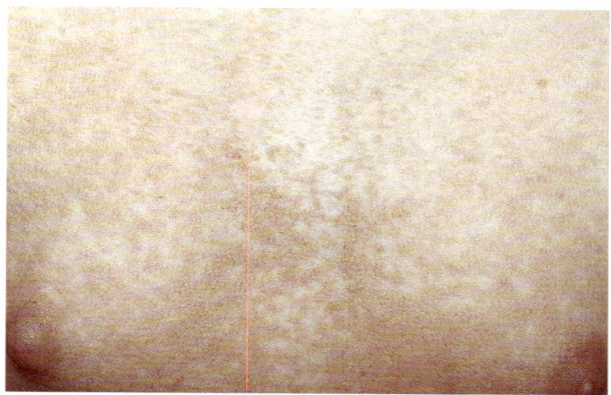

Figure 14.75

Lesions tend to coalesce to form large plaques (Figure 14.76).

Laboratory findings

Conventional histology shows orthokeratotic hyperkeratosis, tenting and mild acanthosis (Figure 14.80).

Genetics and pathogenesis

Of the above five described cases, two were sisters with asymptomatic parents, suggesting autosomal recessive inheritance. One of the described cases had a segmental distribution pattern, without CNS involvement.

This syndrome must be considered as a new neurocutaneous syndrome.

Follow-up and therapy

- Search for CNS involvement
- Topical or systemic retinoids
- Keratolytic agents

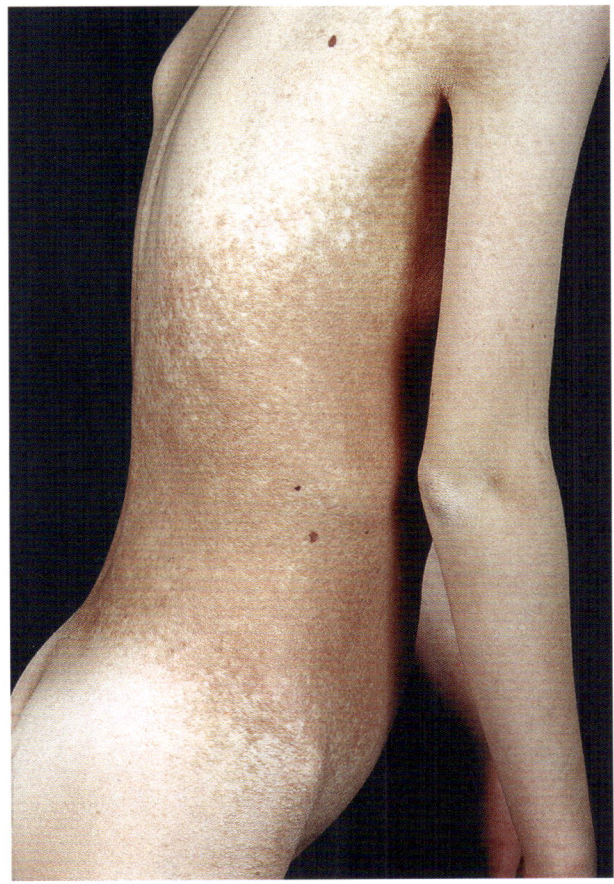

Figure 14.77

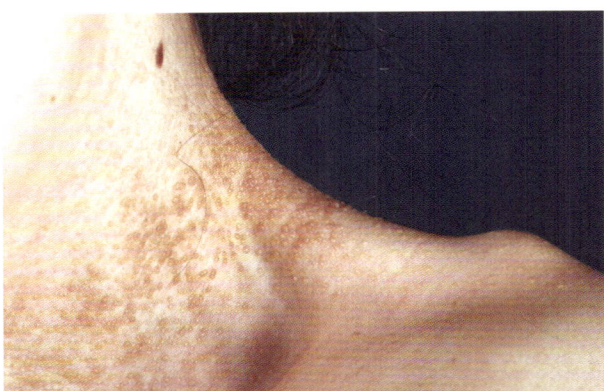

Figure 14.78

Differential diagnosis

- Gougerot–Carteaud syndrome
- Papular epithelial hamartomas with neurologic abnormalities (PEHANA) syndrome

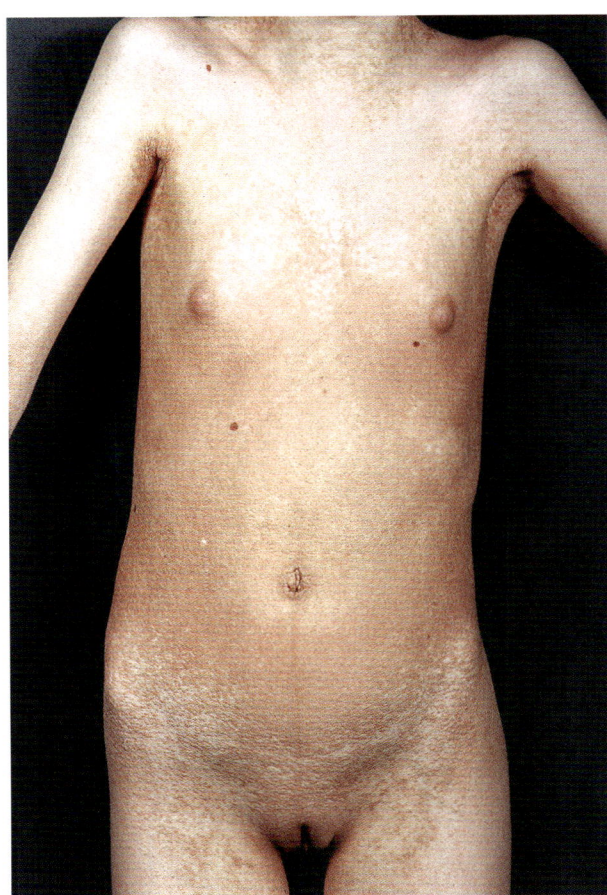

Figure 14.76

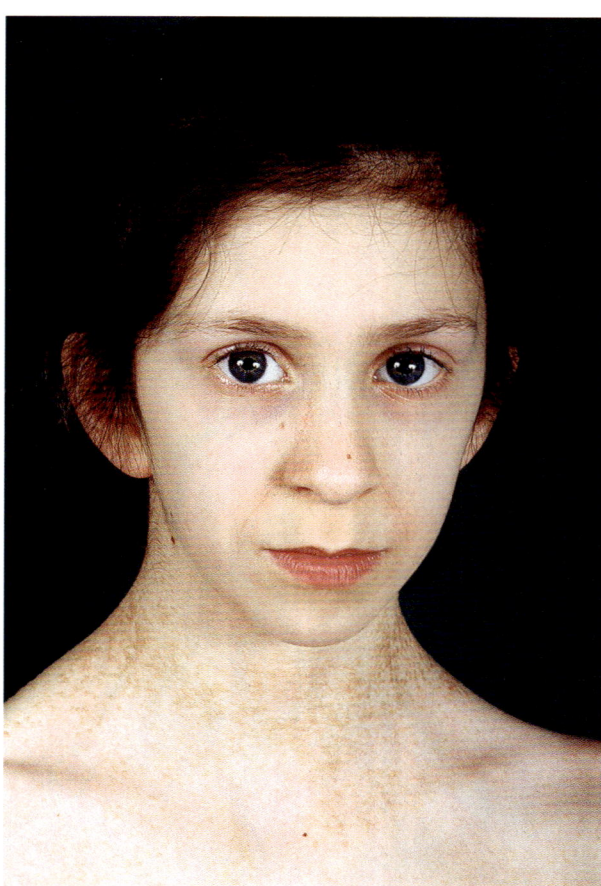

Figure 14.79

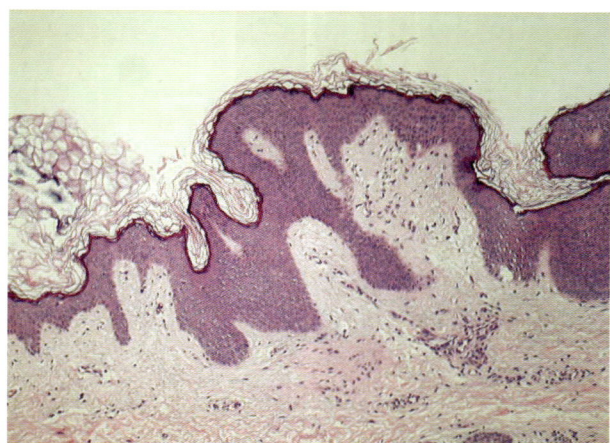

Figure 14.80

REFERENCES

Coleman R, Malone M, Handfield-Jones S, et al. Waxy keratoses of childhood. Clin Exp Dermatol 1994; 19: 173–6

Mehrabi D, Thomas JE, Selim MA, Prose NS. Waxy keratoses of childhood in a segmental distribution. Pediatr Dermatol 2001; 18: 415–16

PAPULAR EPITHELIAL HAMARTOMAS AND NEUROLOGIC ABNORMALITIES SYNDROME

Synonym

- PEHANA syndrome

Epidemiology

This is an undescribed syndrome. We have observed three cases in a 10-year survey.

Age of onset

- At birth

Clinical findings

- Small keratotic firm papules (2–5 mm) first isolated (Figures 14.81 and 14.82) then merging to form plaques of 2–3 cm in dimension, randomly distributed on the body (Figures 14.83–14.84)
- Papules and plaques are not arranged in a known mosaic pattern
- Lesions are slightly pruritic
- Normal hair and nails
- Normal sweating

Extracutaneous findings

- Mild mental retardation
- Cephalea and late-onset epilepsy (absences and neurovegetative symptoms)
- Maybe a certain degree of dolichocephaly and hypertelorism configuring a 'facies'
- Normal vision and hearing

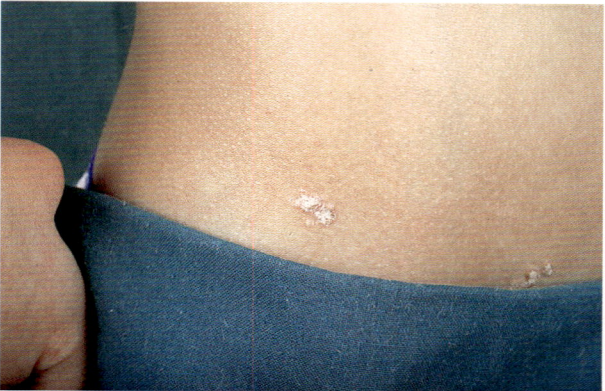

Figure 14.81

Course and prognosis

Cutaneous lesions tends to grow slowly until adolescence and then stabilize.

Neurologic abnormalities are usually not severe and are well managed by pharmacological therapy and neurologic follow-up.

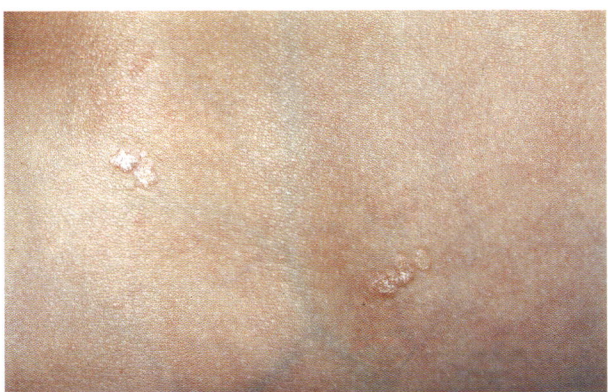

Figure 14.82

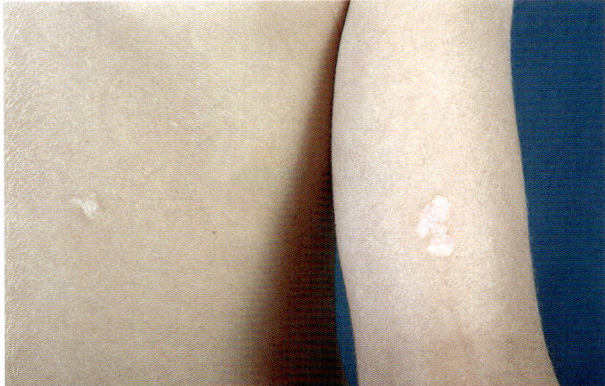

Figure 14.83

Laboratory findings

- Histologic examination shows basaloid acanthosis with orthokeratotic hyperkeratosis, associated with keratin-plugged acrosyringia
- Ultrastructural examination shows aspecific signs of hyperproliferation

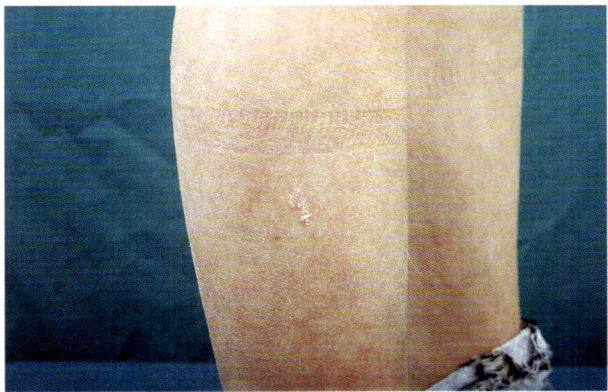

Figure 14.84

- EEG in one of the above cases showed aspecific abnormalities
- MRI did not show any major brain abnormality

Genetics and pathogenesis

All three above patients were sporadic cases from unrelated families. No consanguinity was reported.

The association of epithelial 'hamartomas' and neurological abnormalities led us to conclude a common derivation of symptoms with a genetic defect involving two ectodermal derivates, configuring a previously undescribed neurocutaneous syndrome.

Follow-up and therapy

- Skin lesions are almost asymptomatic
- Neurological examination is mandatory to detect early manifestation of the disease (seizures, eventual EEG abnormalities)
- Pharmacological therapy for seizures
- School/psychological support

Differential diagnosis

- Warts
- Epidermal nevus
- Waxy dermatosis of childhood

PROTEUS SYNDROME

Age of onset

- At birth or during first years of life

Clinical findings

Skin manifestations

- Cerebriform or nodular gross thickening of palms and soles (Figures 14.85 and 14.86)
- Linear verrucous epidermal nevi (distributed along Blaschko's lines) (Figure 14.87)
- Hamartomatous masses of subcutaneous tissue consisting of adipose tissue or various combinations of adipose and lymphatic–angiomatous tissue (Figure 14.88)
- Port-wine stains
- Café-au-lait macules
- Hypopigmented spots

Extracutaneous manifestations

- Progressive and asymmetric macrodactyly (Figure 14.89)
- Macrocephaly and skull exostosis
- Body hemihypertrophy (Figure 14.88)
- Scoliosis and spinal-canal stenosis
- Ocular abnormalities

Course and prognosis

The disease is slowly progressive and dependent on the extent and severity of extracutaneous lesions.

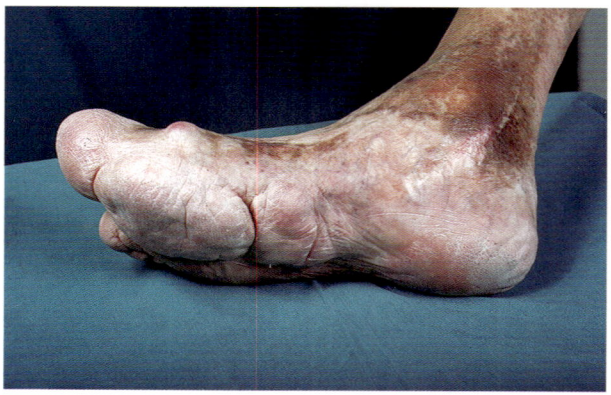

Figure 14.86

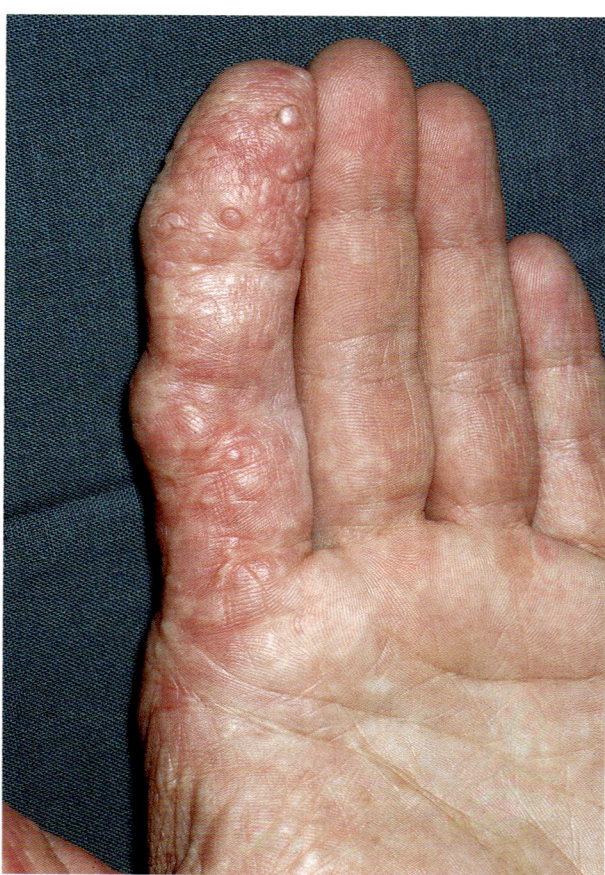

Figure 14.85

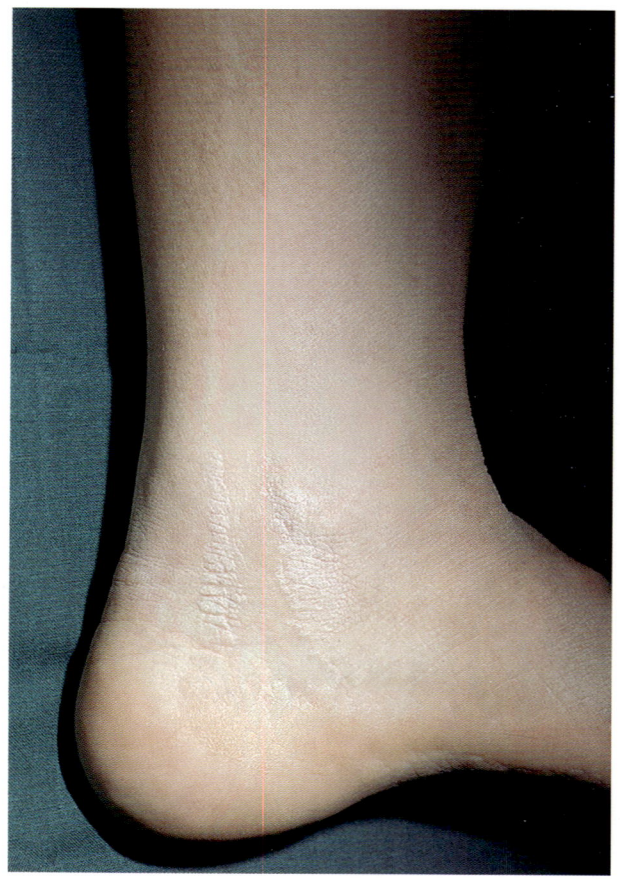

Figure 14.87

Neurocutaneous syndromes

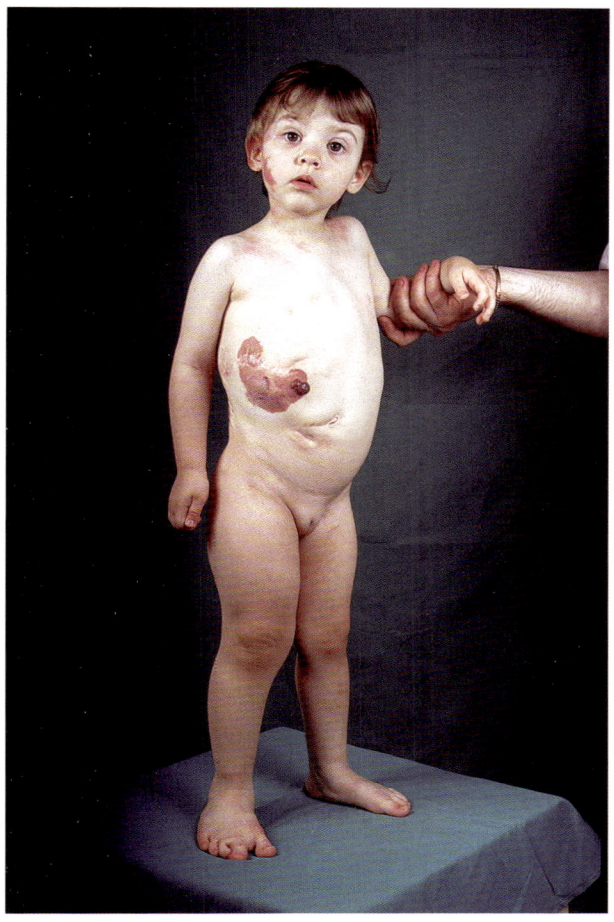

Figure 14.88

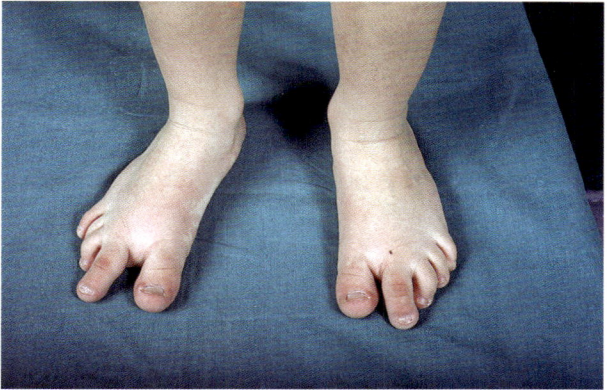

Figure 14.89

Laboratory findings

Radiography shows bone and soft tissue hypertrophies.

Genetics and pathogenesis

Almost all sporadic cases are probably due to a somatic mutation, lethal in the non-mosaic state, with an alteration in local production of tissue growth factors.

Paradominant inheritance is possible (see Chapter 25 'Cutaneous mosaicism').

Linkage to PTEN gene has not been confirmed by recent studies.

Follow-up and therapy

- Great variability between extremely severe forms and milder ones
- Propensity for neoplastic changes
- Normal mental function
- Surgical approach for gigantism
- Orthopedic intervention

Differential diagnosis

- Neurofibromatosis
- Klippel–Trénaunay–Weber syndrome
- Maffucci syndrome
- Epidermal nevus syndrome

REFERENCES

Child FJ, Werring DJ, Du Vivier AWP. Proteus syndrome: diagnosis in adulthood. Br J Dermatol 1998; 139: 132–6

Nazzaro V, Cambiaghi S, Montagnani A, et al. Proteus syndrome. Ultrastructural study of linear verrucous and depigmented nevi. J Am Acad Dermatol 1991; 25: 377–83

Samlaska CP, Levin SW, James WD, et al. Proteus syndrome. Arch Dermatol 1989; 125: 1109–14

CHAPTER 15

Ectodermal dysplasias and related disorders

15.1 Ectodermal dysplasias

Definition

Ectodermal dysplasia defines a disease that involves primary defects in hair, sweat glands, nails and teeth, i.e. ectodermally derived structures.

This is a vast, heterogeneous group of genetically transmitted diseases that has historically been classified following the famous Freire–Maya and Pinheiro classification that encompasses more than 190 different clinical pictures and is based only on clinical evidence. We think that this is rather an old-fashioned way to order and study these diseases, and we accept a more recently proposed classification based on clinical pictures strictly related to molecular and functional genetic findings.

HYPOHIDROTIC ECTODERMAL DYSPLASIA

Synonyms

- Anhidrotic ED
- Christ–Siemens–Touraine syndrome

Epidemiology

Incidence is estimated at 1:100 000. In Italy, patients with 'pure' anhidrotic ectodermal dysplasia number about 100 out of 57 million inhabitants.

Clinical findings

- Abnormalities of the epidermis and adnexa are extremely variable

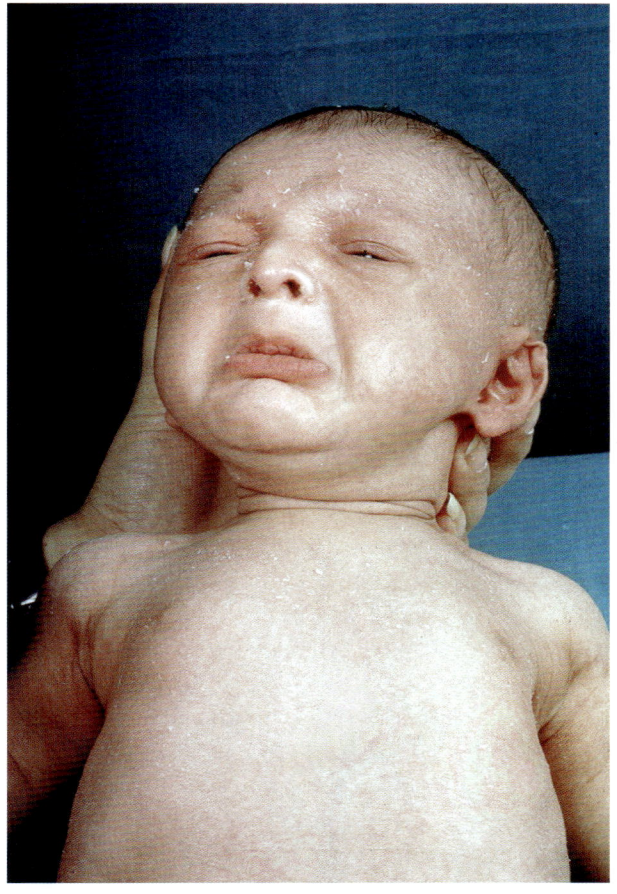

Figure 15.1

- Babies may be born with a 'post-mature' ichthyotic presentation, rarely as a classic 'collodion-baby' presentation with medium-sized lamellae and slight underlying erythema (Figure 15.1)

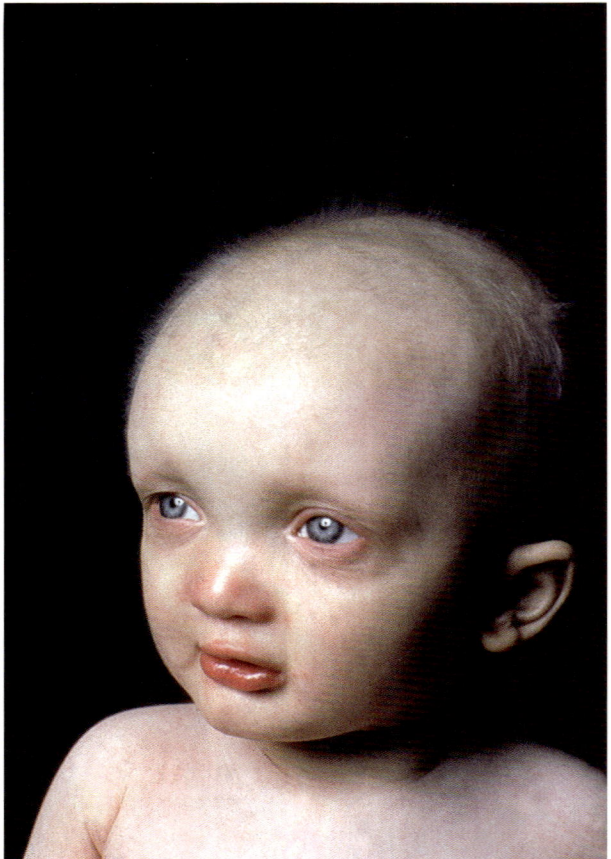

Figure 15.2

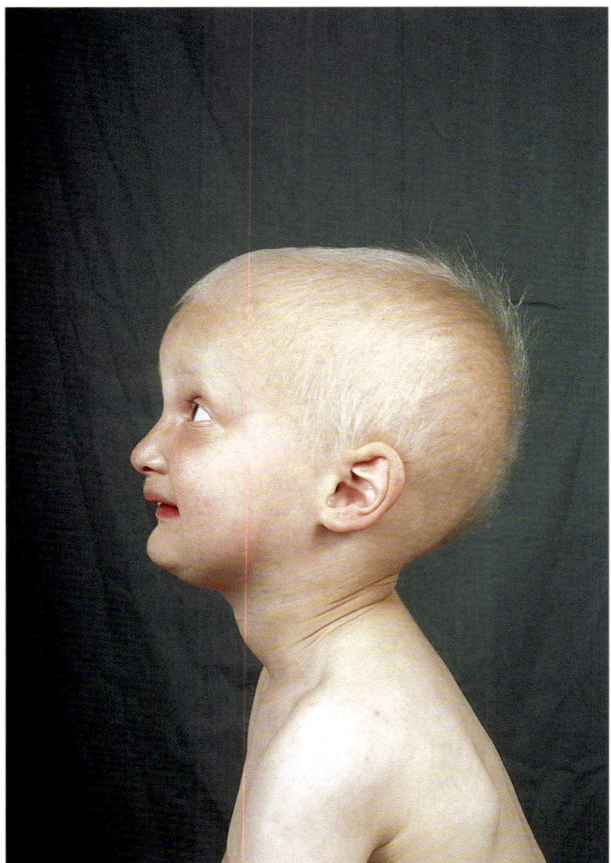

Figure 15.3

- Peculiar facies characterized by frontal bosses, mild hypertelorism with antimongolian slants, malar region hypoplasia with small saddle-shaped nose and hypoplastic alae, O-shaped mouth with prominent lips and possibly a pointed chin. External ears may be low-placed and hypotrophic (Figures 15.2 and 15.3)
- Epidermis is dry, fine and smooth with xerotic patches and eczematous areas (Figure 15.2)
- Body hair follicles are diminished or absent
- Hair is usually blond, fine and scanty, even if partial or total alopecia or hypotrichosis may be present (Figure 15.4)
- Eyebrows and eyelashes may be rudimentary or absent (Figures 15.2–15.4)
- Nails are usually less involved in hypohidrotic ectodermal dysplasia (HED), but some degree of dystrophy can be noted as split, fragmented, striated and discolored laminae. Less frequently, nails are thickened (Figure 15.5)
- Eccrine sweat glands are dramatically dimished, hypoplastic or even absent, with extreme heat intolerance
- Absent or rudimentary oral mucous glands and salivary glands lead to xerostomia

- Apocrine glands are hypoplastic
- Female carriers may present minimal or discrete signs of the disease such as partial alopecia, abnormal dentition (Figure 15.6), hypodontia, some degree of the 'facies' and streaks of epidermis without appendages along Blaschko's lines (Figures 15.7 and 15.8) that are more visible with the 'starch–iodine' test to evaluate sweat gland function (Figure 15.9)

Extracutaneous symptoms

- Hypo- or anodontia is the hallmark of the disease, with abnormal and defective dentition
- Conical or rudimentary teeth are present and caries is very common (Figure 15.10)
- Lacrimal glands are rudimentary or hypoplastic
- The dense texture of nasal secretions promotes mucous stasis with uncomfortable crust formation in the choanae and subsequent infection of the paranasal sinuses
- Hypoplasia of ear mucus glands leads to cerumen impaction and chronic otitis media
- Mucus glands are diminished or hypoplastic in the entire respiratory tract, leading to susceptibilty to

Ectodermal dysplasias and related disorders

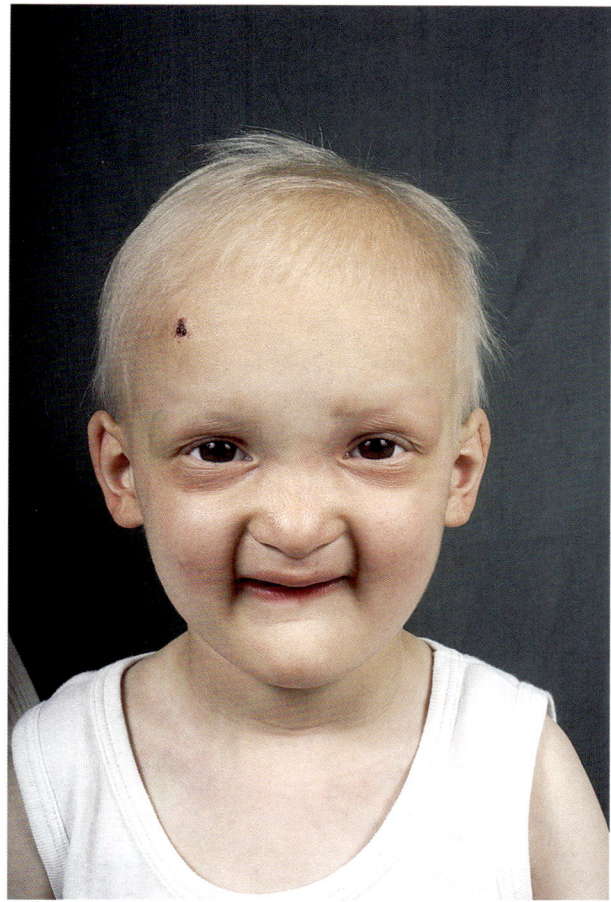

Figure 15.4

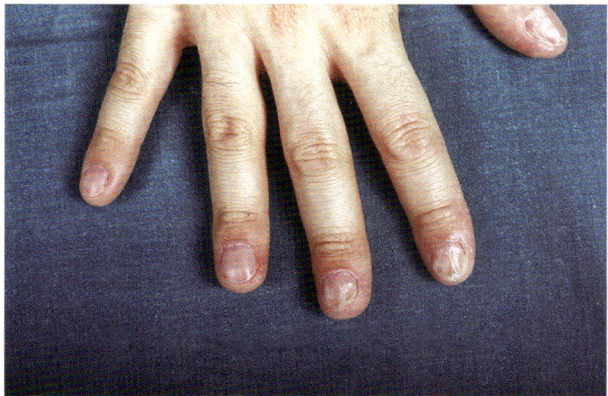

Figure 15.5

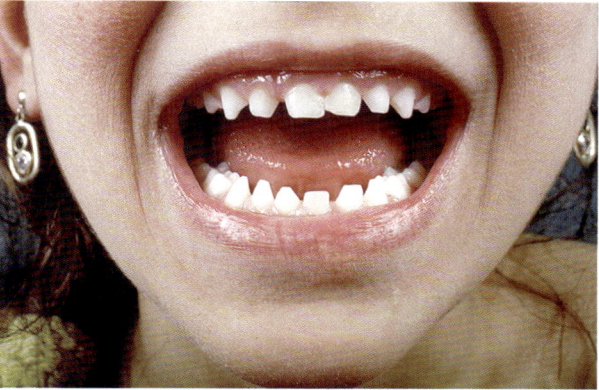

Figure 15.6

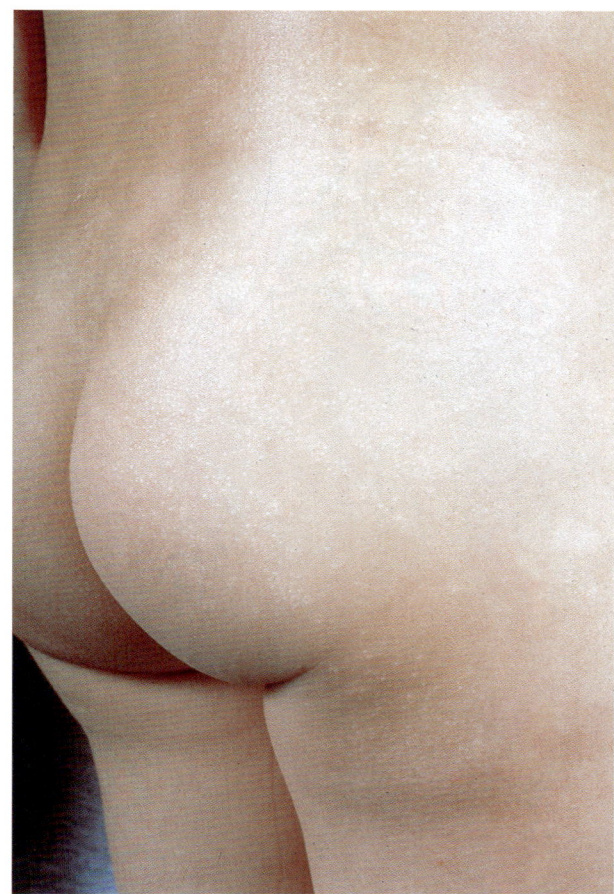

Figure 15.7

recurrent infections of both upper and lower sections
- Dysphagia and stypsis are common symptoms in these patients and are due to extreme hypofunction of mucous glands in the whole gastrointestinal system
- Mammary glands may be absent
- Abnormalities in immune function, both humoral and cellular, have been reported
- Mental retardation is reported in some cases

Course and complications

- Unexplained recurrent fever and extreme heat intolerance during hot weather may lead to seizures and coma, especially during the first year of life
- Recurrent infections of the upper respiratory tract and otitis media may become chronic
- Hypoanodontia is linked to diminished intake of food, anemia and failure to thrive

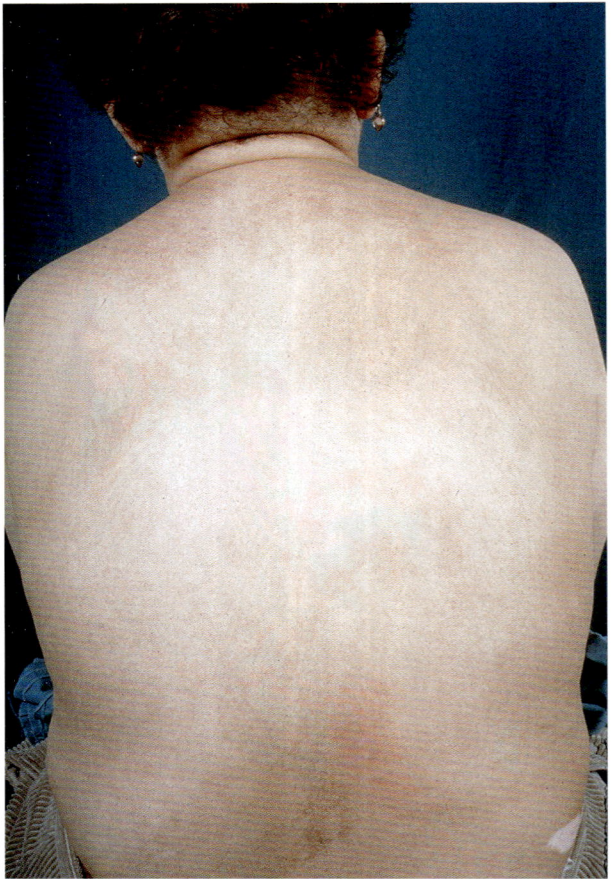

Figure 15.8

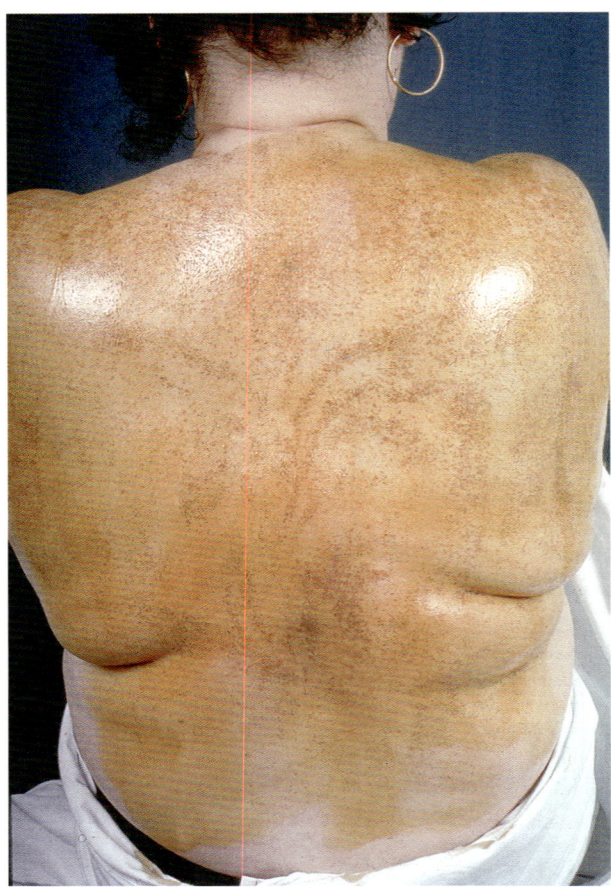

Figure 15.9

- Atopic dermatitis is frequently associated
- Stypsis

Female carrier cases of hypohydrotic ectodermal dysplasia is often misdiagnosed in neonatal age and in early infancy.

The disease is steady during life in males. Uneventful amelioration is reported in some cases, especially in female carriers.

Laboratory findings

- Histology shows a decrease or absence of eccrine and apocrine glands
- The starch–iodine test demonstrates the absence of functioning eccrine glands in male subjects and is used to detect female carriers
- Humoral and cellular immunity is revealed by blood examination
- Total IgE and specific IgE test to detect allergic patients
- Bacteriological examination of nasal and auricolar smears is needed

Genetics and pathogenesis

HED is highly genetically heterogeneous. Nevertheless, even if the X-linked HED form is by far the more frequent genotype, five different subtypes of HED have been demonstrated by genetic studies:

- X-linked form due to mutations in ectodysplasin gene (EDA) (Figure 15.11)
- Autosomal dominant form due to mutations in the gene that encodes the receptor for ectodysplasin (EDAR)
- Autosomal recessive form, the same EDAR gene (Figure 15.12)
- Autosomal recessive form due to mutations in a gene encoding an adaptor factor of the EDA/EDAR signaling system (EDARADD)

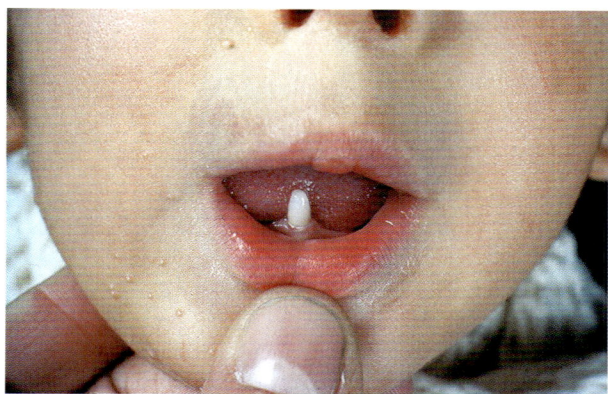

Figure 15.10

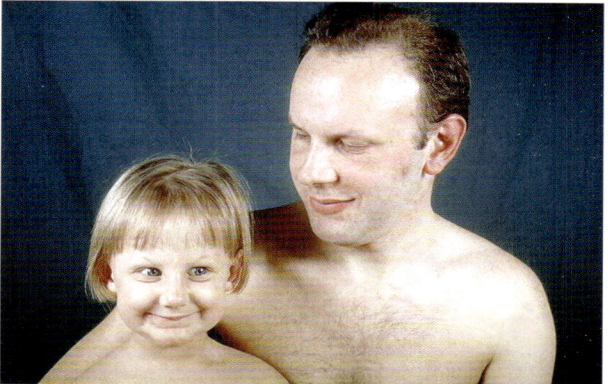

Figure 15.12

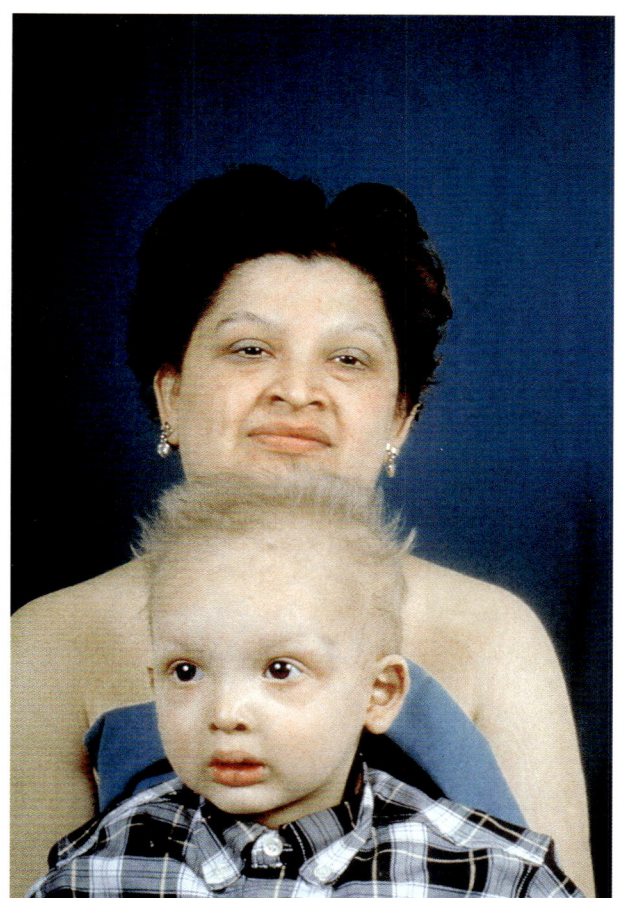

Figure 15.11

- HED phenotype with severe immunodeficiency is related to mutations in the NEMO gene that conversely cause incontinentia pigmenti

All the above four different molecules converge on the system of nuclear factor (NF)-κB molecule activity, which plays a key role in the control of apoptosis, immune response, differentiation and proliferation of tissues of ectodermal derivation during embryogenesis.

Unfortunately, there is not sufficient experience to detect clinically the different forms, and molecular genetic studies are complex and even uneventful in some cases.

It is mandatory to detect female carriers using the starch–iodine test before genetic testing, and genetic counseling should take into account this complex genetic heterogeneity.

Differential diagnosis

- Ichthyoses with collodion baby presentation
- Other complex ectodermal dysplasia
- IFAP syndrome (ichthyosis follicularis with atrichia and photophobia)
- Milder cases of trichothiodystrophy

REFERENCES

Itin PH, Fistarol SK. Ectodermal dysplasias. Am J Med Genet 2004; 131C: 45–51

Lamartine J. Towards a new classification of ectodermal dysplasias. Clin Exp Dermatol 2003; 28: 351–5. Review

Priolo M, Lagana C. Ectodermal dysplasias: a new clinical-genetic classification. J Med Genet 2001; 38: 579–85

Priolo M, Silengo M, Lerone M, Ravazzolo R. Ectodermal dysplasias: not only 'skin' deep. Clin Genet 2000 58: 415–30. Review

RAPP–HODGKIN–AEC, EEC SYNDROME, LIMB–MAMMARY DISEASE, ADULT-SPECTRUM ECTODERMAL DYSPLASIA

Synonyms

This 'complex' includes at least five diseases that were considered exclusive until molecular biology discovered a unique pathogenesis for all of them in the p63 gene.

We propose the term 'p63-related ectodermal dysplasia' or 'p63rED'.

Epidemiology

p63-related ectodermal dysplasias are very rare. There is no established study or registry available.

Clinical findings

This group of diseases comprises the following 'old' definitions:

Ectrodactyly, ectodermal dysplasia, cleft lip with or without cleft palate syndrome (EEC): (Figures 15.13 and 15.14):

- Various degrees of brachydactyly–ectrodactyly, especially rays II and III
- Cleft lip–palate
- Blond thin hair
- Lacrimal duct anomalies
- Conductive deafness

Ankyloblepharon, ectodermal dysplasia, cleft lip/palate syndrome (AEC) + Rapp–Hodgkin syndrome (Figures 15.15–15.19):

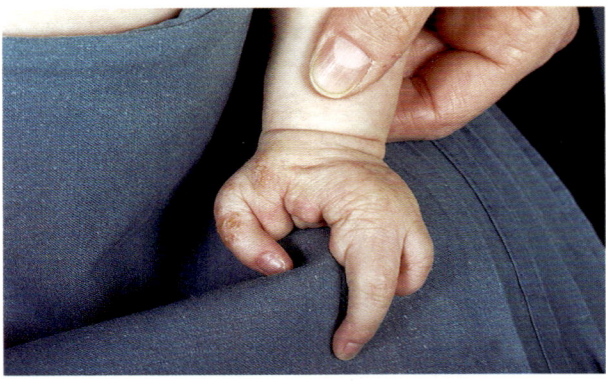

Figure 15.14

- Large areas of eroded skin on the vertex at birth and residual alopecia
- Ankyloblepharon and lacrimal duct anomalies
- Nail dystrophies
- Typical facies with beak-like nose, malar hypoplasia
- Hypodontia
- Hypohidrosis
- Cleft lip and palate
- Hypospadias
- Remember that CHAND syndrome is a further variant of AEC complex

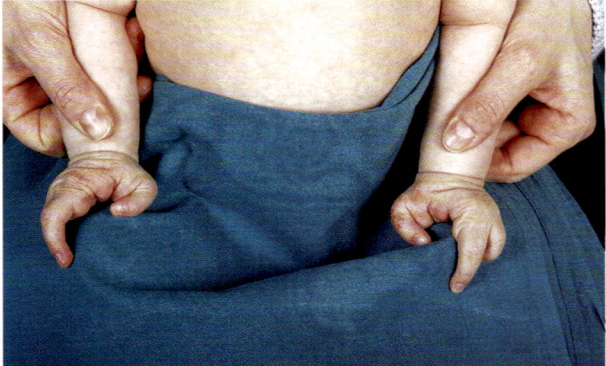

Figure 15.13

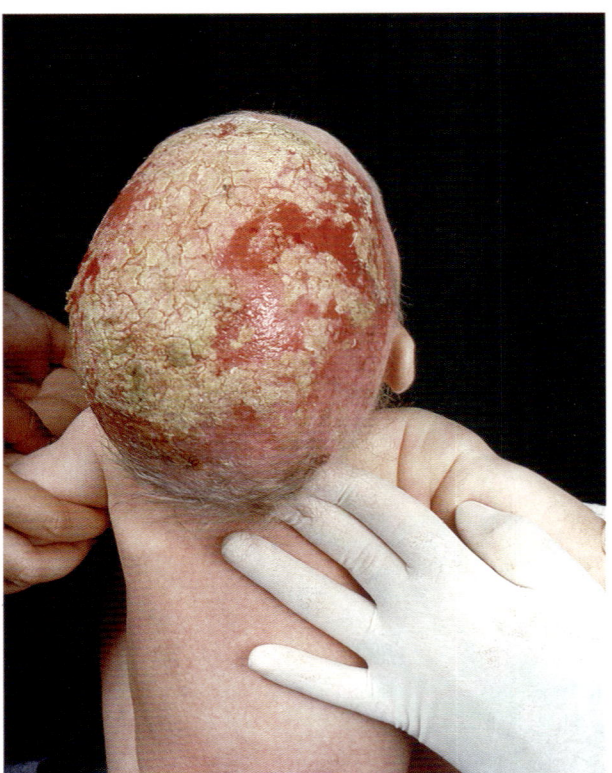

Figure 15.15

Ectodermal dysplasias and related disorders 209

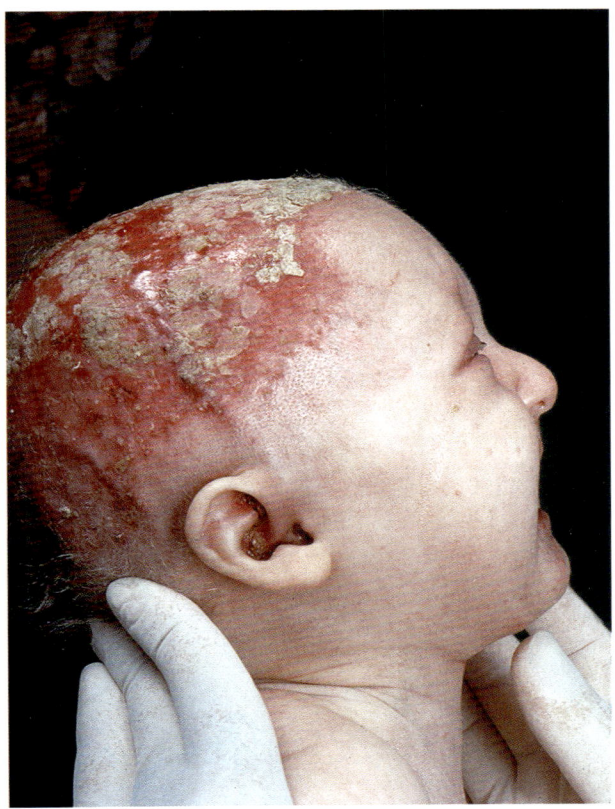

Figure 15.16

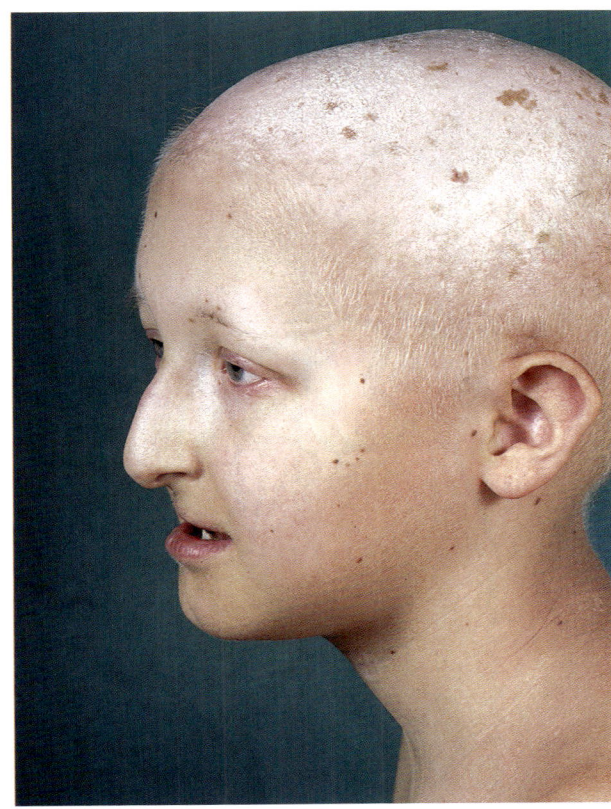

Figure 15.18

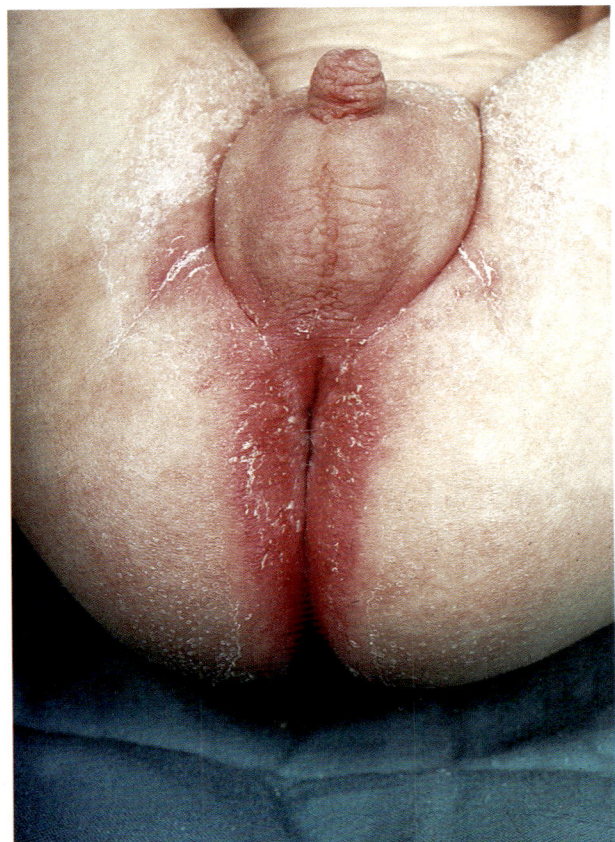

Figure 15.17

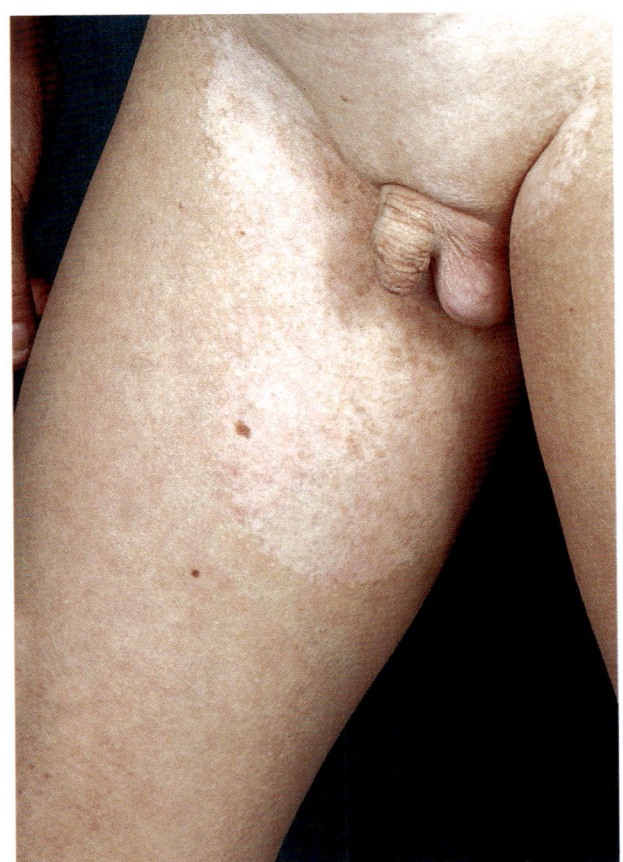

Figure 15.19

Acral-dermato-ungual-lacrimal-tooth syndrome (ADULT) (Figures 15.20 and 15.21)

- Ectrodactyly
- Excessive freckling
- Onychodysplasia
- Lacrimal duct anomalies
- Hypodontia

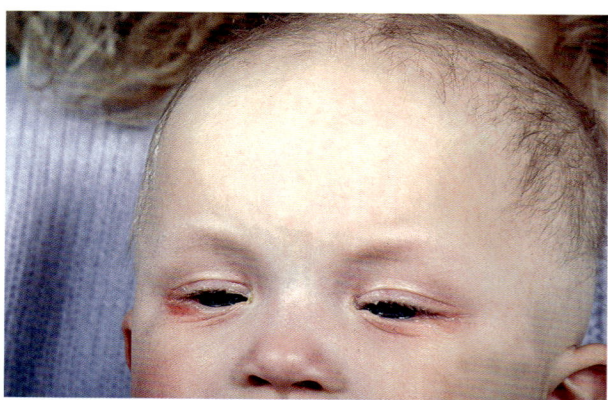

Figure 15.20

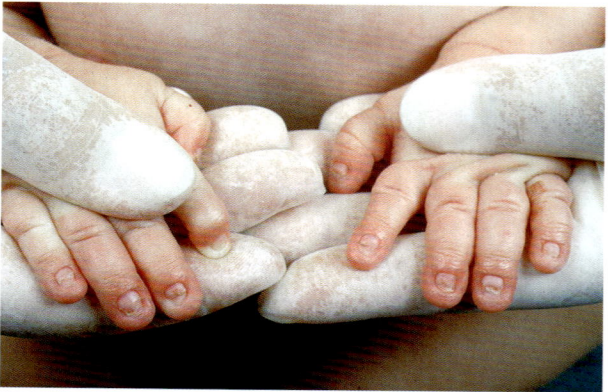

Figure 15.21

Limb–mammary disease (Figures 15.22–15.25):

- Mammary glands and nipples may be hypotrophic or absent
- Limb anomalies
- Hair and onychodysplasia
- Mental retardation

All these diseases herald common features and are caused by mutations in the same gene. For most, a genotype–phenotype relationship is well demonstrated. In fact, specific mutations of the p63 gene cause specific phenotypes.

It must be recorded that AEC and Rapp–Hodgkin have been considered the same disease by many authors in the past, and that there is a described case of an 'RH phenotype mother with an EEC phenotype son with ankyloblepharon'!

Course

The course is chronic and without great discrepancy in the various periods of life.

Susceptibility to infections may shorten the life span.

Laboratory findings

- The sweat test (starch–iodine test) may be strongly altered

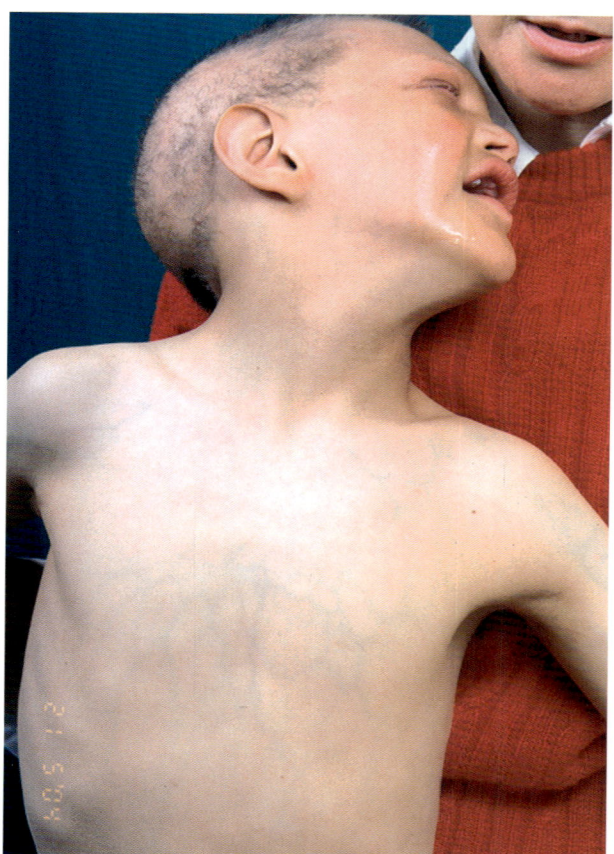

Figure 15.22

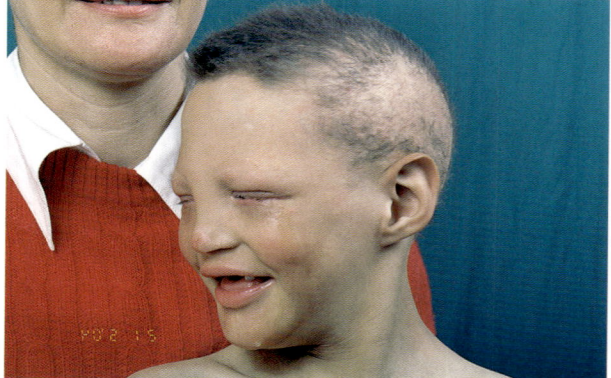

Figure 15.23

Ectodermal dysplasias and related disorders

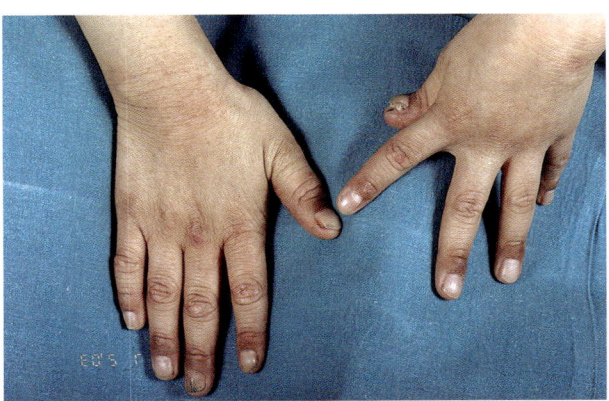

Figure 15.24

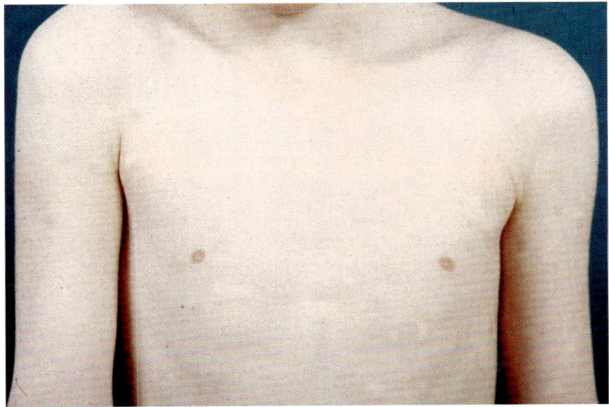

Figure 15.25

- Scanning electron microscopy reveals aspecific and various abnormalities of the hair shaft, such as pili canaliculi and pili torti

Genetics and pathogenesis

All the diseases included in this group are inherited as an autosomal dominant trait.

The gene involved in pathogenesis is p63 (a p53 homolog), which is a regulator of gene transcription and expression that leads to a defect in the epithelial–mesenchymal interaction.

Differential diagnosis

- Hypohidrotic ectodermal dysplasia
- Goltz's syndrome (ectrodactyly)
- Trichothiodystrophy (brittle hair and subject to central nervous system (CNS) involvement)
- IFAP (alopecia)
- Other syndromes with cleft lip–palate

Follow-up

- In patients with major limb defects such as severe ectrodactyly, physiotherapy and specific devices are suggested
- Oral hygiene and prevention of caries is advised
- Neurologist/psychologist support for patients and family and school personnel

Therapy

- Hand surgery when possible to correct minor defects of ectrodactyly
- Orthodontic devices are mandatory to ensure correct food intake and better facial development
- Cleft lip/palate surgery

REFERENCES

Barrow LL, van Bokhoven H, Daack-Hirsch S, et al. Analysis of the p63 gene in classical EEC syndrome, related syndromes, and non-syndromic orofacial clefts. J Med Genet 2002; 39: 559–66

Hamada T, Chan I, Willoughby CE, et al. Common mutations in Arg304 of the p63 gene in ectrodactyly, ectodermal dysplasia, clefting syndrome: lack of genotype–phenotype correlation and implications of mutation detection strategies. J Invest Dermatol 2002; 119: 1202–3

Kantaputra PN, Hamada T, Kumchai T, McGrath JA. Heterozygous mutation in the SAM domain of p63 underlies Rapp–Hodgkin ectodermal dysplasia. J Dent Res 2003; 82: 433–7

Tsutsui K, Asai Y, Fujimoto A, et al. A novel p63 sterile alpha motif (SAM) domain mutation in a Japanese patient with ankyloblepharon, ectodermal defects and cleft lip and palate (AEC) syndrome without ankyloblepharon. Br J Dermatol 2003; 149: 395–9

van Bokhoven H, Hamel BC, Baamshad M, et al. p63 Gene mutations in EEC syndrome, limb–mammary syndrome, and isolated split hand–split foot malformation suggest a genotype–phenotype correlation. Am J Hum Genet 2001; 69: 481–92

TRICHO-DENTO-OSSEOUS SYNDROME

Age of onset

- At birth

Epidemiology

The disease is rare, even among ectodermal dysplasias. About 100 cases are described in the literature.

Clinical findings

- Kinky and curly, uncombable, whitish hair that tends to be less marked with age (Figure 15.26)
- Brittle nails with superficial peeling and transverse banding
- Dystrophic eyebrows and eyelashes (Figure 15.27)
- Xerosis

Extracutaneous symptoms

- Teeth are usually small (taurodontism) with visible enamel defects and discolorations
- Increased bone density of the skull base with dolichocephaly and frontal bossing (Figure 15.28), but without CNS defects and with normal psychomotor development
- Tall stature
- Decreased pneumatization of sinuses

Complications

Early caries, suppurative periodontitis and premature loss of teeth can occur.

Course and progress

This is a lifelong disease.

- Hair tends to straighten in the third decade
- Tendency towards caries and dental abscesses
- Prognathism after puberty

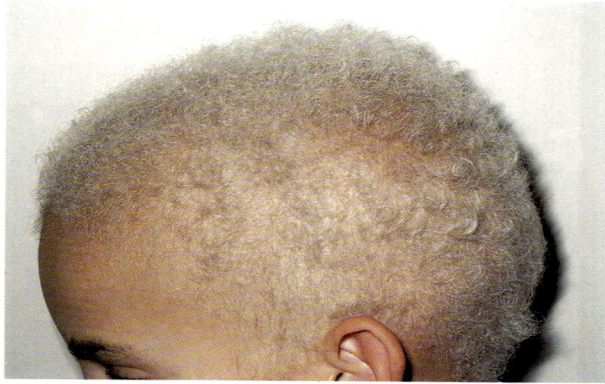

Figure 15.26

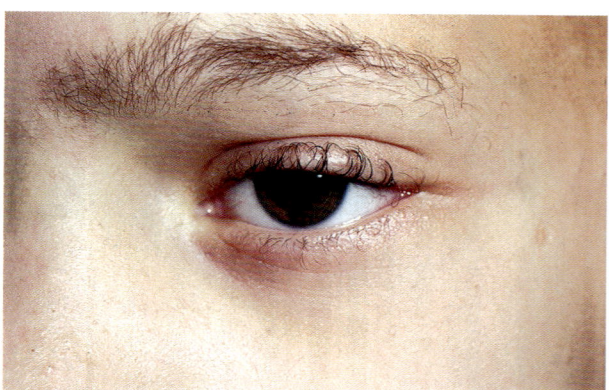

Figure 15.27

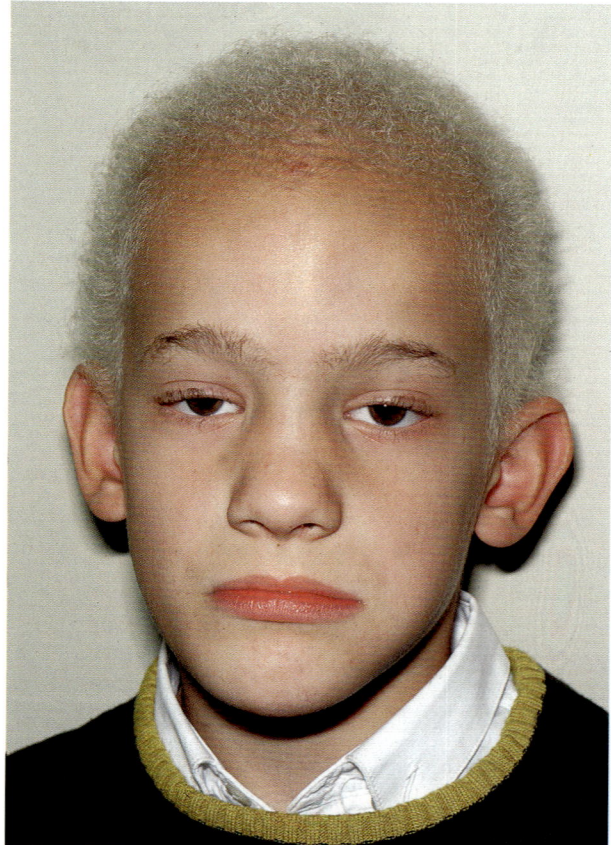

Figure 15.28

Laboratory findings

- Scanning electron microscopy shows aspecific alterations in the hair shaft
- Computed tomography (CT) shows increased deposition of mineralized bone at the skull base. In some, sclerotic bones are visible upon radiography

Genetics and pathogenesis

The disease is inherited as an autosomal dominant trait and there is a high clinical heterogeneity, even in the same family.

The causative gene of tricho-dento-osseous syndrome is DLX3, a homeodomain transcription factor.

This factor is expressed preferentially during tooth and hair follicle development, giving rise to a perturbed epithelial–mesenchymal interaction.

Complex interactions with other proteins such as MSX (see 'Witkop's disease', below) and indirectly with Cbfa1, an osteoblast differentiation factor, explain the increased bone density in this syndrome.

Differential diagnosis

- Other brittle hair syndromes such as trichothiodystrophy
- Isolated uncombable curly hair

Follow-up

- Odontostomatological assessment for caries and periodontitis prevention

Therapy

- Dental prostheses

REFERENCES

Price JA, Bowden DW, Wright JT, et al. Identification of a mutation in DLX3 associated with trichodento-osseous (TDO) syndrome. Hum Mol Genet 1998; 7: 563–9

Price JA, Wright JT, Kula K, et al. A common DLX3 gene mutation is responsible for trichodento-osseous syndrome in Virginia and North Carolina familes. J Med Genet 1998; 35: 825–8

Spangler GS, Hall KI, Kula K, et al. Enamel structure and composition in the trichodento-osseous syndrome. Connect Tissue Res 1998; 39: 165–75; discussion 187–94

WITKOP'S SYNDROME

Synonym

- Tooth and nail syndrome

Age of onset

- At birth

Clinical findings

- Koilonychia and thin laminae (Figure 15.29)
- Toenails more severely affected than fingernails (Figure 15.30)
- Anonychia is reported
- Rarely, hair shaft anomalies

Extracutaneous findings

- An almost physiologic primary dentition is not followed by the permanent dentition, partially or totally, with consequent retained primary teeth
- Facies and sweating are normal

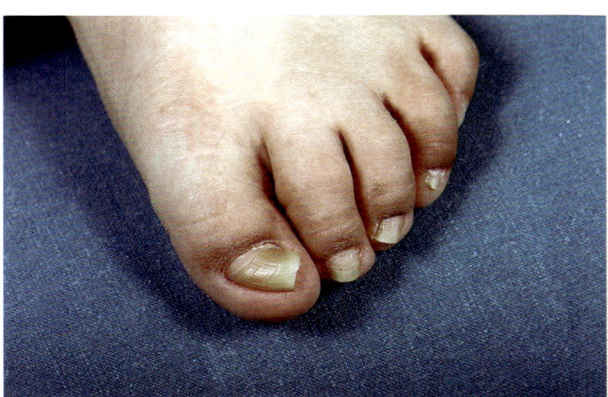

Figure 15.29

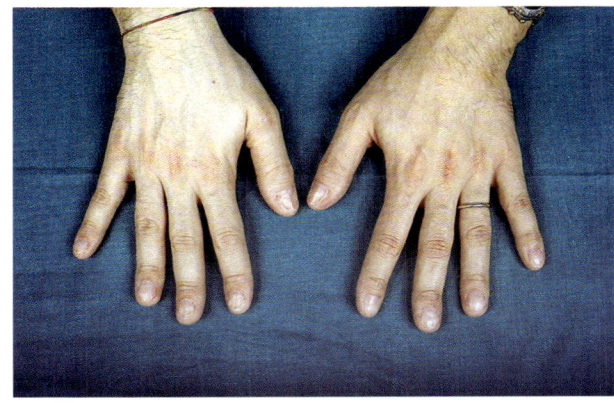

Figure 15.30

Complications

Orthodontic problems may lead to a pathologic maxillary–mandibular relationship.

Course

Teeth abnormalities are not visible until school age; nail abnormalities may improve with age.

Laboratory findings

Orthopantomography shows partial or total absence of the permanent teeth.

Genetics and pathogenesis

Mutations in the MSX1 gene result in Witkop's disease. The MSX1 gene is also mutated in familial tooth agenesis with or without cleft lip/palate, demonstrating that the MSX1 gene is crucial for tooth development. Expression studies have demonstrated that it is also crucial for nail development. The MSX1 gene, as well as other transcription factors related to ectodermal dysplasia, is expressed at the epithelial–mesenchymal interface, in this case at the mesenchymal side.

As already reported, the MSX and DLX genes interact in regulating other nuclear transcription factors that are important for morphogenesis during embryonic development (see also 'Tricho-dento-osseous syndrome').

Differential diagnosis

- Hypohidrotic ectodermal dysplasia

Follow-up

- Orthodontic consultations

Therapy

- Dentist and orthodontist to treat caries and provide protheses when needed

REFERENCES

Hodges SJ, Harley KE. Witkop tooth and nail syndrome: report of two cases in a family. Int J Paediatr Dent 1999; 9: 207–11

Jumlongras D, Bei M, Stimson JM, et al. A nonsense mutation in MSX1 causes Witkop syndrome. Am J Hum Genet 2001; 69: 67–74

ELLIS–VAN CREVELD–WEYERS ACRODENTAL DYSOSTOSIS COMPLEX

Synonym

- Chondroectodermal dysplasia

Age of onset

- At birth

Epidemiology

This disease is very rare; there are no data available.

Clinical findings

- Nails are dysplastic (hypoplastic) and koilonychia is present; anonychia is rare (Figure 15.31)
- Fine and sparse hair in some patients

Extracutaneous findings

This complex is characterized by:

- Disproportionate dwarfism with short distal extremities and less severe proximal anomalies
- Short ribs with narrow thorax
- Pelvis with hypoplastic iliac bones
- Postaxial polydactyly
- Neonatal teeth, hypoanodontia and delayed eruption for both primary and permanent dentitions and obliteration of upper oral vestibules (Figures 15.32 and 15.33)
- Congenital heart defects (almost always septal, present in about 50% of patients)
- Cryptorchidism and hypospadias
- Mental retardation of variable degree in some patients

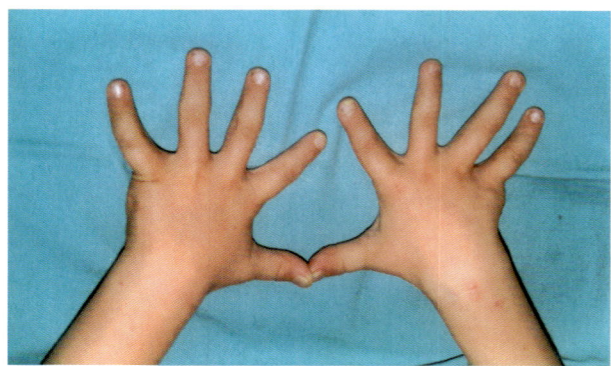

Figure 15.31

Complications

Heart failure may be lethal or life-threatening in the first year of life.

Course

The life span is reduced.

Laboratory findings

Cone-shaped epiphyses of the hand bones are pathognomonic on conventional radiography.

Genetics and pathogenesis

The Ellis–van Creveld–Weyers acrodental dysostosis (EvC–WAD) – complex is due to mutations in a gene, called the EVC gene, encoding a 992 amino-acid protein. This gene is expressed in developing bone, heart, kidney and lung. In bones it is overexpressed in the distal portion, reflecting the clinical aspects of the disease. It is highly expressed in both atrial and ventricular septa.

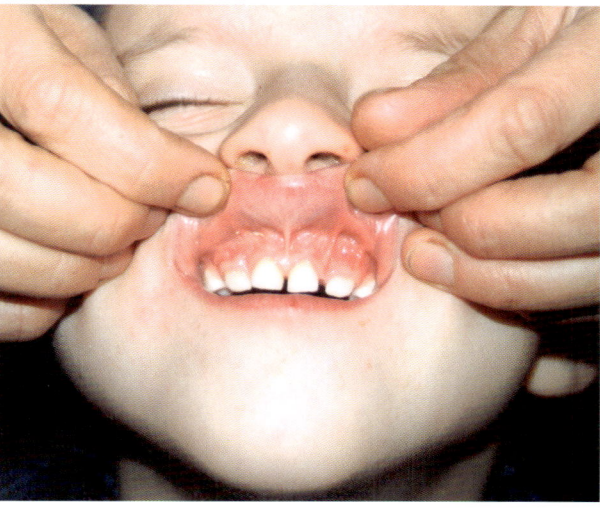

Figure 15.33

EvC disease and WAD, once classified as separate entities, now represent the same entity, inherited recessively for EvC phenotypes (homozygous loss of function mutations) and as a dominant mutation causing WAD, occurring in the same gene as discovered by molecular biology investigations.

Differential diagnosis

- Other rarest chondrodysplasias with or without ectodermal dysplasia

Follow-up

- Consultations for cardiologic and maxillofacial abnormalities

Therapy

- Restoration of interatrial and interventricular septa
- Oral and limb prostheses when needed

REFERENCES

Arya L, Mendiratta V, Sharma RC, Solanki RS. Ellis–van Creveld syndrome: a report of two cases. Pediatr Dermatol 2001; 18: 485–9

Galdzicka M, Patnala S, Hirshman MG, et al. A new gene, EVC2, is mutated in Ellis–van Creveld syndrome. Mol Genet Metab 2002; 77: 291–5

Ruiz-Perez VL, Tompson SE, Blair HJ, et al. Mutations in two nonhomologous genes in a head-to-head configuration cause Ellis–van Creveld syndrome. Am J Hum Genet 2003; 72: 728–32

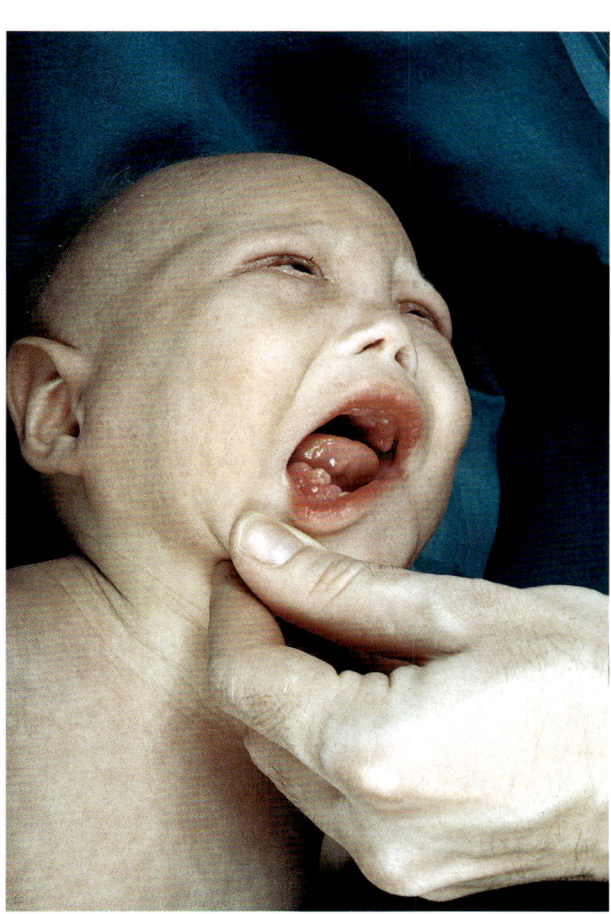

Figure 15.32

CLEFT LIP–PALATE WITH ECTODERMAL DYSPLASIA SYNDROME

Synonyms

This definition may encompass several entities, such as Margarita Island ED, Zlotogora–Ogur syndrome, Rosselli–Giulienetti syndrome and cleft lip–palate with mental retardation and syndactyly.

Epidemiology

This group of diseases is very rare.

Clinical findings

- Hypohidrosis
- Fine and woolly hair, fine eyebrows and eyelashes
- Aspecific nail changes with reported toenail hypoplasia
- Occasional palmoplantar keratoderma

Extracutaneous findings

- Cleft lips
- Cleft palate (Figure 15.34)
- Hypo-oligodontia
- Frontal bossing and malar hypoplasia
- Pterygia and syndactyly
- External genitalia malformation
- Mental retardation of variable degree in some pedigrees

Complications

There is an absence of major complications.

Course

The disease is lifelong.

Laboratory findings

- Radiography (conventional) reveals defects in facial bones and tooth development
- Sweat starch–iodine test may be helpful to detect hypohidrosis

Genetics and pathogenesis

The cleft lip–palate with ectodermal dysplasia (CLPED1) group of diseases is caused by mutations in a gene called PVRL1 that encodes a cell–cell adhesion molecule and herpes virus receptor. It has an immunoglobulin-like membrane receptor denominated nectin 1, which is important for the binding of several other proteins, such as afadin and ponsin, that are necessary for the maintenance of cell membrane stability, and is thought to be important in linkage to cytoskeleton proteins such as the cadherin–catenin system.

The diseases are probably inherited as an autosomal recessive trait.

Differential diagnosis

- Other ectodermal dysplasias with hypohidrosis
- Ectodermal dysplasia with cleft lip–palate

Follow-up

- Consultation with maxillofacial surgeon

Therapy

- Correction of cleft lip–palate malformations

REFERENCE

Cobourne MT. The complex genetics of cleft lip and palate. Eur J Orthodont 2004; 26: 7–16

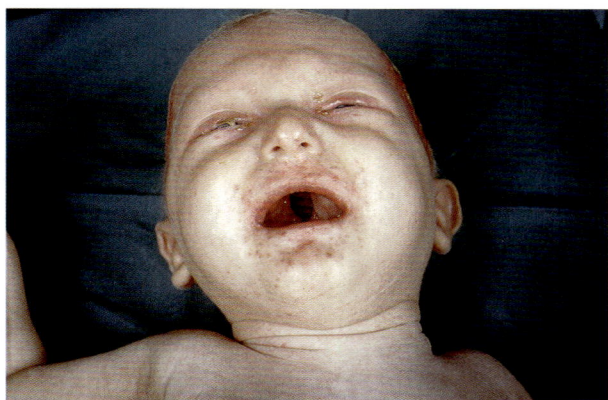

Figure 15.34

CLOUSTON'S DISEASE

Synonym

- Hidrotic ectodermal dysplasia

Epidemiology

The disease is rare. There are no data available on prevalence and incidence.

Clinical findings

- Palmoplantar keratoderma, severe diffuse form (Figures 15.35 and 15.36)
- Mild hypohidrosis
- Scalp hypotrichosis of variable degree, from mild cases (fragile curly hair) to complete alopecia (Figure 15.37)
- Scanty eyebrows and eyelashes that may be absent (Figure 15.38)
- Sparse or absent body hair
- Nail dystrophy of variable severity, to thickened, discolored, short laminae to scarring and total absence (Figures 15.39 and 15.40)
- Hyperkeratotic plaques in oral and jaw mucosa
- Occasionally hyperpigmentation of the skin over joints
- Xerosis and ichthyotic-like skin (Figure 15.40)

Extracutaneous findings

- Mental retardation (50% of patients)
- Congenital cataracts, pterygia and diminished lacrimation

Course and complications

- Progressive hair loss
- Nail and skin signs worsen with age
- Rarely, malignant degeneration in palmoplantar areas is reported
- Conjunctivitis and blepharitis

Laboratory findings

Electroencephalography may reveal abnormalities.

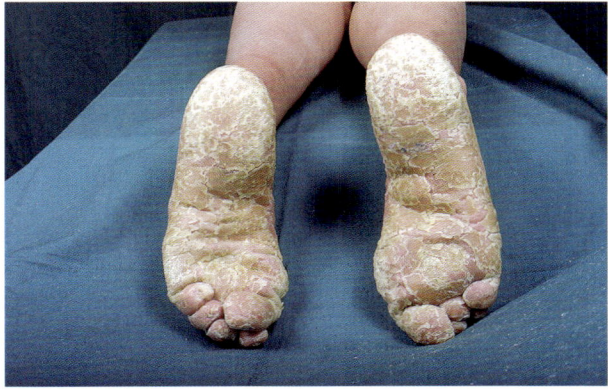

Figure 15.35

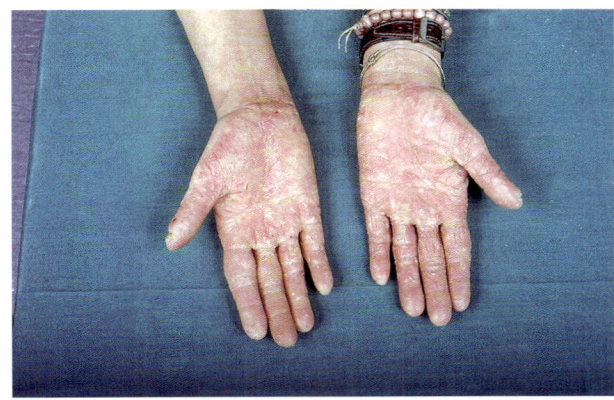

Figure 15.36

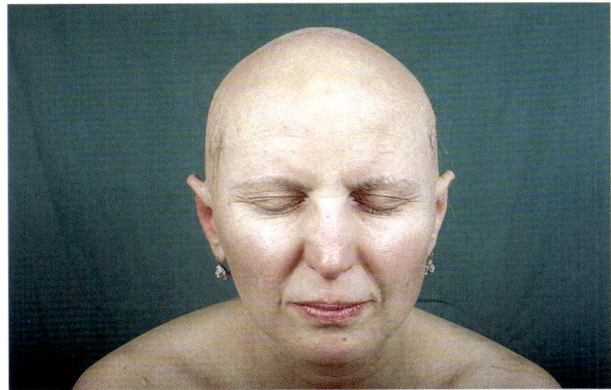

Figure 15.37

Genetics and pathogenesis

Connexin 30 is mutated in Clouston's patients. This gene encodes a gap junction protein that is highly expressed in ectodermal derivates such as brain and skin. Connexins are responsible for correct cell to cell signaling during morphogenesis.

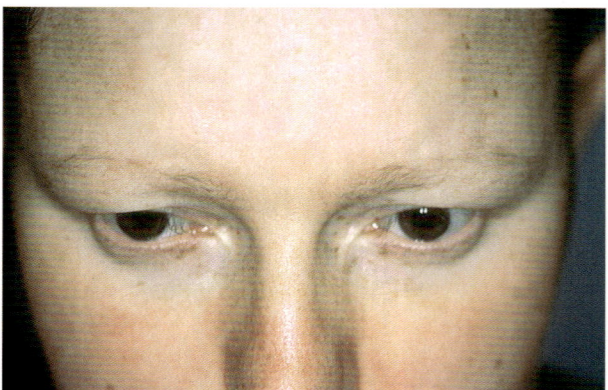

Figure 15.38

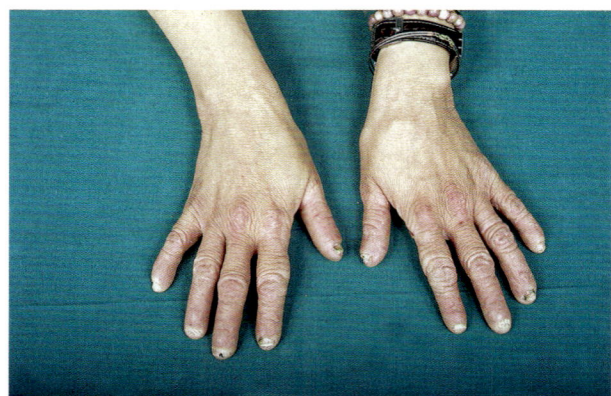

Figure 15.40

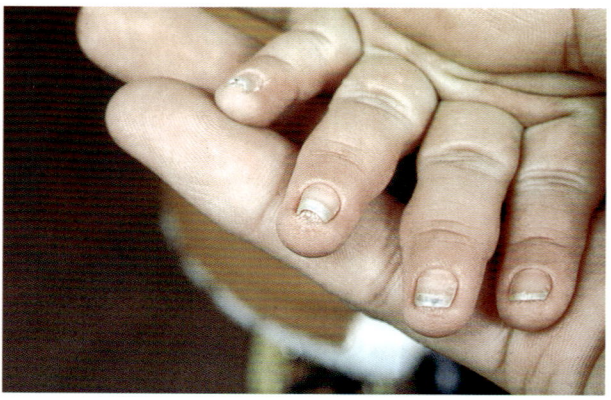

Figure 15.39

It must be noted that different connexins are mutated in diseases that have palmoplantar keratoderma and/or deafness as a major feature, such as KID (keratitis, ichthyosis and deafness) syndrome, Vohwinkel's syndrome (palmoplantar keratoderma of the mutilating type and deafness), twenty-nail leukodystrophy and deafness (personal observation) and erythrokeratodermia variabilis (diffuse figurated-like ichthyosis).

Differential diagnosis

- KID syndrome
- Pachyonychia congenita

Follow-up

- Periodic dermatological and neurological consultations

Therapy

- Psychological support for school and job
- Hair prosthesis when claimed
- Keratolytic agents for palmoplantar keratoderma
- Ablative surgery for malignant degeneration of palmoplantar keratoderma

REFERENCES

Kibar Z, Dube MP, Powell J, et al. Clouston hidrotic ectodermal dysplasia (HED): genetic homogeneity, presence of a founder effect in the French Canadian population and fine genetic mapping. Eur J Hum Genet 2000; 8: 372–80

Smith FJ, Morley SM, McLean WH. A novel connexin 30 mutation in Clouston syndrome. J Invest Dermatol 2002; 118: 530–2

Zhang XJ, Chen JJ, Yang S, et al. A mutation in the connexin 30 gene in Chinese Han patients with hidrotic ectodermal dysplasia. J Dermatol Sci 2003; 32: 11–17

ECTODERMAL DYSPLASIA–SKIN FRAGILITY SYNDROME

Epidemiology

The disease is very rare, accounting for ten cases described to date.

Clinical findings (Figures 15.41 and 15.42)

- Widespread blisters at birth (Figure 15.41)
- Trauma-induced blisters on pressure points
- Short and sparse hair
- Thickened and dystrophic nails (Figure 15.42)
- Hyperkeratotic plaques of palms and soles in adulthood (15.42)

Complications

Walking is slow owing to the painful plantar hyperkeratosis.

Course

The continuing formation of blisters on trauma points leads to the formation of hyperkeratotic plaques, especially on palms and soles. These lesions are painful and disabling.

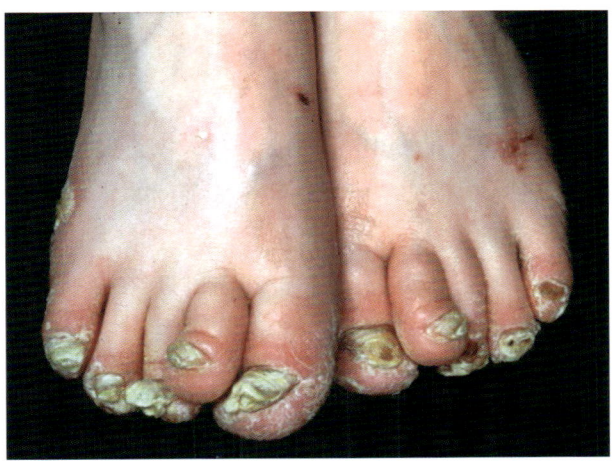

Figure 15.42

Laboratory findings

Electron microscopy reveals poorly formed or rudimentary desmosomes with a disorganized keratin filament network and cytolysis (Figure 15.43).

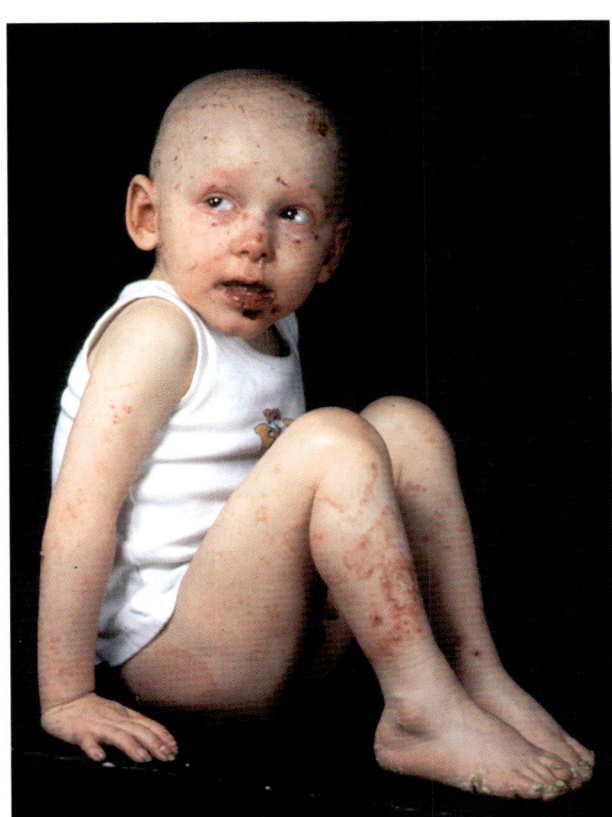

Figure 15.41

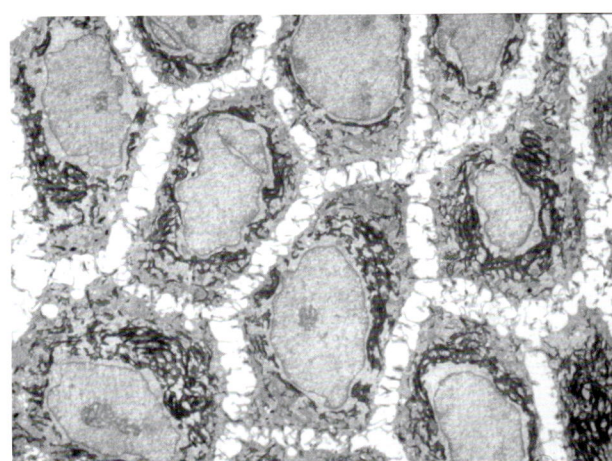

Figure 15.43

Genetics and pathogenesis

This disorder is autosomal recessive. The involved gene is called PKP1 and encodes a major component of the desmosomal structure, namely plakophilin 1. Mutations on this gene lead to defective cell–cell adhesion and interactions as well as abnormal architecture of the keratin network.

Follow-up and therapy

- Even babies must avoid minimal trauma
- Topical antibiotics are needed to avoid infections in the blister sites
- Keratolytic agents are suggested to manage palms and soles with painful hyperkeratoses

Differential diagnosis

- Epidermolytic epidermolysis bullosa (Dowling–Meara)
- Epidermolytic hyperkeratosis at birth

REFERENCES

Hamada T, South AP, Mitsuhashi Y, et al. Genotype–phenotype correlation in skin fragility–ectodermal dysplasia syndrome resulting from mutations in plakophilin 1. Exp Dermatol 2002; 11: 107–14

McMillan JR, Haftek M, Akiyama M, et al. Alterations in desmosome size and number coincide with the loss of keratinocyte cohesion in skin with homozygous and heterozygous defects in the desmosomal protein plakophilin 1. J Invest Dermatol 2003; 121: 96–103

Thornhill AR, Pickering SJ, Whittock NV, et al. Preimplantation genetic diagnosis of compound heterozygous mutations leading to ablation of plakophilin-1 (PKP1) and resulting in skin fragility ectodermal dysplasia syndrome: a case report. Prenat Diagn 2000; 20: 1055–62

PURE HAIR–NAIL ECTODERMAL DYSPLASIA

Epidemiology

There are five described pedigrees.

Age of onset

- At birth

Cutaneous findings

- Hair is dark and curly with areas of alopecia in frontal and temporal regions (Figures 15.44 and 15.45)
- Decalvans folliculitis (Figure 15.46)
- Onychodystrophy (Figure 15.47)

Extracutaneous findings

- Beak-like nose
- Normal sweating and teeth
- Normal neurological development

Course and prognosis

The disease is steady throughout life.

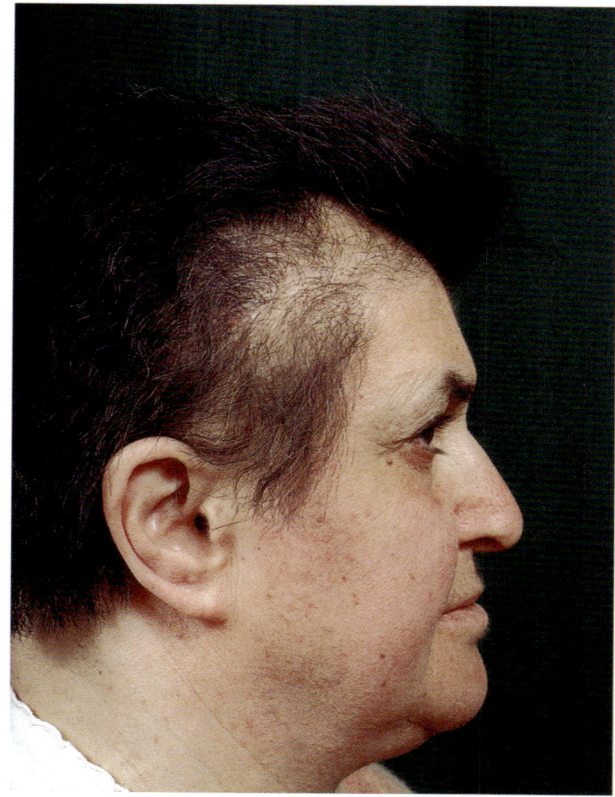

Figure 15.44

Ectodermal dysplasias and related disorders

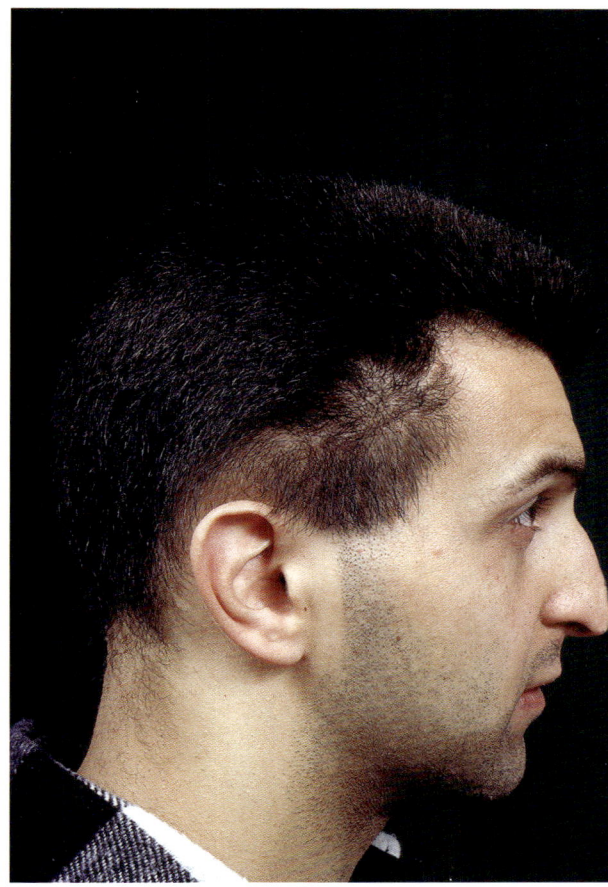

Figure 15.45

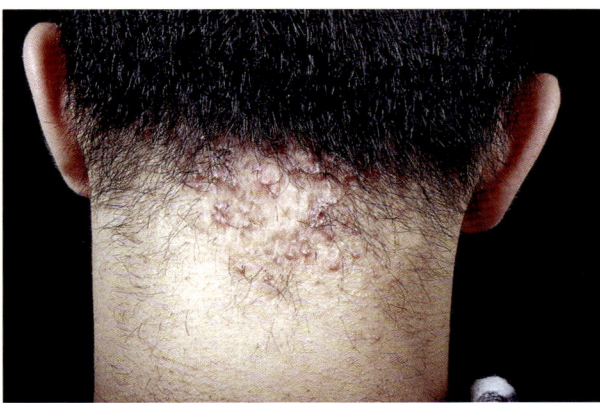

Figure 15.46

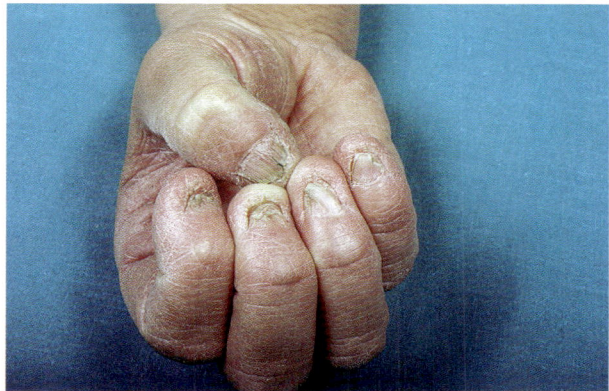

Figure 15.47

Laboratory investigations

Scanning electron microscopy shows twisted hair with abnormal cuticle.

Genetics and pathogenesis

- Autosomal dominant disease
- Unknown gene

Follow-up and therapy

- Local steroids for inflammatory folliculitis

Differential diagnosis

- Decalvans folliculitis
- Other ectodermal dysplasias with hair and nail dysplasia

REFERENCES

Barbareschi M, Cambiaghi S, Crupi AC, Tadini G. Family with 'pure' hair-nail ectodermal dysplasia. Am J Med Genet 1997; 72: 91–3

Pinheiro M, Freire-Maia N. Hair–nail dysplasia – a new pure autosomal dominant ectodermal dysplasia. Clin Genet 1992; 41: 296–8

INCONTINENTIA PIGMENTI

Synonym

- Bloch–Sulzberger syndrome

Age of onset

- At birth

Epidemiology

Incontinentia pigmenti is a rare disease, with an estimated prevalence of 1 : 300 000.

Clinical findings

It is classically described as a four-stage disease:

- The vesicobullous or inflammatory stage (present at birth) comprises vesicles and blisters distributed along Blaschko's lines, arising on an erythematous base. Lesions can be seen anywhere, but preferential sites are arms, legs and trunk. These lesions undergo involution in days or weeks and can be replaced by verrucous–squamous lesions. First-stage lesions may relapse throughout infancy, elicited by intercurrent disease or sun exposure (Figures 15.48 and 15.49)
- Verrucous–squamous stage is the mode of healing of the first stage. A linear portion can heal, with hyperkeratotic lesions that do not persist for long. In severe diffuse cases, such lesions can be seen at birth, as a result of an intrauterine vesicobullous stage (Figures 15.50 and 15.51)
- The hyperpigmented stage is characterized by pigmentary, brown to grayish linear lesions following Blaschko's lines, more usually located on the trunk and extremities. Linear parallel lesions are connected to each other by short perpendicular pigmented features, creating a particular picture defined as 'rail-sleepers', giving a reticulate appearance. Pigmented lesions disappear in many patients during childhood or adolescence, but sometimes can persist throughout life (Figures 15.52 and 15.53)
- The atrophic–hypopigmented stage is represented by white translucent stripes of atrophic skin characterized by the absence of hair follicles (histology and starch–iodine test also reveal the

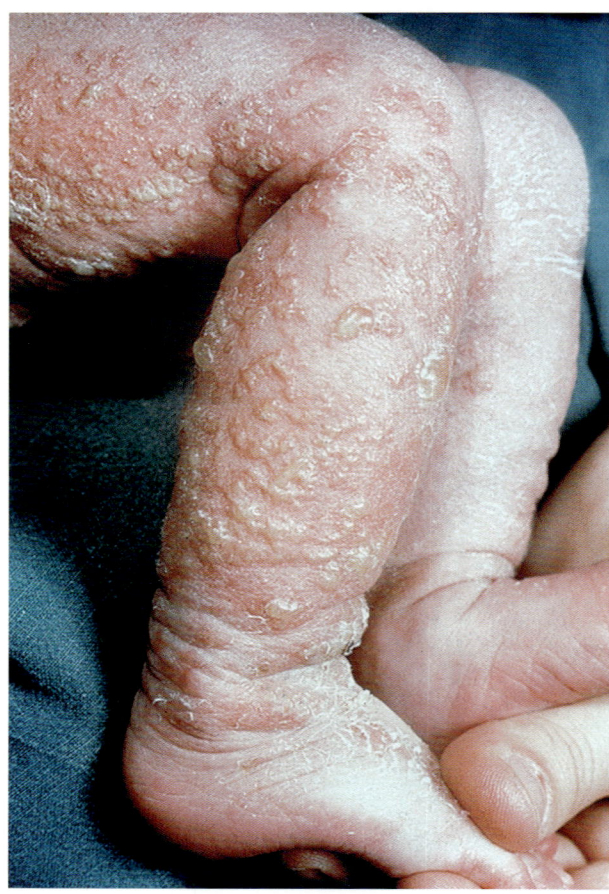

Figure 15.49

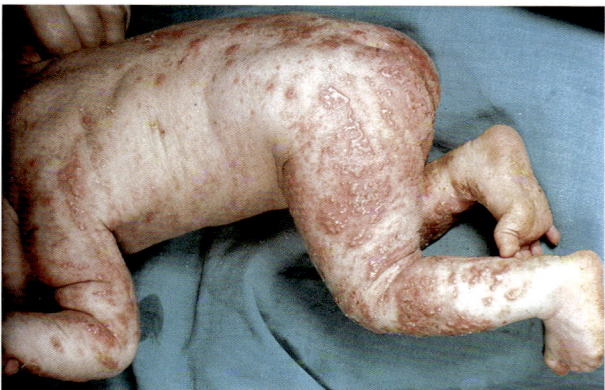

Figure 15.48

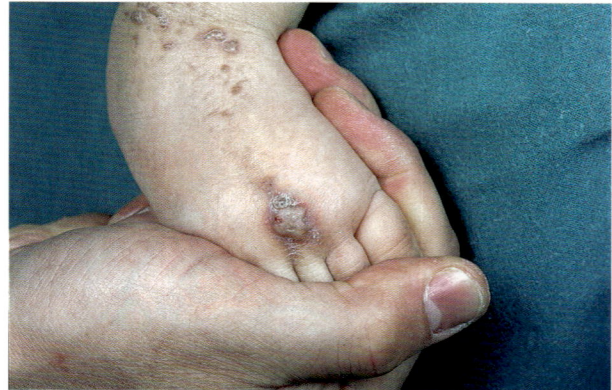

Figure 15.50

absence of sweat glands). They maintain the reticulate appearance described for the third stage, and can be the unique detectable symptom of incontinentia pigmenti in adult patients (Figures 15.54 and 15.55)

It must be remembered that all the stages can fade rapidly or be absent or underestimated by the patient.

Scarring alopecia is also present at the vertex as a result of the inflammatory initial stage (Figure 15.56).

Nail dystrophy is visible in 40% of patients and ranges from mild pitting to onychogryphosis with variable expression in the same subject, reflecting the presence of linear Blaschko line-associated inflammatory lesions (Figure 15.57).

Extracutaneous symptoms and complications

CNS manifestations are present in about 25% of patients:

- Severe mental retardation or oligophrenia
- Seizures
- Hemiplegia, spastic tetraplegia
- Microcephaly and hydrocephaly

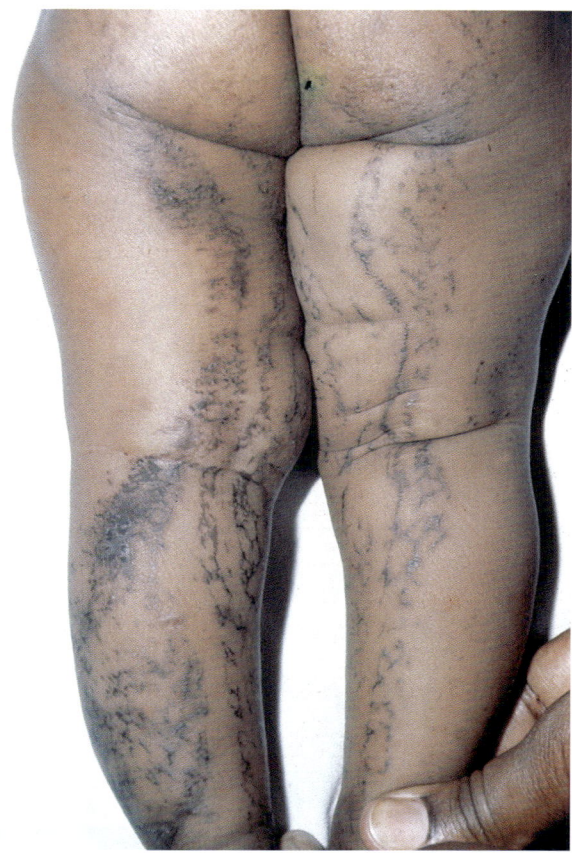

Figure 15.52

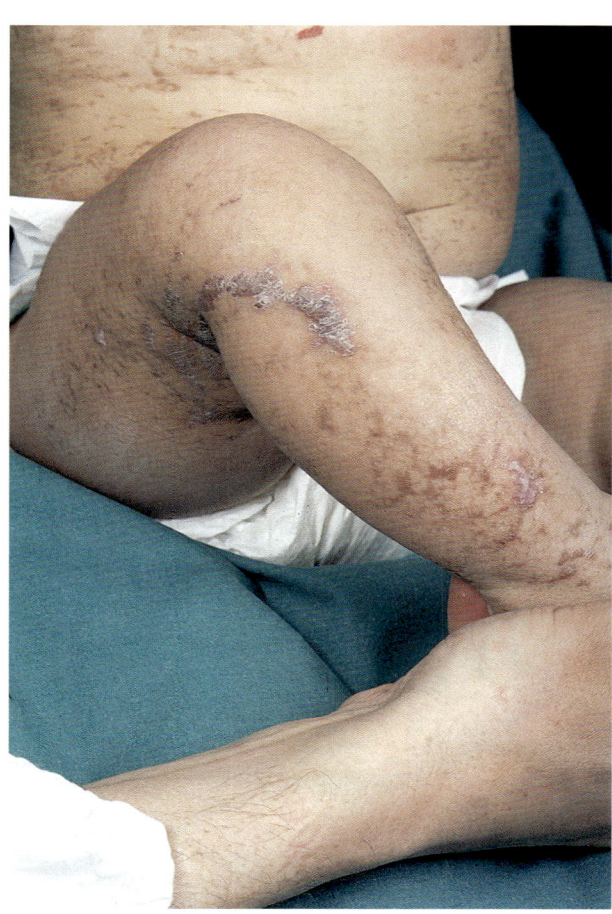

Figure 15.51

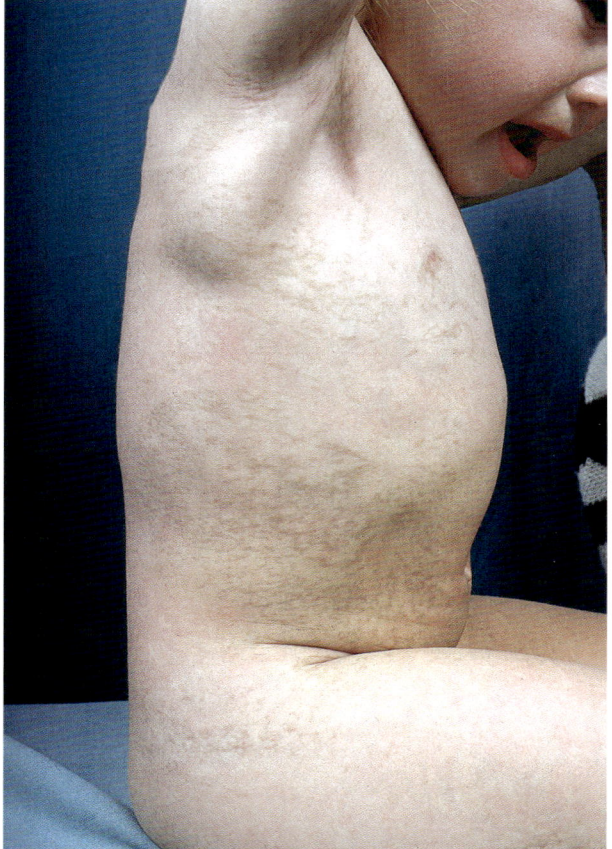

Figure 15.53

Ocular symptoms

Ophthalmological manifestations are present in 30% of patients:

- Usually monolateral and rare in patients without CNS symptoms
- Ischemic lesions of the retinal blood vessels that lead to neoangiogenesis and subsequent hemorrhages (retinal or vitreous) and to retractions with retinal detachments and partial blindness

- Foveal or peripheral retinal epithelium pigmentary linear anomalies
- Optic nerve atrophy
- Non-retinal symptoms: cataracts, corneal opacities, uveitis, nystagmus, myopia, blue sclerae and strabismus
- Microanophthalmia is described in rare cases

Odontoiatric symptoms

- Present in over 70% of patients
- Defects of decidual and permanent dentitions, such as partial anodontia, late dentition, malformed teeth, in particular hypoplastic teeth, conical or peg-shaped teeth (Figure 15.58)

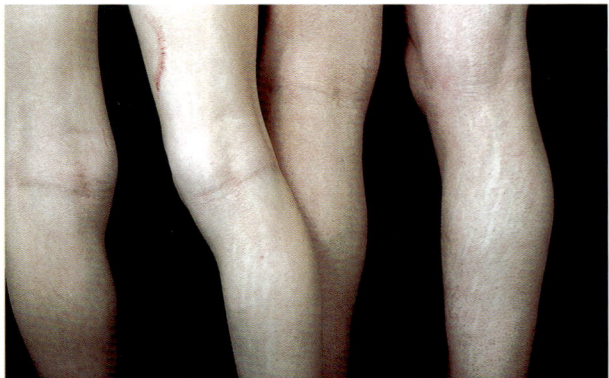

Figure 15.54

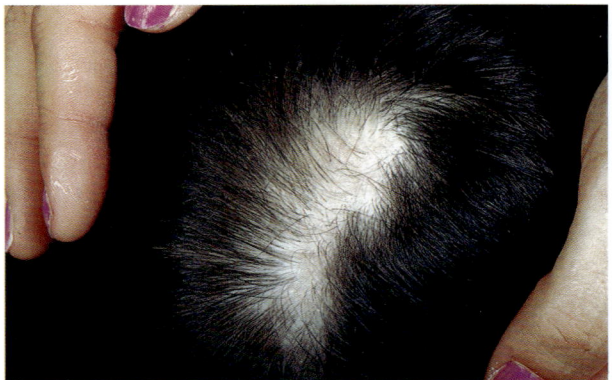

Figure 15.56

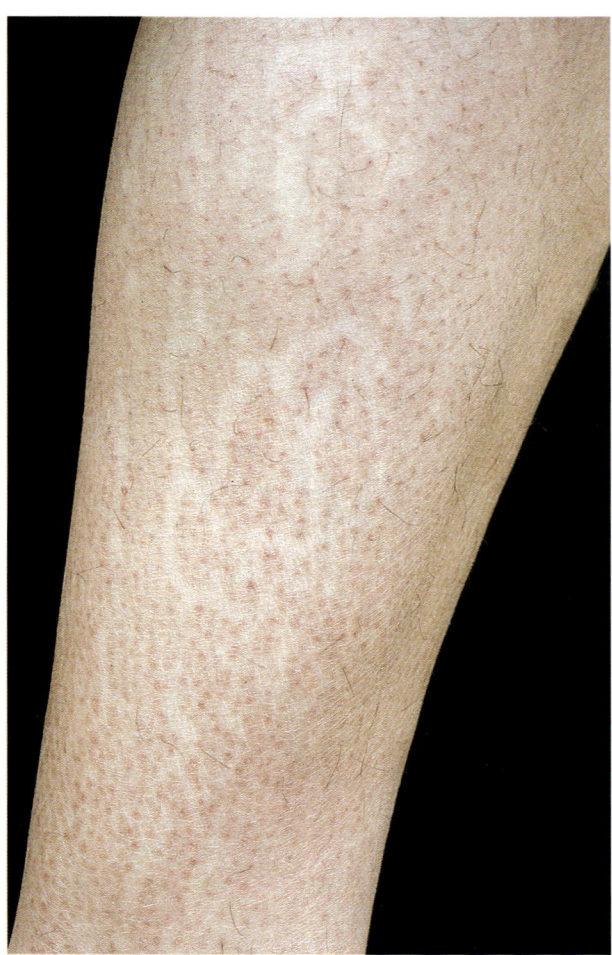

Figure 15.55

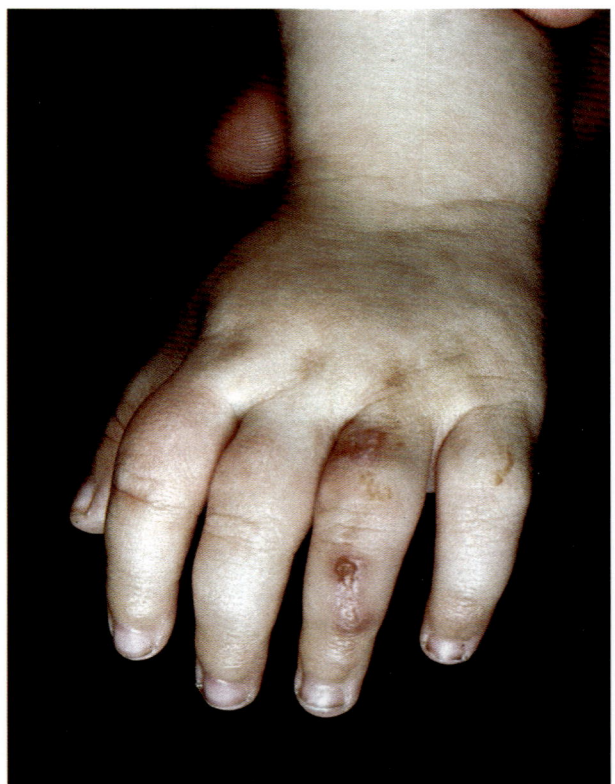

Figure 15.57

Such lesions persist throughout life and may be the only sign (as for fourth-stage lesions) of incontinentia pigmenti (IP) in adulthood.

In severe cases body hemihypotrophy is visible, strictly related to the side of skin lesions, reflecting a non-random X-inactivation process (Figure 15.59).

Course

The disease is lifelong.

In the majority of patients without CNS or ocular involvement the epidermal lesions may heal completely, leaving just fourth-stage atrophic linear lesions.

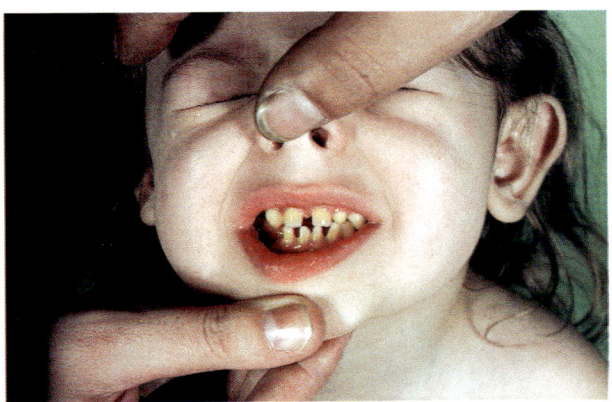

Figure 15.58

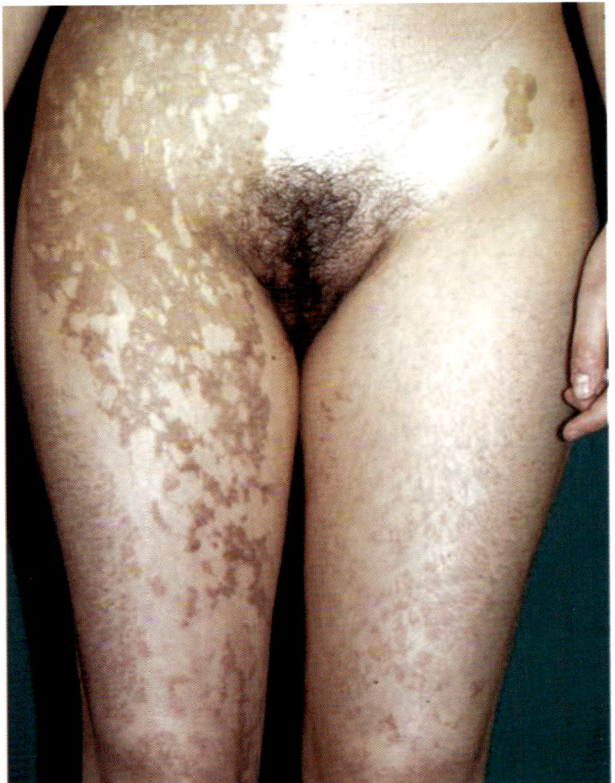

Figure 15.59

These lesions, together with isolated conical teeth, must be searched for in the mother and grandmothers of the neonate propositus patient to help in diagnosis. Characteristically, IP-affected parents of a young patient do not report any symptoms even if fourth-stage lesions are clearly visible.

In the same family, clinical variability is possible, hindering prognostic counseling for futher pregnancies.

Laboratory findings

- Leukocytosis (over 40 000 white blood cells/mm³)
- Eosinophilia is present wthin the first month of life in 75% of patients, ranging from 20% to even 65% of white blood cells
- Electroencephalogram, CT and magnetic resonance imaging (MRI) anomalies when CNS is involved
- Histology is useful in milder cases to confirm the clinical diagnosis in the first stages, revealing intraepidermal vesicles, surrounded by a massive eosinophilic infiltrate, spongiosis and apoptotic signs in the basal layer

Genetics and pathogenesis

Incontinentia pigmenti is an X-linked dominant disease. Usually this pattern is lethal for affected males, and females are variably affected. Females are affected along Blaschko's lines following a skewed or 'non-random X-inactivation' that favors the healthy X chromosome and explains the high clinical variability of the disease. It is highly probable that the IP defect is lethal even for female subjects if, as a rule, the normal 'random' X-inactivation is adopted, without selection of the normal allele (lyonization).

The gene for IP, called NEMO (NF-κB essential modulator), is located on Xq28, and the related protein plays a pivotal role in the modulation of an

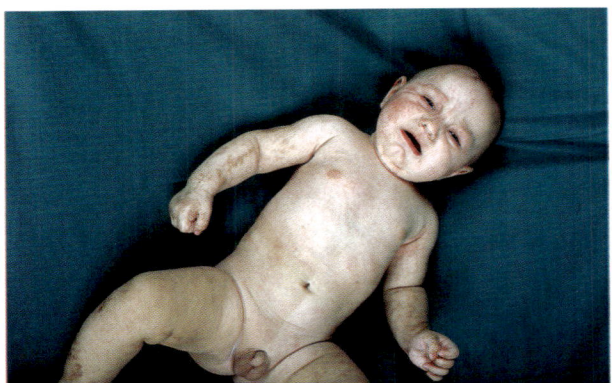

Figure 15.60

ancestral nuclear transcription system (NF-κB) that is responsible for the regulation of several functions, such as tumor necrosis factor (TNF)-mediated apoptosis, immune response, inflammatory response, differentiation of ectoderm-derived tissues and their proliferation. Lack of NEMO protein means altered control of NF-κB functions, and as a consequence, IP cells are highly sensitive to proapoptotic signals that lead to the clinical phenotype.

The NEMO gene encompasses ten exons. Some 80% of patients (female) suffer from a gene rearrangement that 'cuts' the gene from exon 4 to exon 10. The remaining 20% of patients have point mutations.

Male subjects (Figure 15.60) survive in three circumstances:

- Mosaic postzygotic mutations
- Mutations in exon 10 known as hypomorphic mutations
- XXY males

Finally, it must be remembered that HED genes act via the NEMO gene pathway to the same target NF-Kβ and that IP and HED show identical linear atrophic and 'adnexa-free' lesions along Blaschko's lines. Partial overlap between these two ectodermal dysplasias exists in the literature (osteopetrosis, lymphedema, hypohidrotic ectodermal dysplasia and IP with immunodeficiency).

Differential diagnosis

First stage:

- Epidermolysis bullosa, epidermolytic Dowling–Meara subtype
- Bullous mastocytosis
- Epidermolytic hyperkeratosis
- Bullous impetigo
- Herpes simplex and varicella

Second stage:

- Linear epidermal nevus
- Lichen striatus
- Linear Darier's disease

Third stage:

- Nevus hyperpigmentosus linearis
- Whorled hypermelanosis

Fourth stage:

- Linear hypomelanosis (including hypomelanosis of Ito)
- Female carriers of HED
- Goltz's syndrome

Follow-up

- Neurological examination in patients with signs of delayed development using CT scan, MRI, electroencephalography
- Odontostomatologic supervision for prosthesis adaptation to growth
- Dermatological consultations for relapses

Therapy

- Dermatological: infections of the first stage
- Odontostomatology: prostheses and caries
- Ophthalmology: laser therapy for retinal detachment and cataracts or corneal lesions
- Neurology: assesment for mental retardation and major CNS lesions at pediatric age
- Genetic counseling: detection of the affected female, elucidation of the risk of recurrence. Any affected mother has a 25% risk of abortion and half of her daughters being affected, without the chance to predict the prognosis (high interfamilial heterogeneity). In male patients, study of mutation of exon 10 or mosaic condition or karyotype for detection of 47XXY.

REFERENCES

Bardaro T, Falco G, Sparago A, et al. Two cases of misinterpretation of molecular results in incontinentia pigmenti, and a PCR-based method to discriminate NEMO/IKKgamma gene deletion. Hum Mutat 2003; 21: 8–11

Berlin AL, Paller AS, Chan LS. Incontinentia pigmenti: a review and update on the molecular basis of pathophysiology. J Am Acad Dermatol 2002; 47: 169–87

Dupuis-Girod S, Corradini N, Hadj-Rabia S, et al. Osteopetrosis, lymphedema, anhidrotic ectodermal dysplasia, and immunodeficiency in a boy and incontinentia pigmenti in his mother. Pediatrics 2002; 109: e97

Erickson RP. Somatic gene mutation and human disease other than cancer. Mutat Res 2003; 543: 126–36

Yamamoto Y, Gaynor RB. Role of the NF-kappaB pathway in the pathogenesis of human disease states. Curr Mol Med 2001; 1: 287–96

15.2 'Ectomesodermal' dysplasias

GOLTZ'S SYNDROME

Synonym

- Focal dermal hypoplasia

Epidemiology

There are about 250 cases reported in the literature.

Age of onset

- At birth

Clinical findings

- Erythematous streaks are visible at birth, distributed along the lines of Blaschko, especially on arms and legs (Figures 15.61 and 15.62)
- Lesions are non-homogeneous, often fragmented, and may be formed by a sequence of pinpoint or guttate, rough and patchy 'depressions', in which mosaic-like patterns are almost always recognizable, even when the streaks are short (Figures 15.62 and 15.63)
- On the face patterned peribuccal and perinasal streaks of red papules are visible (Figures 15.64 and 15.65)

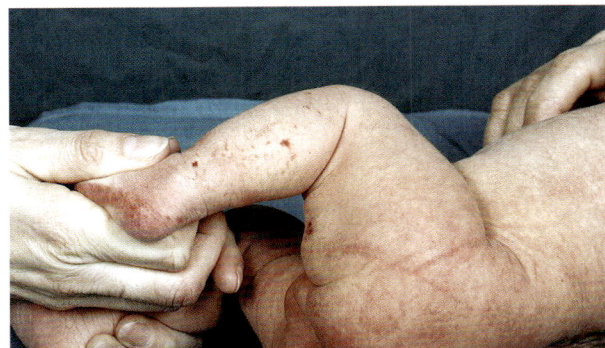

Figure 15.61

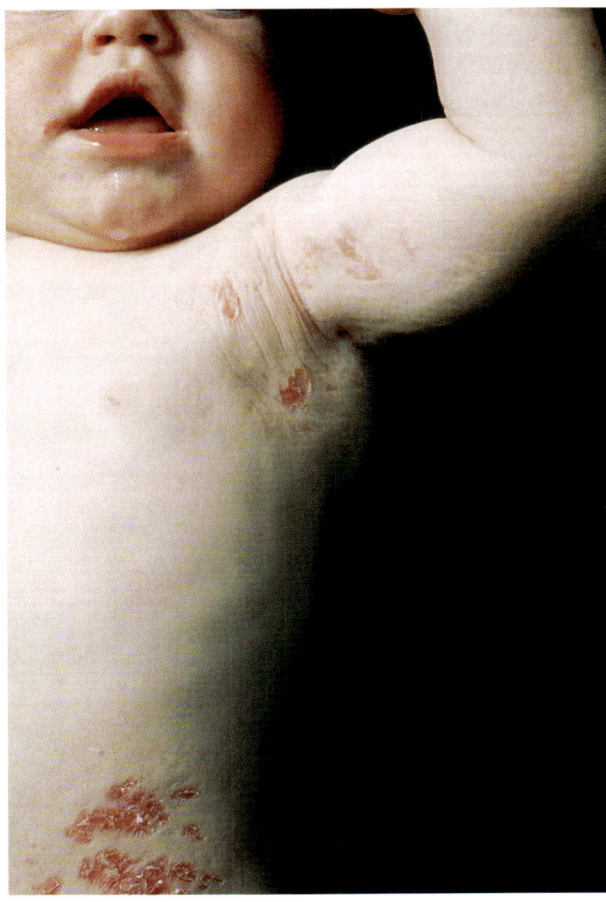

Figure 15.62

- Small, papillomatous-like lesions may be present in genital and perianal areas and major folds (Figures 15.66 and 15.67)
- Hypopigmented and hyperpigmented lesions along the Blaschko lines are present in over 50% of patients (Figures 15.67 and 15.68)
- Less frequently, the atrophic lesions are so severe that the skin is composed of an elementary two-layer border (atrophic epidermis and basal membrane), rendering the subcutaneous fatty tissue easily visible (these lesions have been described as 'herniations of the fatty tissue') (Figures 15.62 and 15.69)

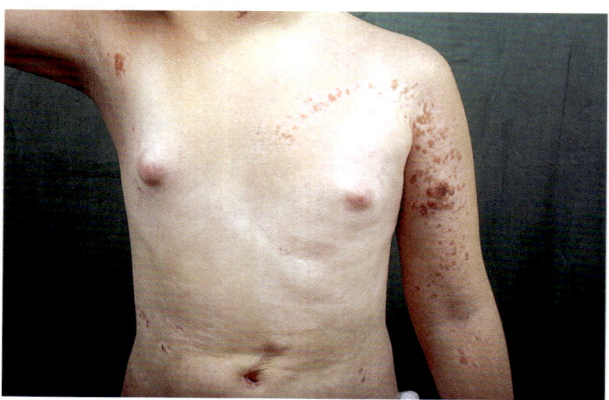

Figure 15.63

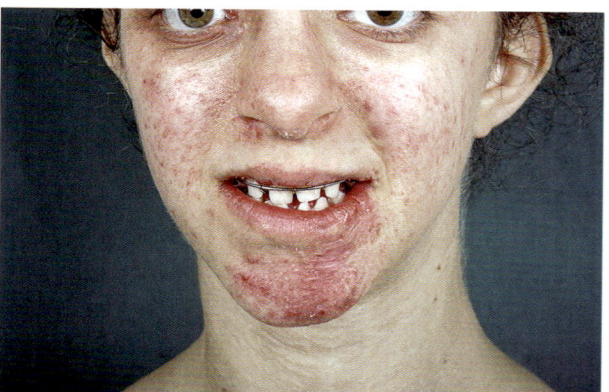

Figure 15.64

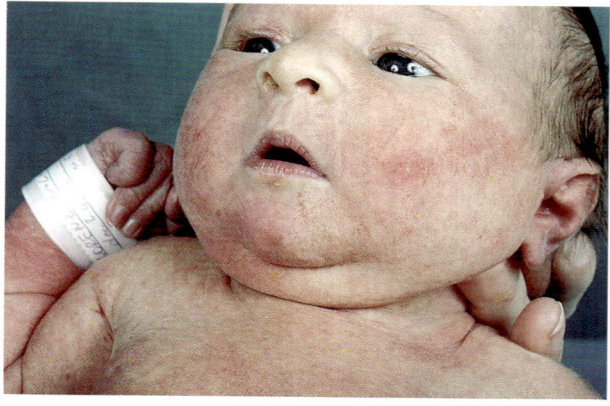

Figure 15.65

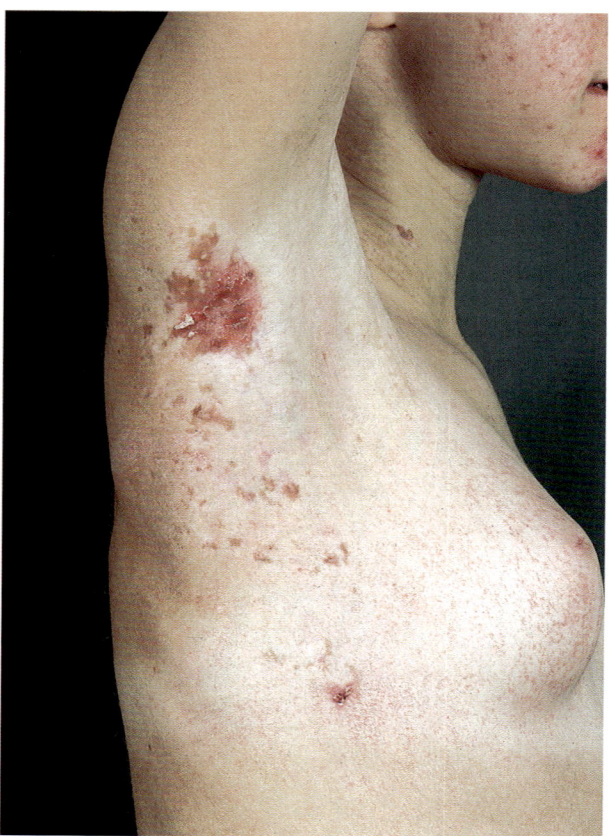

Figure 15.66

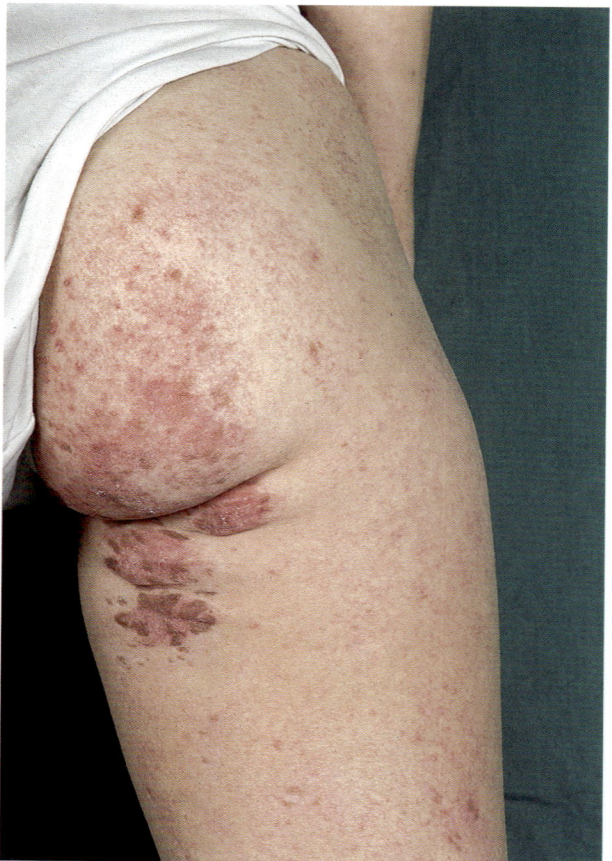

Figure 15.67

- Hypohidrosis distributed in a mosaic pattern
- 'Aplasia cutis'-like lesions and scarring alopecia (Figure 15.70), together with onychodysplasia, complete the clinical picture

Extracutaneous findings

- A particular 'facies' with thin nose, and hypotelorism, pointed chin and asymmetry may be present (Figures 15.64 and 15.65)
- Microphthalmia, nystagmus and strabismus may be associated with retinal defects
- Delayed dentition, hypo-oligodontia and enamel defects
- Cleft lip/palate and tongue
- Papillomatous lesions may be detected in the oral cavity and esophagus
- Mental retardation of variable degree in half of patients
- Hearing loss is rare
- True or pseudosyndactyly, together with hypo-aplasia of the II, III and IV rays of hands, metacarpal bones and toes, is highly characteristic (Figure 15.71); lobster-claw appearance is rare

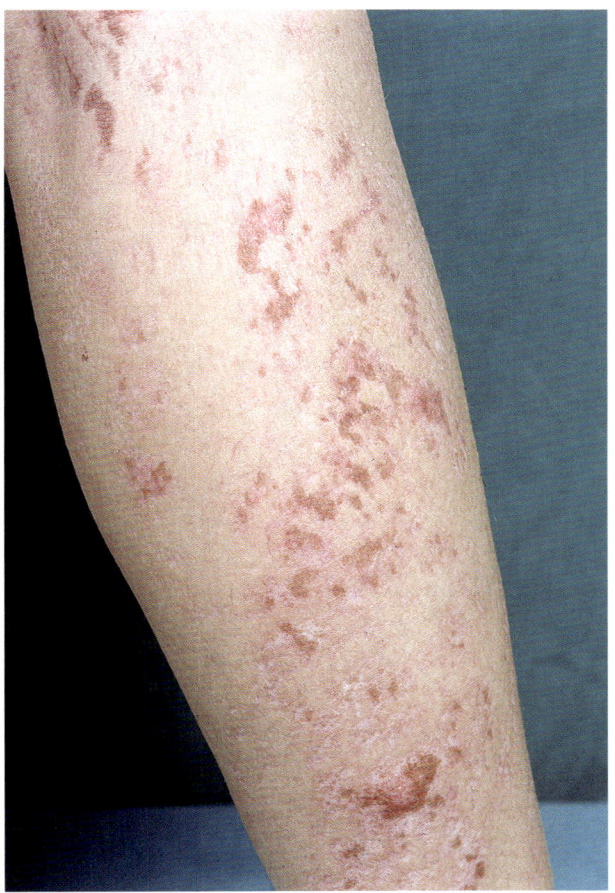

Figure 15.68

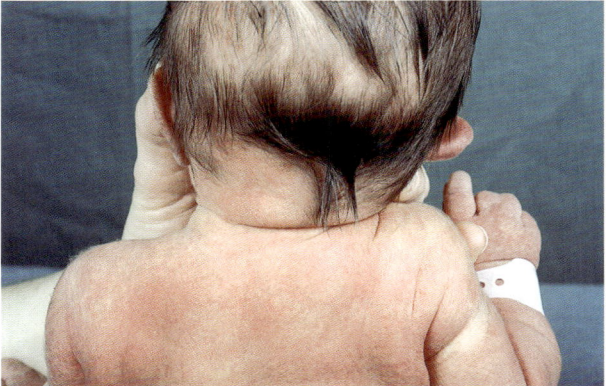

Figure 15.70

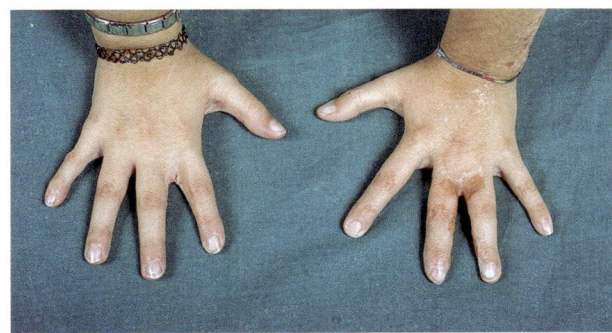

Figure 15.71

- Short stature with asymmetry is frequent
- Septal cardiac defects, abdominal wall defects and renal malformations have been reported
- Amenorrhea and delayed sexual development

Course and complications

We believe that Goltz's syndrome represents the 'mesodermal–ectodermal variant' of incontinentia pigmenti. Strong similarities between these two X-linked dominant diseases are easily detectable. As occurs in IP, the cutaneous lesions in Goltz's may represent a sequence of lesions and not a true list of symptoms.

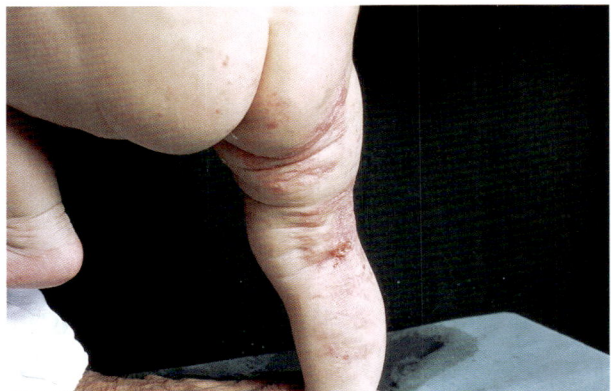

Figure 15.69

Stage I may be represented by erythematous depressed streaks and papillomatous lesions and herniations (variable severity of the genetic defect and different areas explaining the different phenotypes).

Stage II may be represented by hypo- and/or hyperpigmented lesions.

Life expectancy is normal.

Laboratory findings

Radiography shows 'osteopathia striata' that is characteristic of Goltz's syndrome.

Genetics and pathogenesis

The disease is X-linked dominant. Few male subjects survive.

Unfortunately, the gene has not been mapped, but as already discussed, the similarities between the group of diseases that are linked to the NEMO gene (mosaic pattern, inheritance, atrophic lesions with hypohidrosis, microphthalmia and CNS involvement, syndactyly and malformations of hands and feet, teeth defects, cleft lip and palate) strongly argue in favor of the inclusion of Goltz's syndrome under the heading 'ectomesodermal dysplasias'.

We could hypothesize that Goltz's syndrome may be due to a gene that has NEMO-like functions, expressed not only in the ectoderm but also in the mesoderm-derived structures.

Follow-up and therapy

- Once the diagnosis is established through the cutaneous signs, a multidisciplinary approach is mandatory to detect eye and ear abnormalities as well as internal organ involvement
- Plastic surgery of face lesions has been performed with success in many patients
- Hand surgery for bone defects and syndactyly

Differential diagnosis

- Incontinentia pigmenti
- EEC complex syndrome (ectrodactyly, ectodermal dysplasia, cleft lip/palate)

REFERENCES

Fryssira H, Papathanassiou M, Barbounaki J, et al. A male with polysyndactyly, linear skin defects and sclerocornea. Goltz syndrome versus MIDAS. Clin Dysmorphol 2002; 11: 277–81

Hancock S, Pryde P, Fong C, et al. Probable identity of Goltz syndrome and Van Allen–Myhre syndrome: evidence from phenotypic evolution. Am J Med Genet 2002; 110: 370–9

Kanitakis J, Souillet AL, Butnaru C, Claudy A. Melanocyte stimulation in focal dermal hypoplasia with unusual pigmented skin lesions: a histologic and immunohistochemical study. Pediatr Dermatol 2003; 20: 249–53

MIDAS SYNDROME

Synonyms

- Microphthalmia, dermal aplasia, sclerocornea syndrome
- Microphthalmia and linear skin defects

Epidemiology

There are no data. The disease is very rare.

Age of onset

- At birth

Clinical findings

- Atrophic, linear, scar-like lesions exclusively of the face and neck, distributed along Blaschko's lines (Figure 15.72)
- Aplasia cutis of the face and scalp areas

Clinical findings

The disease has a steady evolution. Life expectancy is related to the degree of CNS lesions.

Extracutaneous findings

- Microphthalmia, colobomas and strabismus (Figure 15.72)
- Cranial and CNS malformations
- Mental retardation

Course and complications

The disease has a steady evolution. Life expectancy is related to the degree of CNS lesions.

Genetics and pathogenesis

- X-linked dominant form
- Mapped to X22.1–22.3

Follow-up and therapy

- MRI to exclude CNS involvement
- Plastic surgery for facial lesions

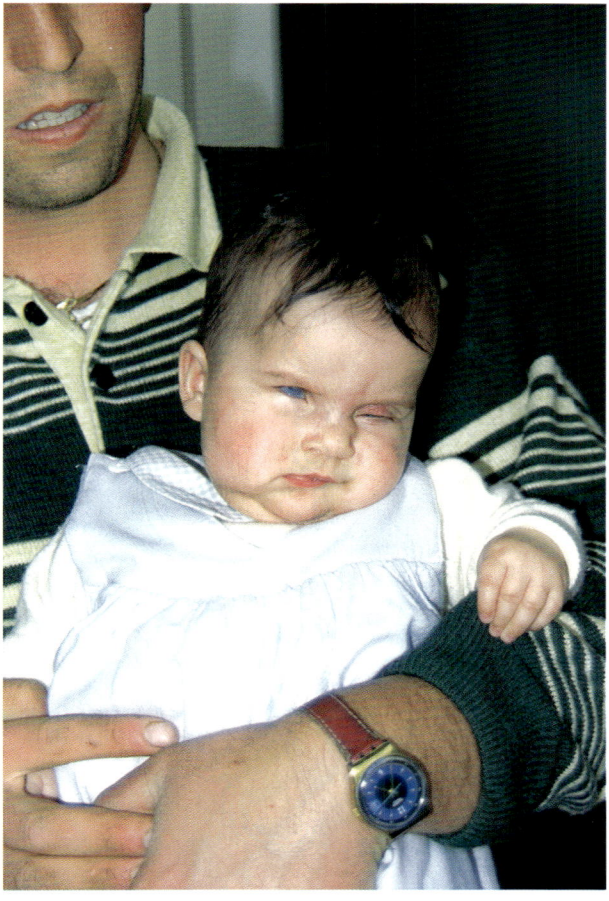

Figure 15.72

- Ophthalmological consultations for eventual corneal transplant

Differential diagnosis

Some authors hypothesize that MIDAS could be a partial form of Goltz's syndrome.

REFERENCES

Anguiano A, Yang X, Felix JK, Hoo JJ. Twin brothers with MIDAS syndrome and XX karyotype. Am J Med Genet 2003; 119A: 47–9

Fryssira H, Papathanassiou M, Barbounaki J, et al. A male with polysyndactyly, linear skin defects and sclerocornea. Goltz syndrome versus MIDAS. Clin Dysmorphol 2002; 11: 277–81

CHAPTER 16

Fatty tissue anomalies

LAUNOIS–BENSAUDE SYNDROME

Synonyms

- Familial symmetric lipomatosis
- Madelung disease

Epidemiology

A few reports exist in the literature, leading to an estimated number of a maximum 100 cases described.

Age of onset

- From the third decade

Clinical findings

- Slowly enlarging and disfiguring lipomas on the upper trunk, and neck but also arms and legs (Figures 16.1 and 16.2)
- Lesions also may be nodular or create a diffuse hypertrophy of the body fat, giving the appearance of a 'body-builder'

Extracutaneous findings

- Glucose intolerance, diabetes and related peripheral neuropathy
- Hyperlipidemia
- Gout and renal acidosis
- Alcohol abuse is noted in many of the reported patients

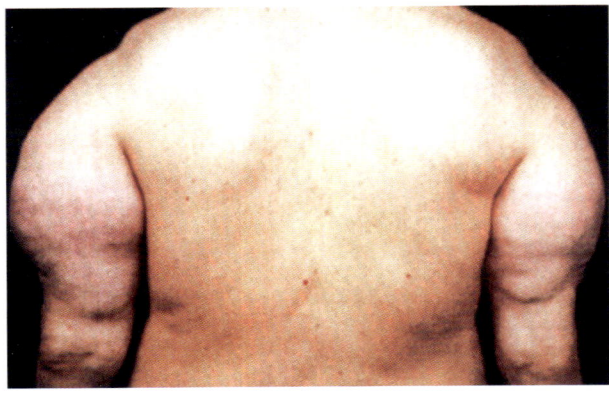

Figure 16.1

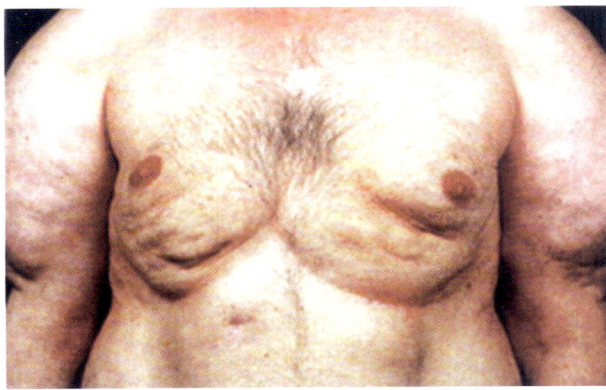

Figure 16.2

Course and prognosis

- Cutaneous lesions are slowly progressive
- Prognosis depends on the severity of related metabolic abnormalities

Laboratory findings

On conventional microscopy, lipomas appear well circumscribed and encapsulated.

Genetics and pathogenesis

- Majority of sporadic cases
- Few pedigrees described (autosomal dominant?)
- The causative gene is unknown

Follow-up and therapy

- Check for metabolic abnormalities
- Prevention of alcohol abuse
- Surgery when mandatory

Differential diagnosis

- Other lipomatoses
- Sebocystomatosis

REFERENCES

Bojanic P, Simovic I. Launois–Bensuade syndrome (Madelung's disease). Dermatol Online J 2001; 7: 9

Harsch IA, Schahin SP, Fuchs FS, et al. Insulin resistance, hyperleptinemia, and obstructive sleep apnea in Launois–Bensaude syndrome. Obes Res 2002; 10: 625–32

Preisz K, Karpati S, Horvath A. Launois–Bensuade syndrome and Bureau–Barriere syndrome in a psoriatic patient: successful treatment with carbamazepine. Eur J Dermatol 2002; 12: 267–9

TOTAL LIPODYSTROPHY

Synonyms

- Congenital generalized lipodystrophy
- Seip–Lawrence syndrome
- Berardinelli's syndrome

Age of onset

- At birth or during early infancy

Clinical findings

Cutaneous and mucosal manifestations

- Hypertrichosis (Figures 16.3 and 16.4)
- Acanthosis nigricans (Figure 16.5)
- Scrotal tongue (Figure 16.6)
- Hypotrophy of subcutaneous fat

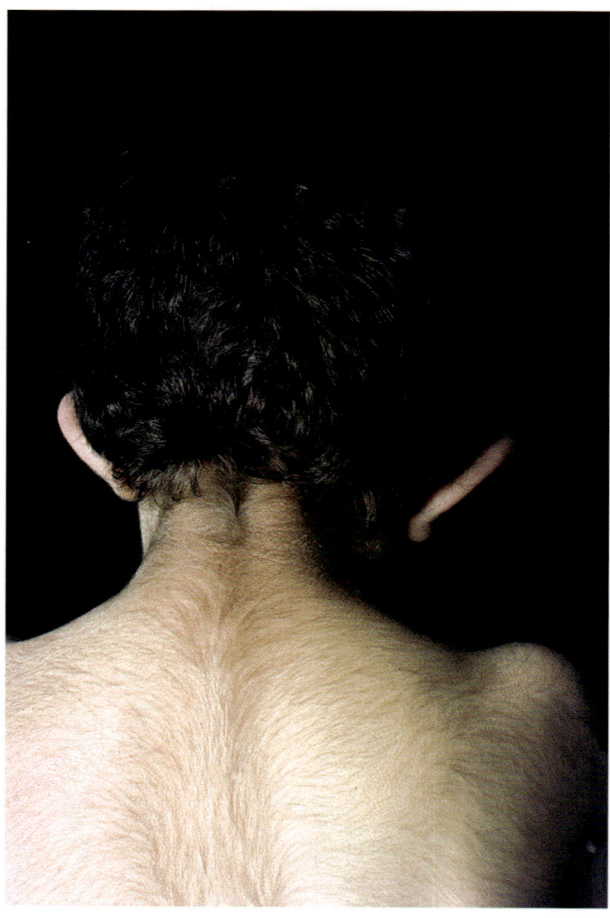

Figure 16.3

- Curly scalp hair
- Hypertrophy of external genitalia (Figure 16.5)

Extracutaneous manifestations

- Insulin-resistant diabetes
- Characteristic facies with prominent zygomatic bones, hollowed temples, sunken cheeks and prominent ears
- Prominent superficial and scalp veins
- Protuberant abdomen
- Hepatomegaly
- Severe mental retardation
- Cardiac, ovarian, skeletal and ocular anomalies

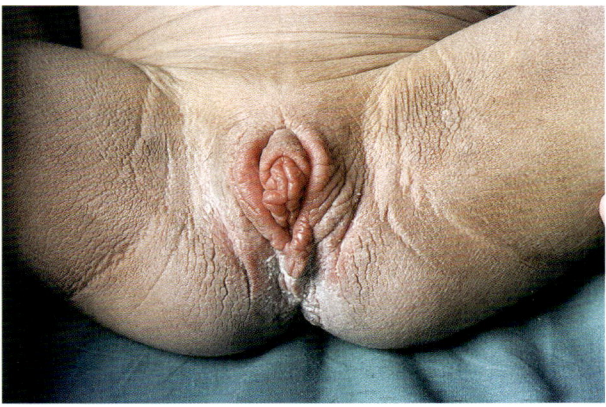

Figure 16.5

Course and prognosis

This disease is slowly progressive.

Life-expectancy is greatly reduced, mainly due to diabetes and its complications.

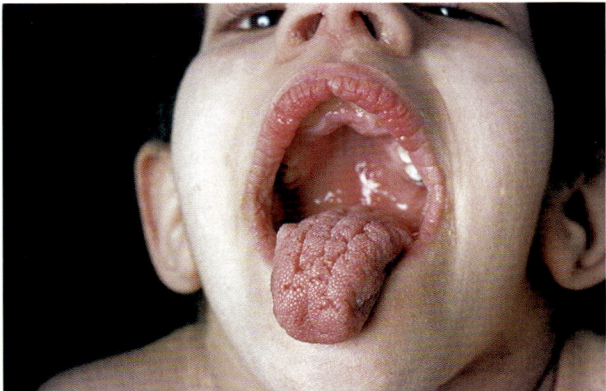

Figure 16.6

Laboratory investigations

- Persistent hyperglycemia and severe glycosuria
- Hyperlipidemia
- Abnormal liver function
- Advanced skeletal maturation radiographically

Genetics and pathogenesis

- Autosomal recessive inheritance
- Gene locus on chromosome 9q34 (?) with insulin receptor mutations
- Two possible mechanisms suggested to produce lipoatrophy: failure to deposit fat in the subcutaneous fat-storage cells or an overactive fat-mobilizing system

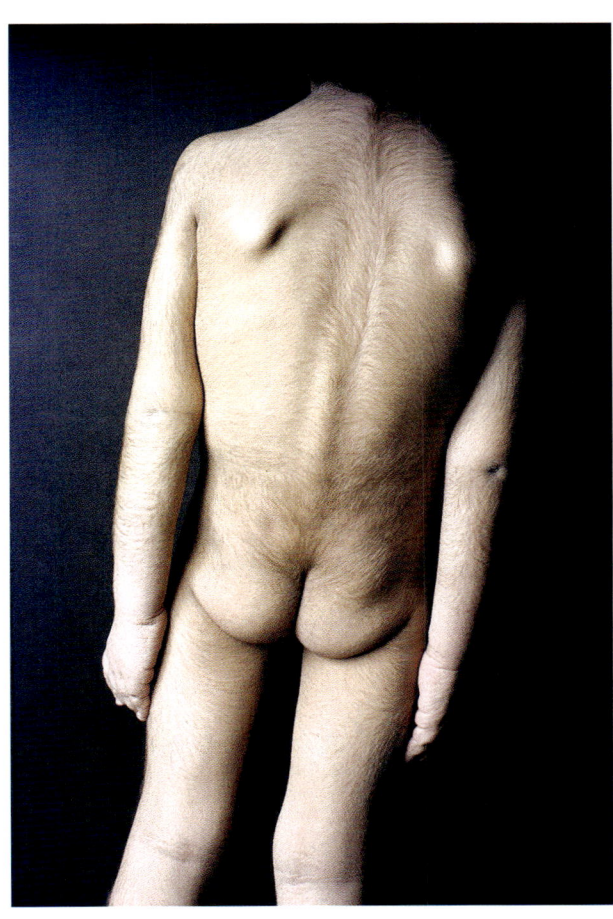

Figure 16.4

Differential diagnosis

- Leprechaunism
- Cockayne's syndrome
- Rabson–Mendenhall syndrome

Follow-up and therapy

- Control of metabolic alterations
- Troglitazone, rosiglitazone and pioglitazone may be useful in controlling hyperglycemia and increasing adipose tissue mass

REFERENCES

Agarwal AK, Simha V, Oral EA, et al. Phenotypic and genetic heterogeneity in congenital generalized lipodystrophy. J Clin Endocrinol Metab 2003; 88: 4840–7

Brubaker MM, Vevan NE, Collipp PJ. Acanthosis nigricans and congenital total lipodystrophy. Arch Dermatol 1965; 91: 320–5

Janaki VR, Premelatha S, Raghyveeza Rao N, et al. Lawrence–Seip syndrome. Br J Dermatol 1980; 103: 693–6

Joffe BI, Pauz VR, Rael F. From lipodystrophy syndromes to diabetes mellitus. Lancet 2001; 357: 1379–81

Requena Caballero C, Angel Navarro Mira M, Bosch IF, et al. Barraquer–Simons lipodystrophy associated with antiphospholipid syndrome. J Am Acad Dermatol 2003; 49: 768–9

PARTIAL LIPODYSTROPHY

Synonyms

- Familial lipodystrophy of limbs and lower trunk
- Kobberling–Dunnigan syndrome

Age of onset

- Childhood

Clinical findings

Cutaneous manifestations

- Loss of subcutaneous fat restricted to the extremities or affecting limbs and trunk (Figure 16.7)
- Acanthosis nigricans
- Xanthomas

Extracutaneous manifestations

- Prominent musculature and veins
- Insulin-resistant diabetes mellitus
- Hyperlipoproteinemia

Course

The disease is slowly progressive.

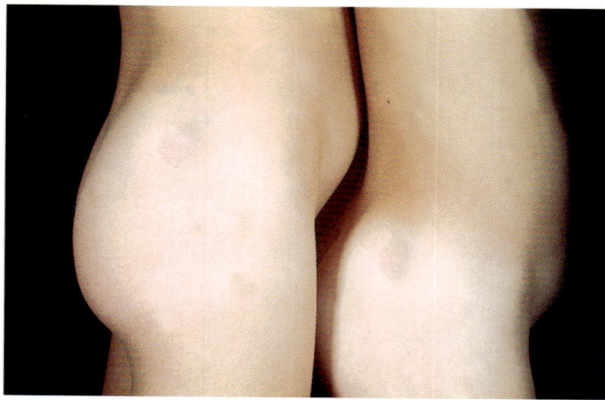

Figure 16.7

Genetics and pathogenesis

- X-linked dominant inheritance
- Seen only in females and linked to a mutation in the gene for lamin A/C, which encodes two nuclear laminar proteins

Differential diagnosis

- Acquired lipodystrophy
- Scleroderma

Therapy

No treatment is available.

REFERENCES

Burn J, Baraitser M. Partial lipoatrophy with insulin resistant diabetes mellitus and hyperlipidemia (Dannigan syndrome). J Med Genet 1986; 23: 128–30

Joffe BI, Panz VR, Raal FJ. From lipodystrophy syndromes to diabetes mellitus. Lancet 2001; 357: 1379–81

Kobberling J, Dunnigan MG. Familial partial lipodystrophy: two types of an X-linked dominant syndrome, lethal in the hemizygous state. J Med Genet 1986; 23: 120–7

CHAPTER 17

Disorders of connective tissue

EHLERS–DANLOS SYNDROMES

Ehlers–Danlos syndrome type I

Synonym

- Ehlers–Danlos syndrome gravis

Age of onset

- Birth to infancy; birth is frequently premature

Clinical findings

Cutaneous manifestations

- Skin soft, velvety and extremely elastic; after stretching and releasing it returns immediately to normal position (Figure 17.1)
- Increased skin fragility with resultant formation of atrophic scars with papyraceous aspect, mostly situated over bony prominences and extensor surfaces of joints (Figure 17.2)
- Slow healing of wounds; surgical sutures repeatedly fail to hold (Figure 17.3)
- The skin bruises easily and hematomas form frequently
- Development of blue-gray spongy tumors (molluscoid pseudotumors) in areas of trauma due to abnormal accumulations of collagenous and adipose tissue (Figure 17.4)
- Painful piezogenic pedal papules
- Elastosis perforans serpiginosa

Extracutaneous manifestations

- Hyperextensibility of joints may induce dislocations, genu recurvatum, hallux valgus, leading to difficulty in walking (Figure 17.5)
- Distinctive facies with wide nasal bridge, thin lips, hypertelorism, epicanthic folds, lop ears, blue sclerae (Figure 17.6)
- Cardiovascular changes: mitral valve prolapse, aortic aneurysm, varicose veins
- Gastrointestinal changes: inguinal and umbilical hernias, diverticula, hematemesis and melena

Course and complications

- Rupture of colon, uterus and arteries
- Premature rupture of fetal membranes
- Physical and mental development is normal, but complications may shorten life expectancy

Laboratory investigations

- In general, routine laboratory investigations reveal no abnormalities
- On electron microscopy collagen fibers are larger and irregularly shaped

Genetics and pathogenesis

- Autosomal dominant inheritance
- Molecular defect consists of COL5A1 and COL5A2 mutations

240 Atlas of Genodermatoses

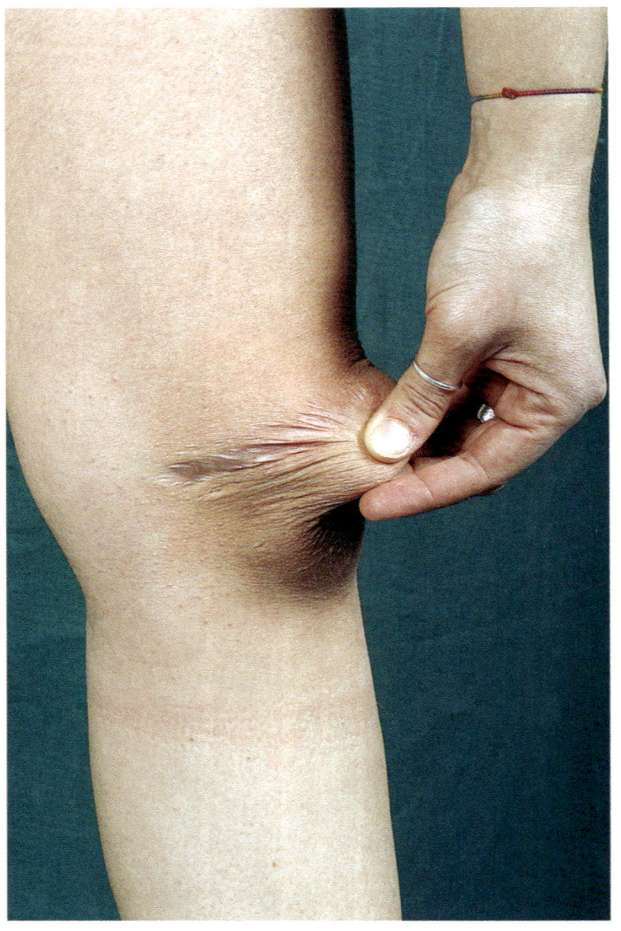

Figure 17.1

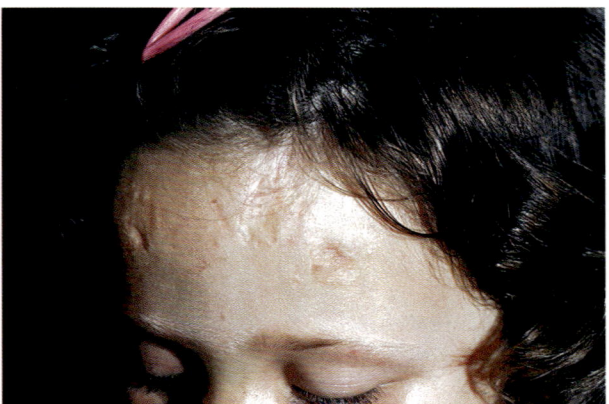

Figure 17.2

Differential diagnosis

- Cutis laxa
- Pseudoxanthoma elasticum

Follow-up and therapy

- Protection from trauma
- A strict obstetric observation during pregnancy

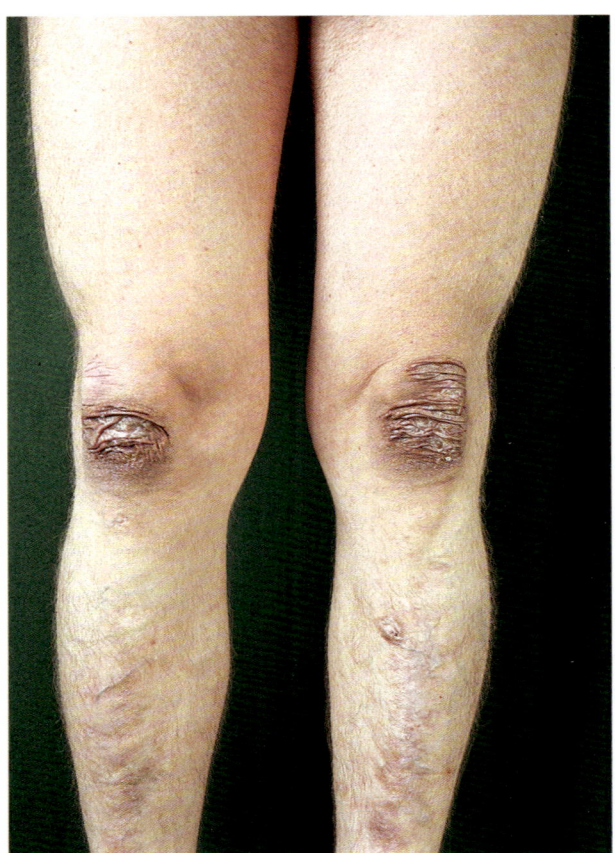

Figure 17.3

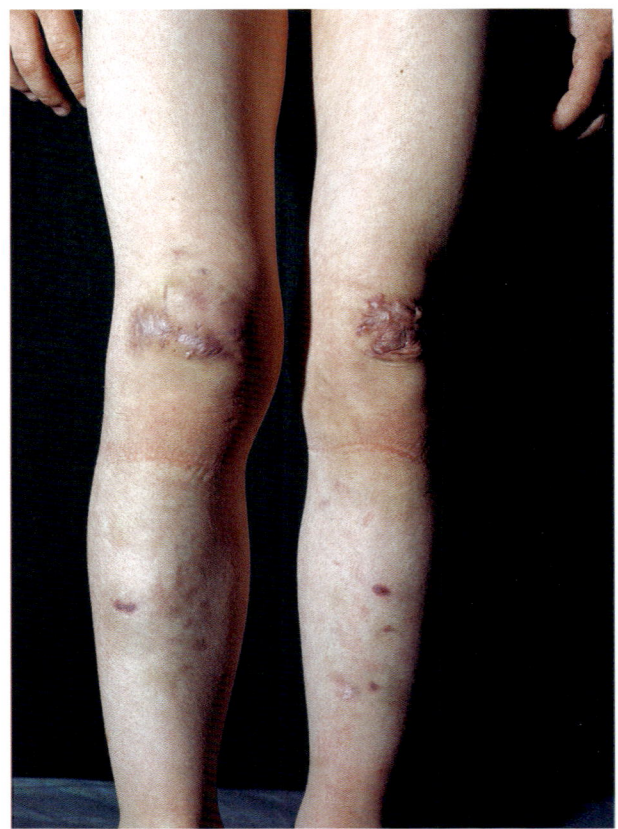

Figure 17.4

Disorders of connective tissue

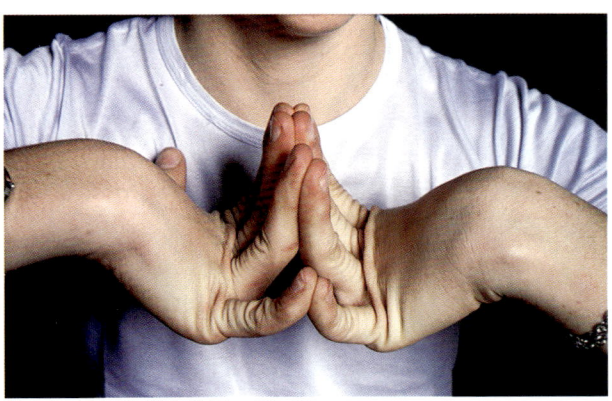

Figure 17.5

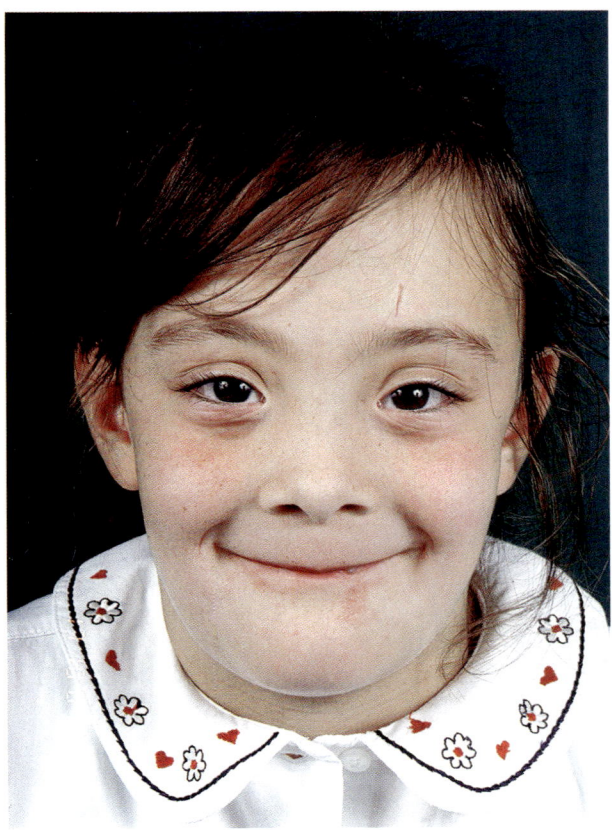

Figure 17.6

REFERENCES

Burrows NP, Nicholls AC, Richards AJ, et al. A point mutation in an intronic branch site results in aberrant splicing of COL5A1 and Ehlers–Danlos syndrome in two British families. Am J Hum Genet 1998; 63: 390–8

Burrows NP. The molecular genetics of the Ehlers–Danlos syndrome. Exp Dermatol 1999; 24: 99–106

De Paepe A, Nuytinck L, Hausser I, et al. Mutations in the COL5A1 gene are causal in the Ehlers–Danlos syndromes I and II. Am J Hum Genet 1997; 60: 547–54

Ehlers–Danlos syndrome type II

Synonym

- Ehlers–Danlos syndrome mitis

Age of onset

- Birth to infancy; prematurity is not a feature of this form

Clinical findings

The clinical features are similar to those of Ehlers–Danlos type I but much milder (Figures 17.7–17.9).

Genetics and pathogenesis

- Autosomal dominant inheritance
- Mutations in the COL5A1 and COL5A2 genes

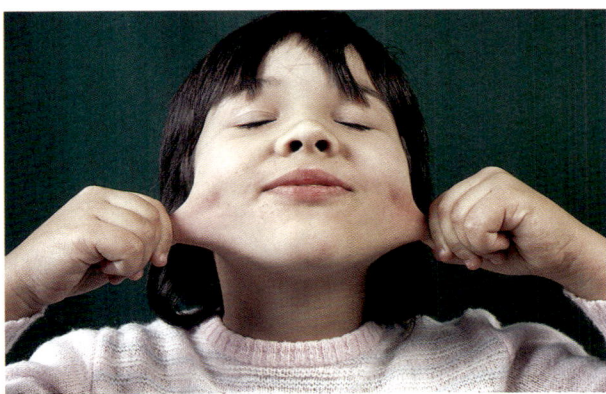

Figure 17.7

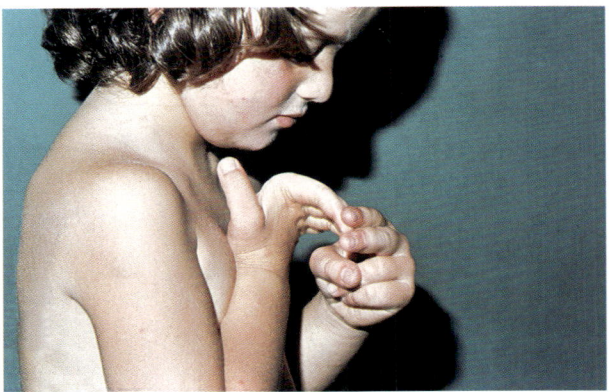

Figure 17.8

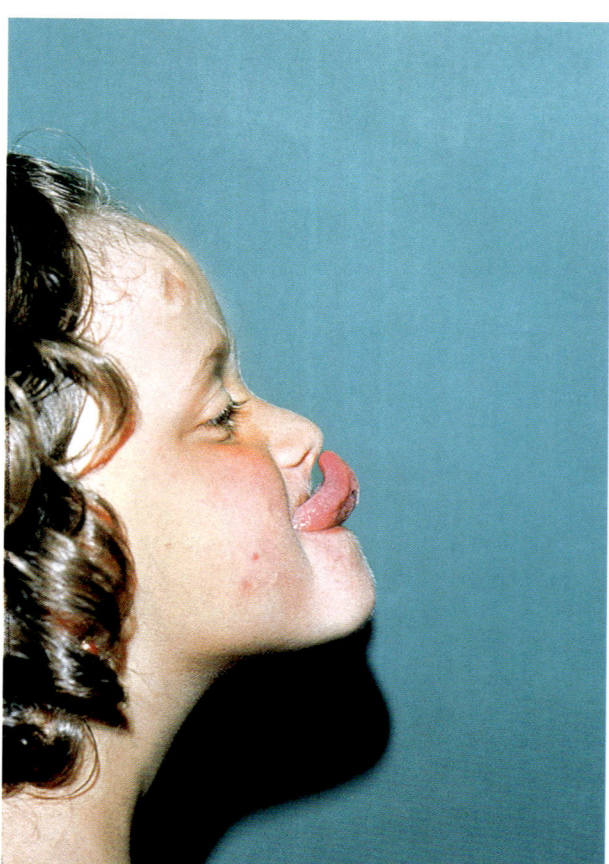

Figure 17.9

Ehlers–Danlos syndrome type III

Synonym

- Ehlers–Danlos benign hypermobile

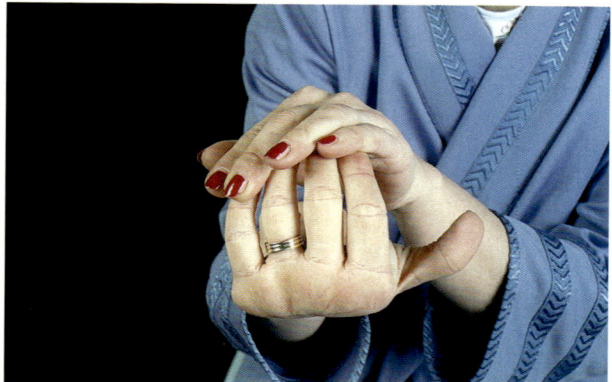

Figure 17.10

Clinical findings

- Minimal skin findings with mild hyperextensibility and fragility
- Severe hyperextensibility of joints resulting in frequent dislocations and difficult walking (Figure 17.10)
- Occasionally mitral valve prolapse

Genetics and pathogenesis

- Autosomal dominant inheritance
- Molecular defect in COL3A1

Therapy

- Avoid physical contact sports
- Referral to orthopedics

REFERENCES

Inrassich S, Rocco D, Aurelia A. Type III Ehlers–Danlos syndrome: correlations among clinical signs, ultrasound, and histologic findings in a study of 35 cases. Int J Dermatol 2001; 3: 175–8

Narcisi P, Richards AJ, Ferguson SD, et al. A family with Ehlers–Danlos syndrome type III/articular hypermobility syndrome has a glycine 637 to serine in type III collagen. Hum Med Genet 1994; 3: 1617–20

REFERENCES

Beighton P, De Paepe A, Steinmann B, et al. Ehlers–Danlos syndromes: revised nosology. Villefranche 1997. Am J Med Genet 1998; 77: 31–7

Loughin J, Irven C, Hardwick LJ, et al. Linkage of the gene than encodes the α1 chain of type V collagen (COL5A1) to type II Ehlers–Danlos syndrome (EDS II). Hum Mol Genet 1995; 4: 1649–51

Richards AJ, Martin S, Nicholls AC, et al. Single base mutation in COL5A2 causes Ehlers–Danlos type II. J Med Genet 1998; 35: 846–8

Ehlers–Danlos syndrome type IV

Synonyms

- Ehlers–Danlos syndrome ecchymotic type
- Ehlers–Danlos syndrome arterial type

Clinical findings

Cutaneous manifestations

- Thin, translucent, extremely fragile skin
- Subcutaneous veins
- Large ecchymoses (Figure 17.11)
- Tendency to form keloids (Figure 17.12)

Extracutaneous manifestations

- Minimal joint laxity
- Fragility of blood vessels with formation of aneurysms and arteriovenous fistulas; increased incidence of ruptures
- Visceral perforations
- Uterine rupture
- Face and lips are 'slim', giving these patients an acrogeric aspect

Course and complications

There is a decreased life span with premature death due to complications.

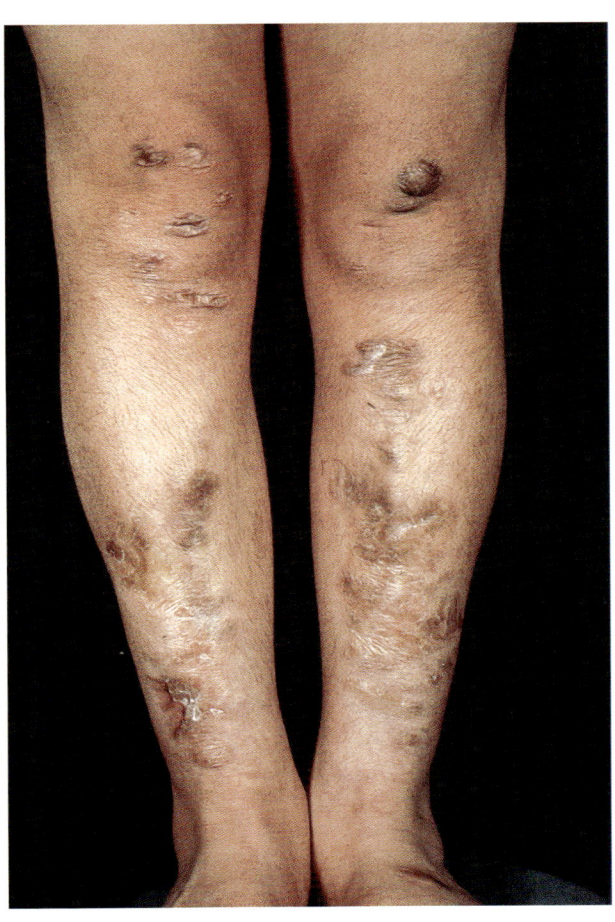

Figure 17.11

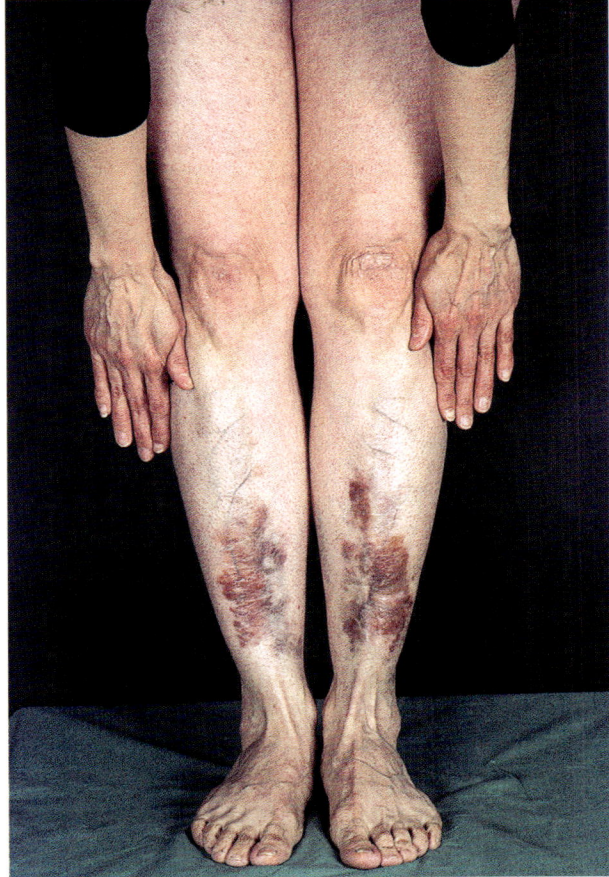

Figure 17.12

Pregnancy and delivery carry a high risk of uterine rupture and arterial hemorrhages.

Laboratory investigations and data

- Lack or decrease of type III collagen formation in cultured fibroblasts
- Skin biopsy for protein and molecular analysis
- Measurement of serum amino terminal propeptide of type III procollagen

Genetics and pathogenesis

- Autosomal dominant inheritance (type A: acrogeric; and type C: ecchymotic)
- Autosomal recessive (type B: acrogeric)
- All types due to COL3A1 mutations inducing alteration in type III collagen synthesis

Follow-up and therapy

- Accurate dermatologic, cardiologic, gastroenterologic and gynecologic surveillance
- Ehlers–Danlos type IV represents 4% of all forms and the higher mortality rate
- Genetic counseling is crucial because of the risk of premature rupture of membranes, severe hemorrhagic episodes and maternal mortality (25%)

REFERENCES

Pepini M, Schzarze V, Superti-Furga A, et al. Clinical and genetic features of Ehlers–Danlos type IV, the vascular type. N Engl J Med 2000; 342: 673–80

Pope FM, Narcisi P, Nicholls AC, et al. COL3A1 mutations cause variable clinical phenotypes including acrogeria and vascular rupture. Br J Dermatol 1996; 135: 163–81

Pyeritz RE. Ehlers–Danlos syndrome. N Engl J Med 2000; 342: 730–2

The following Ehlers-Danlos subtypes are very rare and with poor dermatological interest; they are listed only for didactic reasons.

Ehlers–Danlos syndrome type V

Synonym

- Ehlers–Danlos syndrome X-linked

Clinical findings

- Cutaneous lesions type II, but ecchyimoses are more marked
- Mild hypermobility, short stature, herniae

Genetics and pathogenesis

- Inherited in an X-linked fashion
- Molecular defect unknown; lysyl oxidase deficiency reported

REFERENCES

Beighton P. X-linked recessive inheritance in the Ehlers–Danlos syndrome. Br Med J 1968; 2: 409–11

Beighton P, Curtis D. X-linked Ehlers–Danlos syndrome type V: the next generation. Clin Genet 1985; 27: 472–8

Pope FM, Burrows NP. Ehlers–Danlos syndrome has varied molecular mechanism. J Med Genet 1997; 34: 400–10

Ehlers–Danlos syndrome type VI

Synonyms

- Ehlers–Danlos syndrome ocular type
- Ehlers–Danlos syndrome hydroxylysine-deficient type

Clinical findings

- Cutaneous manifestations
- Soft, fragile skin with moderate hyperextensibility

Extracutaneous manifestations

- Ocular involvement: scleral and corneal fragility with intraocular hemorrhage, keratoconus, blue sclerae, retinal detachment, ocular rupture, blindness
- Severe kyphoscoliosis, marked joint laxity

Laboratory investigations and data

- Reduced lysyl hydroxylase activity in cultured fibroblasts
- Ophthalmologic examination

Genetics and pathogenesis

- Autosomal recessive inheritance
- Mutations in exon 14 of the lysyl hydroxylase gene induce lysyl hydroxylase deficiency and alterations of collagen type I and type III

Therapy

The administration of ascorbic acid, which regulates collagen biosynthesis, may be useful.

REFERENCES

Hantala T, Heikkinen J, Kivirikko KI, et al. A large duplication in the gene for lysyl hydroxylase accounts for the type VI variant of Ehlers–Danlos syndrome in two siblings. Genomies 1993; 15: 399–404

Pousi B, Heikkinen J, Schroter J, et al. A non sense codon of exon 14 reduces lysyl hydroxylase in RNA and leads to aberrant RNA splicing in a patient with Ehlers–Danlos syndrome type VI. Mutat Res 2000; 432: 33–7

Walker LC, Marini JC, Grange DK, et al. A patient with Ehlers–Danlos syndrome type VI is homozygous for a premature termination codon in exon 14 of the lysyl hydroxylase 1 gene. Mol Genet Metab 1999; 67: 74–82

Ehlers–Danlos syndrome type VII

Synonym

- Arthrochalasis multiplex congenita

Clinical findings

- Moderate skin hyperextensibility and fragility
- Extreme hypermobility of all joints, with dislocations, congenital dislocation of hips, short stature

Genetics and pathogenesis

- Autosomal dominant and recessive inheritance
- Mutations in COL1A1 and COL1A2 genes which encode the $\alpha 1$ and $\alpha 2$ chains of type I procollagen with defective conversion of procollagen to collagen

REFERENCES

Burrows NP. The molecular genetics of the Ehlers–Danlos syndrome. Clin Exp Dermatol 1999; 24: 99–106

Giunta C, Superti-Furga A, Sparger S, et al. Ehlers–Danlos syndrome type VII: clinical features and molecular defects. J Bone Joint Surg Am 1999; 81: 225–38

Lichtenstein JR, Martin GR, Kohn LD, et al. Defect in conversion of procollagen to collagen in a form of Ehlers–Danlos syndrome. Science 1973; 182: 298–9

Ehlers–Danlos syndrome type VIII

Synonym

- Ehlers–Danlos syndrome periodontosis type

Clinical findings

- Hyperelastic fragile skin, ecchymoses, pigmented pretibial plaques
- Mild joint hypermobility
- Severe periodontitis with gum resorption and premature loss of permanent teeth

Genetics and pathogenesis

- Autosomal dominant inheritance
- Collagen III deficiency

REFERENCES

Cunnif C, Williamson-Kruse L. Ehlers–Danlos syndrome type VIII presenting with periodontitis and prolonged bleeding time. Clin Dysmorphol 1995; 4: 145–9

Karrer S, Landthaler M, Schmalz G. Ehlers–Danlos type VIII. Review of the literature. Clin Oral Invest 2000; 4: 66–9

Nelson DL, King RA. Ehlers–Danlos syndrome type VIII. J Am Acad Dermatol 1981; 5: 297–303

Ehlers–Danlos syndrome type IX

Synonym

- Ehlers–Danlos syndrome occipital horn type

Clinical findings

- Mild skin hyperextensibility
- Curious exostoses protruding from the occiput inferiorly (occipital horns), mild joint laxity, embryologic bone defects in the elbow and wrist
- Inguinal herniae
- Bladder diverticula

Laboratory investigations and data

- Bone radiography
- Decreased levels of serum copper and ceruloplasmin

Genetics and pathogenesis

- X-linked recessive inheritance
- Lysyl oxidase deficiency due to altered copper metabolism

REFERENCES

Kuivaniemi H, Tromp G, Prockop DJ. Mutations in fibrillar collagens (types I, II, III and XI), fibril-associated collagen (type IX) and network-forming collagen (type X) cause a spectrum of diseases of bone, cartilage and blood vessels. Hum Mutat 1997; 9: 300–15

Peltonen L, Kuivaniemi H, Palotie A, et al. Alteration in copper metabolism in the Menkes' syndrome and a new subtype of Ehlers–Danlos syndrome. Biochemistry 1983; 22: 6156–63

Ehlers–Danlos syndrome type X

Synonym

- Ehlers–Danlos syndrome fibronectin-deficient type

Clinical findings

- Mild skin hyperextensibility, high incidence of cutaneous striae atrophicans
- Joint laxity
- Abnormal platelet aggregation due to a defect in fibronectin

Genetics and pathogenesis

- Autosomal recessive inheritance
- Abnormal function of plasma fibronectin

REFERENCES

Anstey AV, Winter H, Pope FM. Platelet and coagulation studies in Ehlers–Danlos syndrome. Br J Dermatol 1991; 125: 155–63

Arneson MA, Hemmerschmidt DE, Furcht LT, et al. A new form of Ehlers–Danlos syndrome: fibronectin corrects defective platelet function. J Am Acad Dermatol 1980; 244: 144–7

CUTIS LAXA

Synonyms

- Generalized elastolysis
- Dermatochalasis

Age of onset

- Birth to infancy

Clinical findings

Skin manifestations

- Loose and sagging skin with reduced resilience and elasticity leading to pendulous skin folds (Figures 17.13–17.15)
- Premature aged appearance with 'hound dog' facies (Figure 17.16)
- Checkerboard pattern in acquired cutis laxa (Figure 17.17)

Extracutaneous findings

- Vocal cord laxity: deep voice
- Pulmonary emphysema

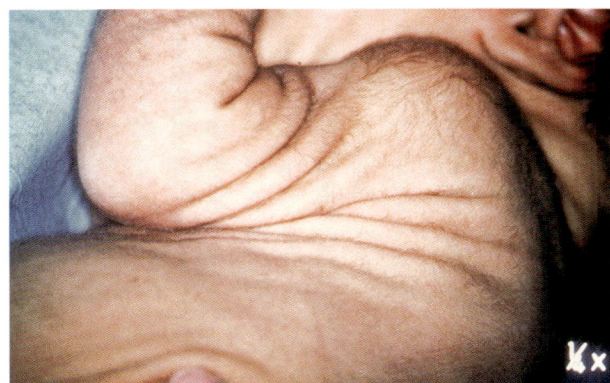

Figure 17.13

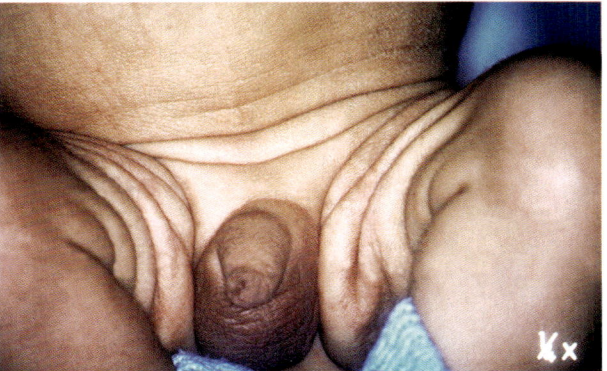

Figure 17.14

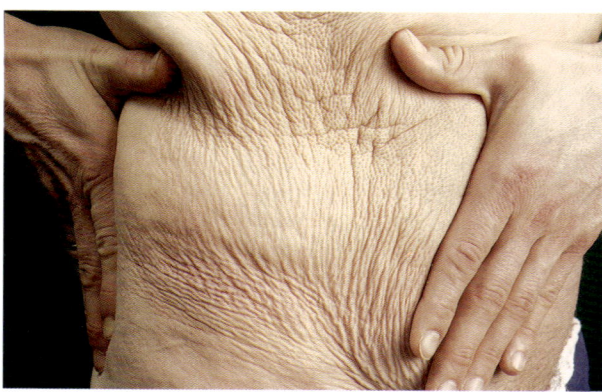

Figure 17.15

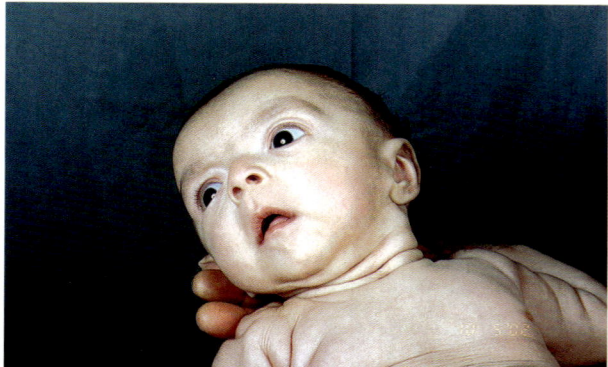

Figure 17.16

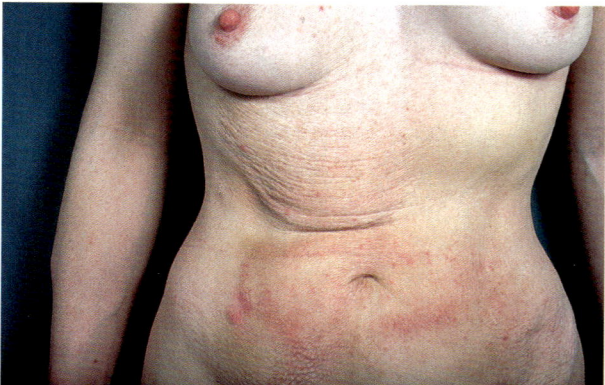

Figure 17.17

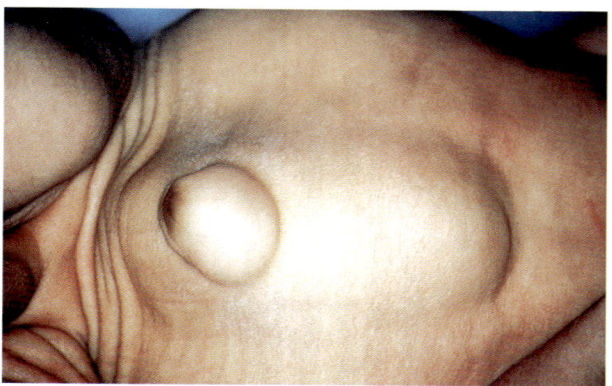

Figure 17.18

- Intestinal and bladder diverticuli
- Abdominal, inguinal and diaphragmatic herniae (Figure 17.18)
- Structural cardiac abnormalities
- Hooked nose
- Oligohydramnios

Course and complications

- Cardiovascular complications
- Liability to chest infection
- Benign in autosominal dominant forms, usually confined to the skin
- In autosomal recessive forms with evident serious internal manifestations, disease worsens with age and leads to death in childhood

Laboratory examinations

- Histopathologic findings: reduced number of elastic fibers which are pigmented and granular

Genetics and pathogenesis

- Autosomal dominant form: due to mutations in elastin gene
- Autosomal recessive form: due to mutations in fibulins (FBLMS) gene
- X-linked form is very rare, associated with a disorder of copper transport
- The abnormality of dermal connective tissue seems to be related to an increased collagenase expression of fibroblasts

Differential diagnosis

- Ehlers–Danlos syndrome
- Pseudoxanthoma elasticum

Follow-up and therapy

- Normal life span if there is no cardiac or pulmonary involvement
- Solar elastosis tends to aggravate the skin conditions
- Cutaneous chemical, electrocardiographic and echocardiographic monitoring is necessary
- Plastic surgery
- Sun protection
- Radiography and functional screenings of cardiovascular and respiratory systems

REFERENCES

Jung K, Veberhan U, Hausser I, et al. Autosomal recessive cutis laxa syndrome. Acta Dermatol Venereol 1996; 76: 298–31

Lambert D, Beer F, Jeannin-Magnificat C, et al. Cutis laxa généralisée congénitale. Ann Dermatol Venereol 1983; 110: 129–38

Litzman J, Buckova H, Ventruba J, et al. A concurrent occurrence of cutis laxa, Dandy–Walker syndrome and immunodeficiency in a girl. Acta Paediatr 2003; 92: 861–4

Markova D, Zou Y, Ringpfeil F, et al. Genetic heterogeneity of cutis laxa: a heterozygous tandem duplication within the fibulin-5 (FBLN5) gene. Am J Hum Genet 2003; 72: 998–1004; Epub 2003; Feb 28

Rodriguez-Revenga L, Iranzo P, Badenas C, et al. A novel elastin gene mutation resulting in an autosomal dominant form of cutis laxa. Arch Dermatol 2004; 140: 1135–9. Review

Sarkar R, Kaur C, Kanwar AJ, et al. Cutis laxa in seven members of a north Indian family. Pediatr Dermatol 2002; 19: 229–31

PSEUDOXANTHOMA ELASTICUM

Synonym

- Gronblad–Strandberg syndrome

Age of onset

- Second decade of life

Clinical findings

Cutaneous and mucous membrane manifestations

- Lemon yellow, xanthoma-like papules confluent in soft and lax plaques leading to a 'plucked-chicken skin' appearance (Figures 17.19–17.21)
- Symmetrical distribution on the sides of the neck and the flexural folds (axillae, antecubital, inguinal, popliteal regions) (Figures 17.22–17.25)
- Occasionally lesions of elastosis perforans serpiginosa (perforating pseudoxanthoma elasticum)
- Rarely mucous membrane involvement: yellow papules on the inner aspect of the lower lip and palate

Extracutaneous manifestations

- Ocular changes:
  - Angioid streaks consisting of bilateral gray lines radiating from the optic disk and lying among the retinal vessels (60–80% of patients) as a result of breakdown of the elastic lamina of Bruch's membrane (Figure 17.26)
  - Ocular hemorrhages with decreased visual acuity
  - Peculiar pigmentary retinal changes
  - Macular degeneration

- Cardiovascular changes due to arterial calcification:
  - Gastrointestinal bleeding
  - Intermittent claudication
  - Hypertension
  - Angina pectoris and myocardial infarction

Course and prognosis

This is a progressive systemic disorder, with separate courses for cutaneous, ocular and vascular changes.

There is reduced life span secondary to cardiovascular involvement.

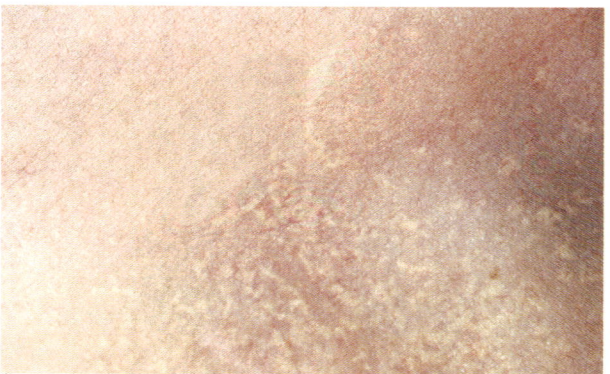

Figure 17.19

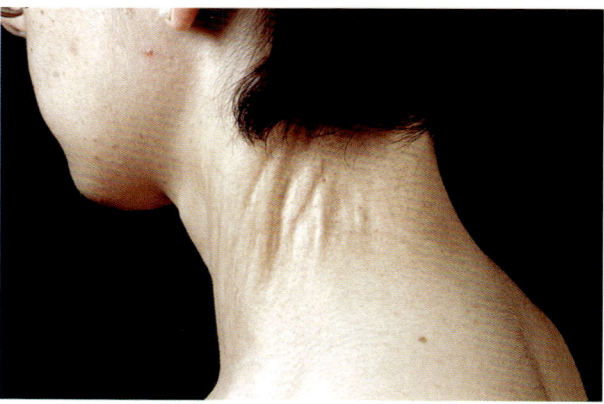

Figure 17.22

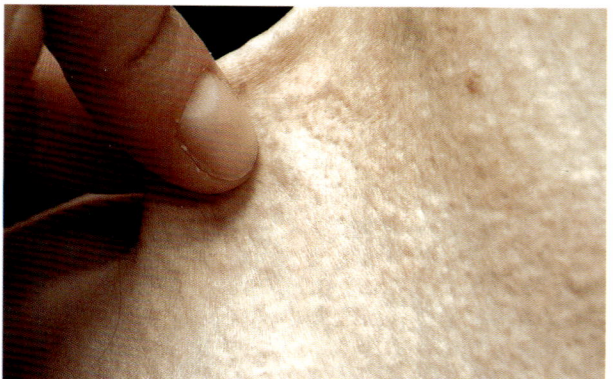

Figure 17.20

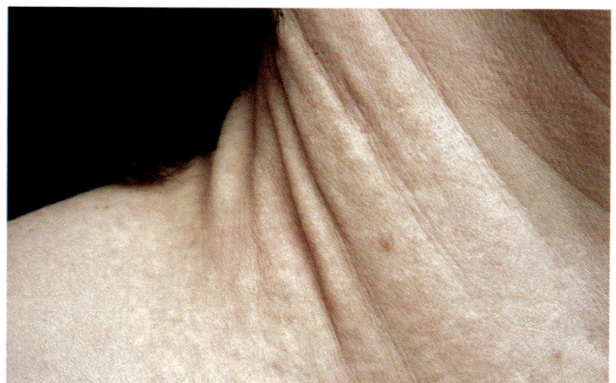

Figure 17.23

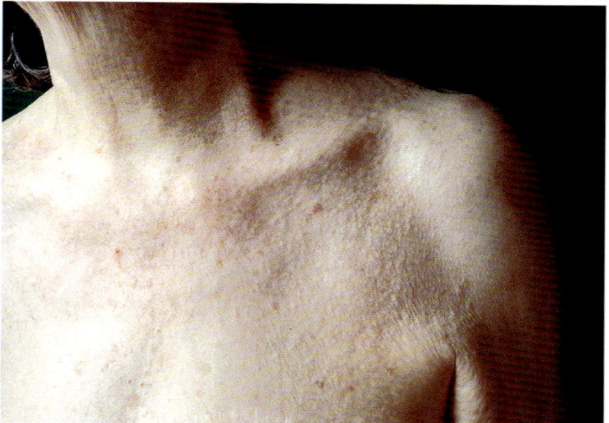

Figure 17.21

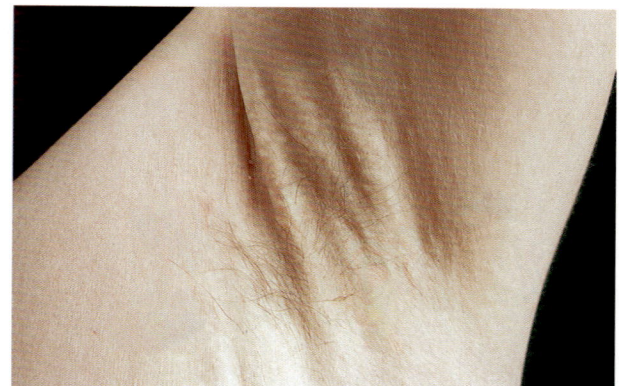

Figure 17.24

Laboratory investigations

- Histopathologic findings: fragmentation, clamping and calcification of elastic fibers in mid- and lower dermis, in subretinal elastic layer and in elastic lamina of arteries
- Radiography to demonstrate soft tissue and vascular calcification
- Fundoscopy

Genetics and pathogenesis

- Most commonly autosomal recessive inheritance; occasionally autosomal dominant
- The gene responsible is the ABCC 6 gene residing on the chromosomal locus 16p13.1
- The related protein plays an important role modulating the intracellular storage of calcium. Early deposition of crystals within the collagen fibrils is the first pathogenetic step of the disease

Disorders of connective tissue

Differential diagnosis

- Ehlers–Danlos syndrome
- Cutis laxa
- Actinic elastosis

Follow-up and therapy

- Plastic surgery for cosmetic correction
- Laser photocoagulation for retinal hemorrhage
- Reduce potential contributing factors (smoking, traumas, pregnancy, etc.)
- Periodic cardiovascular and ophthalmologic surveillance is absolutely necessary

REFERENCES

Le Saux O, Martin L. Genetique moléculaire du pseudoxanthome élastique. Ann Dermatol Venereol 2001; 128: 943–6

Martin L, Le Saux O. Actualités du pseudoxanthome élastique. Ann Dermatol Venereol 2001; 128: 938–42

Sherer DW, Sapadin AN, Lebwohl MG. Pseudoxanthoma elasticum: an update. Dermatology 1999; 199: 3–7

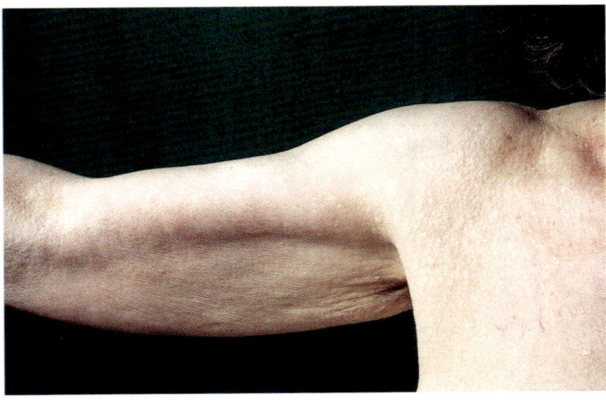

Figure 17.25

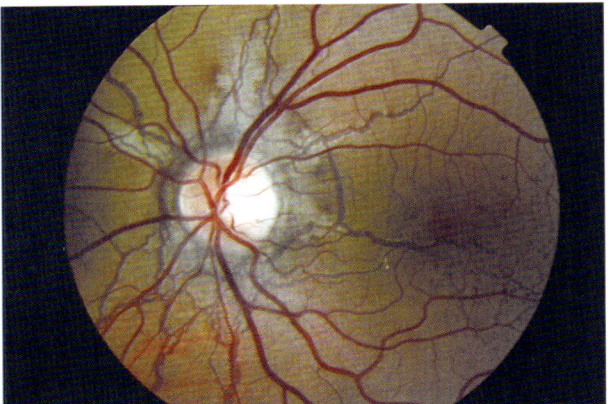

Figure 17.26

MARFAN'S SYNDROME

Epidemiology

Estimated frequency is 1 : 10 000

Age of onset

- First signs are visible during late childhood, full-blown picture after puberty

Clinical findings

Cutaneous findings

- Striae distensae (25% of patients) located on pectoral, deltoid and thigh areas
- Xerosis
- Occasionally elastosis perforans serpiginosa

Extracutaneous findings

- Elongated facies with dolichocephaly, high arched palate
- Height greater than 90th centile, poor muscular tone
- Arachnodactyly (Figures 17.27 and 17.28)
- Joint hyperextensibility
- Pectus carinatum or excavatum (Figure 17.29)
- Ectopia lentis (main feature: 75%), myopia and retinal detachment
- Aortic enlargement (main feature) resulting in aortic insufficiency, dissection, aneurysm and rupture; mitral valve prolapse
- Spontaneous pneumothorax

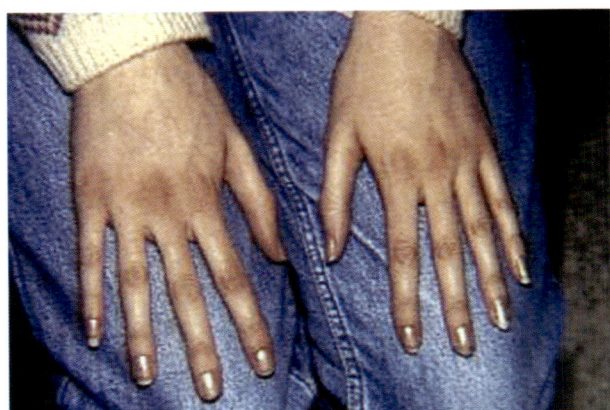

Figure 17.27

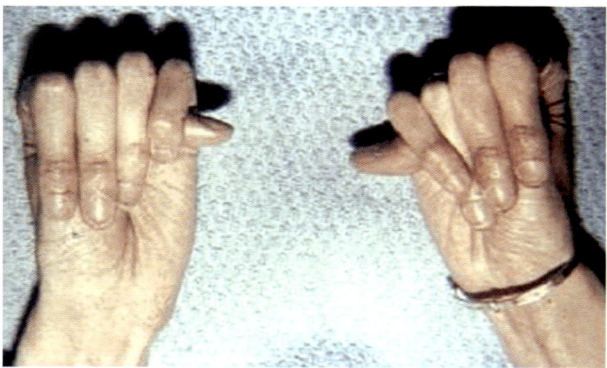

Figure 17.28

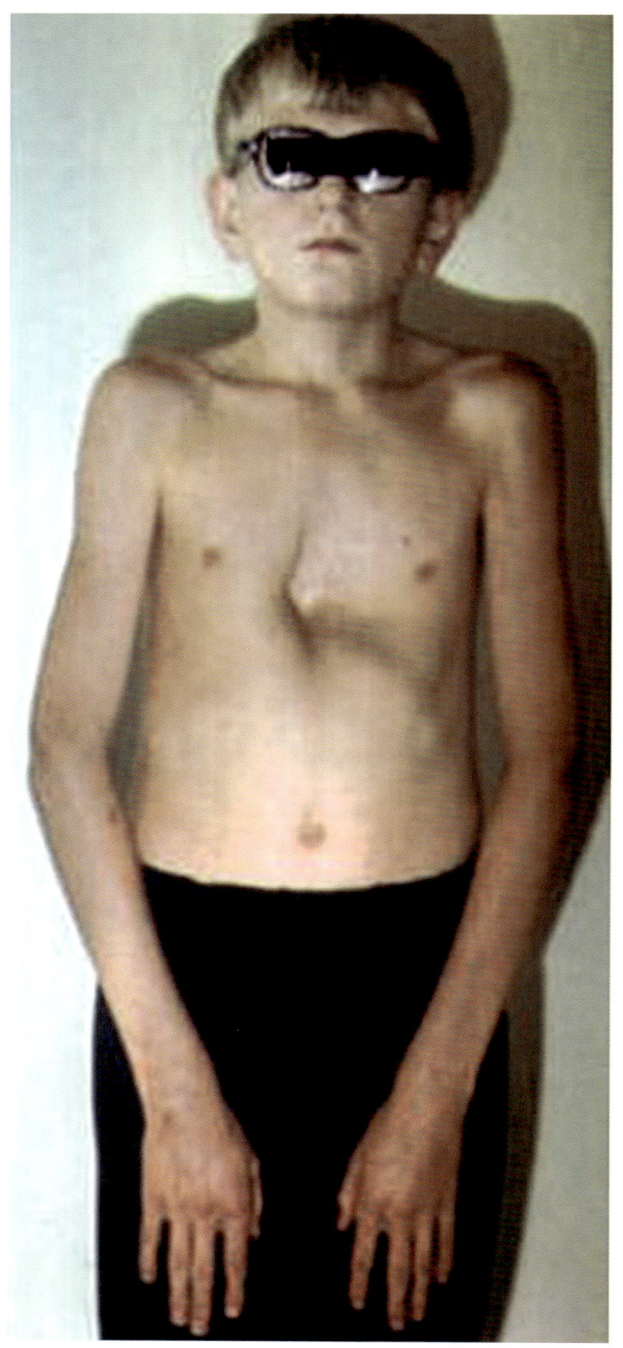

Figure 17.29

Course and prognosis

- Cardiovascular abnormalties may worsen with age, requiring surgery
- Aortic dissection
- Life span is normally reduced in severe cases to 30–40 years

Laboratory investigations

- Electrocardiogram and echocardiogram
- Measurement of body proportions
- Slit lamp examination of fully dilated pupils
- Chest radiography

Genetics and pathogenesis

- Autosomal dominant disease with high penetrance
- About 20% sporadic cases
- Mutations in the gene encoding fibrillin I have been found in affected patients, inducing lack of fibrillin responsible for the ocular, cardiovascular and musculoskeletal defects
- Mosaic conditions have been reported
- Genetic heterogeneity is possible (gene of laminin B1?)
- No clear genotype–phenotype correlation exists

Follow-up and therapy

- Echographic evaluation reveals cardiac defects
- Radiography to detect skeletal abnormalities
- Ophthalmologic assessment

Differential diagnosis

- Ehlers–Danlos syndrome (dermatological)
- Homocystinuria

REFERENCES

Cohen PR, Schneiderman P. Clinical manifestations of Marfan syndrome. Int J Dermatol 1989; 28: 291–9

Loeys BL Matthys DM, de Paepe AM. Genetic fibrillinopathies: new insights inmolecular diagnosis and clinical management. Acta Clin Belg 2003; 58: 3–11

Wang B, Hu D, Xia J, et al. FBN1 mutation in Chinese patients with Marfan syndrome and its gene diagnosis using haplotype linkage analysis. Chin Med J (Engl) 2003; 116: 1043–6

Disorders of connective tissue 253

CONNECTIVE TISSUE NEVI AND BUSCHKE–OLLENDORFF SYNDROME

Age of onset

- Rarely visible at birth, these nevi may be detected within the first decade

Epidemiology

These lesions do not appear frequently in our consultations. No epidemiological data are available in the literature.

Clinical findings

'Pure' connective tissue (collagenic) nevi or hamartomas are represented by papules or nodules that are rarely isolated, but more often grouped lesions or plaques of various dimensions located anywhere on the skin (Figures 17.30 and 17.31). More 'mixed' hamartomas may be associated with hypertrichosis (Figure 17.32). Mucinous nevi are described as histologic findings.

Buschke–Ollendorff syndrome represents the association of disseminated lenticular connective tissue with osteopoikilosis (Figure 17.33a,b). In a recent paper, a family with both Buschke–Ollendorff syndrome and nail–patella syndrome is described, configuring a genetic heterogeneity giving two different phenotypes (see Chapter 11).

Usually in this category are also included the nevus lipomatosus (Figure 17.34) and nevi occurring in tuberous sclerosis in the form of shagreen patches and angiofibrolipomatous nevi (see Figures 14.40 and 14.41).

Extracutaneous findings

Usually connective tissue nevi do not show any association (except for Buschke–Ollendorff syndrome).

Course and prognosis

Nevi may enlarge slowly but are usually steady throughout life.

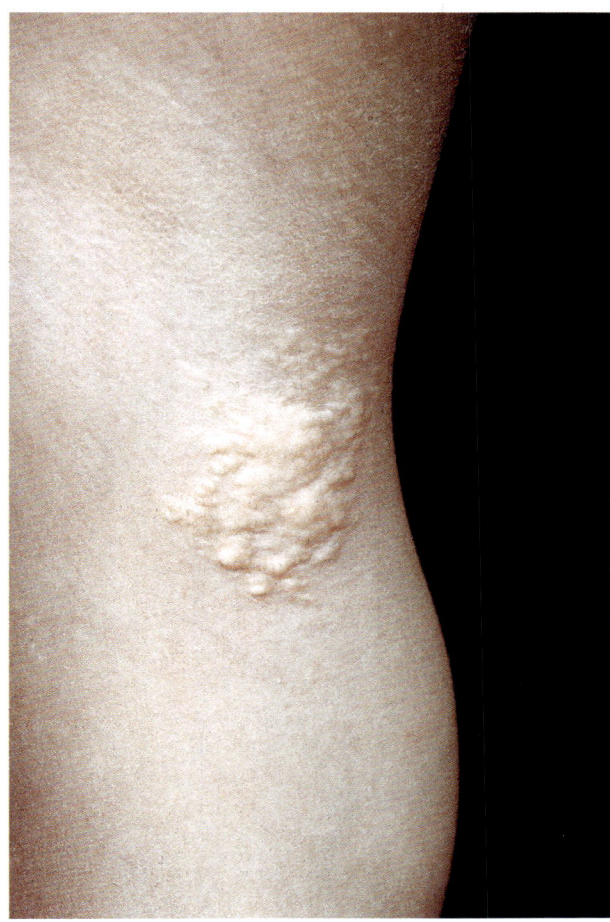

Figure 17.31

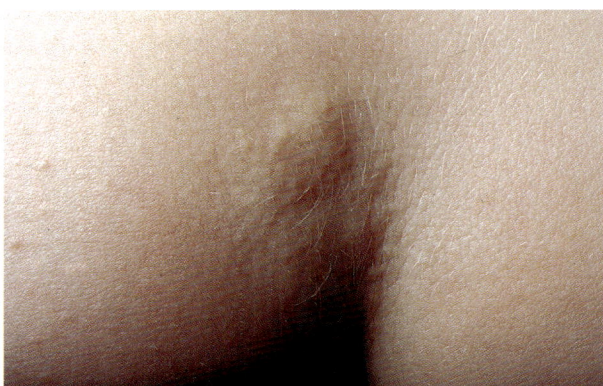

Figure 17.30

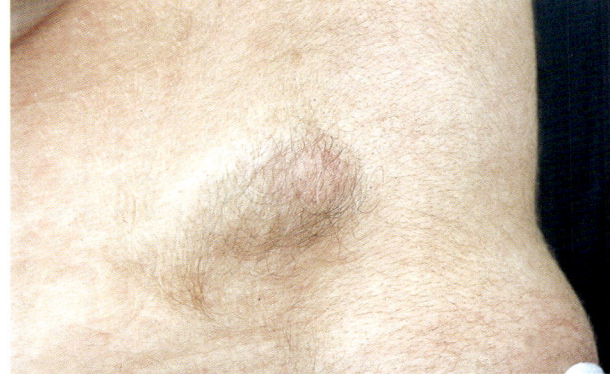

Figure 17.32

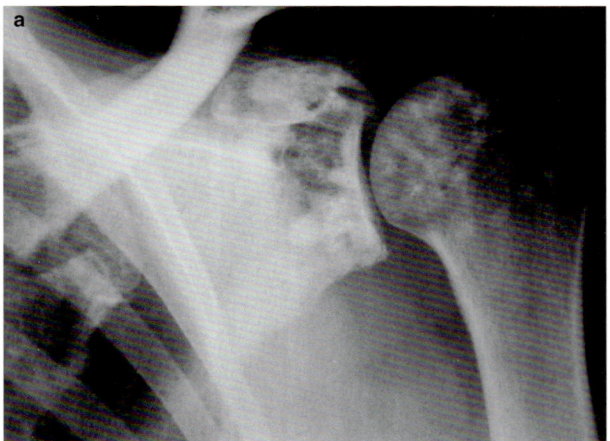 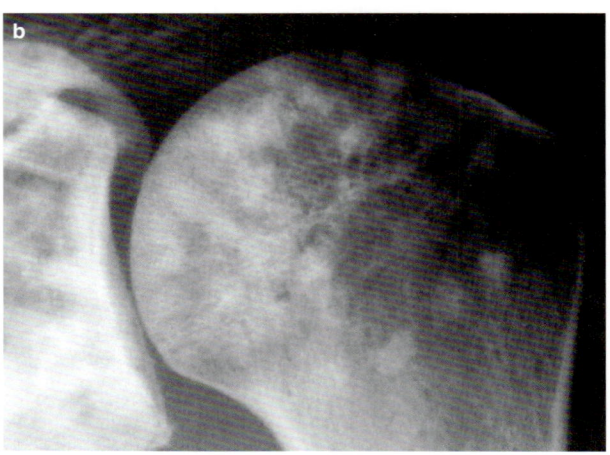

Figure 17.33

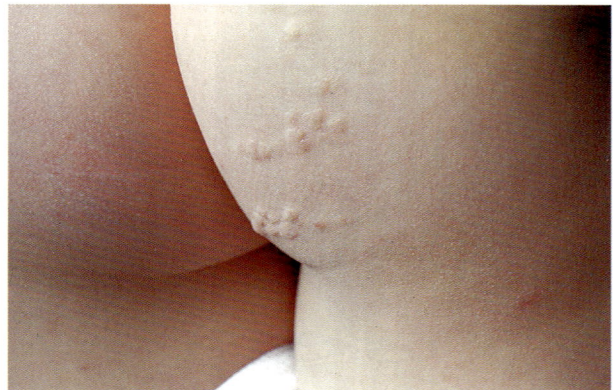

Figure 17.34

Laboratory findings

Histologically these nevi may be well differentiated, following cellular populations and specific patterns.

Genetics and pathogenesis

All these nevi represent clones of undifferentiated cells deriving from postzygotic mutations, distributed randomly without a specific distribution pattern.

Follow-up and therapy

- Investigations to exclude internal associations
- Rarely these nevi require surgery

Differential diagnosis

- Epidermal nevi
- Leiomyomas

REFERENCES

Drouin CA, Grenon H. The association of Buschke–Ollendorf syndrome and nail–patella syndrome. J Am Acad Dermatol 2002; 46: 621–5

Reymond JL, Stoebner P, Beani JC, Amblard P. Buschke–Ollendorf syndrome. An electron microscopy study. Dermatologica 1983; 166: 64–8

ELASTOSIS PERFORANS SERPIGINOSA

Synonym

- Lutz–Miescher disease

Age of onset

- From 6 to 20 years

Clinical findings

Skin manifestations

Skin colored or slightly erythematous keratotic papules, 2–5 mm in diameter arranged in arcuate or serpiginous configuration and located predominantly on the neck, upper part of the trunk, face and extremities (Figures 17.35 and 17.36).

This phenomenon may be seen in different diseases, namely:

- Marfan's syndrome
- Ehlers–Danlos syndrome
- Pseudoxanthoma elasticum
- Down's syndrome
- Osteogenesis imperfecta

Course and prognosis

- Usually persistent with development of new lesions
- Spontaneous involution reported, leaving atrophic scars

Laboratory investigations

Histopathologic findings include the presence of narrow epidermal sinus tracts containing elastotic material, cellular debris and keratin.

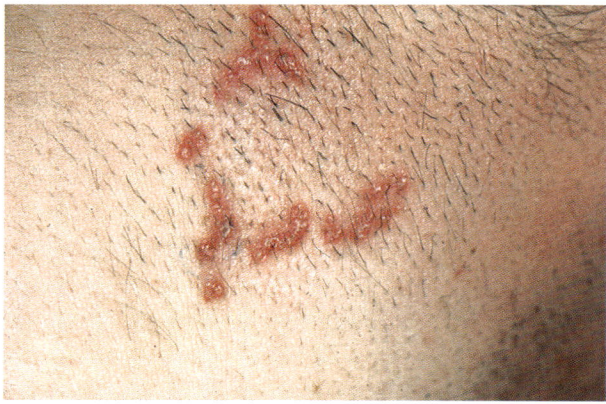

Figure 17.35

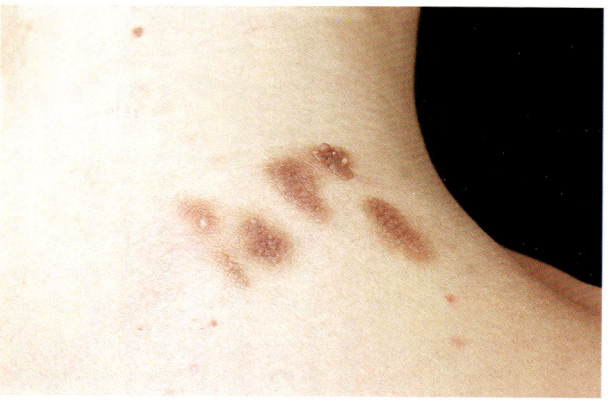

Figure 17.36

Genetics and pathogenesis

- Autosomal dominant and autosomal recessive patterns of inheritance
- Gene locus unknown
- 67-kDa elastin receptors have been detected in the epidermis, eliminating altered elastic fibers (elastin–keratinocyte interaction)

Differential diagnosis

- Kyrle's disease
- Granuloma annulare
- Annular sarcoidosis
- Porokeratosis of Mibelli

Follow-up and therapy

- Oral retinoids
- CO_2 laser

REFERENCES

Fujimoto N, Akagi A, Tajima S, et al. Expression of the 67-kDa elastin receptor in perforating disorders. Br J Dermatol 2002; 146: 74–9

Mehregan AH. Elastosis perforans serpiginosa. A review of the literature and report of 11 cases. Arch Dermatol 1968; 97: 381–93

Mehta RK, Burrows NP, Rowland-Payne CME, et al. Elastosis perforans serpiginosa and associated disorders. Clin Exp Dermatol 2001; 26: 521–4

COSTELLO'S SYNDROME

Epidemiology

The disease is very rare; since the first description in 1971, there have been about 40 described cases.

Age of onset

- At birth

Cutaneous findings

- Cutis laxa-like skin in all areas (Figure 17.37)
- Palmoplantar thickened skin without hyperkeratosis
- Papillomas and acrochordons usually on the face, but visible anywhere else
- Onychodystrophies

Extracutaneous findings

- Coarse face with hypertelorism, large nasal bridge with anteverted nostrils, thick lips (Figure 17.37) and short neck
- Joint hypermobility
- Mental retardation of various degrees
- Cardiac defects

Course and prognosis

- Acanthosis nigricans may develop on the major folds
- The degree of mental retardation influences life expectancy

Laboratory findings

There are none specific.

Genetics and pathogenesis

- Autosomal recessive
- Gene unknown

Follow-up and therapy

- Cardiac evaluation
- Neurological assessment for mental retardation

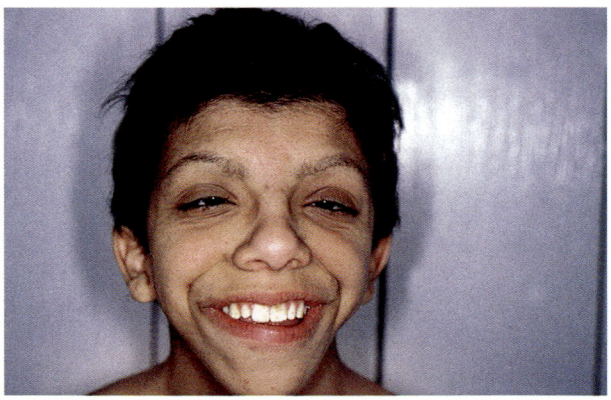

Figure 17.37

Differential diagnosis

- Cutis laxa
- The complex of syndromes with insulin resistance, lipoid proteinosis (Seip's syndrome, leprechaunism)

REFERENCES

Cakir M, Arici C, Tacoy S, Karayalcin U. A case of Costello with parathyroid adenoma and hyperprolactinemia. Am J Med Genet 2004; 124A: 196–9

Hinek A, Braun KR, Liu K, et al. Retrovirally mediated over-expression of versican v3 reverses impaired elastogenesis and heightened proliferation exhibited by fibroblasts from Costello syndrome and Hurler disease patients. Am J Pathol 2004; 164: 119–31

Kerr B, Einaudi MA, Clayton P, Gladman G, et al. Is growth hormone treatment beneficial or harmful in Costello syndrome? J Med Genet 2003; 40: e74

Kerr B, Mucchielli ML, Sigaudy S, et al. Is the locus for Costello syndrome on 11p? J Med Genet 2003; 40: 469–71

Lin A, Harding C, Silberbach M. Hand it to the skin in Costello syndrome. J Pediatr 2004; 144: 135

Troger B, Kutsche K, Bolz H, et al. No mutation in the gene for Noonan syndrome, PTPN11, in 18 patients with Costello syndrome. Am J Med Genet A 2003; 121: 82–4

MICHELIN TIRE BABY

Age of onset

- At birth

Clinical findings

- Generalized or localized (limbs) folding of the skin giving an appearance resembling the tire company's famous symbol (Figure 17.38)
- Occasionally hypertrichosis

Course

The disease is lifelong; there is rarely spontaneous improvement.

Laboratory findings and data

Histopathologic findings include underlying nevus lipomatosus, smooth muscle hamartoma or abnormal elastic fibers.

Genetics and pathogenesis

There is autosomal dominant inheritance; sporadic cases have been reported.

Differential diagnosis

- Cutis laxa
- Lymphedema

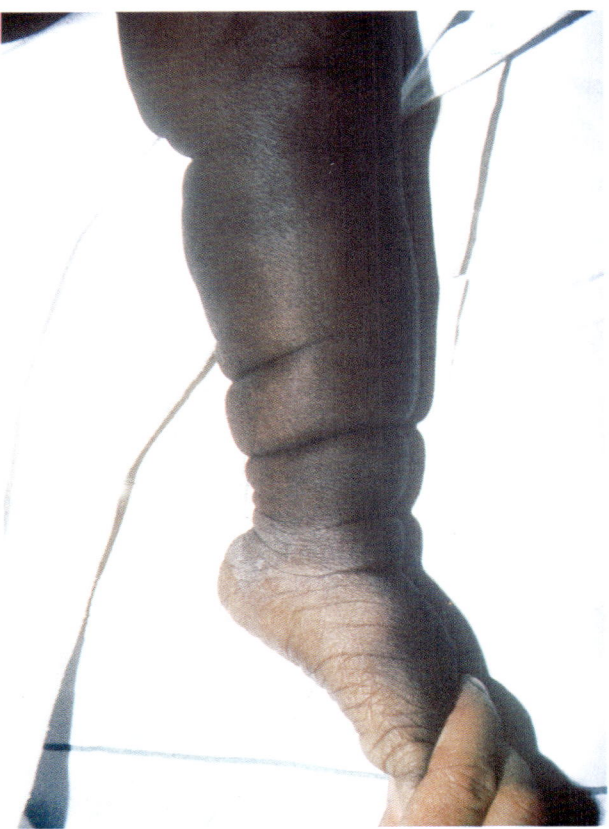

Figure 17.38

REFERENCES

Glover MT, Malone M, Atherton DJ. Michelin-tire baby syndrome resulting from diffuse smooth muscle hamartoma. Pediatr Dermatol 1989; 6: 329–31

Sato M, Ishikawa O, Miyachi Y, et al. Michelin tire syndrome: a congenital disorder of elastic fibre formation? Br J Dermatol 1997; 136: 583–6

Wallach D, Sorm M, Saurat J-H. Nevus musculaire généralisé avec aspect clinique de 'bebé Michelin'. Ann Dermatol Venereol 1980; 107: 923–7

JUVENILE HYALINE FIBROMATOSIS

Synonyms

- Fibromatosis hyalinica multiplex
- Infantile systemic hyalinosis

Age of onset

- Between 3 months and 4 years of age

Clinical findings

Skin lesions

- Small fleshy, pearly-white papules on face and neck
- Translucent nodules of gelatinous consistency on fingers, ears and nose (Figures 17.39 and 17.40)
- Large subcutaneous tumors on scalp, trunk and limbs (Figure 17.41)

(All three types of lesion may occur in the same patient.)

- Hyperhidrosis
- Gingival hypertrophy: this is an expected finding and may be severe. The teeth may be overlapped and may be malaligned (Figure 17.42)

Extracutaneous findings

- Flexion contractures of large joints: this is the first and more constant finding

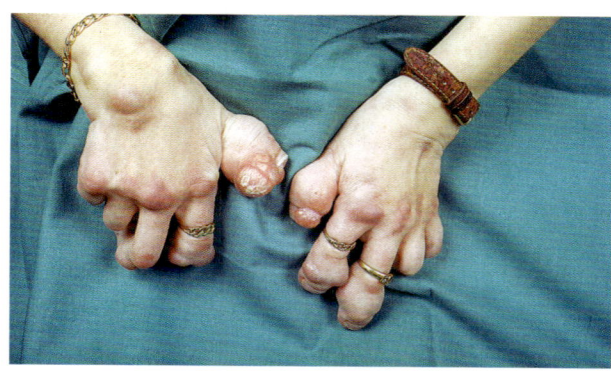

Figure 17.40

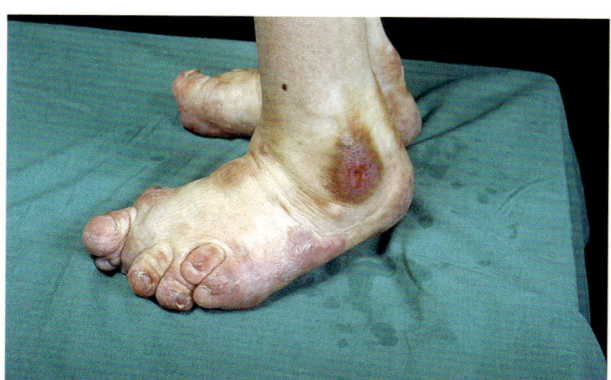

Figure 17.41

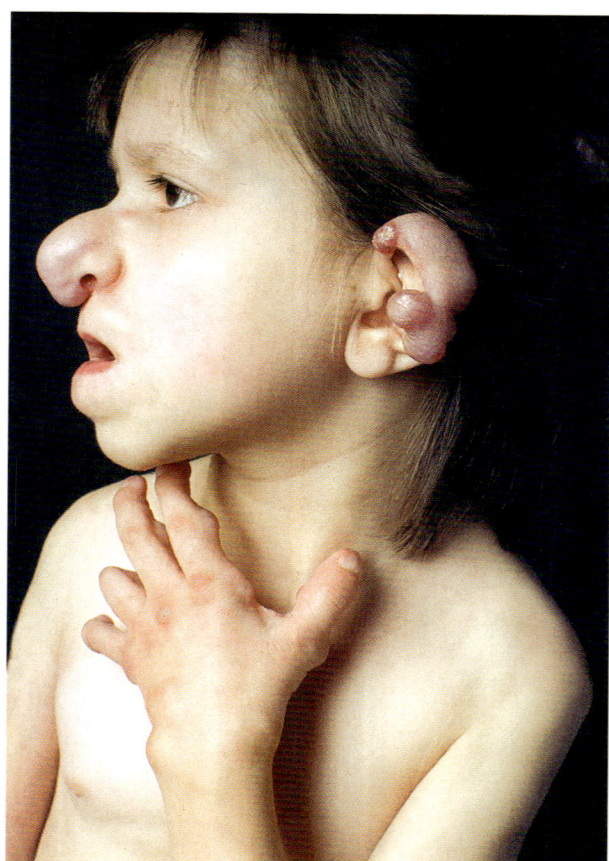

Figure 17.39

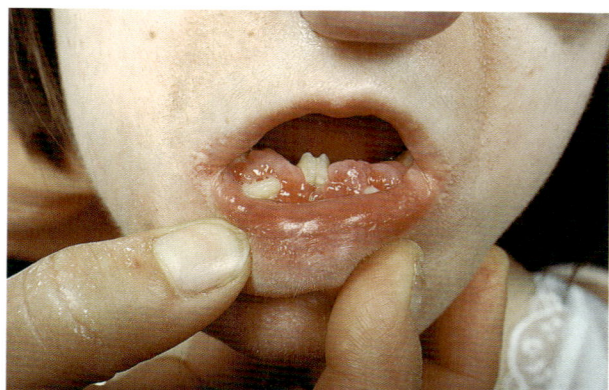

Figure 17.42

- Myopathy
- Short stature

Course and complications

- Susceptibility to superficial infections
- Dental caries

The disease is progressive. Motor development is delayed due to physical deformities.

Laboratory findings

- Radiography: osteolytic lesions, osteoporosis, calcification of soft tissue
- Histopathologic features: closely packed thick bundles of collagen, increased number of oval and spindle-shaped fibrocytes, homogeneous eosinophilic material (PAS (periodic acid–Schiff) positive, diastase resistant)

Genetics and pathogenesis

- Autosomal recessive mode of inheritance
- Abnormal production and accumulation of glycosaminoglycans and glycoproteins
- Defect in collagen synthesis

Differential diagnosis

- Winchester's syndrome
- Congenital generalized fibromatosis

Follow-up and therapy

Patients with juvenile hyaline fibromatosis may stay alive and well in adulthood and are intellectually normal. The term infantile systemic hyalinosis is used in those affected patients who die in early childhood.

Therapy is unsatisfactory. Excision of cutaneous lesions is followed by recurrences. Transient improvement of joint contractures can be obtained with systemic corticosteroids or capsulotomy.

REFERENCES

Kan AE, Rogers M. Juvenile hyaline fibromatosis: an expanded clinicopathologic spectrum. Pediatr Dermatol 1989; 6: 68–75

Kitano Y, Horiki M, Aoki T, et al. Two cases of juvenile hyaline fibromatosis. Arch Dermatol 1972; 106: 877–83

Larralde M, Santos-Muñoz A, Calb I, et al. Juvenile hyaline fibromatosis. Pediatr Dermatol 2001; 18: 400–2

CUTANEOUS MASTOCYTOSIS

Synonym

- Familial urticaria pigmentosa

Age of onset

- In infancy or childhood

Clinical findings

- Most frequently, lesions of urticaria pigmentosa (~50 families): macules, papules or nodules irregularly scattered on the skin with positive Darier's sign (Figure 17.43)
- Less frequently, lesions of telangiectasia macularis eruptiva perstans (three families)

Laboratory investigations

- Histopathologic findings: various degrees of mast cell infiltration
- Occasionally elevated levels of histamine metabolites in blood or urine

Genetics and pathogenesis

- Autosomal dominant pattern with incomplete penetrance
- Familial mastocytosis seems to be due to an increased expression of mast cell growth factors without activating mutations of the stem cell factor c-*kit*

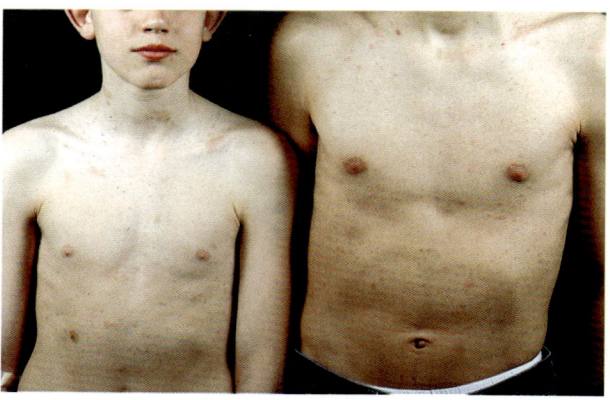

Figure 17.43

Therapy

- Avoidance of mediator-releasing agents
- Symptomatic

REFERENCES

Anstey A, Lowe DG, Kirby JD, et al. Familial mastocytosis: a clinical, immunophenotypic, light and electronmicroscopic study. Br J Dermatol 1991; 125: 583–7

Chang A, Tung RC, Schlesinger T, et al. Familial cutaneous mastocytosis. Pediatr Dermatol 2001; 18: 271–6

Hartmann K, Henz BM. Mastocytosis: recent advances in defining the disease. Br J Dermatol 2001; 144: 682–95

CUTANEOUS LEIOMYOMATOSIS

Synonym

- Familial leiomyomata

Age of onset

- From infancy to middle age

Clinical findings

- Multiple (from a few lesions to several hundreds) firm, smooth, dusky red or brown dermal papules or nodules mainly located on the extensor surfaces of extremities, face and trunk (Figures 17.44 and 17.45)
- Distribution is usually bilateral, although not symmetrical; in one-third of cases it is unilateral with a mosaic pattern arising from postzygotic mutations (Figure 17.46)
- Characteristic feature is pain (aching, stabbing or burning) triggered by tactile or cold thermal stimulation

Associations

- Multiple uterine leiomyomata (Reed's syndrome)
- Dermatitis herpetiformis
- Endocrine neoplasia

Course

There are consecutive outbreaks and then stabilization.

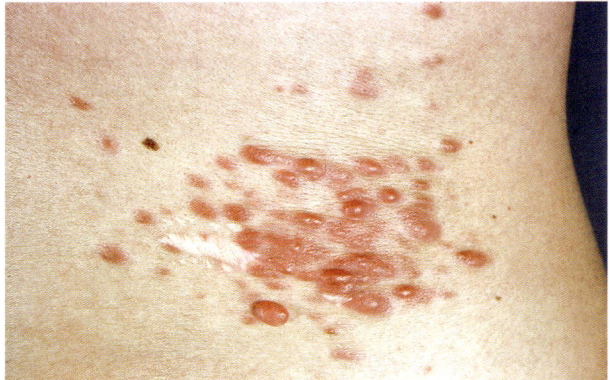

Figure 17.44

Laboratory findings

Histopathologic findings include an ill-defined dermal tumor composed of interlacing smooth muscle fibers with collagen bundles interspersed.

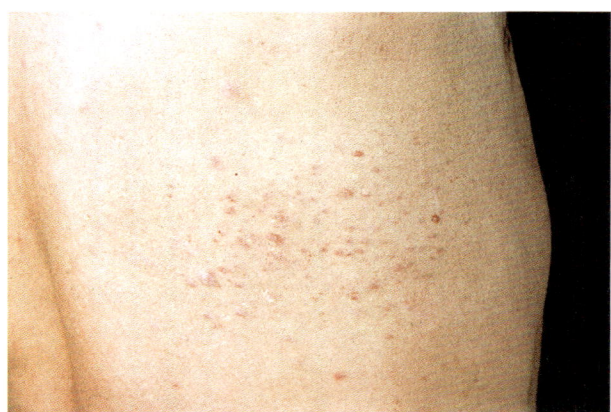

Figure 17.45

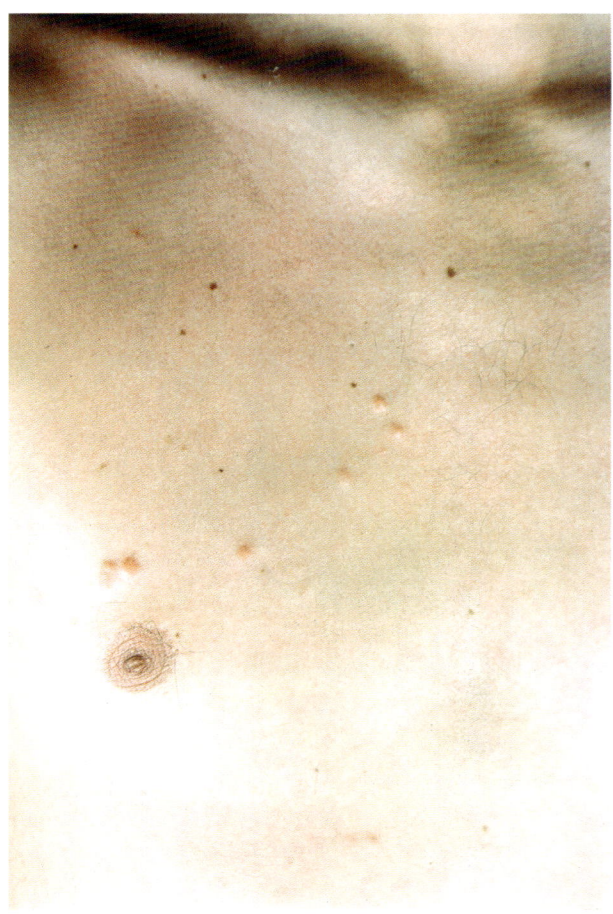

Figure 17.46

Genetics and pathogenesis

- Autosomal dominant inheritance with poor penetrance
- Gene locus unknown
- The lesions consist of piloleiomyomas arising from the arrector muscle of hair

Differential diagnosis

- Neurinomas
- Eccrine spiradenoma
- Granular cell tumor

Follow-up and therapy

- Genetic counseling is important in female patients to control uterine conditions
- Analgesics for control of pain
- Selective surgical excision, frequently followed by relapses

REFERENCES

Fearfield LA, Smith JR, Bunker CB, et al. Association of multiple familial cutaneous leiomyoma with a uterine symplastic leiomyoma. Clin Exp Dermatol 2000; 25: 44–7

Fernandez-Pugnaire MA, Delgado-Florencio V. Familial multiple cutaneous leiomyomas. Dermatology 1995; 191: 295–8

Vellanki LS, Camisa C, Steck WD. Familial leyomiomata. Cutis 1996; 58: 80–2

RESTRICTIVE DERMOPATHY

Synonym

- FADS (fetal akinesia deformation syndrome)

Epidemiology

The disease is very rare. There are fewer than 30 published cases.

Age of onset

- At birth

Clinical findings

- Skin is taut, thin, firm and translucent (Figures 17.47 and 17.48)
- Erosion in major folds and erythema and scaling may be present (Figure 17.49)

Extracutaneous findings

- Facies with open mouth and pinched nose
- Arthrogryposis
- Flexion contractures of joints
- Pulmonary insufficiency
- FADS sequence is represented by polyhydramnios, reduced fetal movements, dysmorphic facies

Course and prognosis

Restrictive dermopathy may be lethal perinatally (respiratory insufficiency), or usually within the first weeks of life due to major pulmonary complications.

Laboratory findings

- Flattening of dermoepidermal junction and thinning of dermis seen on conventional microscopy

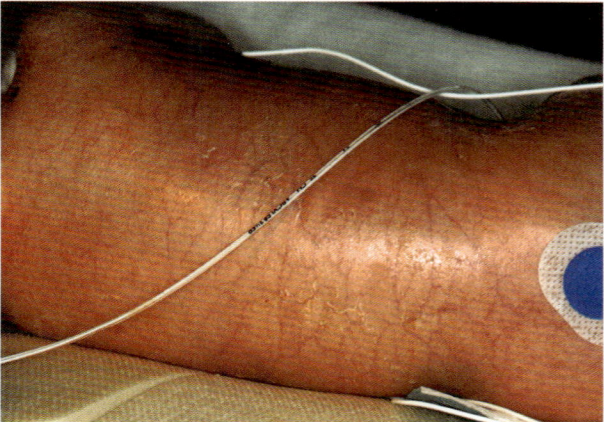

Figure 17.47

- Ultrasound during pregnancy may reveal characteristic features of FADS

Genetics and pathogenesis

- Autosomal recessive
- A mouse model may exist with related skin features and mutations in fatty-acid transport protein (Fatp 4-Slc 27a4)
- Lamin-A mutations have been recently reported

Differential diagnosis

- Harlequin fetus and collodion presentations
- Epidermolysis bullosa

REFERENCE

Nijsten TE, De Moor A, Colpaert CG, et al. Restrictive dermopathy: a case report and a critical review of all hypotheses of its origin. Pediatr Dermatol 2002; 19: 67–72

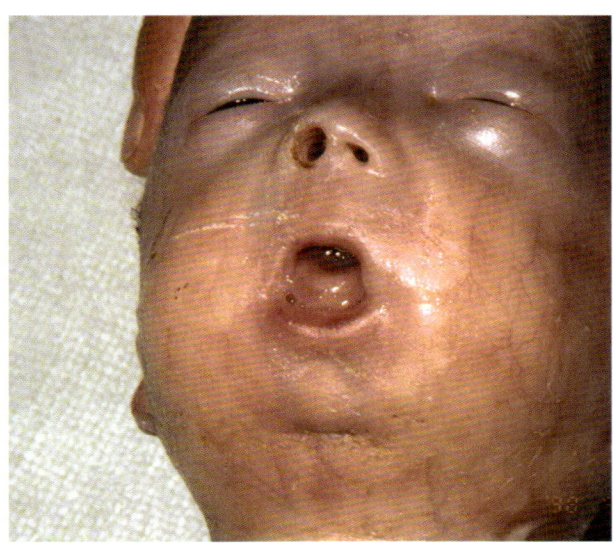

Figure 17.48

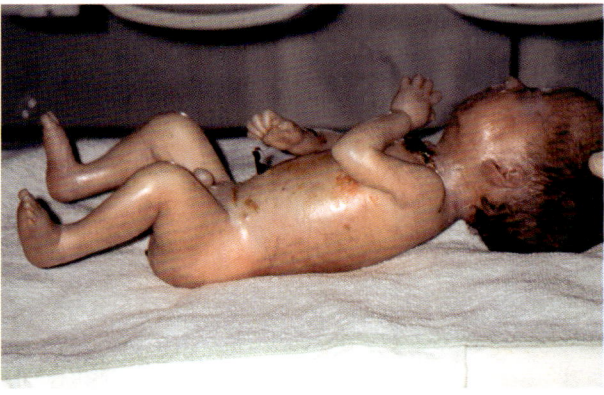

Figure 17.49

DERMOCHONDROCORNEAL DYSTROPHY

Synonym

- François' syndrome

Age of onset

- Childhood or adolescence

Clinical findings

Skin and mucosal lesions

- Firm white grey papulonodular lesions symmetrically distributed on the back of the hands and on the face (nose and ears) (Figures 17.50 and 17.51)
- Hyperplasia of gingival and palatal mucous membranes (Figure 17.52)

Extracutaneous findings

- Osteochondrodystrophy of bones of hands and feet: subluxations and tendinous contractures with limitations of movement
- Corneal dystrophy: bilateral superficial, central white opacities

Course

The disease is slowly progressive.

Molecular biology and laboratory findings

- Increased urinary excretion of hydroxyproline
- Histopathology: strong fibrotic reaction and presence of vacuolized cells (spongiocytes)

Genetics and pathogenesis

- Autosomal recessive disease
- Multitissue proliferation of anomalous fibroblasts with hyperproduction of type III collagen

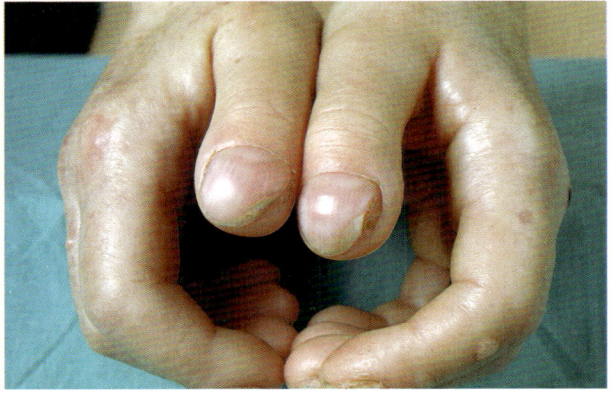

Figure 17.50

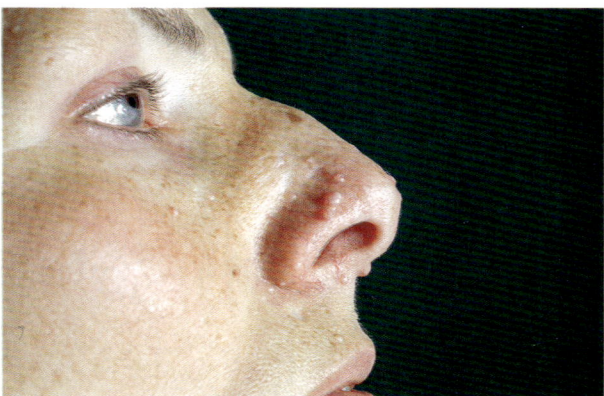

Figure 17.51

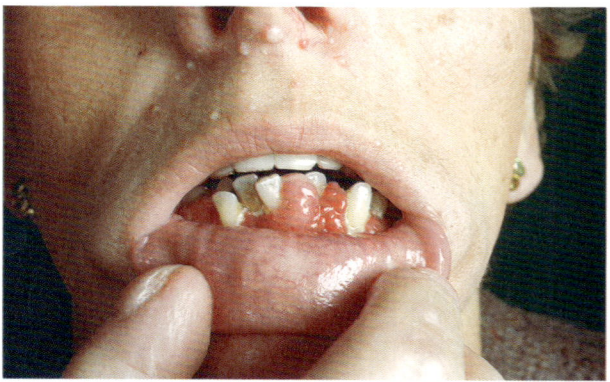

Figure 17.52

Differential diagnosis

- Familial histiocytic dermoarthritis
- Multicentric reticulohistiocytosis
- Fibroblastic rheumatism
- Juvenile hyaline fibromatosis

Follow-up

- Multiple surgical operations by ophthalmologists and dentists to correct gingival hyperplasia and pterygoid
- Corneal transplants

Therapy

- Papulonodular lesions may be excised

REFERENCES

Caputo R, Sambvani N, Monti M, et al. Dermochondrocorneal dystrophy (François syndrome). Arch Dermatol 1988; 124: 424–8.

Maldonado R, Tamayo L, Velazquez E. Dystrophie dermochondro-cornéenne familiale (syndrome de François). Ann Dermatol Venereol 1977; 104: 475–8.

PROGRESSIVE OSSEOUS HETEROPLASIA

Epidemiology

There are fewer than 40 cases reported in the literature; the sex ratio is equal.

Age of onset

- Initial lesions may be noted in the first year of life

Clinical findings

- Initial lesions are small, firm red-purplish papules and nodules, palpable and randomly dispersed (Figure 17.53)
- Plaques may be visible later as a consequence of coalescing subcutaneous lesions, with a red-brownish discoloration (Figures 17.54–17.56)
- Head and face are usually spared
- Phenotype is very variable and there is evidence of different clinical expression within the same family

Extracutaneous findings

- Low birthweight
- Growth retardation
- Normal intelligence

Course and prognosis

- Smaller lesions merge into larger plaques that may result in extensive ossification, ankylosis of affected joints leading to limb-length asymmetries, growth retardation of limbs and limitation of movement
- Ulceration of lesions is possible, with discharge of bony material and infections
- Even if pain is the major referred symptom, milder cases are reported
- The sparse number of cases renders the long-term prognosis difficult to define

Laboratory findings

- Upon conventional microscopy, mature bone formation is visible on the dermis and subcutaneous fat ('osteoma cutis'); later, involvement of fascia, tendon and even muscle is found
- Radiography reveals heterotopic bone in soft subcutaneous tissues
- Thyroid function tests and parathyroid hormone levels are normal, as well as vitamin D levels

Disorders of connective tissue 265

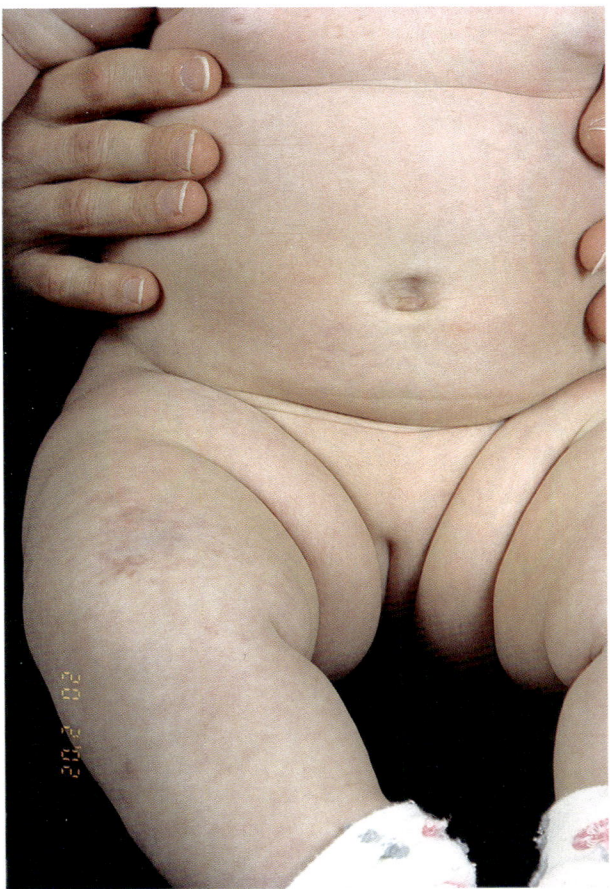

Figure 17.53

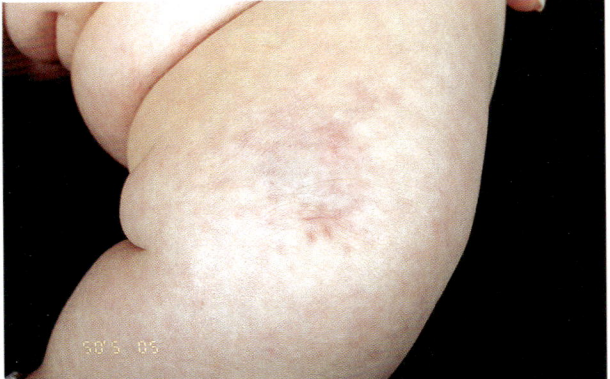

Figure 17.54

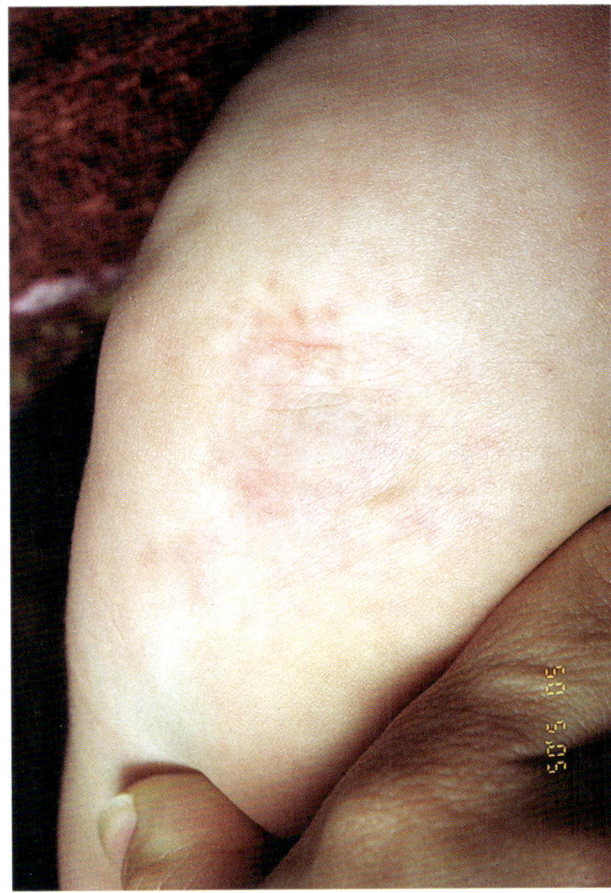

Figure 17.55

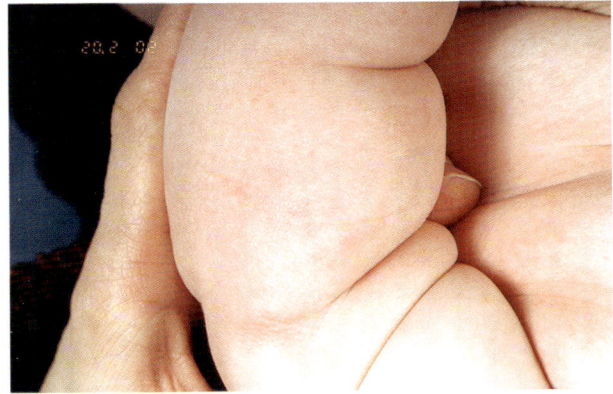

Figure 17.56

Genetics and pathogenesis

- The disease is autosomal dominant
- Recently, paternally inherited mutations of GNAS1 (stimulatory G protein of adenyl cyclase) gene have been found in patients with progressive osseous heteroplasia (POH), although some sporadic cases ('*de novo*' mutations) have been reported
- These latter may be true sporadic cases or germline mosaicisms
- Interestingly, GNAS1 gene shows imprinting: maternally derived mutations result in Albright's hereditary osteodystrophy with pseudohypothyroidsm, whereas paternal mutations may give POH or Albright's hereditary osteodystrophy with pseudopseudohypothyroidism

- GNAS1 gene is thought to be a critical negative modulator in ectopic ossification

Follow-up and therapy

- Orthopedic advice is mandatory to plan surgery for smaller lesions and for eventual corrective devices for limb asymmetries and growth retardation
- Echotomographic examination may be helpful
- Analgesic drugs for pain and discomfort in severe cases
- Antibiotics for skin ulcerations
- Genetic counseling for families, bearing in mind the 'imprinting' of GNAS1 gene and the related different diseases

Differential diagnosis

- Solitary osteoma cutis (post-traumatic or post-inflammatory)
- Epithelioma of Malherbe
- Albright's osteodystrophies
- Scleroderma

REFERENCES

Aynaci O, Mujgan Aynaci F, Cobanoglu U, Alpay K. Progressive osseous heteroplasia. A case report and review of the literature. J Pediatr Orthop B 2002; 11: 339–42

Chan I, Hamada T, Hardman C, et al. Progressive osseous heteroplasia resulting from a new mutation in the GNAS1 gene. Clin Exp Dermatol 2004; 29: 77–80

Faust RA, Shore EM, Stevens CE, et al. Progressive osseous heteroplasia in the face of a child. Am J Med Genet 2003; 118A: 71–5

CUTIS VERTICIS GYRATA

Epidemiology

The familial occurrence is rare and often associated with pachydermoperiostosis (see chapter 7).

Age of onset

- At puberty, rarely during childhood

Clinical findings

- The term 'cutis verticis gyrata' is used to describe a pattern of deep, redundant, linear skin folds in the scalp (Figure 17.57)
- The hypertrophy of these skin folds mimics the brain's 'gyri'
- Usually these deep lines are anteroposteriorly oriented but 'horizontal' patterns are described, as well as the presence of hypertrophic skin folds on the forehead

Extracutaneous findings

- Mental retardation
- Seizures
- Schizophrenia

Course and prognosis

- The disease slowly progress with age

Laboratory findings

- At histological examination, connective tissue may be normal with some degree of adnexal hypertrophy

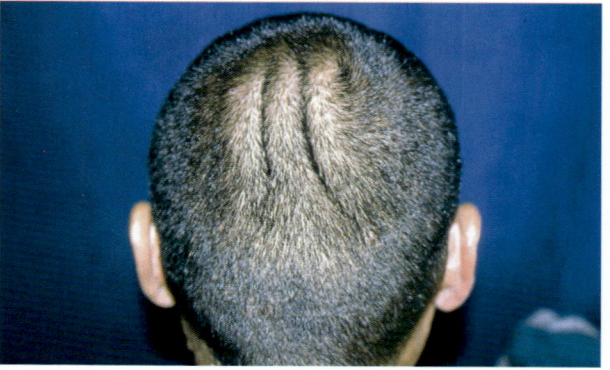

Figure 17.57

Follow-up and therapy

- Exclusion of associated diseases
- Surgery in disfiguring cases

Differential diagnosis

- Genetic diseases presenting with CVG:
  - Pachydermoperiostosis
  - Acromegaly
  - Ehlers-Danlos
  - Cutis laxa
  - Acanthosis nigricans (insulin-resistance syndromes)
  - Costello syndrome
  - Sotos syndrome
  - Turner, Klinefelter and X-fragile syndrome
- Inflammatory skin diseases with CVG
- Amyloidosis
- Myxedema
- Chronic eczema
- Psoriasis

REFERENCES

Nguyen NQ. Cutis verticis gyrata. Dermatol Online J 2003; 9: 32

Ramos-e-Silva M, Martins G, Dadalti P, Maceira J. Cutis verticis gyrata secondary to a cerebriform intradermal nevus. Cutis 2004; 73: 254–6

Schenato LK, Gil T, Carvalho LA, Ricachnevsky N, et al. [Essential primary cutis verticis gyrata] J Pediatr (Rio J). 2002; 78: 75–80 [Portuguese]

CHAPTER 18

Aplasia cutis

Epidemiology

There are no data available.

Age of onset

- At birth

Clinical findings

- Total (full thickness, ulcerated) (Figure 18.1) or partial (membranous) (Figure 18.2) absence of skin components, frequently focal and single, but may more rarely be multiple (Figure 18.3)
- Largely, the preferred site is the scalp (vertex), but all areas may be involved (Figures 18.4 and 18.5)
- Lesions are round or oval and usually small (1–4 cm diameter)
- Larger and irregular lesions are rare (Figure 18.6)
- Often on the scalp a collarette of darker and even hair is present around the aplastic lesion (Figure 18.7)
- Lesions heal in a few months, leaving atrophic and alopecic scars (Figure 18.8)
- Large irregular and deforming scars on the abdomen and trunk are associated with intra-uterine twin death, with fetus papyraceus and placental thrombosis (Figures 18.9 and 18.10)
- A single case of aplasia cutis distributed along the Blaschko lines is reported
- Cutis marmorata telangiectatica congenita is statistically more frequent in patients with aplasia cutis congenita
- Epidermal–sebaceous nevus of the head and face can be associated

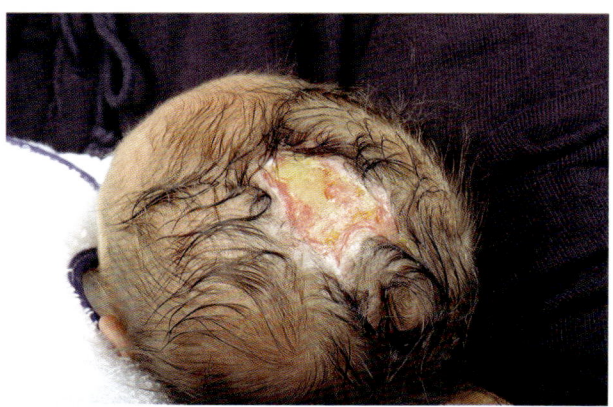

Figure 18.1

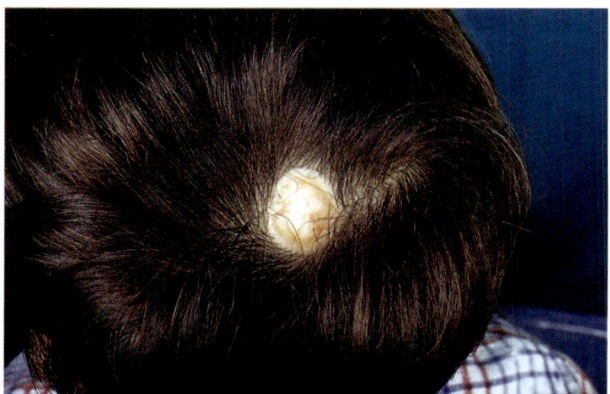

Figure 18.2

270 Atlas of Genodermatoses

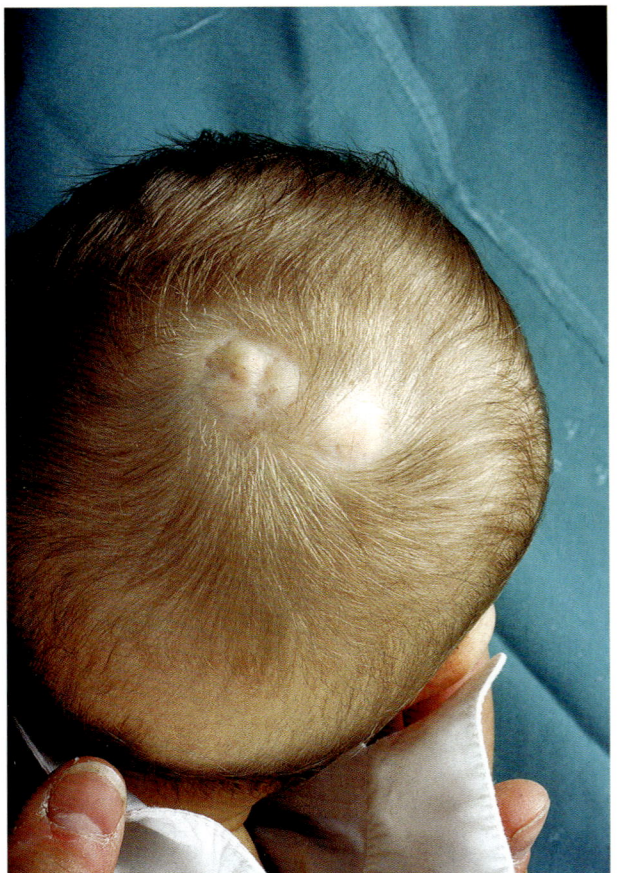

Figure 18.3

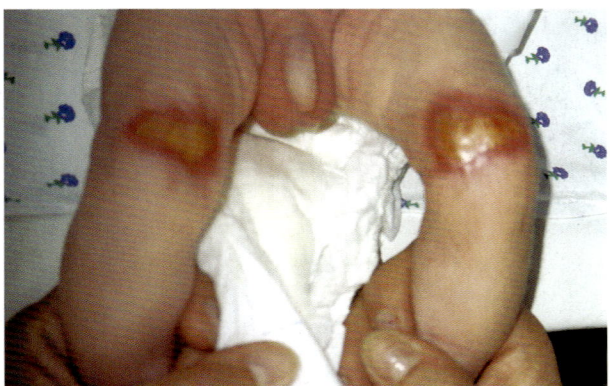

Figure 18.4

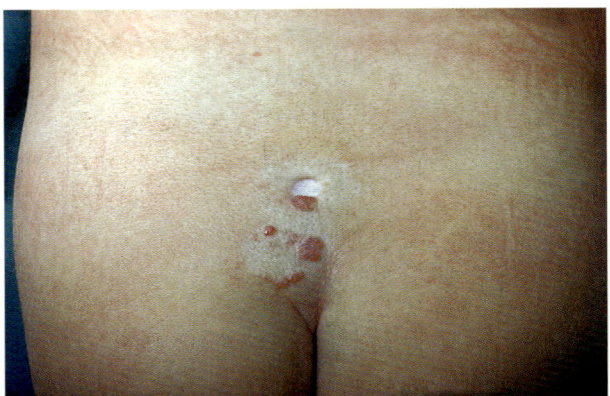

Figure 18.5

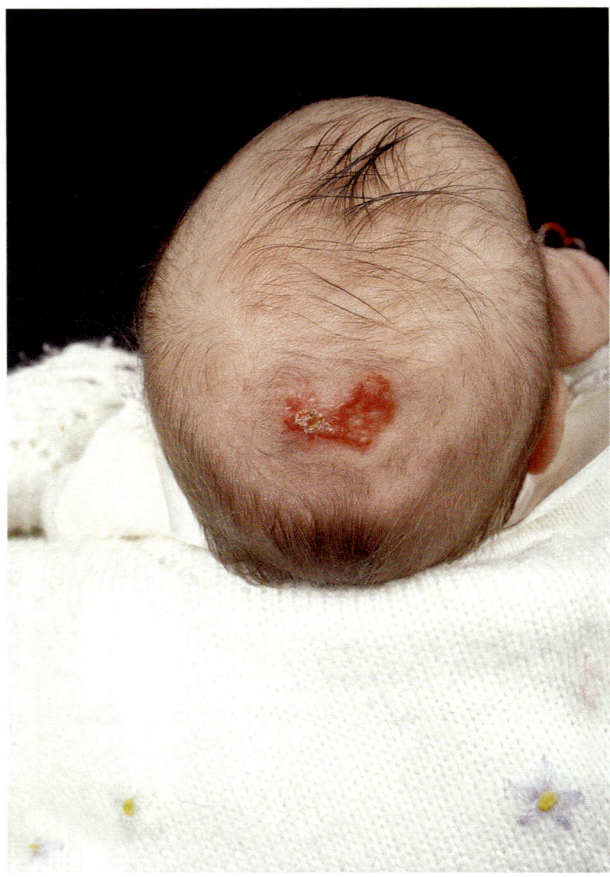

Figure 18.6

Extracutaneous findings

- Skull defects and meningeal exposure are associated with severe ulcerated lesions of aplasia cutis
- Vertebral midline closure defects and meningocele
- More rarely severe central nervous system (CNS) malformations are associated
- Limb defects (anomalies of fingers) appear to be genetically heterogeneous and are relatively frequent (10–20%) as distal phalangeal aplasia, ectrodactyly and sindactyly

Laboratory findings

Echotomography (Figure 18.11) is diagnostic, especially for large lesions: fetus papyraceus-associated

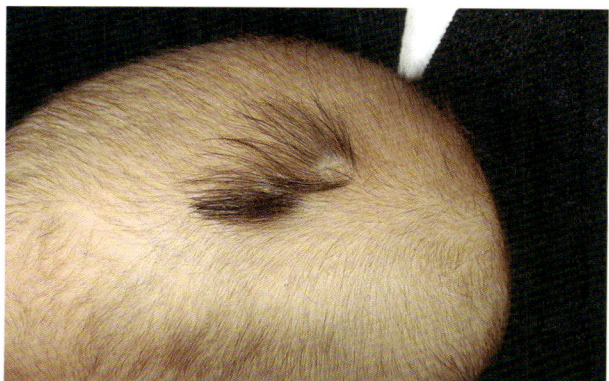

Figure 18.7

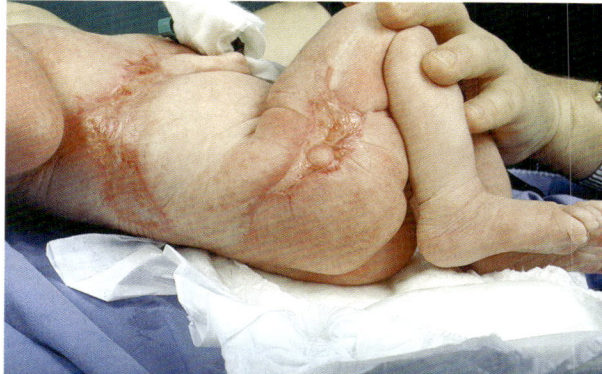

Figure 18.9

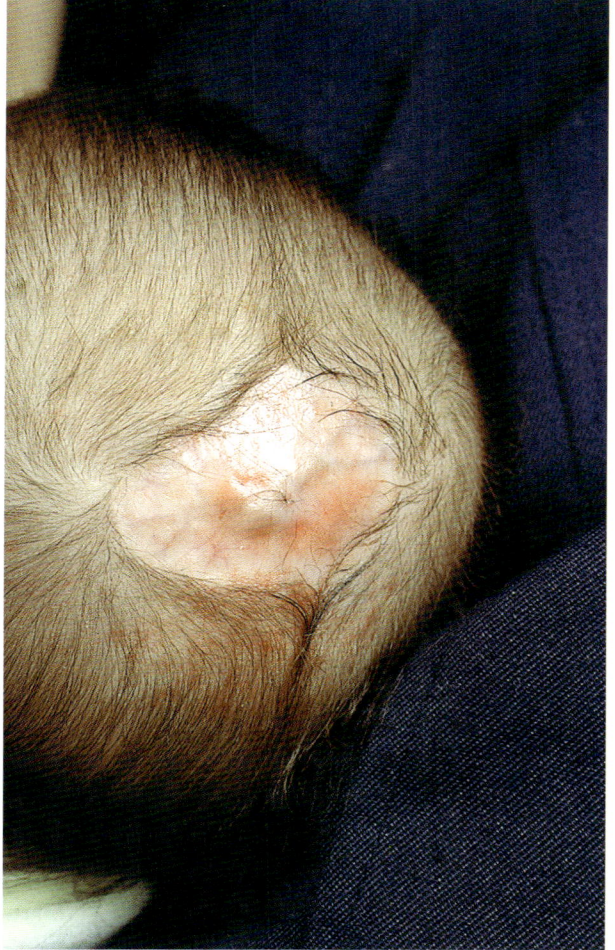

Figure 18.8

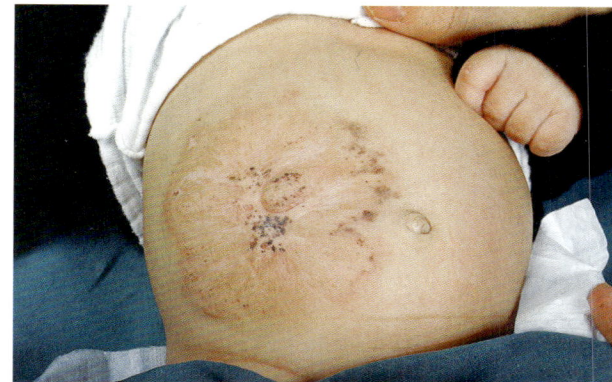

Figure 18.10

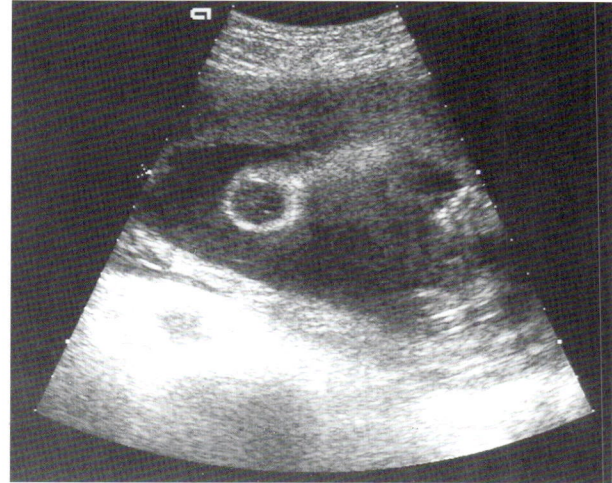

Figure 18.11

aplasia cutis and forms associated with severe CNS and medullary malformations.

Genetics and pathogenesis

Most cases are sporadic, but dominant (Figure 18.12) and less frequently recessive and mosaic forms have been documented.

Aplasia cutis seems to be related to closure defects during embryo development (midline in the scalp is represented by a 'camera obturator' mechanism, and these defects explain the round or oval shape of aplasia cutis lesions at the vertex).

Trisomy 13 is associated with aplasia cutis.

Aplasia cutis may be due to the teratogenic effects of some drugs taken during pregnancy (methimazole), or determined by herpes virus diseases contracted during gestation.

Follow-up and therapy

- Diagnostic images are useful to follow the spontaneous healing of full-thickness lesions
- Neurologic and orthopedic advice for CNS lesions and limb defects

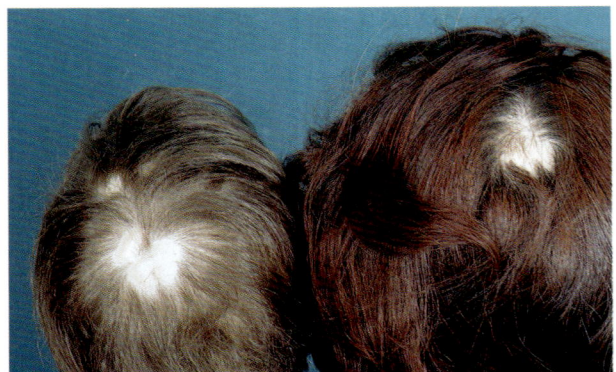

Figure 18.12

Differential diagnosis

- **Adams–Oliver** syndrome (aplasia cutis, heart anomalies, limb and finger defects, cutis marmorata telangiectatica congenita, severe scarring form) (Figures 18.13–18.15)

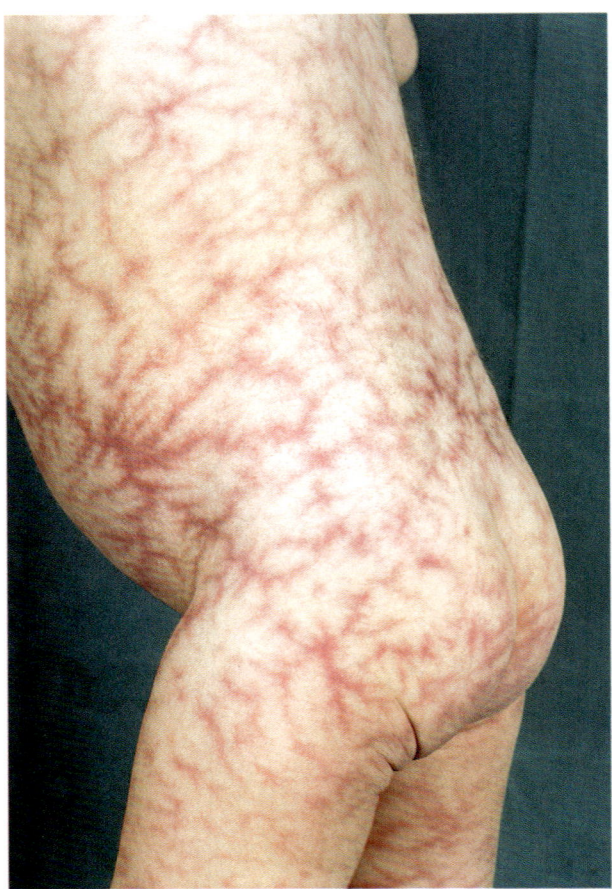

Figure 18.14

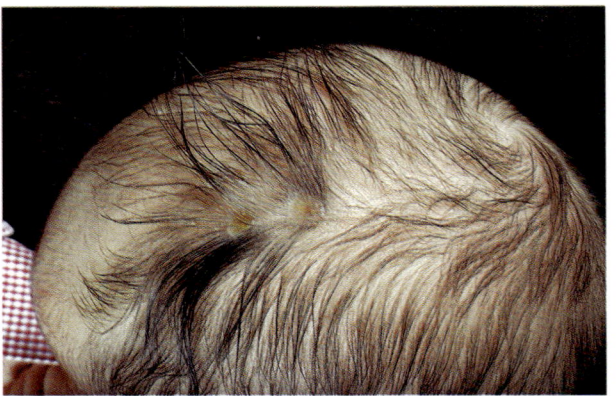

Figure 18.13

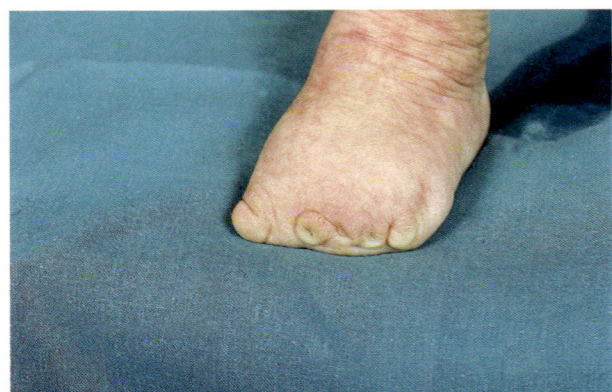

Figure 18.15

- **Setleis disease** (bilateral forceps marks and aplasia cutis) (Figure 18.16)

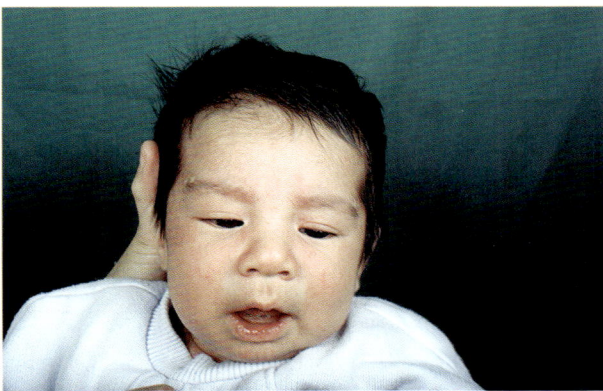

Figure 18.16

- **Delleman's syndrome** or oculocerebrocutaneous syndrome and 'drop-like' lateral aplasia cutis (Figure 18.17)

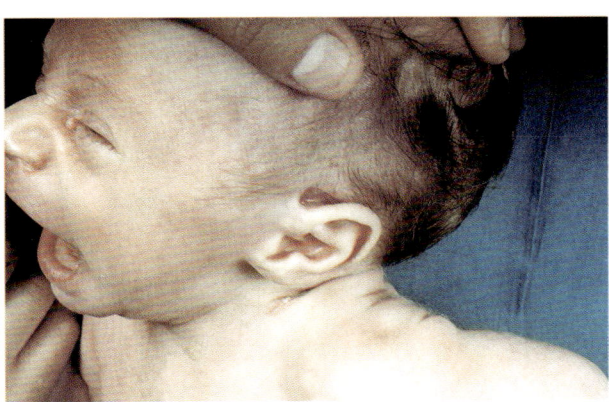

Figure 18.17

- EEC–Rapp–Hodgkin syndrome group (p63 defect-related ectodermal dysplasia) (see Chapter 15.1)
- Goltz's syndrome (see Chapter 15.2)
- In all three forms of epidermolysis bullosa at birth, even large areas of the body (abdomen, arms and legs) may be denuded (formerly known as Bart's syndrome) owing to the specific defects of each form (Figure 18.18)
- Johansson–Blizzard syndrome (beak-like nose, mental retardation, aplasia cutis, skin dimples, hair anomalies)
- Amniotic rupture sequence

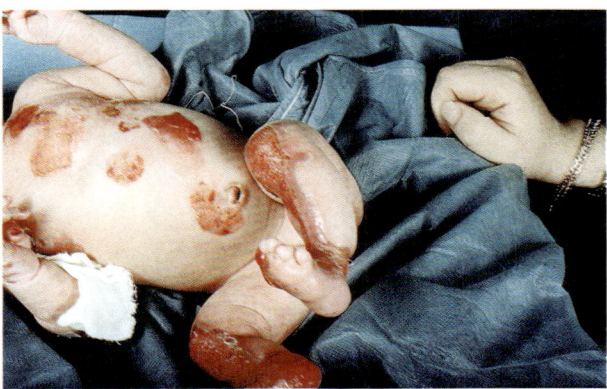

Figure 18.18

REFERENCES

Freiden IJ. Aplasia cutis congenital: a clinical review and proposal for classification. J Am Acad Dermatol 1986; 14: 646–60

Rosenberg JG, Drolet BA. Setleis syndrome. Pediatr Dermatol 2004; 21: 82–3

Tambe KA, Ambekar SV, Bafna PN. Delleman (oculocerebrocutaneous) syndrome: few variations in a classical case. Eur J Paediatr Neurol 2003; 7: 77–80

Tan HH, Tay YK. Familial aplasia cutis congenita of the scalp: a case report and review. Ann Acad Med Singapore 1997; 26: 500–2

Tanabe A, Kusumoto K, Suzuki K, Ogawa Y. Treatment of Setleis syndrome. Case report. Scand J Plast Reconstr Surg Hand Surg 2001; 35: 107–11

Verdyck P, Holder-Espinasse M, Hul WV, Wuyts W. Clinical and molecular analysis of nine families with Adams–Oliver syndrome. Eur J Hum Genet 2003; 11: 457–63

CHAPTER 19

Disorders of pigmentation

OCULOCUTANEOUS ALBINISMS

Oculocutaneous albinism type 1

Synonym

- Tyrosinase-negative albinism, OCA1 types A and B

Epidemiology

OCAs have an estimated frequency of 1 : 20 000.

Age of onset

- At birth

Clinical findings

- Wide spectrum of presentations, depending on genotype–phenotype correlation
- From total absence of melanin in skin, hair and eye (the classic 'albino' features, or OCA1 type A) (Figures 19.1 and 19.2) to milder cases with hair pigmentation and changes after sun exposure with occurrence of nevi and freckles (Figure 19.3)
- Rarely, in milder cases there is the possibility of a heat-related pattern in the secretion of melanin, as occurs in Siamese cats

Extracutaneous symptoms

- Iris may be pink-red or blue-gray in milder cases and show transluscency on slit lamp examination (Figure 19.1)
- Strabismus (Figure 19.3), nystagmus, photophobia and poor vision

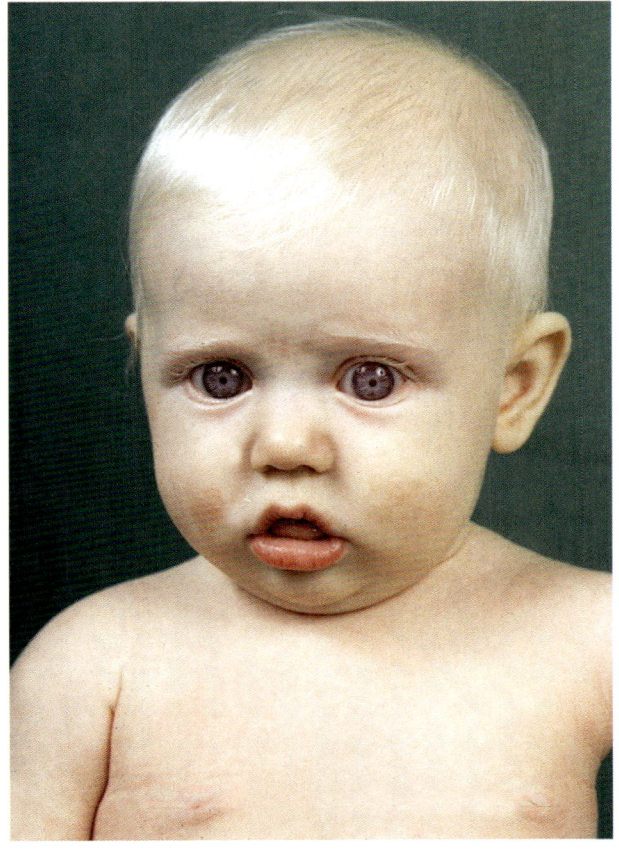

Figure 19.1

- Foveal hypoplasia
- Even auditory evoked response may be abnormal, without hearing impairment

Complications

- Rare amelanotic melanomas

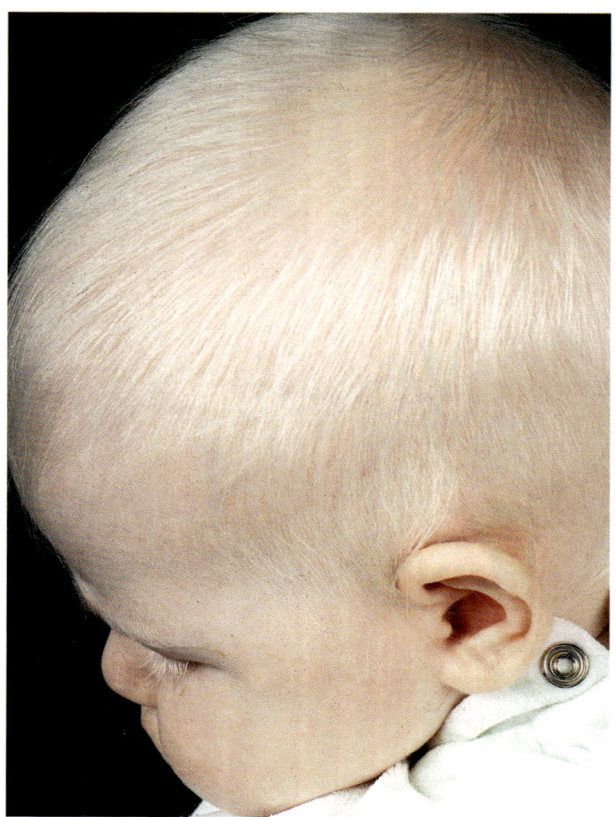

Figure 19.2

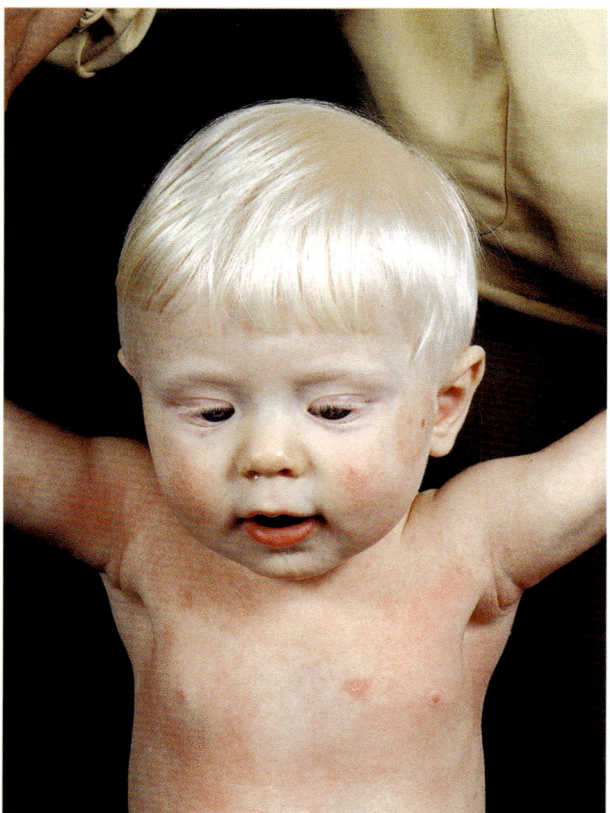

Figure 19.3

- Sunburn, squamous and basal cell carcinomas (UV-induced)

Course

- In milder cases some degree of pigmentation of skin, hair and eye visible during childhood and adolescence
- In the same cases it is common to detect melanocytic nevi, ephelides and lentigines
- Nystagmus may ameliorate with age

Laboratory findings

- On histological examination, skin and hair-bulb structures are normal
- On ultrastructural examination, the first step of development of cytoplasmic organels with melanin-related functions is normal

Genetics and pathogenesis

OCA1 is inherited in a recessive mode and is due to mutations of the tyrosinase gene. There is a wide variability in gene mutations, including stop-codon, missense, splicing, frameshift and deletions, responsible for the wide variation in phenotypes of these patients. A particular missense mutation renders the tyrosinase gene temperature sensitive. Those patients with 'temperature-sensitive cutaneous albinism' develop, after puberty, some degree of pigmentation in the cooler areas of the body, producing the 'Siamese cat' pattern.

Differential diagnosis

- OCA2
- OCA3
- Hermansky–Pudlak syndrome
- Chediak–Higashi syndrome
- Cross–McKusick syndrome: albinism, severe mental retardation, spastic di- or quadriplegia and seizures

Follow-up and therapy

- Ocular assessment is mandatory in the follow-up of these patients
- Prevention of sunburn and UV-derived complications in order to avoid skin cancers

REFERENCES

King RA, Pietsch J, Fryer JP, et al. Tyrosinase gene mutations in oculocutaneous albinism 1 (OCA1): definition of the phenotype. Hum Genet 2003; 113: 2502–13

Rees JL. Genetics of hair and skin color. Annu Rev Genet 2003; 37: 67–90

Oculocutaneous albinism type 2

Synonyms

- OCA2
- Tyrosinase-positive albinism

Epidemiology

OCA2 may be the most common albinism in African and American populations.

Age of onset

- At birth

Clinical findings

- Some amount of pigment is present at birth
- Minimal to moderate pigmentation of hair, skin and eyes from northern Caucasian to Mediterranean population
- Hair may be fairly blond at birth, skin may be creamy (Figure 19.4)
- In African and African-American populations hair is yellow and the skin is very clear

Extracutaneous symptoms

- Iris may be blue-gray or 'sandy' in color with punctate and radial translucency
- Retinal pigmentation is fair
- Visual impairment is common

Course

- During the first two decades of life pigmented nevi and freckles may occur
- No tan develops after sun exposure

Genetics and pathogenesis

The 'P' gene, a human homolog to the mouse pink-eye dilution locus, is mutated in these patients; different types of mutation are present, giving rise to different phenotypes. The 'P' gene product, the 'pink protein', modulates the processing and trafficking of tyrosinase, resulting in abnormal secretion of melanin. This gene is also a strong candidate for determination of human eye color. The disease is inherited in a recessive manner.

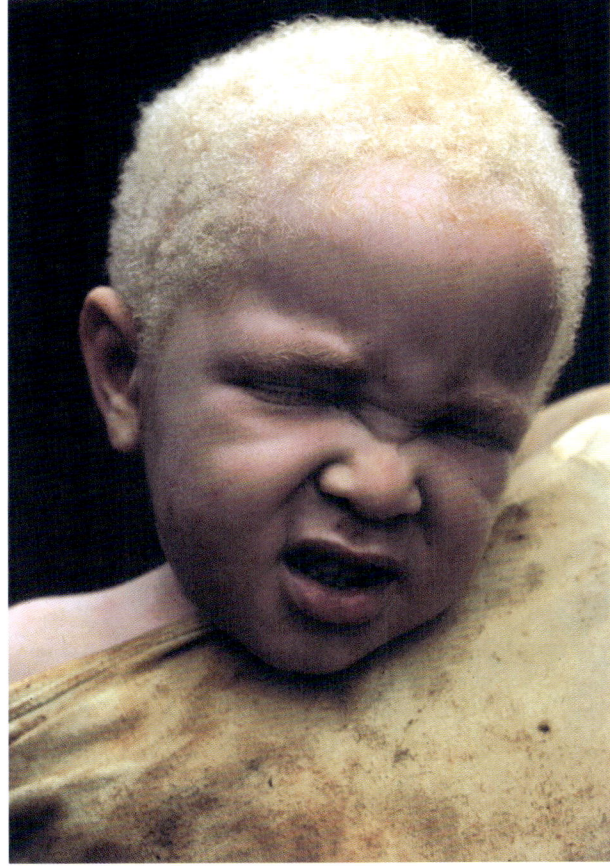

Figure 19.4

Follow-up and therapy

Ophthalmological assessment is mandatory as well as preventive measures to ensure avoidance of UV-induced damage.

Differential diagnosis

- Other OCAs
- Hermansky–Pudlak syndrome

REFERENCE

King RA, Willaert RK, Schmidt RM, et al. MC1R mutations modify the classic phenotype of oculocutaneous albinism type 2 (OCA2). Am J Hum Genet 2003; 73: 638–45

Oculocutaneous albinism type 3

Synonym

- OCA3

Epidemiology

There are no recent data available. This form of OCA seems to be more frequent in the South African native population.

Age of onset

- At birth

Clinical findings

- Light-brown skin and hair (Figure 19.5) to reddish-brown skin and red hair

Extracutaneous symptoms

- Blue-gray iris and nystagmus

Course

There are no consistent changes throughout life.

Laboratory findings

These are aspecific.

Genetics and pathogenesis

The disease is autosomal recessive and is due to mutations in the TRP1 gene. The function of this protein is not fully investigated, but is related to the oxidation process leading to indolequinones in the eumelanin pathway. A further OCA, named **OCA4**, shares a similar clinical pattern to that of the other oculocutaneous albinisms and is due to mutations of the MATP (membrane-associated transporter protein gene) and are thought to function in a parallel pathway to the P gene.

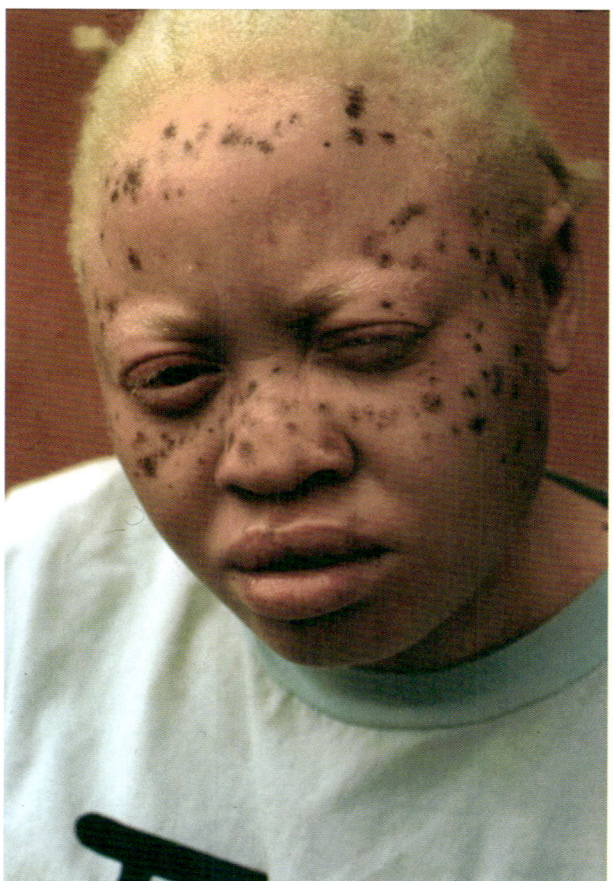

Figure 19.5

Follow-up and therapy

- Ophthalmological survey
- UV protection

REFERENCE

Toyofuku K, Wada I, Valencia JC, et al. Oculocutaneous albinism types 1 and 3 are ER retention diseases: mutation of tyrosinase or Tyrp 1 can affect the processing of both mutant and wild-type proteins. FASEB J 2001; 15: 149–61

HERMANSKY–PUDLAK SYNDROME

Synonym

- Albinism with hemorrhagic diathesis

Epidemiology

The disease is rare. In Puerto Rico there are several families that segregate for Hermansky–Pudlak syndrome (HPS). A few non-Puerto Rican pedigrees are known, especially in large Jewish or Muslim populations. A total of 600–700 patients are estimated.

Age of onset

- At birth

Clinical findings

- Four subtypes of HPS exist, each related to four different genes. They have in common the following signs, with varying severity:
    - Ethnic-dependent hypopigmentation of the skin and hair (albinism) (Figure 19.6)
    - Progressive pigmentation recovery
    - Bruising and ecchymoses

Extracutaneous symptoms

- Different degrees of iris color, red to light-brown
- Red retinal reflex, photophobia and nystagmus
- Hemorrhagic diathesis due to a storage pool platelet defect (menorrhagia, epistaxis)
- Severe pulmonary fibrosis and inflammatory bowel disease in HPS1 Puerto Rican families, absent in HPS2 and HPS3 (mild hypopigmentation and bleeding) mutation-related subjects
- Childhood neutropenia and recurrent upper respiratory infections in some families (HPS2)

Laboratory findings

- Melanocytes contain macromelanosomes and are tyrosinase positive

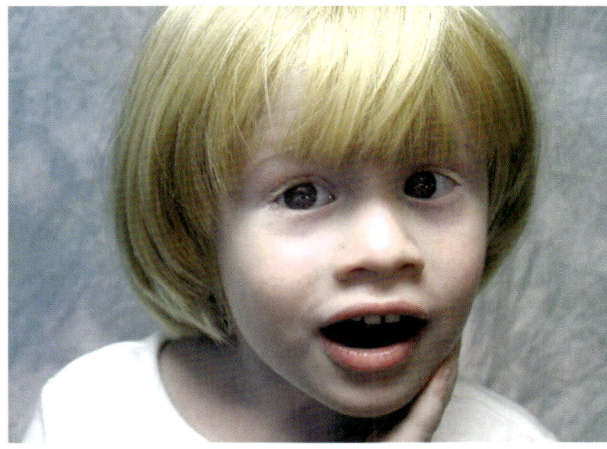

Figure 19.6

- Platelets and monocyte–phagocyte cells show dense bodies and abnormal cytoplasmic pattern and organelles

Genetics and pathogenesis

All four identified genes related to HPS (HPS-1, -3 and -4 and ADTB3A) encode proteins and factors related to the formation of melanosomes, platelet dense bodies and lysosomal compartments ('cytoplasmic vesicular trafficking'), explaining the clinical phenotypes of HPS.

Differential diagnosis

- Oculocutaneous albinism
- Griscelli's disease
- Chediak–Higashi syndrome
- Elejalde's syndrome

REFERENCES

Bennett DC. The colours of mice and men – 100 genes and beyond? Pigment Cell Res 2003; 16: 576–7

Huizing M, Helip-Wooley A, Dorward H, et al. Hermansky–Pudlak syndrome: a model for abnormal vesicle formation and trafficking. Pigment Cell Res 2003; 16: 584

Nguyen T, Wei ML. Characterization of melanosomes in murine Hermansky–Pudlak syndrome: mechanisms of hypopigmentation. J Invest Dermatol 2004; 122: 452–60

HYPOMELANOSIS OF ITO

Synonym

Incontinentia pigmenti acromians is an old denomination that defines hypopigmented nevi + central nervous system (CNS) anomalies.

Epidemiology

The complex of symptoms is rare.

Age of onset

- At birth or within the first 2 years of life

Clinical findings

- Linear, whorled or figured pattern of hypopigmentation in a mosaic distribution (Figures 19.7–19.9)

Extracutaneous symptoms

We believe that is mandatory to define as 'true' hypomelanosis of Ito only those patients having hypomelanotic nevi and associated abnormalities, such as:

- Mental retardation
- Seizures
- CNS structural abnormalities

Course and prognosis

- Skin changes are usually stable
- Neurological symptoms and their evolution are strictly related to the extent of CNS involvement and usually worsen with age

Laboratory findings

- Chromosomal mosaicism is frequent, but may be present also in patients with hypo/hyperpigmented nevi without any sign of CNS involvement
- Magnetic resonance imaging (MRI) for CNS lesions

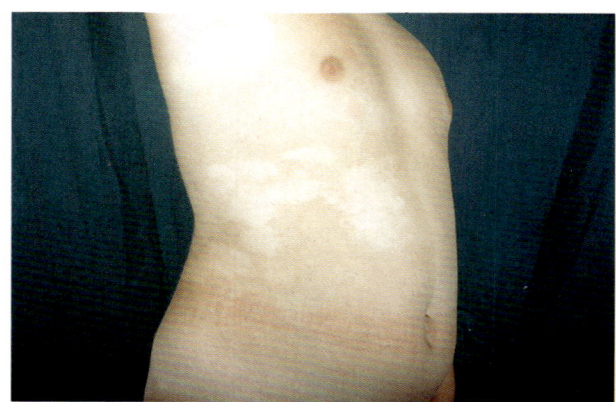

Figure 19.8

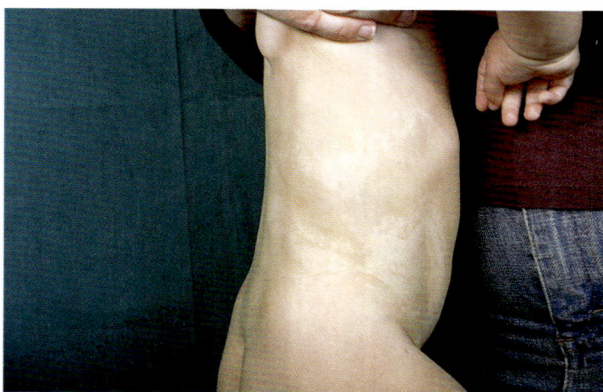

Figure 19.7

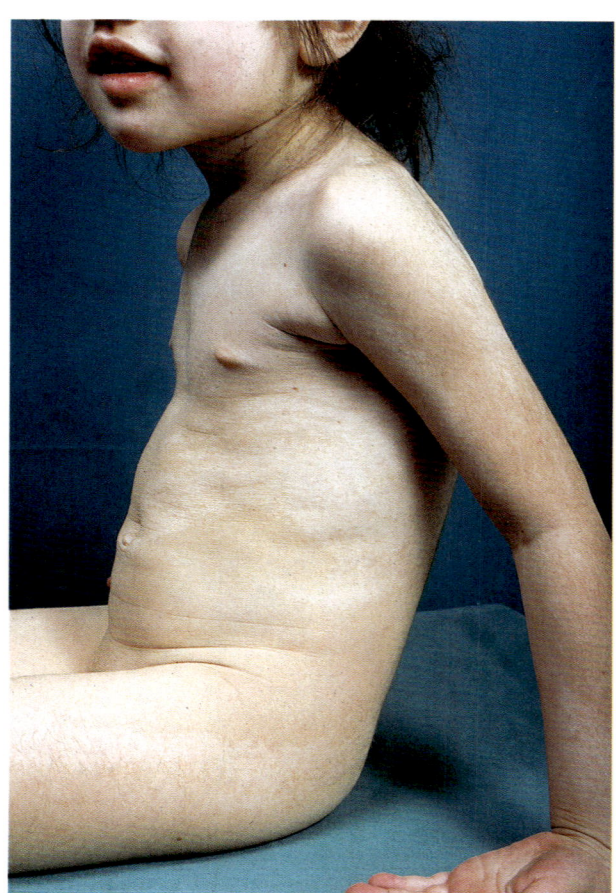

Figure 19.9

Genetics and pathogenesis

Hypomelanosis of Ito is a mosaic disease associated in part with a chromosomal alteration. The involved gene is unknown.

Follow-up and therapy

- Karyotyping
- Neurological evaluation
- Prevention of sun exposure damage in large hypopigmented areas

Differential diagnosis

- Any kind of hypopigmented mosaic nevus
- Vitiligo

REFERENCES

Echenne BP, Leboucq N, Humbertclaude V. Ito hypomelanosis and moyamoya disease. Pediatr Neurol 1995; 13: 169–71

Turleau C, Taillard F, Doussau de Bazignan M, et al. Hypomelanosis of Ito (incontinentia pigmenti achromians) and mosaicism for a microdeletion of 15q1. Hum Genet 1986; 74: 185–7

Vral J, De Smet L, Fabry G. Triphalangeal thumb in Ito's hypomelanosis syndrome. Genet Couns 1991; 2: 217–19

PIEBALDISM

Synonym

- Partial albinism

Epidemiology

There are no data available in the literature.

Age of onset

- At birth

Clinical findings

- Totally depigmented skin patches, especially in midfrontal areas ('diamond-patches') (Figure 19.10) and chin, chest, abdomen, arms and legs (symmetrical distribution) (Figure 19.11)
- Islet of repigmentation within the white patches
- White forelock and involvement of eyebrows and eyelashes

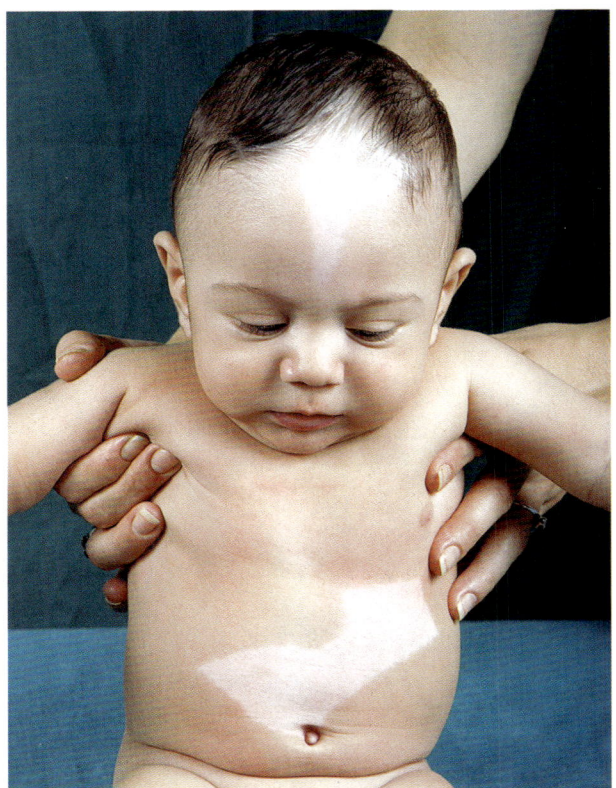

Figure 19.10

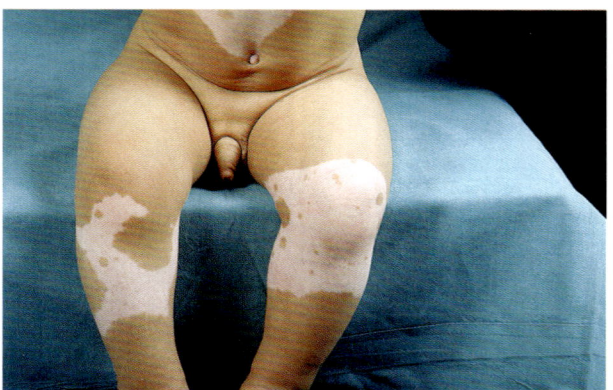

Figure 19.11

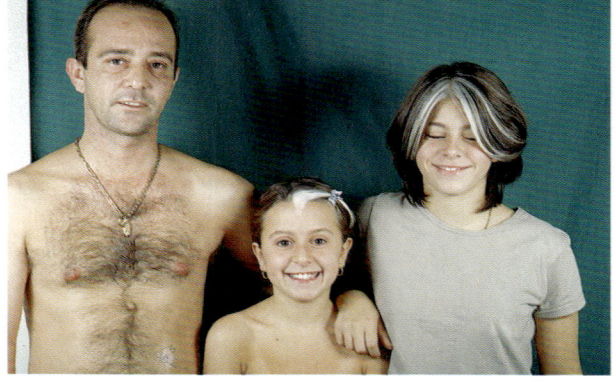

Figure 19.12

Complications and course

Depigmented skin lesions may undergo slight modification in life.

Laboratory findings

- Abnormal melanocyte cytoplasmic pattern
- Decreased Langerhans' cells

Genetics and pathogenesis

The disease is autosomal dominant (Figure 19.12), as in this family with isolated forelock.

Proto-oncogene *c-kit* mutations are responsible for the disease, enabling normal development and migration of melanocytes during embryogenesis.

Differential diagnosis

- Vitiligo
- Waardenburg's syndrome

REFERENCES

Alexeev V, Igoucheva O, Yoon K. Simultaneous targeted alteration of the tyrosinase and c-kit genes by single-stranded oligonucletides. Gene Ther 2002; 9: 1667–75

Ramadevi AR, Naik U, Dutta U, et al. De novo pericentric inversion of chromosome 4, inv(4) (p16q12) in a boy with piebaldism and mental retardation. Am J Med Genet 2002; 113: 190–2

Syrris P, Heathcote K, Carrozzo R, et al. Human piebaldism: six novel mutations of the proto-oncogene KIT. Hum Mutat 2002; 20: 234

WAARDENBURG'S SYNDROME

Synonyms

- Klein–Waardenburg syndrome
- Shah–Waardenburg syndrome

Epidemiology

There are no data available on prevalence and incidence.

Age of onset

- At birth

Clinical findings

- White forelock and white patches randomly distributed on the scalp (Figure 19.13)
- Premature generalized canities
- Patches of white skin on frontal areas
- Synophris

Extracutaneous symptoms

- Iris heterochromia
- 'Dystopia canthorum' and displacement of lower lacrimal duct origin (Figure 19.13)
- Broad nasal root (Figure 19.13)
- Cleft lip and palate with scrotal tongue (Figure 19.14)
- Uni- or bilateral hearing loss
- Hirschsprung's malformation of the gut

Course and complications

Progressive severe intestinal symptoms occur in patients developing megacolon.

Laboratory findings

- No melanocytes visible in affected skin
- Where present, melanocytes show abnormal melanosomes

Genetics and pathogenesis

Clinical and genetic heterogeneities are markers of Waardenburg's syndrome. Three genes are involved in its pathogenesis: PAX3, MITF and EDNRB, which encode two transcription factors and endothelin B receptor, respectively. These defects may be involved in migration defects of the melanocytes and neural cells during embryogenesis.

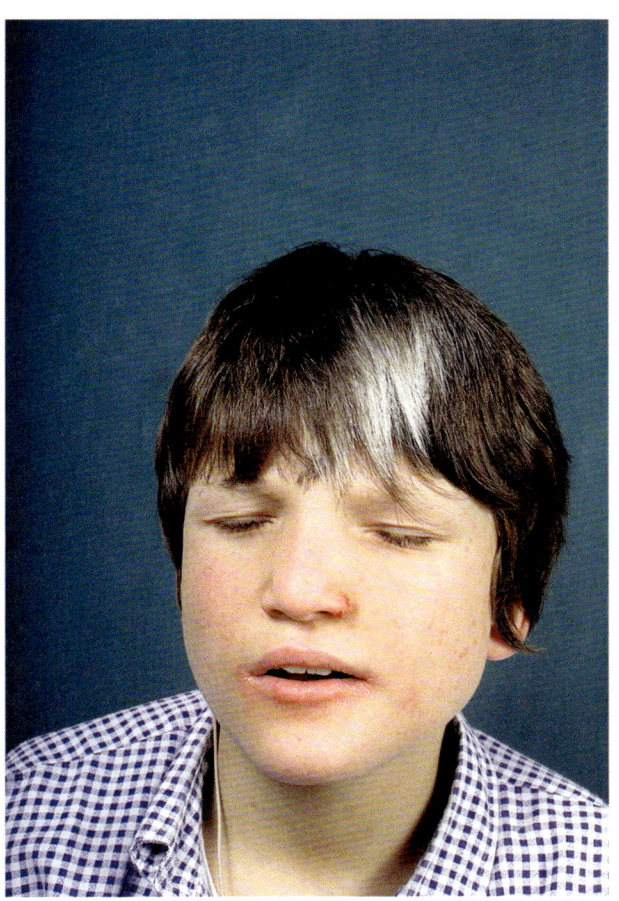

Figure 19.13

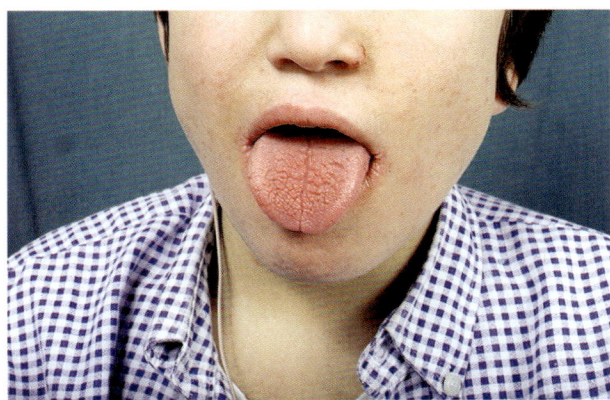

Figure 19.14

Differential diagnosis

- Piebaldism
- Vitiligo
- Isolated white forelock
- True hypomelanosis of Ito
- Isolated 'nevus depigmentosus'
- Mowat–Wilson syndrome: widespread patchy hypopigmented areas, Hirschsprung's disease, severe mental retardation and microcephaly, hypospadias, strikingly upturned earlobes, feeding difficulties. The disease is related to mutation in the zinc finger homeobox B gene

Follow-up and therapy

- Gastroenterological consultations for management of Hirschsprung's disease
- Survey for hearing loss

REFERENCES

Hofstra RM, Osinga J, Tan-Sindunata G, et al. A homozygous mutation in the endothelin-3 gene associated with a combined Waardenburg type 2 and Hirschsprung phenotype (Shah– Waardenburg syndrome). Nature Genet 1996; 12: 445–7

Pingault V, Bondurand N, Kuhlbrodt K, et al. SOX10 mutations in patients with Waardenburg–Hirschsprung disease. Nature Genet 1998; 18: 171–3

Tachibana M, Takeda K, Nobukuni Y, et al. Ectopic expression of NITF, a gene for Waardenburg syndrome type 2, converts fibroblasts to cells with melanocyte characteristics. Nature Genet 1996; 14: 50–4

McCUNE–ALBRIGHT SYNDROME

Synonym

- Polyostotic fibrous dysplasia with café-au-lait spots

Epidemiology

The disease is rare. About 200 cases are reported in the literature.

Age of onset

- At birth or developing progressively during infancy

Clinical findings

- Usually large café-au-lait spots with somewhat dark and different homogeneous pigmentation and irregular borders (Figures 19.15 and 19.16)
- Cutaneous lesions are usually monolateral and distributed in a mosaic pattern
- Trunk and arms are the preferred site; head and face are less frequently involved
- More rarely oral mucosa pigmentation, soft tissue mixomas and epidermal nevi
- Cutaneous lesions are not invariably present

Extracutaneous symptoms

- Pseudocystic long bone fibrous dysplasia ('hockey-stick deformities') with loss of trabeculae that are replaced by fibrous stroma, often homolateral to the cutaneous lesions
- Facial hyperostotic lesions of maxillae, jaws and skull base, often resulting in facial asymmetry in a third of patients (Figure 19.17)
- Precocious puberty and ovarian cysts in females with normal fertility (20–25% of patients)
- Other endocrinopathies (hyperthyroidism (20% of patients), hyperprolactinemia)

Course and complications

- The signs are steady
- Fractures, often multiple and recurrent, of the involved bones (60–70% of patients)
- Malignant transformation of bone cystic–fibrous lesions in fewer than 5% of patients
- Breast cancer reported in a minority of patients
- Rarely mental retardation (secondary to skull development?)

Laboratory findings

- Radiography shows easily the long bone 'polycystic' changes and hyperostotic changes in the maxillofacial region
- Blood tests for hormonal abnormalities

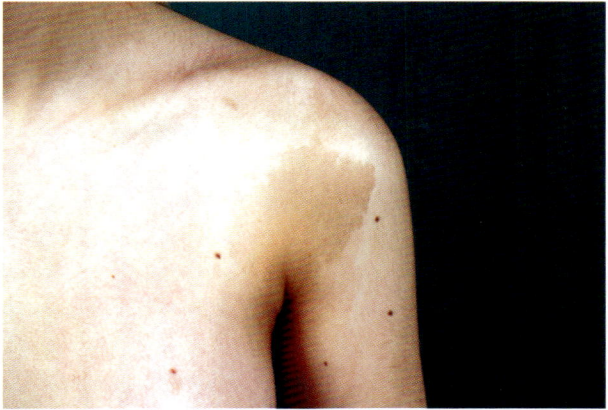

Figure 19.15

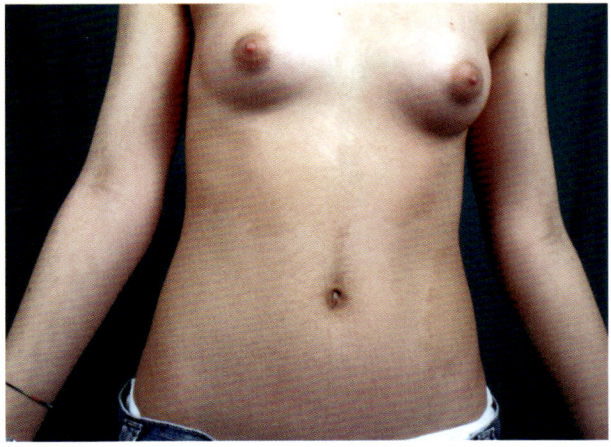

Figure 19.16

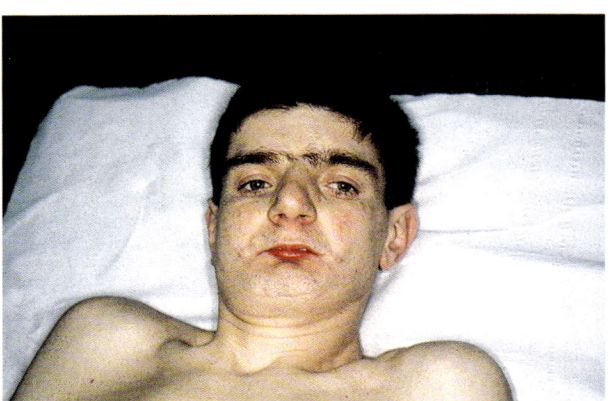

Figure 19.17

Genetics and pathogenesis

In survivors, the condition exists as mosaicism as postulated by Happle in 1985 (postzygotic mutation of an autosomal dominant lethal gene) and confirmed by molecular analysis in 1991 by Weinstein; this paper was the first demonstration of genetic mosaicism causing a mosaic phenotype.

The few familiar cases are due to misdiagnosis (i.e. neurofibromatosis type 1) or may be due to a paradominant inheritance as occurs in Becker's nevus and proteus syndrome.

The related gene is called GNAS1, and encodes the α subunit of the stimulatory G protein that is coupled to two other (β–γ) subunits, forming a signal-transducing protein mediating several hormonal processes (i.e. parathormone) via the activation of adenylate cyclase and synthesis of cyclic adenosine monophosphate (AMP). Mutations of GNAS1 have been found in various percentages of cells in the lesions of involved tissue (mosaic pattern).

GNAS1 is mutated also in progressive osseous heteroplasia of the skin and isolated fibrous dysplasia.

Differential diagnosis

- Neurofibromatosis type 1
- Isolated osseous fibrous dysplasia

Follow-up and therapy

- Osseous lesions may require surgery and/or pain-relieving drugs
- Thyroid metabolism abnormalities require the usual pharmacological or surgical approach

REFERENCES

Pacini F, Perri G, Bagnolesi P, et al. McCune–Albright syndrome with gigantism and hyperprolactinemia. J Endocrinol Invest 1987; 10: 417–20

Stoll C, Alembik Y, Steib JP, De Saint-Martin A. Twelve case with hemihypertrophy: etiology and follow up. Genet Couns 1993; 4: 119–26

LINEAR AND FIGURATED HYPO- AND HYPERPIGMENTED NEVI

Synonyms

- Nevus melanoticus and nevus depigmentosus
- Whorled nevoid hyper-hypomelanosis

Epidemiology

In our experience this condition is not so rare. In a 10-year survey more than 200 cases have been referred to our consultations.

Age of onset

- At birth or during the first months of life

Clinical findings

- Hyperpigmented or hypopigmented lesions, linear, figurated, following the Blaschko lines, arranged sometimes in a vortex-like ('whorled') or checkerboard pattern (Figures 19.18–19.22)
- Lesions may be single or multiple and may involve all of the skin in a fascinating pattern (Figure 19.23)
- Hair may be involved (Figure 19.24)

Extracutaneous symptoms

There are some reports of hyperpigmented nevi with CNS involvement (seizures, mental retardation and autism) and body asymmetry due to osseous abnormalities.

Hypopigmented lesions with associated abnormalities (CNS) are referred to in the literature by the term hypomelanosis of Ito (see above in this chapter).

Course and complications

The lesions may fade with age but usually remain unchanged.

Laboratory findings

- Karyotyping is recommended in all patients bearing this anomaly
- Histological examination shows little change in melanocyte number and pigment distribution
- Ultrastructure is not diagnostic

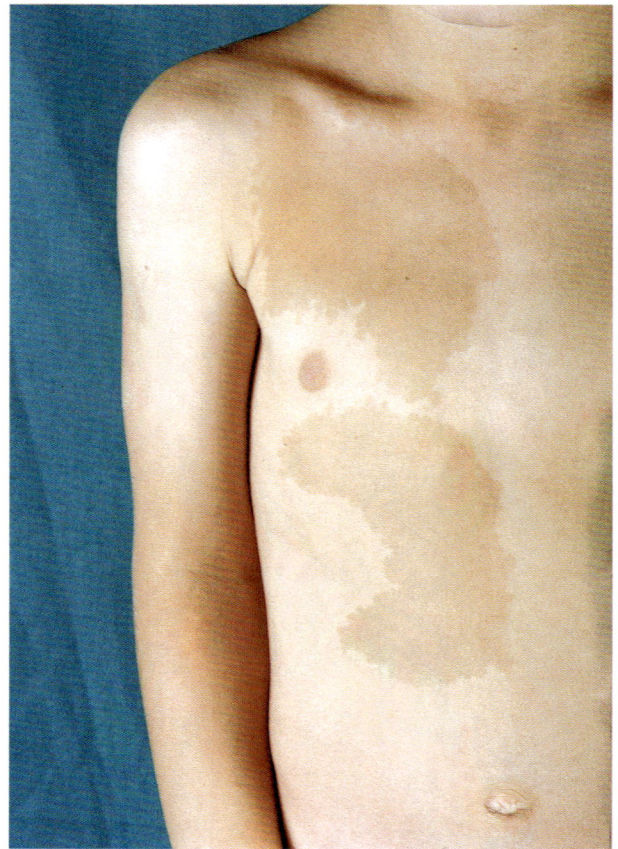

Figure 19.18

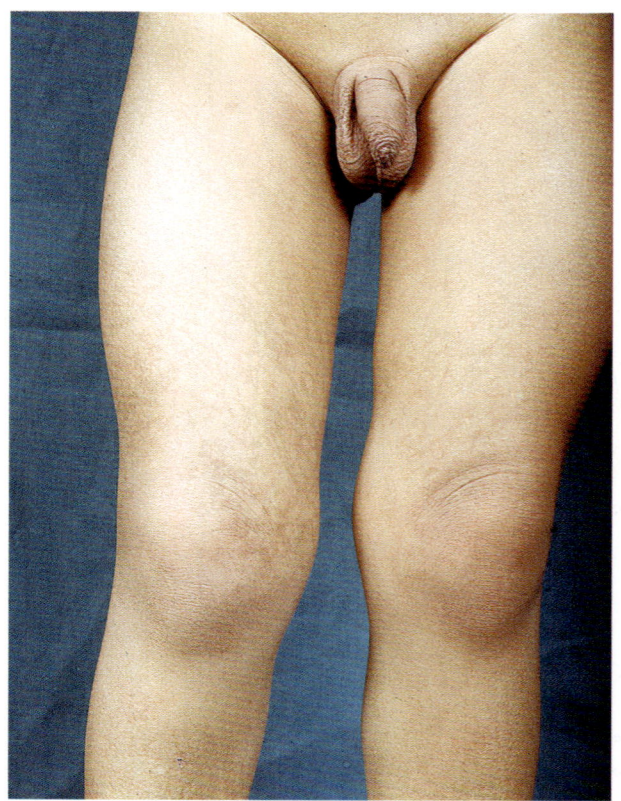

Figure 19.19

Disorders of pigmentation   287

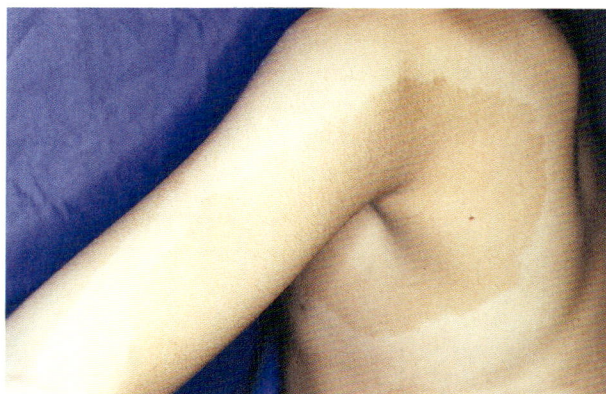

Figure 19.20

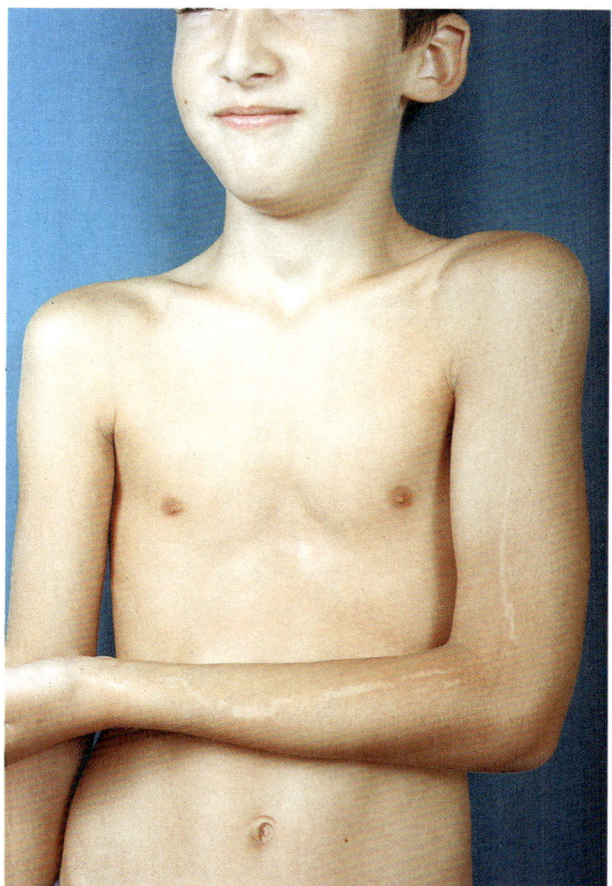

Figure 19.22

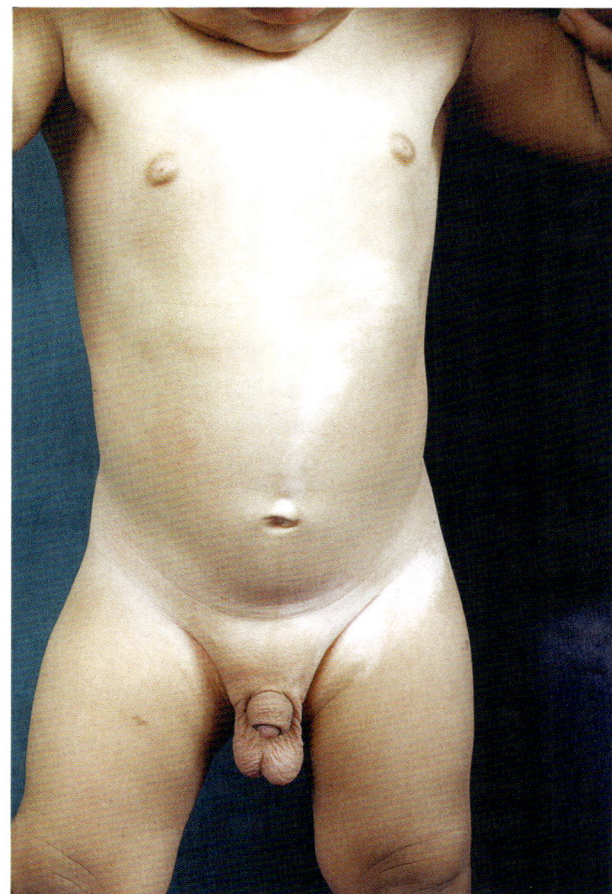

Figure 19.21

- Leaf-shaped pigmented changes referred to by Happle as the 'phylloid' mosaic distribution pattern (see Chapter 25), which seems to be related to anomalies of chromosome 13
- In patients with **MELAS syndrome** (mitochondrial myopathy, encephalopathy, lactic acidosis and stroke-like episodes) due to mutation in the mitochondrial DNA, linear hyperpigmented nevi (Figure 19.25 and 19.26) are frequently a marker of the disease

Whether pigmentation abnormalities distributed along the Blaschko lines are related to a specific anomaly of embryological development of melanocytes, or are due to keratinocyte anomalies that influence melanocyte distribution during embryogenesis, remains to be elucidated.

Genetics and pathogenesis

- Mosaic condition due to postzygotic mutations
- In many patients different chromosomal abnormalities have been found in both hyper- and hypopigmented conditions

Differential diagnosis

- Incontinentia pigmenti (late phases)
- Epidermal nevi (onset phases)
- Lichen striatus (late phases)

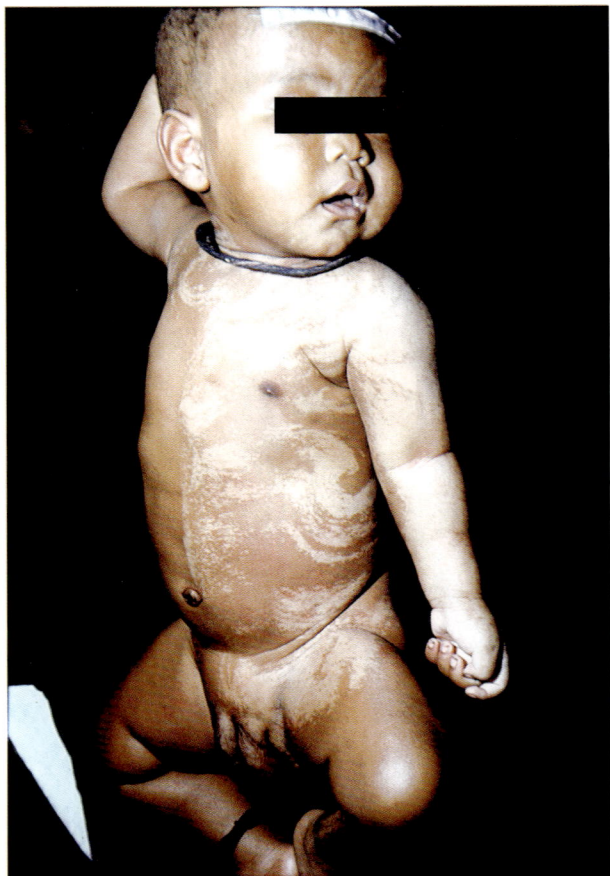

Figure 19.23

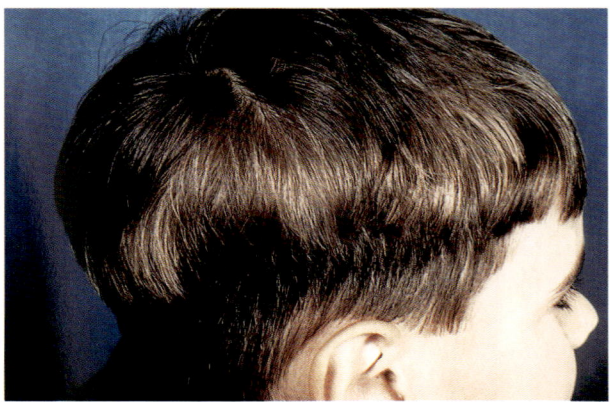

Figure 19.24

Follow-up and therapy

- Pediatric evaluation to find associated neurologic abnormalities

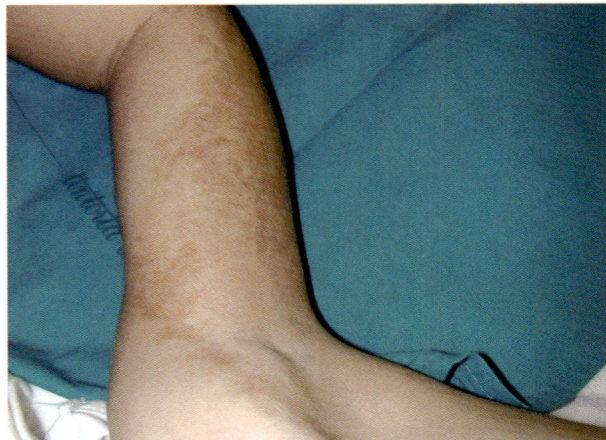

Figure 19.25

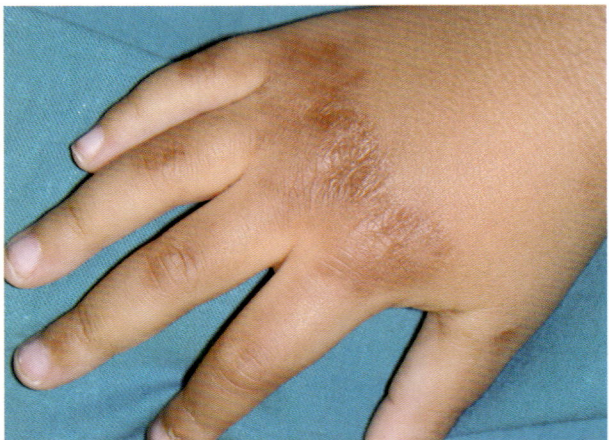

Figure 19.26

REFERENCES

Nehal KS, PeBenito R, Orlow SJ. Anaysis of 54 cases of hypopigmentation and hyperpigmentation along the lines of Blaschko. Arch Dermatol 1996; 132: 1167–70

Verghese S, Newlin A, Miller M, Burton BK. Mosaic trisomy 7 in a patient with pigmentary abnormalities. Am J Med Genet 1999; 87: 371–4

SEGMENTAL LENTIGINOSIS

Synonym

- Lentiginous nevus

Age of onset

- Rarely at birth
- Usually within school age after UV exposure

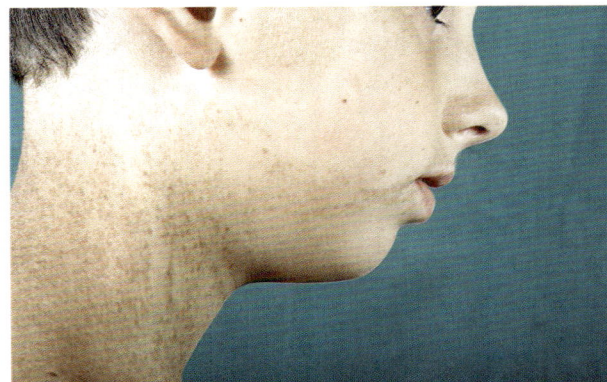

Figure 19.27

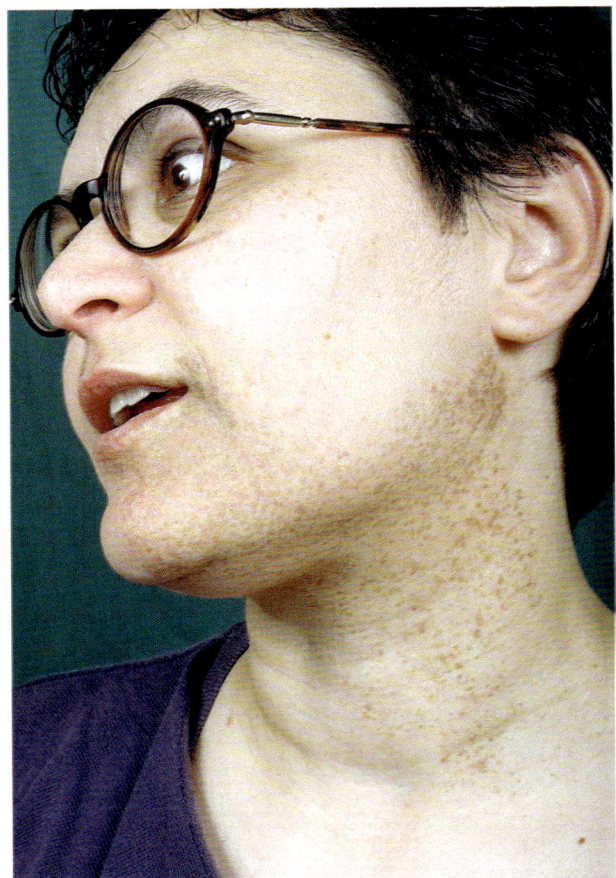

Figure 19.28

Epidemiology

Considered to be rare, we think that the disease is underestimated.

Clinical findings

- Lentigines (pinpoint to small pigmented macules) in a mosaic pattern (checkerboard) located especially in the upper part of the body (Figures 19.27–19.29) with or without intermingled café-au-lait spots (Figure 19.30)
- True melanocytic nevi may be scattered in association with segmental lentiginosis (Figure 19.31)
- Association with speckled lentiginous nevus with histological 'lentigo' pattern (Figures 19.32 and 19.33, same patient)
- Association with classic neurofibromatosis type 1 (NF1) or twin-spot with segmental NF1 (Figure 19.34)

Extracutaneous findings

There is rarely osseous and CNS involvement, configuring a segmental lentiginosis–neurocutaneous syndrome.

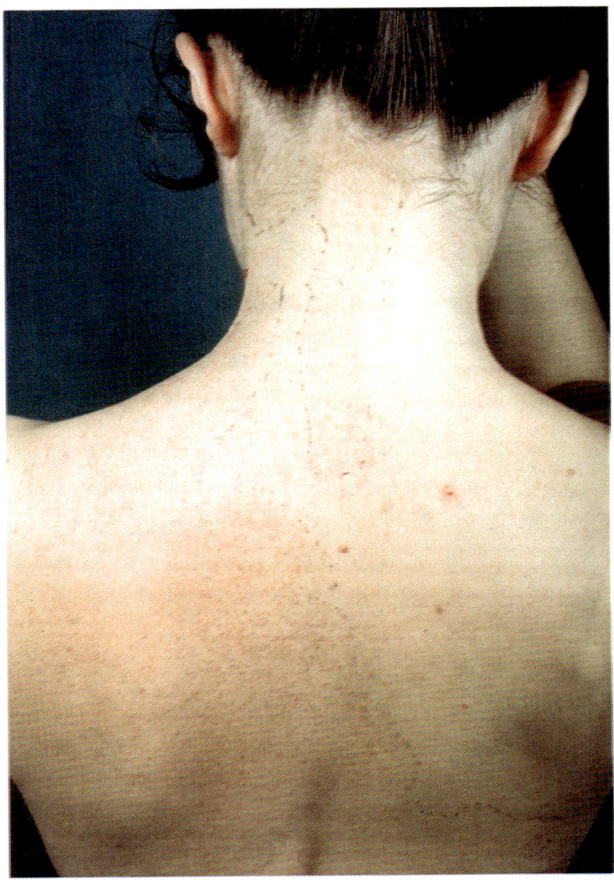

Figure 19.29

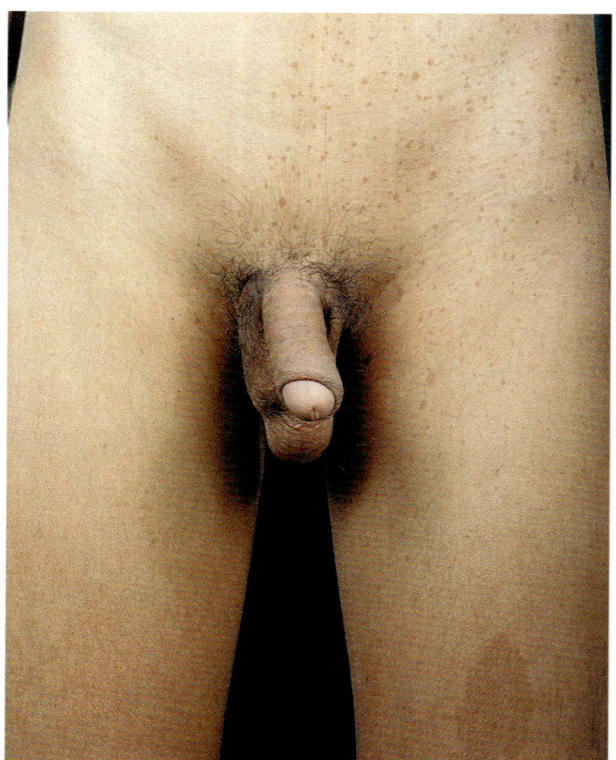

Figure 19.30

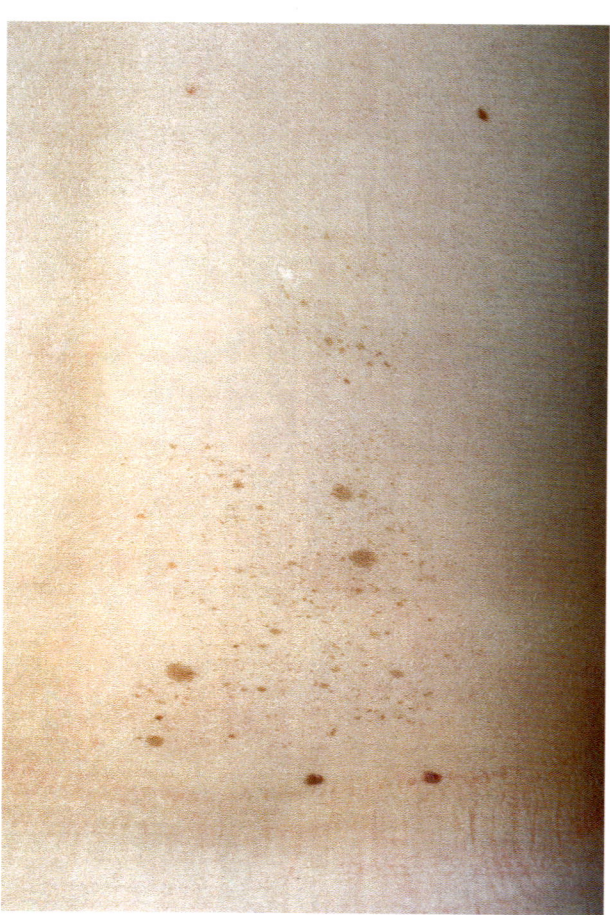

Figure 19.31

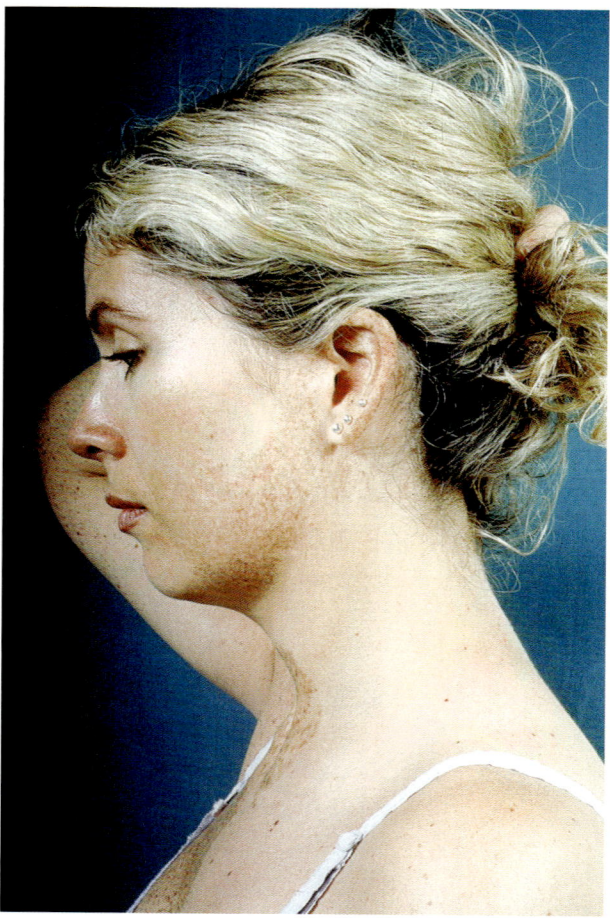

Figure 19.32

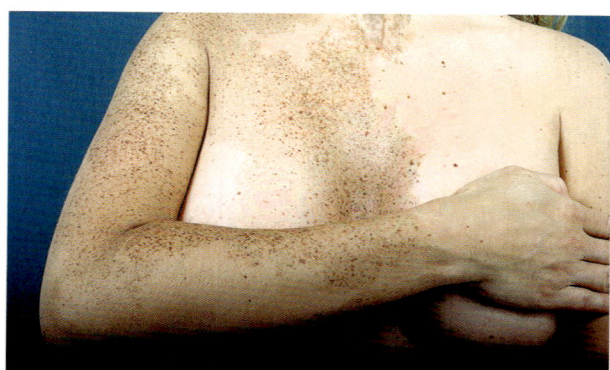

Figure 19.33

Course and prognosis

The disease is modified directly by UV exposure.

Genetics and pathogenesis

- Sporadic cases and rare paradominant inheritance
- Distinction between true lentiginous mosaicism, speckled lentiginous nevus and mosaic forms of NF1 is still to be explained and elucidated by molecular analysis

- It must be remembered that diffuse 'non-syndromic' lentiginosis is possible (Figures 19.35 and 19.36)

Follow-up and therapy

- Detection of associated abnormalities
- Epidiascopy
- UV protection

Differential diagnosis

- Neurofibromatosis type 1
- Speckled lentiginous nevus
- Syndromic lentiginoses (Carney's complex, LEOPARD syndrome, Peutz–Jeghers syndrome)

REFERENCES

Allegue F, Espana A, Fernandez-Garcia JM, Ledo A. Segmental neurofibromatosis with contralateral lentiginosis. Clin Exp Dermatol 1989; 14: 448–50

Lee WS, Yoo MS, Ahn SK, Won JH. Partial unilateral lentiginosis associated with segmental neurofibromatosis. J Dermatol 1995; 22: 958–9

Marchesi L, Naldi L, Di Landro A, et al. Segmental lentiginosis with 'jentigo' histologic pattern. Am J Dermatopathol 1992; 14: 323–7

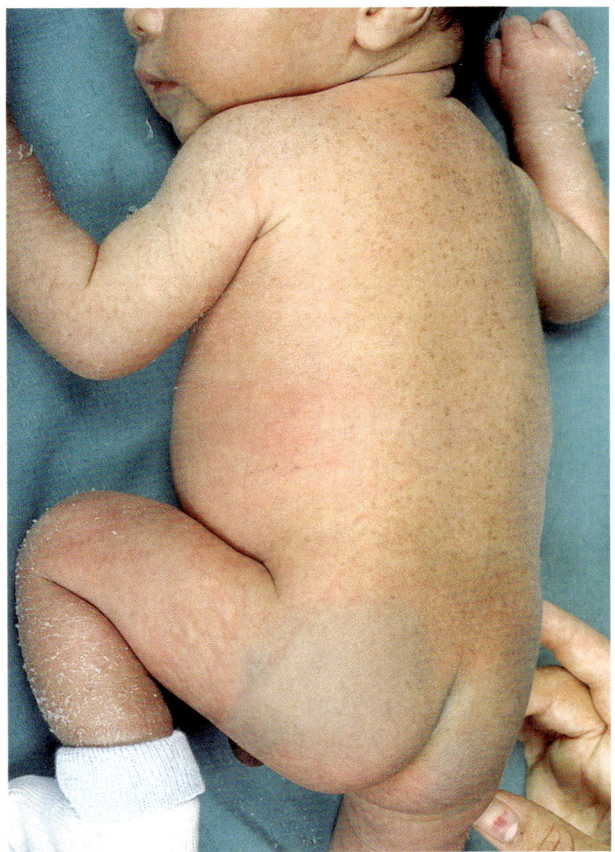

Figure 19.35

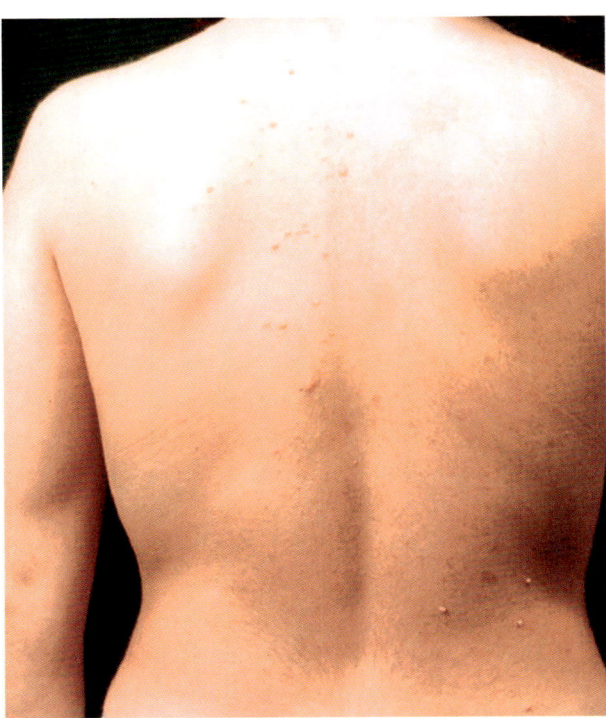

Figure 19.34

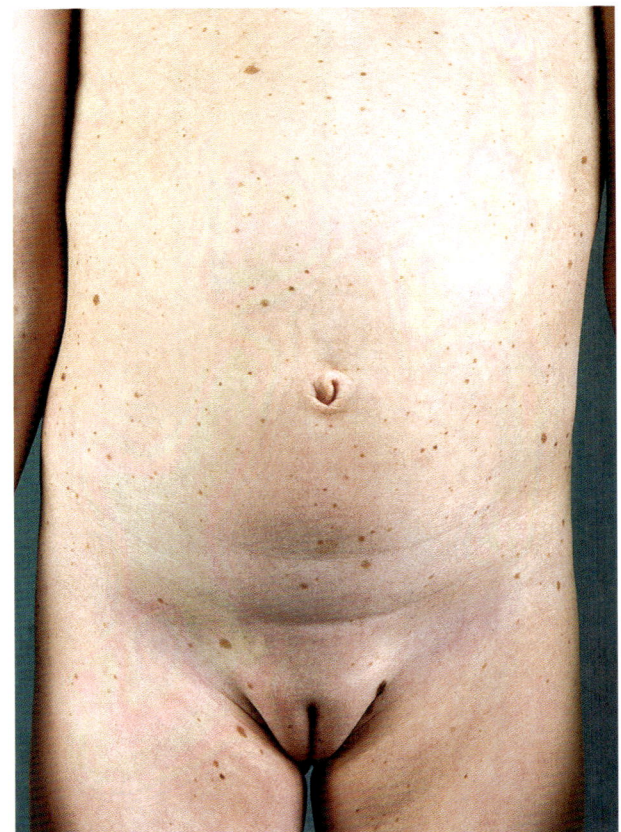

Figure 19.36

LEOPARD SYNDROME

Synonym

- **L**entigines, **E**chocardiographic abnormalities, **O**cular hypertelorism, **P**ulmonary stenosis, **A**bnormal genitalia, **R**etarded growth, **D**eafness

Epidemiology

This disease is very rare; no further data are available.

Age of onset

- Rarely at birth, progressive eruption during first year of life

Clinical findings

- Progressive eruption of lentigines on the upper part of the body surface, especially face and neck (Figures 19.37 and 19.38)
- Palms and soles and genitalia may be involved (Figure 19.39)
- Dark-brown large macules intermingled with lentigines in upper trunk (Figure 19.40)

Extracutaneous symptoms

- Hypertelorism, associated with epicanthus, ptosis and, less frequently, irideal dyspigmentation
- Abnormalities of heart conduction and severe arrhythmias
- Stenosis of pulmonary artery and aorta (15% of patients)
- Cryptorchidism, hypospadias, delayed puberty for both sexes and decreased fertility
- Psychomotor and somatic retardation
- Scoliosis, pectus carinatus
- Sensorineural deafness in 20% of patients

Course and complications

- Pigmented lesion number progresses with age
- Severe arrhythmias may be life-threatening

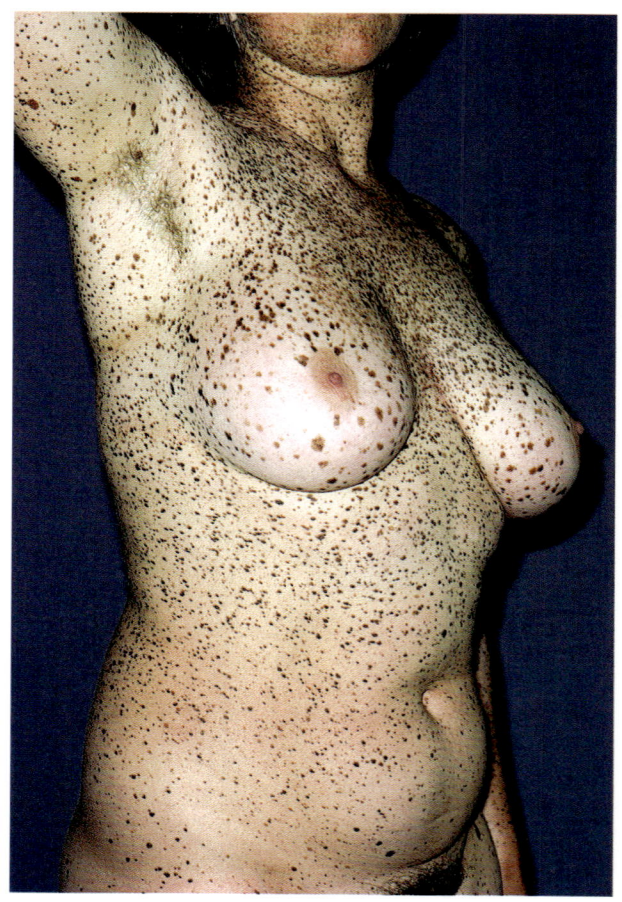

Figure 19.38

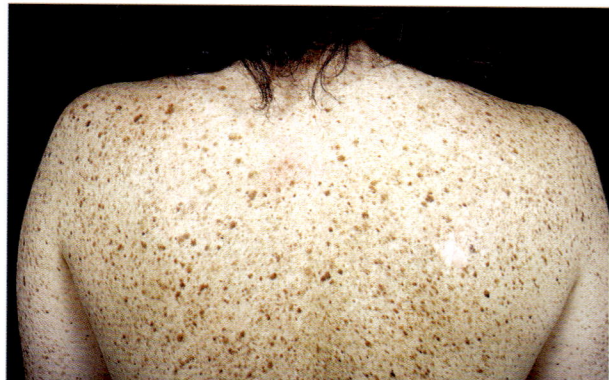

Figure 19.37

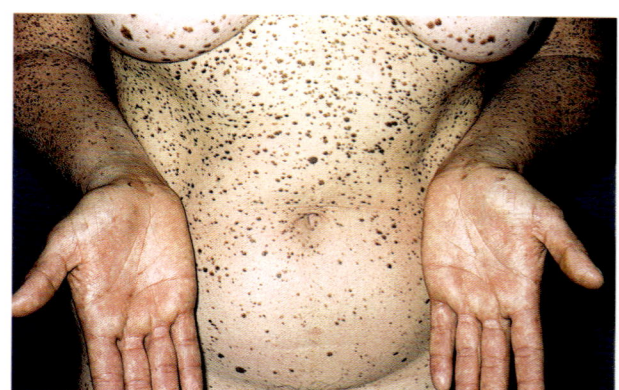

Figure 19.39

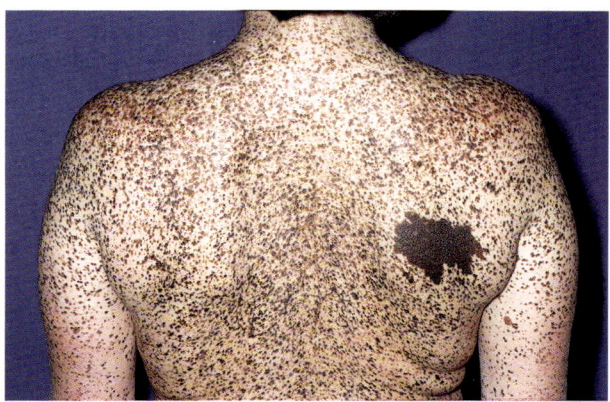

Figure 19.40

Laboratory findings

There is an increased number of melanocytes and of macromelanosomes.

Genetics and pathogenesis

- Autosomal dominant
- The responsible gene is PTPN11, also involved in the pathogenesis of Noonan syndrome
- Variable expression of the disease within the same pedigree

Differential diagnosis

- Carney's complex
- Peutz–Jeghers syndrome
- Centrofacial lentiginosis, isolated or with psychomotor anomalies
- Isolated autosomal dominant lentiginosis
- Watson's syndrome (NF1 and pulmonary artery stenosis)
- Mosaic lentiginoses
- Phakomatosis pigmentovascularis
- Noonan's syndrome

Follow-up and therapy

- Cardiological evaluation and prevention of arrhythmias
- Endocrinological survey for delayed puberty and couple fertility

REFERENCES

Jozwiak S, Schwartz RA, Janniger CK, Zaremba J. Familial occurrence of the LEOPARD syndrome. Int J Dermatol 1998; 37: 48–51

Legius E, Schrander-Stumpel C, Schollen E, et al. PTPN11 mutations in LEOPARD syndrome. J Med Genet 2002; 39: 571–4

Petter G, Rytter M, Haustein UF. [Multiple lentigines (LEOPARD) syndrome. Case reports and review of the literature.] Hautarzt 2002; 53: 403–8

OTA NEVUS

Epidemiology

Asian and Central American native populations are preferentially involved. Ota nevus is less frequently reported in Caucasians.

Age of onset

- Lesions may be visible at birth or later in childhood, or at puberty

Clinical findings

Typical bluish or matt greenish lesions are preferentially distributed on the frontal and temporal areas of the face following a checkerboard pattern with irregular or even polycyclic borders (Figures 19.41 and 19.42).

Extracutaneous symptoms

- Sclera and conjunctiva are characteristically involved, with blue-blackish discoloration
- Rarely, oral and nasal mucosae may be involved as well as external ears and upper digestive and respiratory tracts
- CNS abnormalities may be associated (10%)

Course and prognosis

Rare cases of melanomas arising from ota nevus are reported.

Laboratory findings

Upon histologic examination, dendritic melanocytes are found intermingled between fibroblasts in the lower dermis.

Genetics and pathogenesis

The mosaic lesions are due to postzygotic mutation.

Follow-up and therapy

- Ophthalmological consultations
- Prevention of risk of melanoma

Differential diagnosis

- Melanocytic nevus
- Speckled lentiginous nevus (early phases)
- Epidermal–sebaceous nevus (early phases)

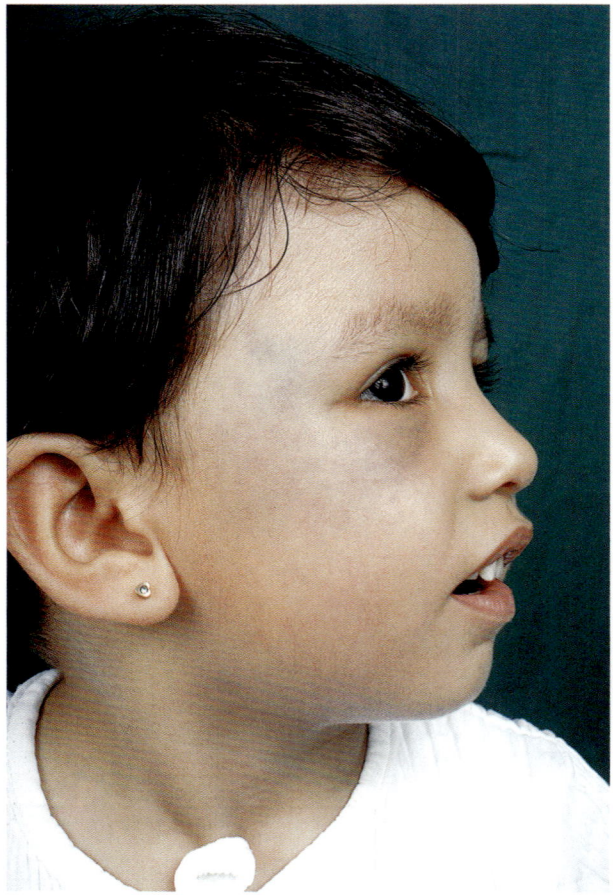

Figure 19.41

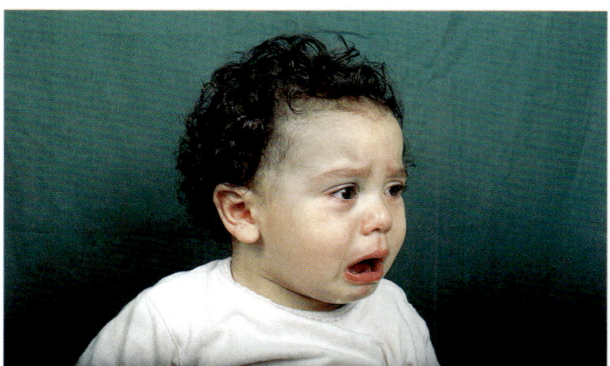

Figure 19.42

REFERENCES

Baroody M, Holds JB. Extensive locoregional malignant melanoma transformation in a patient with oculodermal melanocytosis. Plast Reconstr Surg 2004; 113: 317–22

Kono T, Ercocen AR, Kikuchi Y, et al. A giant melanocytic nevus treated with combined use of normal mode ruby laser and Q-switched alexandrite laser. J Dermatol 2003; 30: 538–42

Ruiz-Villaverde R, Blasco Melguizo J, Buendia Eisman Am Serrano Ortega S. Bilateral ota naevus. J Eur Acad Dermatol Venereol 2003; 17: 437–9

CUTIS TRICOLOR

Epidemiology

Three patients are described in the literature with the complete spectrum of the syndrome.

Age of onset

- At birth

Clinical findings

- Combination of paired hypo- and hyperpigmented lesions arranged in streaks following mosaic distribution with a background of normal skin (Figure 19.43)
- Bushy eyebrows
- Cutaneous abnormalities alone may be present

Extracutaneous symptoms

- Facial asymmetries with dolichocephaly
- Hypoplasia of corpus callosum
- Seizures with electroencephalogram anomalies
- Mental retardation and behavioral disturbances
- Scoliosis and vertebral abnormalities (Figure 19.44)
- Tibial bowing

Course and prognosis

The life span may be reduced owing to the severe associated anomalies.

Laboratory findings

Cytogenetic abnormalities are absent.

Genetics and pathogenesis

This is a further example of the 'twin-spotting' phenomenon due to loss of heterozygosity and somatic recombination during late embryogenesis. The earlier the mutation during embryogenesis, the wider is the involvement of the skin, central nervous system and other structures, and, in contrast, later postzygotic mutations generate only skin involvement.

Follow-up and therapy

- Neurologic and psychiatric supervision for epilepsy and behavioral abnormalities
- Orthopedic devices or surgery for severe scoliosis

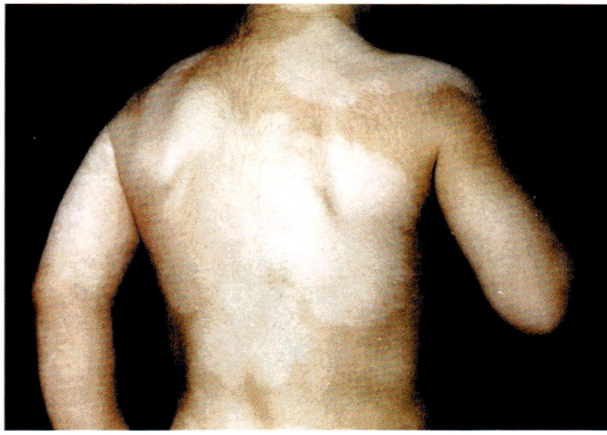

Figure 19.43

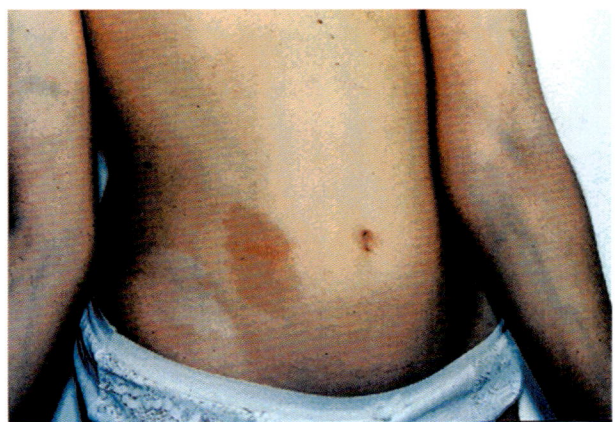

Figure 19.44

Differential diagnosis

- Phakomatosis pigmentovascularis
- Phakomatosis pigmentokeratotica

REFERENCES

Baba M, Seckin D, Akcali C, Happle R. Familial cutis tricolor: a possible example of paradominant inheritance. Eur J Dermatol 2003; 13: 343–5

Ruggieri M, Iannetti P, Pavone L. Delineation of a newly recognized neurocutaneous malformation syndrome with 'cutis tricolor'. Am J Med Genet 2003; 120A: 110–16

Ruggieri M. Cutis tricolor: congenital hyper- and hypopigmented lesions in a background of normal skin with and without associated systemic features: further expansion of the phenotype. Eur J Pediatr 2000; 159: 745–9

DYSCHROMATOSIS SYMMETRICA HEREDITARIA

Synonym

- Acropigmentation symmetrica of Dohi

Epidemiology

The disease is rare, with less than ten families reported in Japanese literature and some sporadic cases in other ethnic groups.

Age of onset

- During childhood

Clinical findings

- Presence of hypo- and hyper-pigmented macules on the dorsal aspects of hands and feet (Figures 19.45 and 19.46)

Extracutaneous findings

- None

Course and prognosis

- The disease is slowly progressive without complications

Laboratory findings

- None specific

Genetics and pathogenesis

- The disease is autosomal dominant
- Mutations of a gene (DSRAD), coding for a double-stranded RNA-specific adenosine deaminase, (one of the RNA-editing enzymes) have been detected in these pedigrees
- The gene may be involved in the migration of melanoblasts from the neural crest to the skin, explaining that the extremities may receive different amount of melanoblasts compared to the other sites of the body. A second speculation may involve a temperature-sensitive mechanism as occurs in OCA4

Follow-up and therapy

- Photoprotection

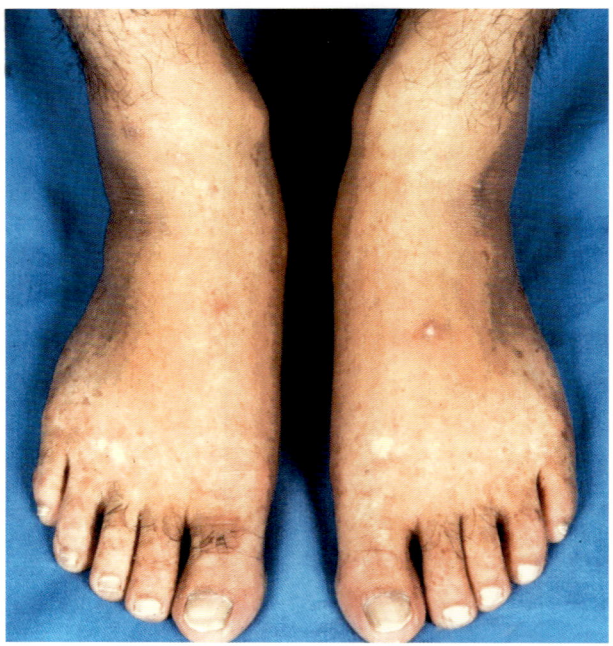

Figure 19.45

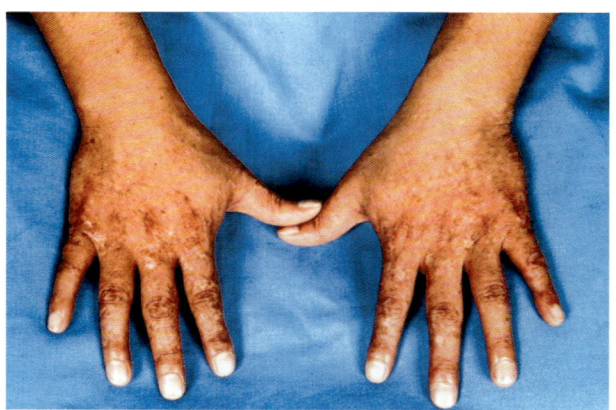

Figure 19.46

Differential diagnosis

- Kitamura disease
- Vitiligo
- Post-lesional pigmentations (burns, sunburns, etc.)

REFERENCES

Suzuki N, Suzuki T, Inagaki K, et al. Mutation analysis of the ADAR1 gene in dyschromatosis symmetrica hereditaria and genetic differentiation from both dyschromatosis universalis hereditaria and acropigmentatio reticularis. J Invest Dermatol 2005; 124: 1186–92

Tomita Y, Suzuki T. Genetics of pigmentary disorders. Am J Med Genet C Semin Med Genet 2004; 131C: 75–81 [Review]

CHAPTER 20

Vascular disorders

COMPLEX OF STURGE–PARKES–WEBER, KLIPPEL–TRÉNAUNAY AND COBB'S SYNDROMES

Definition

Formerly considered as separate entities, these three syndromes have proved to be the same disorder, differentiated only by the sites of involvement of the skin (port-wine stains), subcutaneous tissues and central nervous system (CNS). In fact, in many subjects, all three syndromes may be present simultaneously (Figures 20.1 and 20.2, same patient).

They are mosaic diseases (autosomal dominant disorders surviving by mosaicism) and are distributed following a checkerboard pattern (Figure 20.3) and not, as always reported, following the territories of sensory peripheral innervation. Paradominant inheritance has been demonstrated in some families. Only for didactic reasons are they treated separately here.

STURGE–WEBER SYNDROME

Synonym

- Encephalotrigeminal angiomatosis

Epidemiology

No data are available.

Age of onset

- At birth

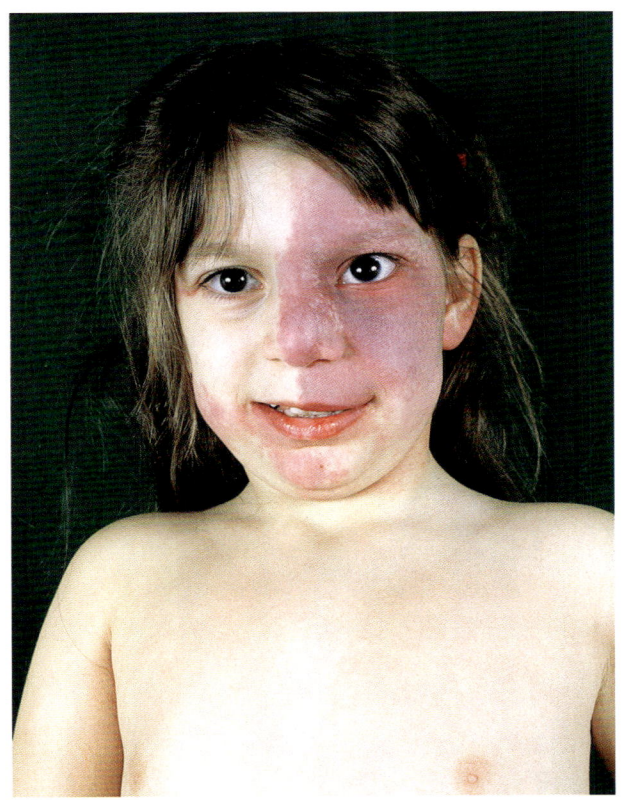

Figure 20.1

Clinical findings

- Port-wine stains (PWS) on the face, distributed in a checkerboard mosaic pattern ('stop at midline') (Figure 20.4)
- PWS are usually unilateral but may be bilateral on the face or involve other areas of the body (neck, trunk) (Figures 20.5 and 20.6)

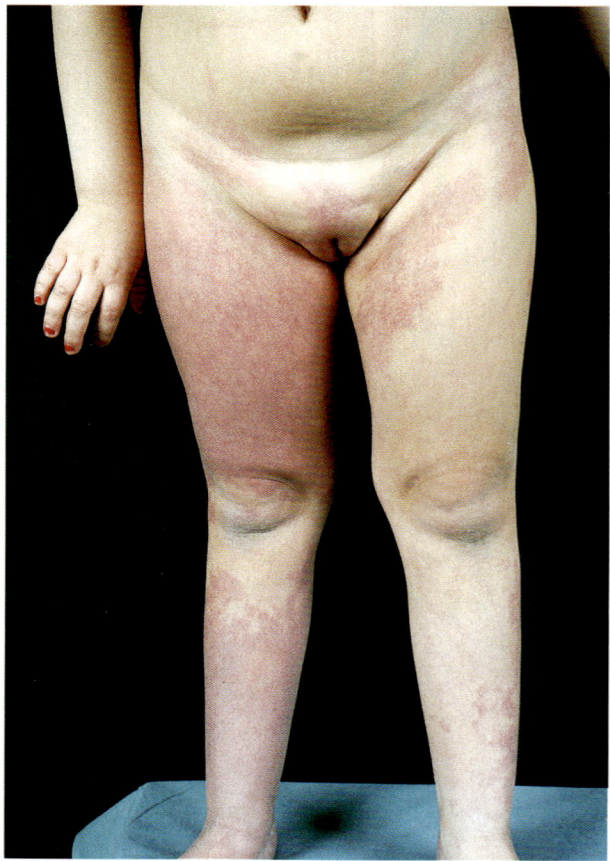

Figure 20.2

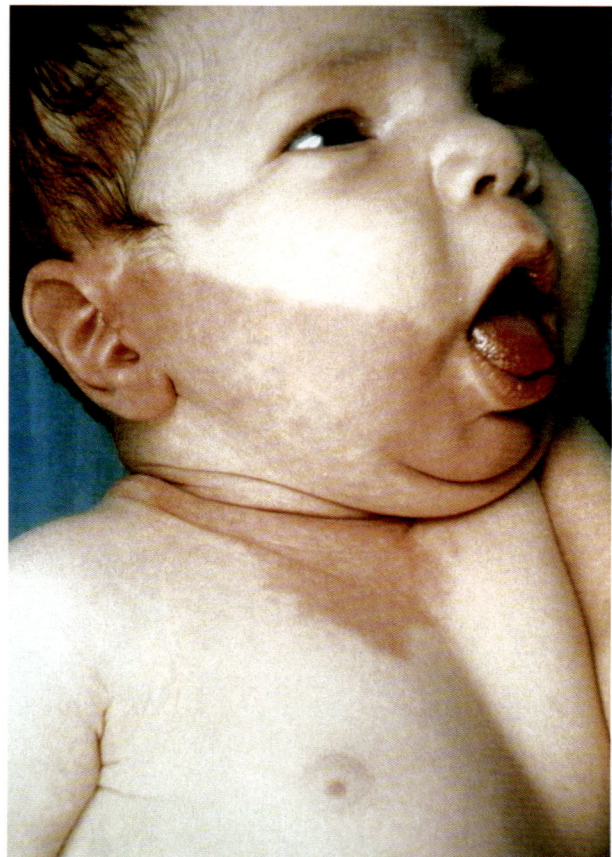

Figure 20.3

- Less frequently there is oral mucosa involvement with angiomas on tongue, gingivae and lips (Figure 20.7)

Extracutaneous findings

- Ipsilateral vascular malformation of the meninges and brain calcifications with epilepsy and hemiplegia
- Mental retardation
- The eye may be involved 'in toto' (conjunctiva and iris, choroid and retina), resulting in congenital glaucoma and major retinal abnormalities leading progressively to blindness
- Facial and body asymmetry

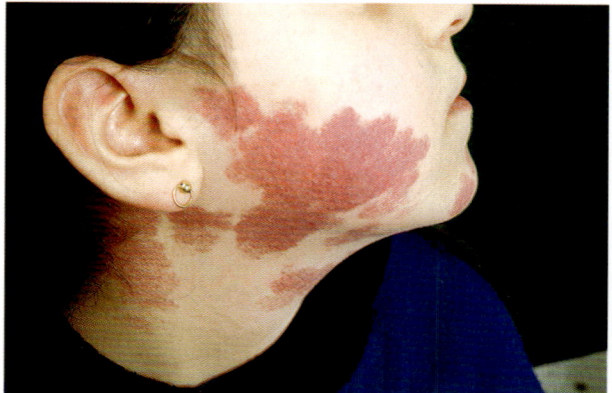

Figure 20.4

Course and complications

The prognosis is directly linked to the severity of CNS involvement. Strokes are rare.

Laboratory findings

Angiomagnetic resonance imaging (MRI) reveals early cerebral calcification and the extent of vascular intracranial lesions.

Genetics and pathogenesis

- Sporadic, paradominant inheritance possible
- Distribution of the lesions evokes mosaic pattern of distribution and postzygotic mutation
- The disease is an example of 'disease surviving by mosaicism'
- Recently, the gene for Parkes–Weber syndrome was located to chromosome 5, CMC1 locus, which

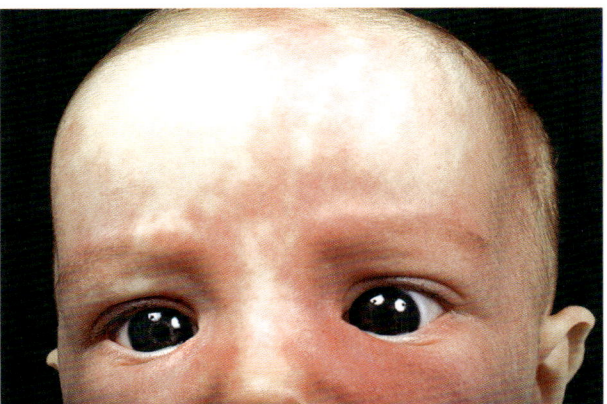

Figure 20.5

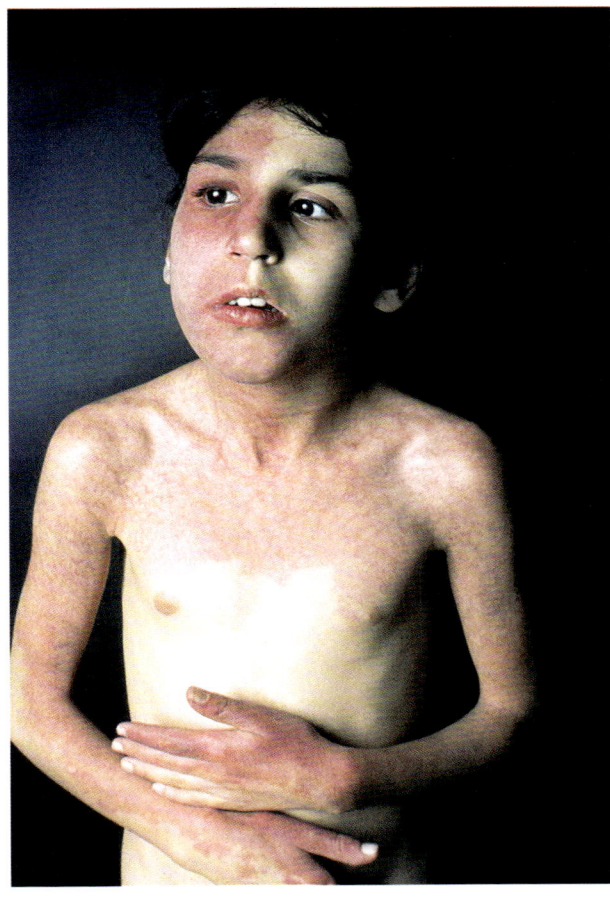

Figure 20.6

is the same locus as for familial port-wine stains and hereditary benign teliangiectasia

Differential diagnosis

- Central facial PWS without CNS involvement
- Overlap with Klippel–Trénaunay syndrome when PWS are diffuse

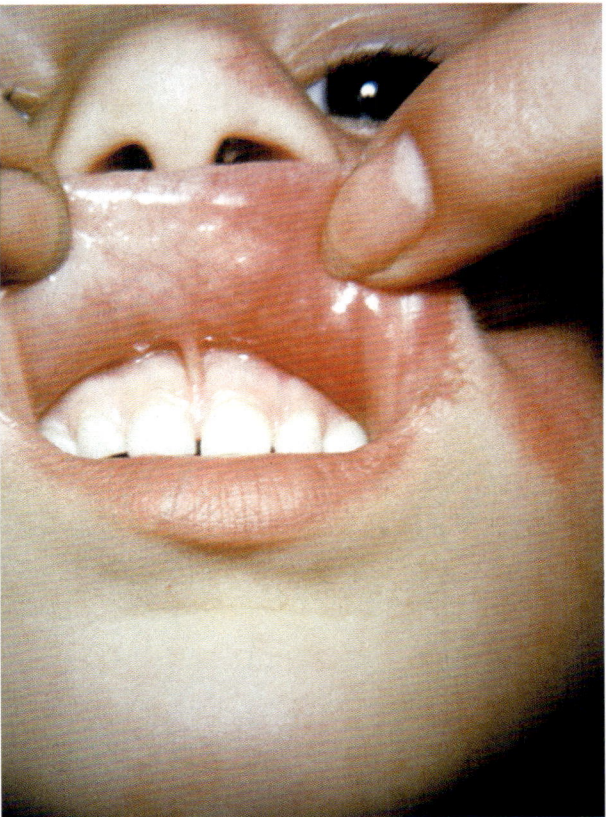

Figure 20.7

Follow-up and therapy

- Angio-MRI is mandatory for the evaluation of CNS damage
- Ophthalmologist can detect early glaucoma and retinal malformation
- Therapy for seizures to avoid progressive mental retardation

REFERENCES

Eerola I, Boon LM, Mulliken JB, et al. Capillary malformation–arteriovenous malformation, a new clinical and genetic disorder caused by RASA1 mutations. Am J Hum Genet 2003; 73: 1240–9

Happel R. Sturge–Weber–Klippel–Trenaunay syndrome: what's in a name? Eur J Dermatol 2003; 13: 223

Vissers W, Van Steensel M. Steijlen P, et al. Klippel–Trenaunay sydnrome and Sturge–Weber syndrome: variations on a theme? Eur J Dermatol 2003; 13: 238–41

KLIPPEL–TRÉNAUNAY SYNDROME

Synonym

- Klippel–Trénaunay–Parkes–Weber syndrome

Epidemiology

The disease is rare; there are no further data available.

Age of onset

- At birth

Clinical findings

- Usually unilateral and extensive port-wine stains, especially on lower legs and less frequently arms and trunk and bilaterally (Figures 20.8 and 20.9)
- Venous and lymphatic malformations, usually associated with hypertrophy of soft tissues (and underlying bones) with leg asymmetry visible at birth (Figure 20.10)
- Diffuse angiokeratomas referred to as 'frog-spawn' appearance
- Lymphangiomas
- Stasis dermatitis

Extracutaneous findings

- As stated above, soft tissue and underlying bone hypertrophy is common
- Arteriovenous fistulae

Course and complications

- The disease is slowly progressive and vascular abnormalities may lead to phlebitis, thrombosis and ulcerations that become chronic

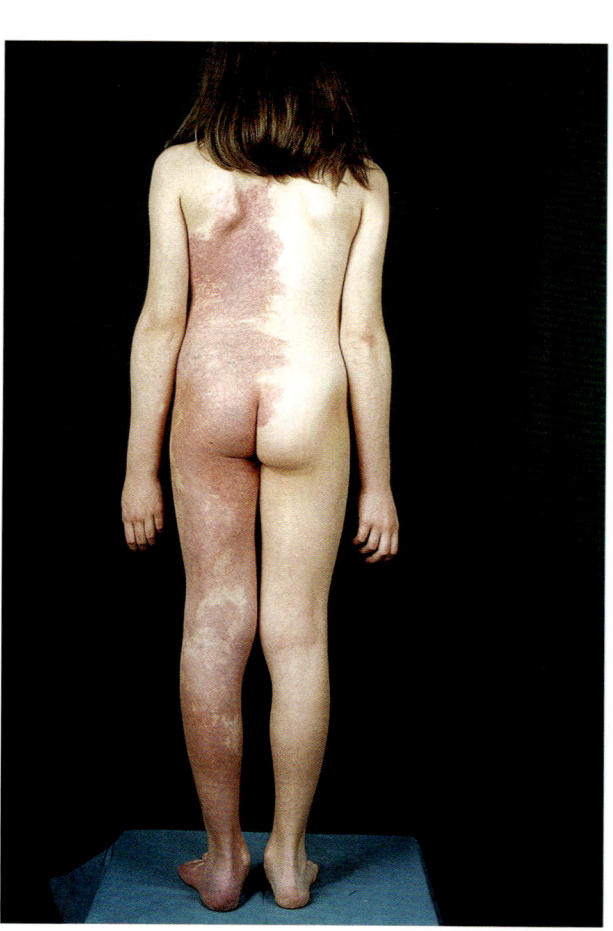

Figure 20.8

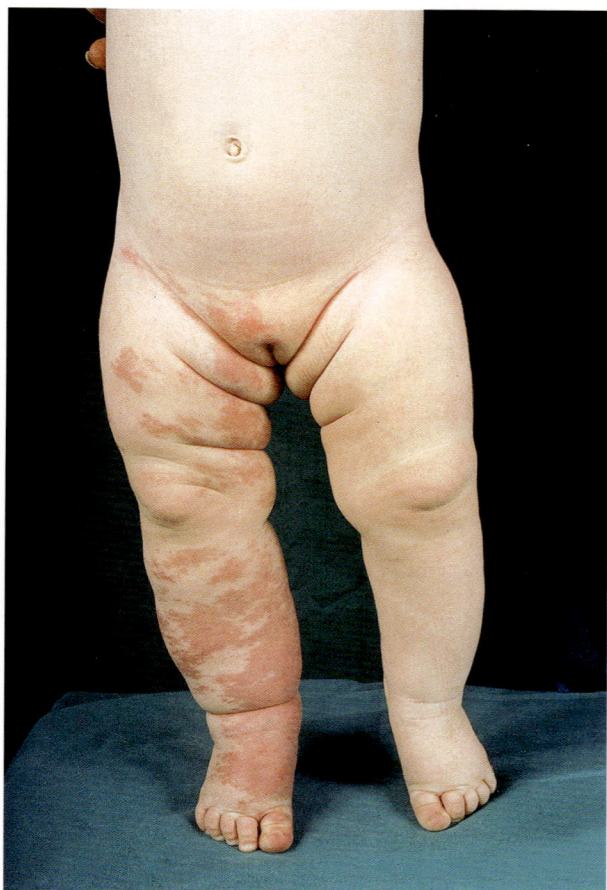

Figure 20.9

Vascular disorders

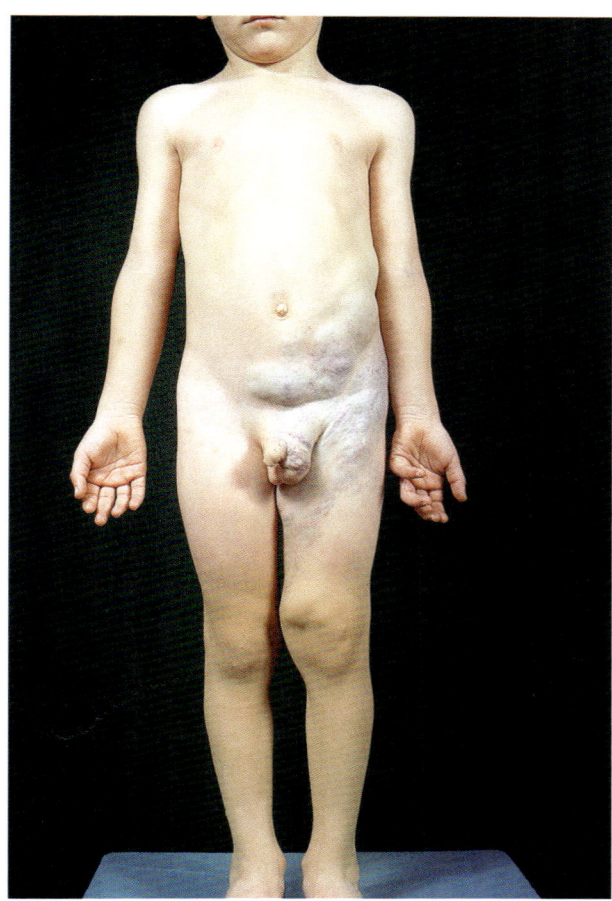

Figure 20.10

- Lymphedema worsens with age
- Walking impairment after puberty is common owing to severe asymmetry of the legs

Laboratory findings

Angio-MRI is used to assess the severity of venous and lymphatic malformations and arteriovenous fistulae.

Genetics and pathogenesis

- Sporadic, paradominant inheritance in some pedigrees
- The gene for the complex is on the CMC1 locus on chromosome 5
- Unilateral involvement argues for a mosaic form due to postzygotic mutation
- Disease surviving in the mosaic form
- The dominant generalized form of this type of disease is incompatible with life, leading to abortion

Differential diagnosis

- Overlap with Sturge–Weber syndrome
- Proteus syndrome
- Beckwith–Wiedemann syndrome

Follow-up and therapy

- Surgical approach to major vascular abnormalities
- Prevention of phlebitis, thrombosis and ulcerations

REFERENCES

Happle R. Sturge–Weber–Klippel–Trenaunay syndrome: what's in a name? Eur J Dermatol 2003; 13: 223

Tian XL, Kadaba R, You SA, et al. Identification of an angiogenic factor that when mutated causes susceptibility to Klippel–Trenaunay syndrome. Nature (London) 2004; 427: 640–5

Vissers W, Van Steensel M, Steijlen P, et al. Klippel–Trenaunay syndrome and Sturge–Weber syndrome: variations on a theme? Eur J Dermatol 2003; 13: 223

COBB'S SYNDROME

Synonym

- Cutaneomeningeal angiomatosis

Epidemiology

The disease is very rare, with no more than 50 cases published.

Age of onset

- At birth

Clinical findings

- PWS overlying spinal defects almost totally located in lumbar region (Figures 20.11 and 20.12)
- Rarely PWS in other areas

Extracutaneous findings

- Spinal septal malformations and angiomatosis
- Meningeal angiomatosis
- Hemiplegia or paraplegia due to vascular malformation defects

Course and prognosis

The course of the disease is directly related to the severity of vascular spinal defects.

Laboratory findings

Angio-MRI provides a tool for both prognosis and therapy.

Genetics and pathogenesis

- Sporadic
- Probably linked to the same locus, CMC1

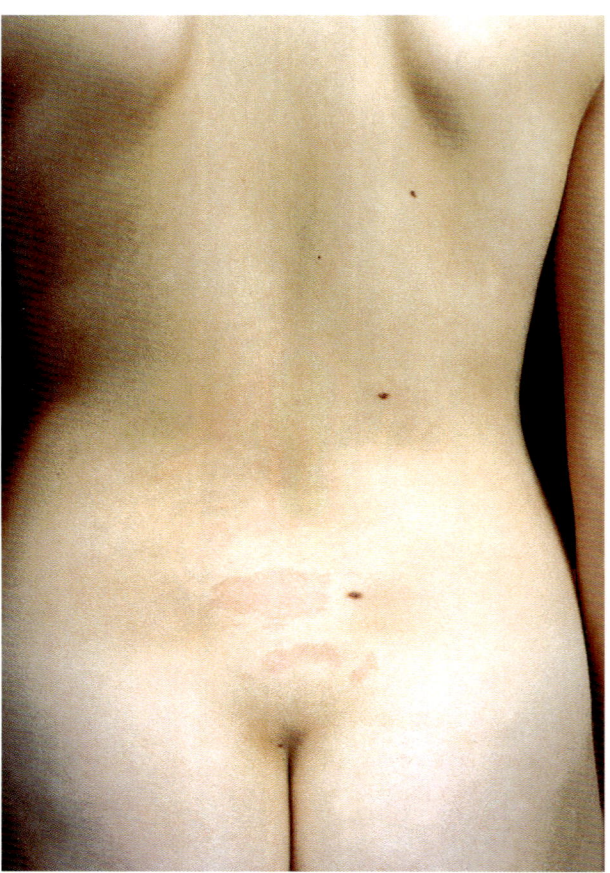

Figure 20.11

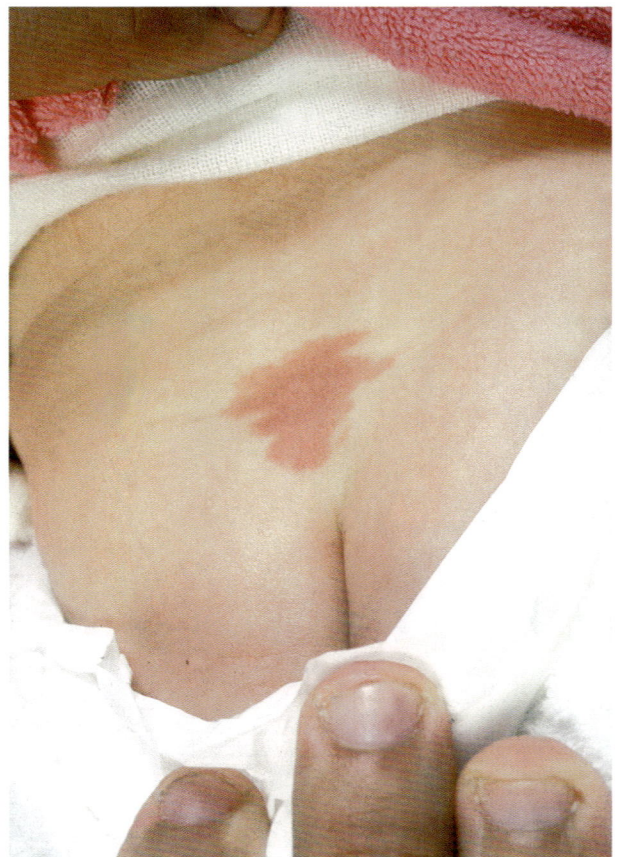

Figure 20.12

Differential diagnosis

- Overlap with Klippel–Trénaunay–Sturge–Weber syndromes
- Spina bifida complex
- Non-syndromic PWS of lumbar areas

Follow-up and therapy

- Neurosurgery when possible

REFERENCES

Gordon-Firing S, Purriel JA, Pereyra D, Brodbek I. [Report of a new case of Cobb syndrome. Meningo-spinal cutaneous angiomatosis.] Acta Neurol Latinoam 1981; 27: 99–111

Mercer RD, Rothner AD, Cook SA, Alfidi RJ. The Cobb syndrome: association with hereditary cutaneous hemangiomas. Cleve Clin Q 1978; 45: 237–40

Rodesch G, Hurth M, Alvarez H, et al. Classification of spinal cord arteriovenous shunts: proposal for a reappraisal – the Bicetre experience with 155 consecutive patients treated between 1981 and 1999. Neurosurgery 2002; 51: 374–9; discussion 379–80

VON HIPPEL–LINDAU SYNDROME

Synonym

- Hemangioblastoma of retina and cerebellum

Epidemiology

Large kindreds are reported in the literature but there is a lack of data on incidence and prevalence.

Cutaneous findings

PWS of the face, occipital and cervical regions occur in 5–20% of patients.

Extracutaneous findings

- Cerebellar and/or spinal hemangioblastomas
- Retinal angiomas in a large percentage of patients
- Less frequently, vascular malformations in internal organs
- Pheochromocytoma and renal polycystic disease and carcinomas

Course and complications

- Rarely, the basic lesions may lead to epilepsy and progressive mental retardation
- High risk for vascular intracranial ruptures

Laboratory findings

Angio-MRI is used to detect the severity of cerebellar and retinal lesions (Figure 20.13).

Genetics and pathogenesis

The disease is inherited as an autosomal dominant trait and is due to mutations on the VHL gene, which may be responsible for the associated neoplasms.

Differential diagnosis

- Non-syndromic intracranial vascular malformations

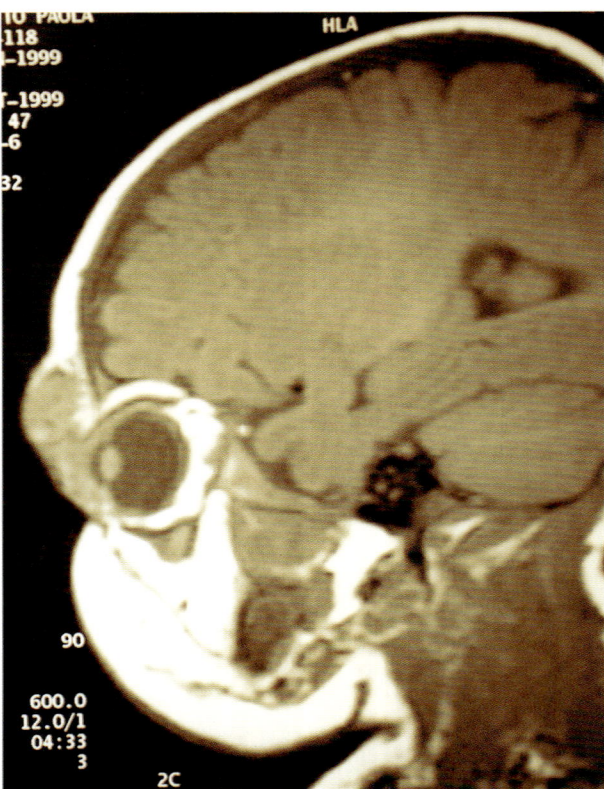

Figure 20.13

Follow-up and therapy

- Angio-MRI
- Neurosurgical approach when applicable

REFERENCES

Iida K, Okimura Y, Takahashi K, et al. A variety of phenotype with R161Q germline mutation of the von Hippel–Lindau tumor suppressor gene in Japanese kindred. Int J Molec Med 2004; 13: 401–4

Kuwai T, Kitadai Y, Tanaka S, et al. Mutation of the von Hippel–Lindau (VHL) gene in human colorectal carcinoma: association with cytoplasmic accumulation of hypoxia-inducible factor (HIF)-1alpha. Cancer Sci 2004; 95: 149–53

Wait SD, Vortmeyer AQ, Lonser RR, et al. Somatic mutations in VHL germline deletion kindred correlate with mild phenotype. Ann Neurol 2004; 55: 236–40

ATAXIA TELANGIECTASIA

Synonym

- Louis–Bar's syndrome

Epidemiology

- At least 200 families with large kindreds are reported
- Prevalence: 1 : 500 000
- Birth frequency: 1 : 300 000

Age of onset

- Very rare at birth
- Common after 3–4 years of age (ataxia and conjunctival signs first, skin lesion onset may be delayed)

Clinical findings

- Telangiectases in a butterfly-like pattern in the mid-portion of the face (Figures 20.14 and 20.15)
- Similar lesions on ears and periorbital areas (Figure 20.16)

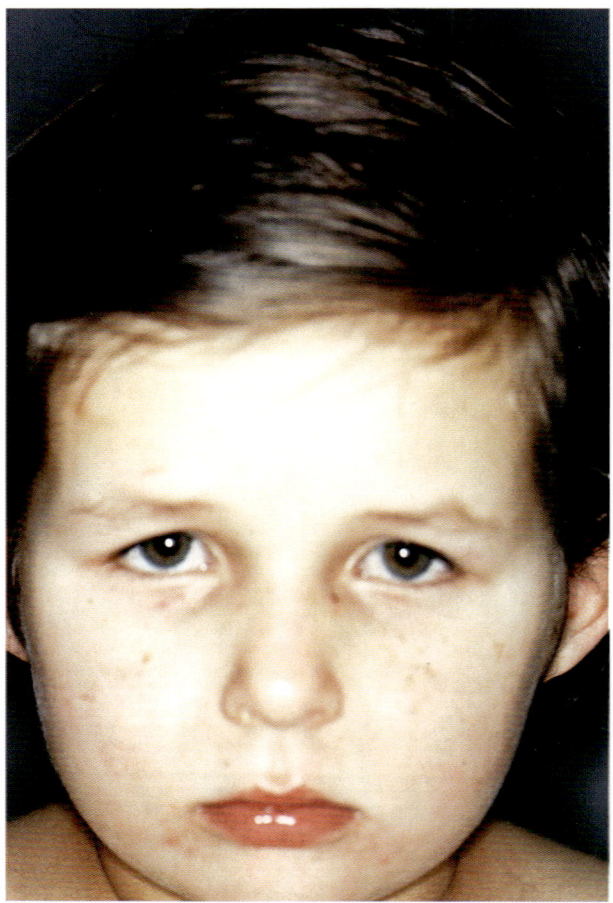

Figure 20.14

Vascular disorders

- Less frequently in other sun-exposed areas or major folds (Figure 20.17)
- In a minor percentage of patients canities or hirsutism are reported, as well as café-au-lait spots and seborrheic dermatitis
- Poikiloderma and sclerodermatous changes in sun-exposed areas are common
- Mucosal involvement

Extracutaneous symptoms

- Conjunctival telangiectases usually precede skin lesions and may be associated with strabismus (Figure 20.15)
- Cerebellar ataxia is the first sign of the disease (onset commonly within the first year of life) (Figure 20.18)
- Choreoathetoid movements (including eyes), dysarthria and tremors
- Hypotonia and muscular atrophy
- Immunodeficiency with recurrent upper respiratory tract infections, lymphadenopathy
- Growth failure
- Insulin-resistant diabetes in a majority of patients

Course and prognosis

- Progressive mental retardation
- Frequently a wheelchair is needed after adolescence
- Recurrent pulmonary infections may become chronic and life-threatening
- High risk of malignancies with age, even for heterozygotes
- Life expectancy greatly reduced

Laboratory findings

- Computed tomography (CT) analysis may reveal cerebral and cerebellar atrophy of white matter
- Immunoglobulins IgA and IgE defects
- Cellular immunity impaired with lymphopenia
- High carcinoembryonic antigen and α-fetoprotein

Genetics and pathogenesis

The disease is linked to mutations in the ATM gene, a tumor suppressor gene that is a modulator of cell

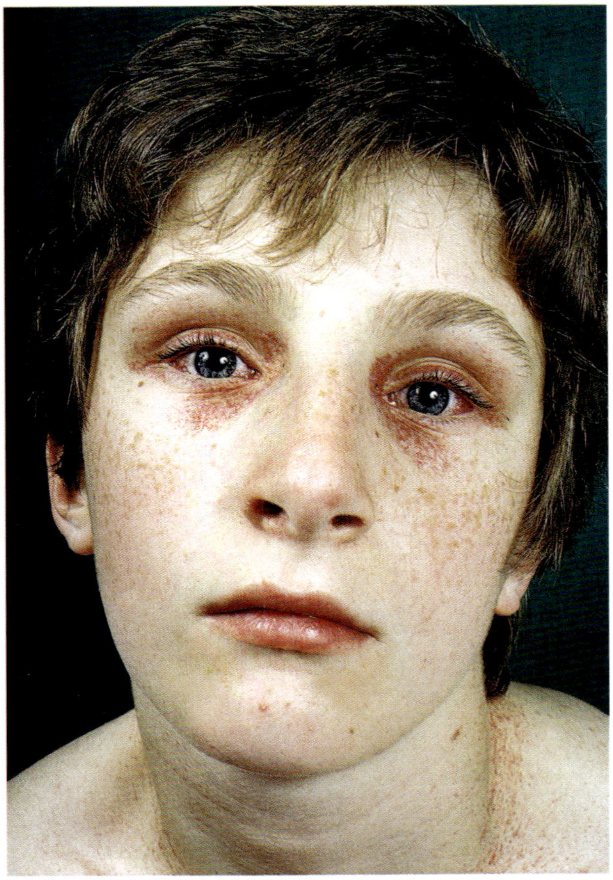

Figure 20.15

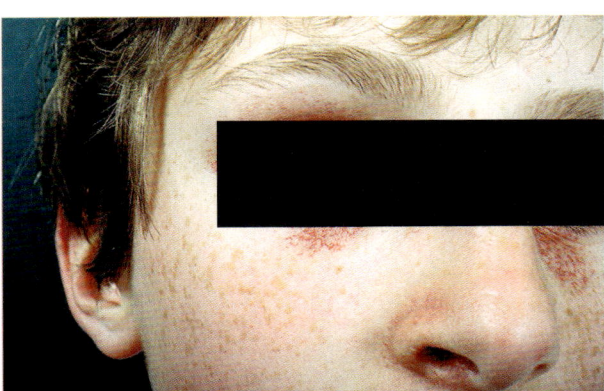

Figure 20.16

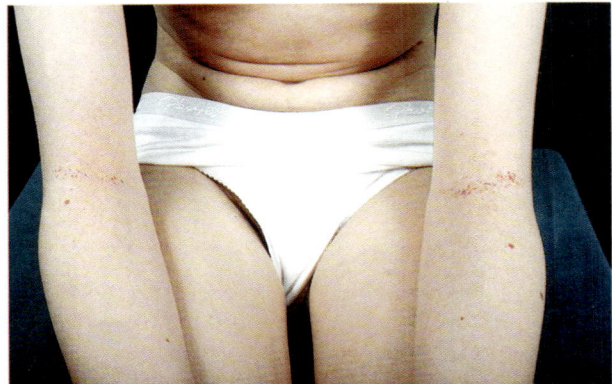

Figure 20.17

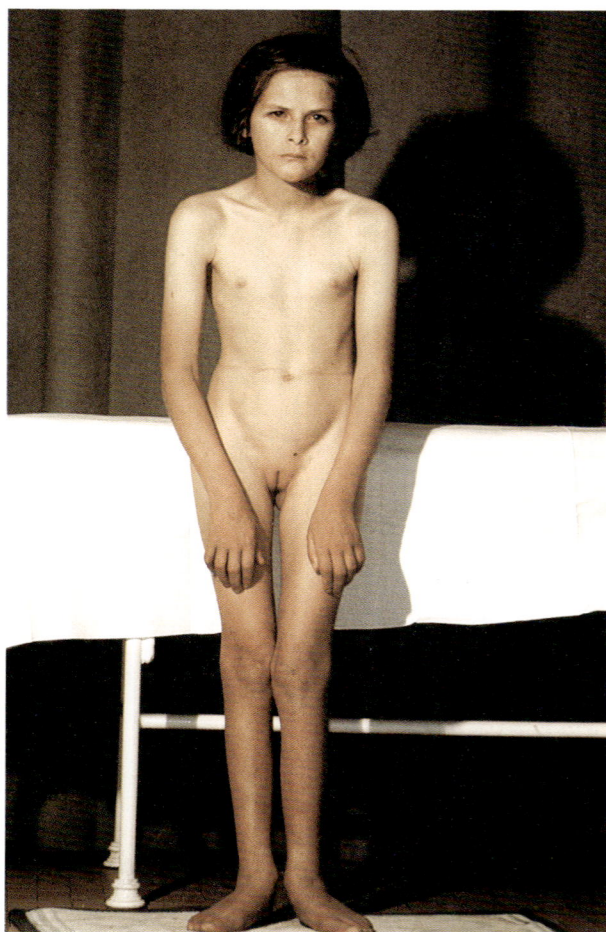

Figure 20.18

cycle arrest, apoptosis and DNA double-strand break repair.

Differential diagnosis

- Bloom's disease
- Rothmund–Thomson syndrome
- Cockayne's syndrome
- Fanconi's disease
- Systemic lupus erythematosus

REFERENCES

Cuneo A, Bigoni R, Rigolin GM, et al. Acquired chromosome 11q deletion involving the ataxia teleangiectasia locus in B-cell non-Hodgkin's lymphoma: correlation with clinicobiologic features. J Clin Oncol 2000; 18: 2607–14

HEMORRHAGIC TELANGIECTASIA

Synonym

- Rendu–Osler syndrome

Epidemiology

No data are available.

Age of onset

- Late first decade

Clinical findings

- Fine telangiectases, macules, palpable papules and small nodules seen progressively on the face, lips, ears, nail beds; vascular lesions may be seen on virtually entire skin area (Figures 20.19–20.21)
- Nasal and oral mucosa (internal lips and tongue) involvement is usual, with similar lesions (Figure 20.22)
- Conjunctival telangiectases

Extracutaneous findings

- Severe nasal bleeding
- Pulmonary involvement with arteriovenous malformations
- CNS and spinal primary vascular malformations
- Gastrointestinal hemorrhages
- Hepatic vascular nodules
- As already noted for the skin, vascular hemorrhagic lesions may be scattered throughout all organs

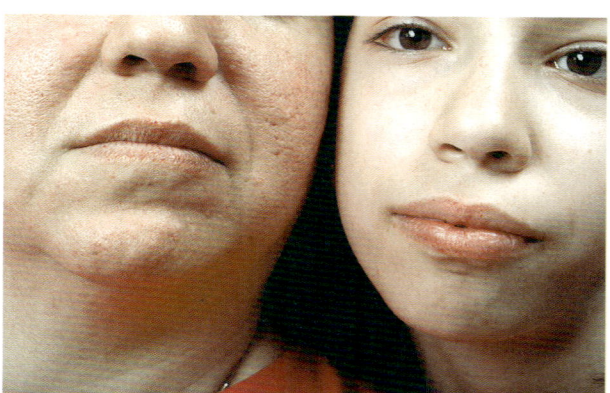

Figure 20.19

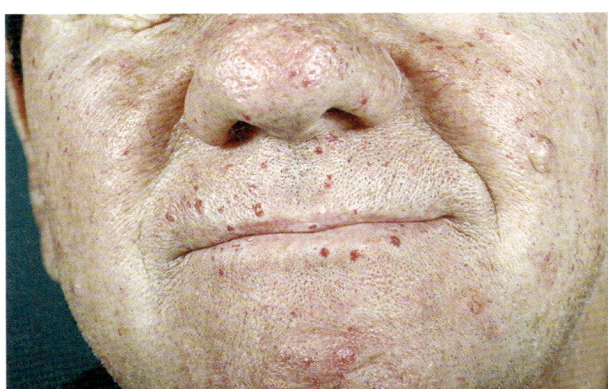

Figure 20.20

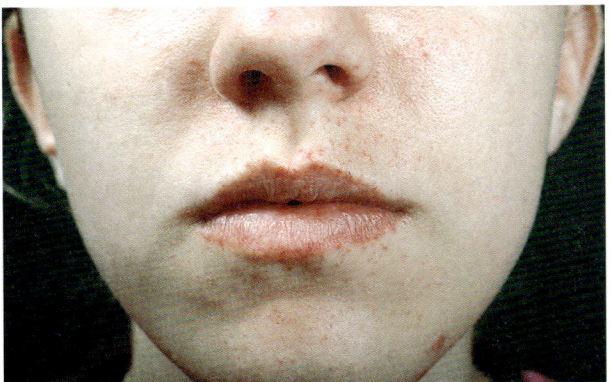

Figure 20.21

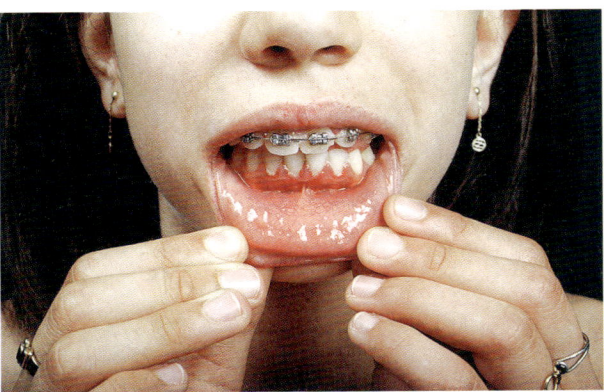

Figure 20.22

Course and complications

- The majority of patients may complain of secondary vascular CNS lesions (strokes) due to embolic episodes from pulmonary bleeding
- Nasal bleeding can be severe and even life-threatening
- Liver lesions may lead to fibrosis and portal hypertension
- Secondary severe anemia
- Recurrent pulmonary infections
- Septic endocarditis

Laboratory findings

- Anemia is easily detected by routine testing
- Coagulation tests are usually normal

Genetics and pathogenesis

The disease is inherited in an autosomal recessive fashion.

The syndrome is due to mutations in two genes: ALK1/ACVRL1 and endoglin.

Differential diagnosis

- Bloom's disease
- Ataxia–telangiectasia
- Hereditary benign telangiectasia
- Fabry's disease

REFERENCES

Begbie ME, Wallace GM, Shovlin CL. Hereditary haemorrhagic telangiectasia (Osler–Weber–Rendu syndrome): a view from the 21st century. Postgrad Med J 2003; 79: 18–24

Kukulj S, Ivanovi-Herceg Z, Slobodnjak Z. Hereditary hemorrhagic telangiectasia or Rendu–Osler–Weber syndrome in the same family. Coll Antropol 2000; 24: 241–7

Rius C, Smith JD, Almendro N, et al. Cloning of the promoter region of human endoglin, the target gene for hereditary hemorrhagic telangiectasia type 1. Blood 1998; 92: 4677–90

CUTIS MARMORATA TELANGIECTATICA CONGENITA

Synonym

- Congenital livedo reticularis

Epidemiology

No data are available.

Age of onset

- At birth

Clinical findings

- Reticulated, marble-like appearance of the skin due to abnormal venous and capillary distribution of skin-associated vessels, generalized or in mosaic arrangement (Figures 20.23–20.25)
- Overlying cutaneous atrophy with crusts and hyperkeratotic lesions with loss of substance, especially on legs (Figure 20.26, patient with Adams–Oliver syndrome)
- Lesions may be more subtle and the pattern of vascular lesions may give a designed tissue appearance to entire skin (Figures 20.27 and 20.28)
- Vascular lesions may be generalized or unilateral or segmental with PWS association (Figures 20.29 and 20.30)
- Secondary hypo- and hyperpigmented residual linear lesions may be visible

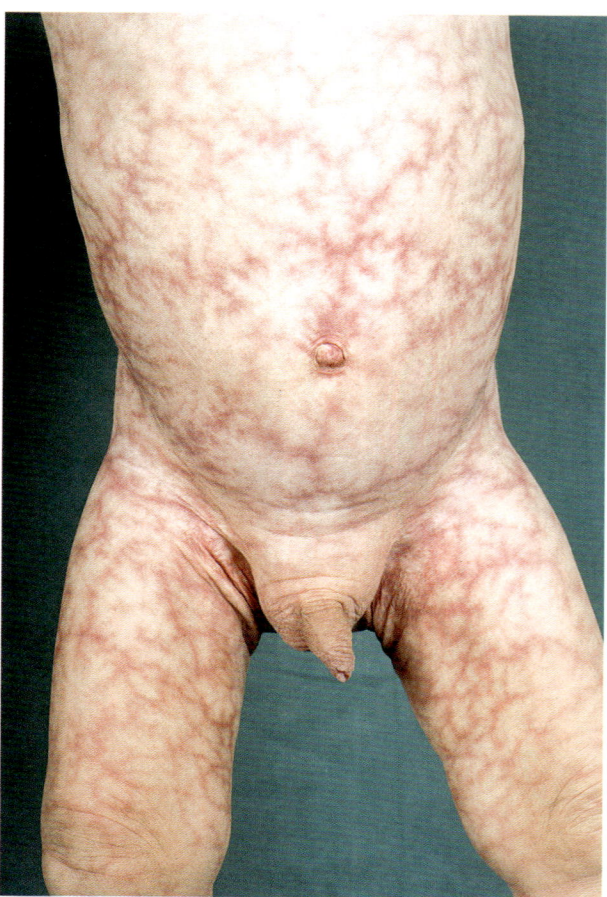

Figure 20.23

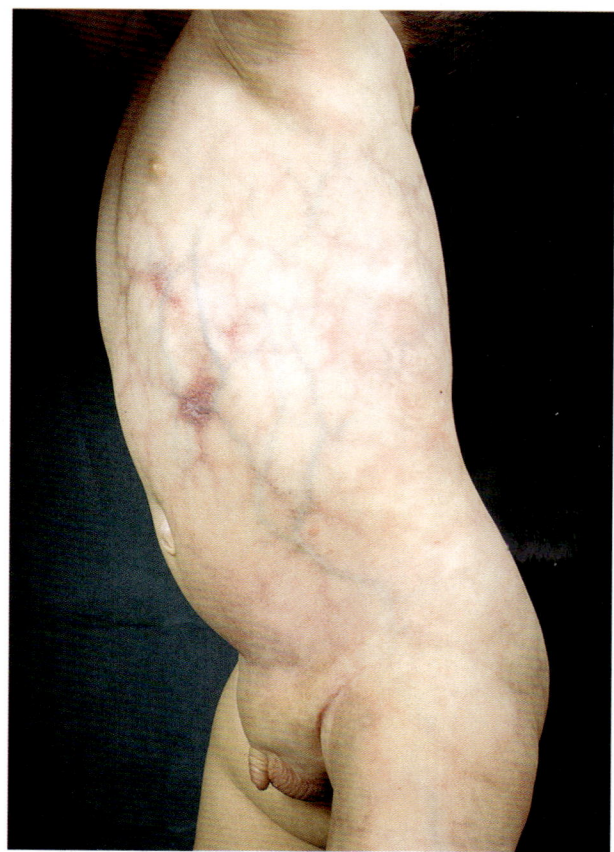

Figure 20.24

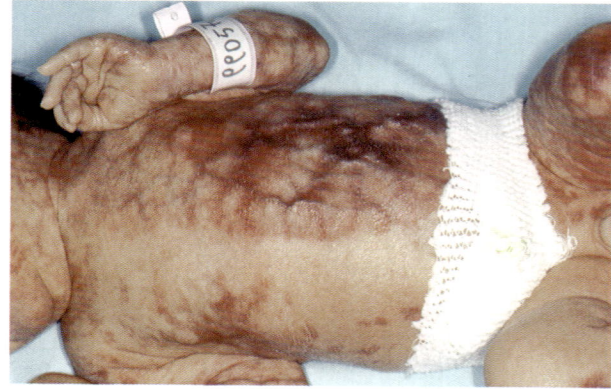

Figure 20.25

Vascular disorders

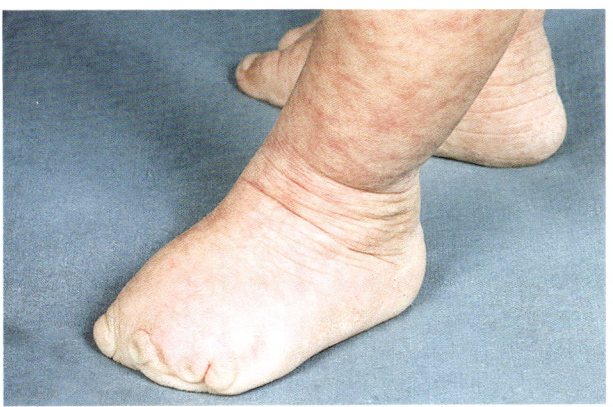

Figure 20.26

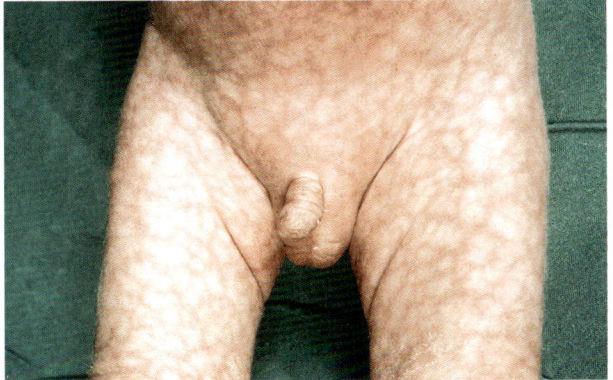

Figure 20.27

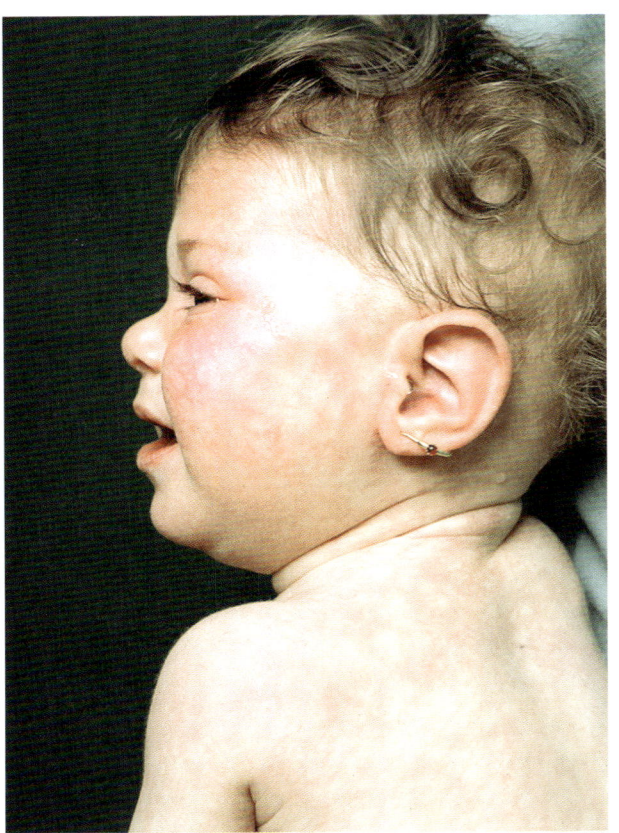

Figure 20.28

Extracutaneous symptoms

- CNS involvement, microcephaly and macrocephaly have been reported, together with severe porencephalic abnormalities and mental retardation (15–20%)
- Craniofacial abnormalities may lead to micrognathia and triangle-shaped facies
- Glaucoma

Course and complications

- Localized necrosis overlying the vascular reticulum (Figures 20.31 and 20.32)
- Loss of substance with hypoatrophy in the related leg or area involved
- Rarely, hemiatrophy of the face
- Usually the cutaneous symptoms improve with age

Laboratory findings

- There are no specific alterations in routine hematological examination
- CT scan can easily detect CNS-associated signs

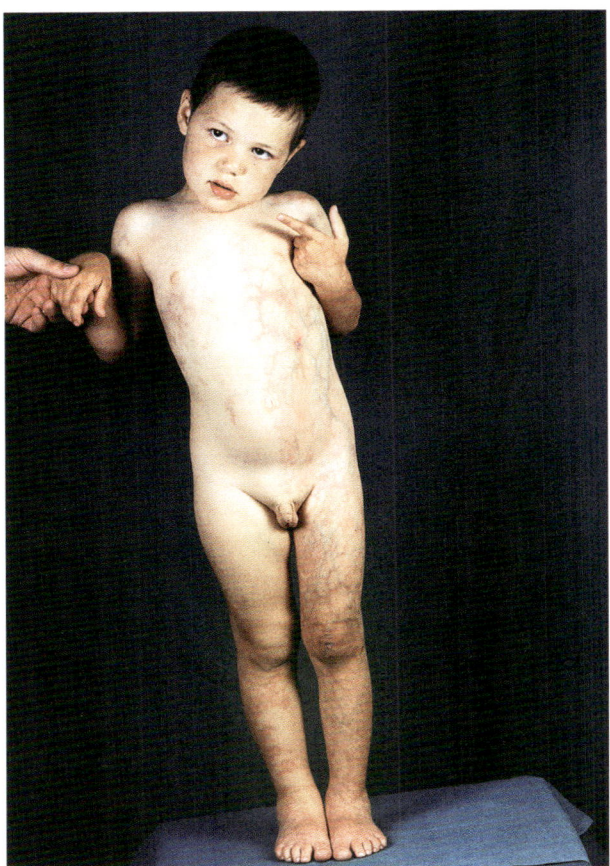

Figure 20.29

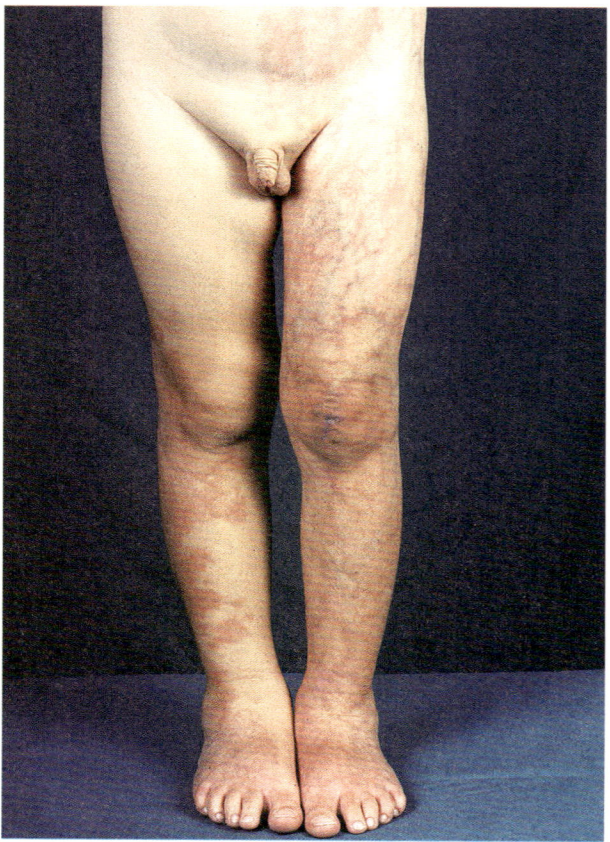

Figure 20.30

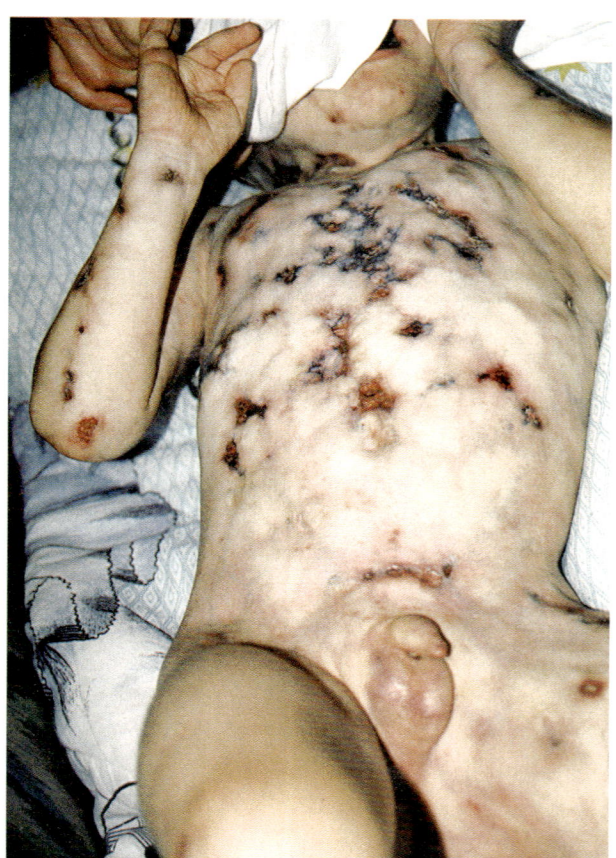

Figure 20.31

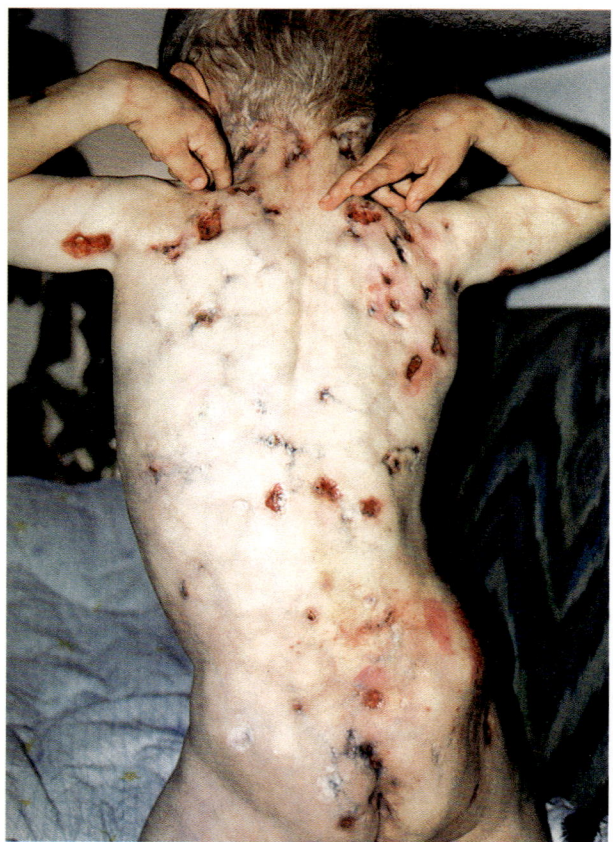

Figure 20.32

Genetics and pathology

- Sporadic and mosaic postzygotic mutations
- There are some confusing reports claiming autosomal dominant transmission

Differential diagnosis

- Aplasia cutis congenita
- Adams–Oliver syndrome
- Down's syndrome
- Normal reactive livedo reticularis in newborns and in infancy

REFERENCES

Hamm H. Cutaneous mosaicism of lethal mutations. Am J Med Genet 1999; 85: 342–5

Krause MH, Bonnekoh B, Weisshaar E, Gollnick H. Coincidence of multiple, disseminated, tardive–eruptive blue nevi with cutis marmorata telangiectatica congenita. Dermatology 2000; 200: 134–8

Rupprecht R, Hundeiker M. [Cutis marmorata telangiectatica congenita. Important aspects for dermatologic practice.] Hautarzt 1997; 48: 21–5

MAFFUCCI SYNDROME

Synonyms

- Enchondromatosis
- Hemangiomatosis

Epidemiology

The disease is rare; fewer than 50 cases are described.

Age of onset

Fewer than 20% of cases are congenital, but usually the disease appears around the age of 5 years; more than three-quarters of cases are visible before puberty.

Clinical findings

- The disease often starts with a swelling of the dorsa of hands and feet (Figure 20.33)
- Soft tissue vascular malformations and cutis marmorata telangiectatica (Figure 20.34) or bluish subcutaneous nodules occur especially on extremities, but they can be present anywhere on the body
- Lymphangiomas and varicosities (less frequently)
- Oral mucosa involvement is possible but rare
- Mosaic forms (unilateral, segmental) are possible

Extracutaneous symptoms

- Enchondromatosis is represented by benign cartilaginous tumors, usually on the hands, but they may be present elsewhere
- Visceral and CNS vascular malformations in some patients with severe disease

Course and complications

- Usually the symptoms progress slowly until the third decade of life
- Vascular malformations may undergo thrombotic evolution and phleboliths may be detected
- Rarely, aneurysms of major vessels may develop
- Malignant transformation (chondrosarcomas) of enchondromas may occur in a quarter of patients
- Tumors of the ovaries and testes, adenocarcinomas and lymphangiosarcomas are described

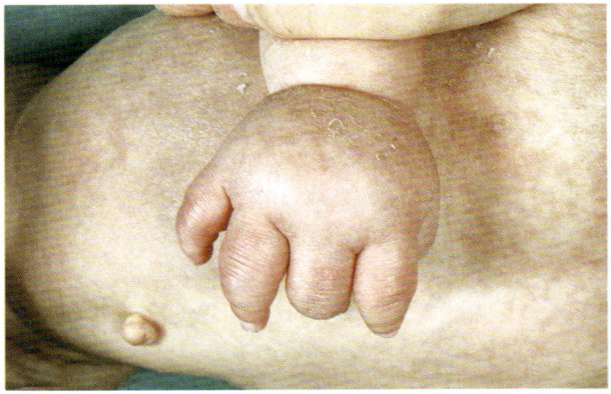

Figure 20.33

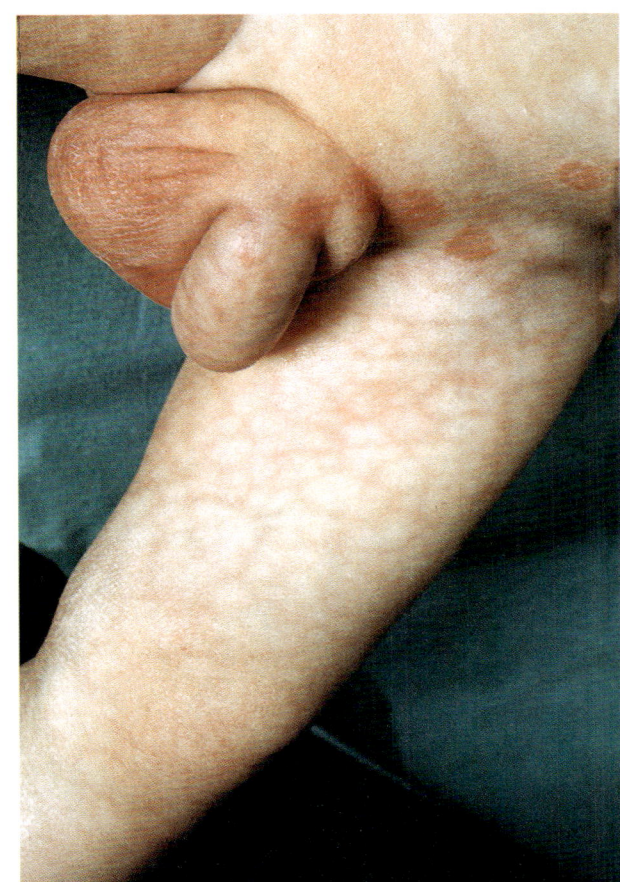

Figure 20.34

- Severe cases may experience severe deformities of extremities that can impair their daily activities

Laboratory findings

Radiography of the hands and feet is used for the detection of early enchondromas.

Genetics and pathogenesis

The disease is caused by a mutant PTH/PTHrP type I receptor causing abnormal control of mesodermal derivates and abnormal proliferation.

Follow-up and therapy

- Radiography of the involved areas
- Surgical treatment of severe lesions
- Special shoes for foot deformities
- Prosthetic devices when amputation is mandatory
- Surgical treatment of malignancies

Differential diagnosis

- Klippel–Trénaunay complex
- Many authors refer to Ollier's disease (isolated dyschondroplasia, cancer proneness) in the spectrum of Maffucci syndrome
- Blue rubber bleb nevus syndrome

REFERENCES

Auyeung J, Mohanty K, Tayton K. Maffucci lymphangioma syndrome: an unusual variant of Ollier's disease, a case report and a review of the literature. J Pediatr Orthop B 2003; 12: 147–50

Colonna G, Ascencio G, Meunier L, Guillot B. [Lymphangioma in a patient with Maffuci syndrome of the lower legs.] J Mal Vasc 2002; 27: 174–6

Hopyan S, Gokgoz N, Poon R, et al. A mutant PTH/PTHrP type 1 receptor in enchondromatosis. Nature Genet 2002; 30: 306–10

BLUE RUBBER BLEB NEVUS SYNDROME

Synonym

- Beau's syndrome

Age of onset

- At birth or in early infancy

Clinical findings

Cutaneous manifestations

- Soft, papulonodular lesions, varying in size from 0.1 to 5 cm in diameter and in number from one to more than 100 that resemble rubber nipples (Figures 20.35 and 20.36)
- The lesions are easily compressible and refill promptly when pressure is released
- Hyperhidrosis is often apparent at the surfaces of lesions
- The blebs may be painful spontaneously or when pressed, mainly during the night
- Sites of predilection: trunk and limbs; occasionally lesions in the oral cavity (Figure 20.37)

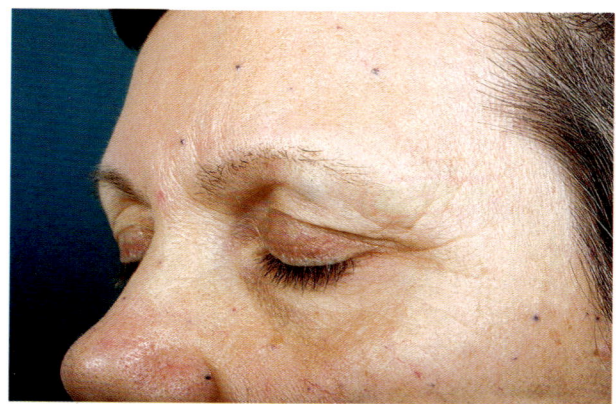

Figure 20.35

Extracutaneous manifestations

- Hemangiomas in the gastrointestinal tract (90%), especially in the small bowel, responsible for various complications
- Rarely lesions may occur in the lungs, urinary tract, liver, spleen, brain, meninges, bones and heart
- Other tumors
- Central nervous system anomalies

Vascular disorders

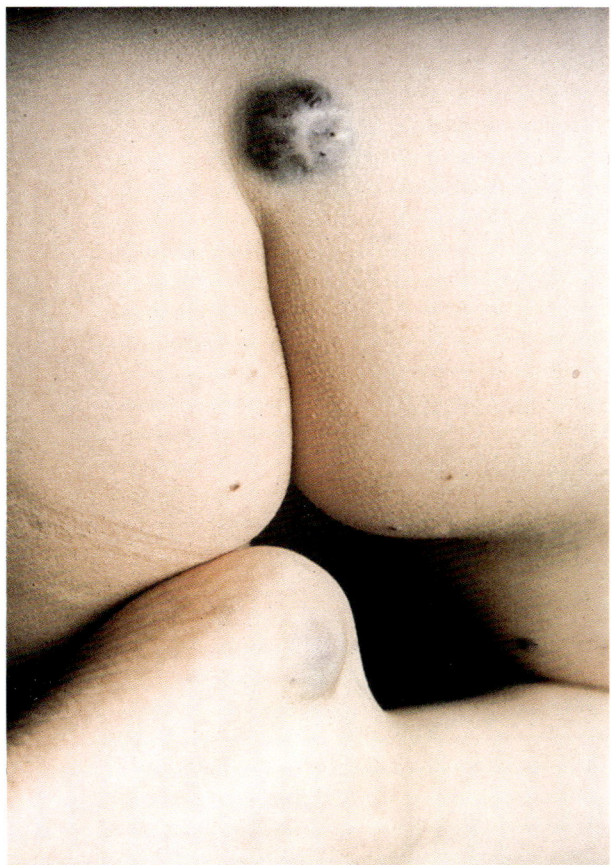

Figure 20.36

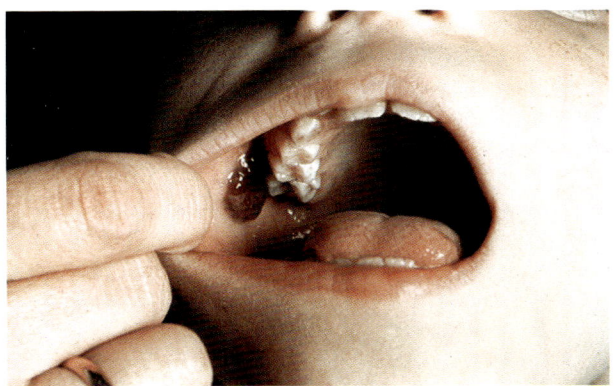

Figure 20.37

Differential diagnosis

- Multiple glomus tumors
- Maffucci syndrome

Therapy

- Mainly symptomatic
- Surgical excision
- CO_2 laser

Complications

- Gastrointestinal bleeding may induce hematemesis, melena, severe iron-deficiency anemia
- Intussusceptions
- Focal neurologic defects

Course

The disease is slowly progressive throughout life.

Laboratory findings and data

- Anemia due to iron deficiency
- Endoscopy
- Complete radiography and MRI of bowel and skull
- Histopathologic findings: very widely dilated vein-like structures in the dermis and subcutaneous fat, some of which may thrombose and become organized

Genetics and pathogenesis

- Sporadic cases in the majority
- Claimed autosomal dominant transmission in one pedigree

REFERENCES

Boente MC, Cordisco MR, Frontini MV, et al. Blue rubber bleb nevus (Beau syndrome): evolution of four cases and clinical response to pharmacologic agents. Pediatr Dermatol 1999; 16: 222–7

Carvalho S, Barbosa V, Santos N, Machado E. Blue rubber-bleb nevus syndrome: report of a familial case with a dural arteriovenous fistula. Am J Neuroradiol 2003; 24: 1916–18

Ertem D, Acar Y, Kotiloglu E, et al. Blue rubber bleb nevus syndrome. Pediatrics 2001; 107: 418–20

DIFFUSE BENIGN TELANGIECTASIA AND PORT-WINE STAINS COMPLEX

Definition

Familial PWS (see also Figures 20.3 and 20.4) and benign telangiectasia are usually considered distinct disorders, based on the clinical presentation of cutaneous lesions. However, overlapping phenotypes have been described in some families (see Figure 20.42), suggesting that both conditions are part of the wide phenotypic spectrum of the same clinical entity. Recent personal linkage studies confirm the clinical observation.

Synonym

- Familial capillary malformation

Epidemiology

At least 50 families are reported.

Age of onset

- At birth

Clinical findings

- PWS: large dark red-purple lesions, found preferentially on the upper part of the body, distributed in a mosaic fashion with checkerboard pattern (Figure 20.38) (see also Figures 20.1 to 20.9)
- Benign telangiectasia: smaller, lighter and multiple lesions (Figure 20.39), located at any site on the body (Figures 20.40 and 20.41)

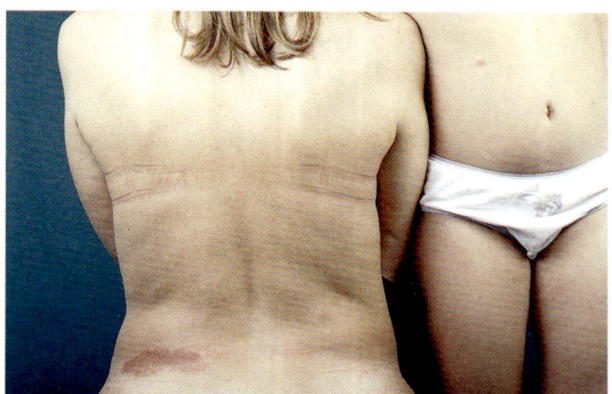

Figure 20.38

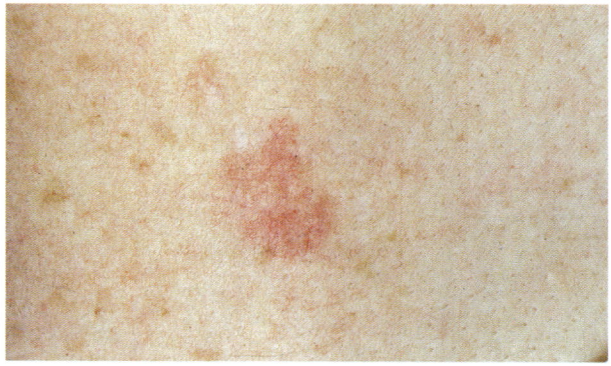

Figure 20.39

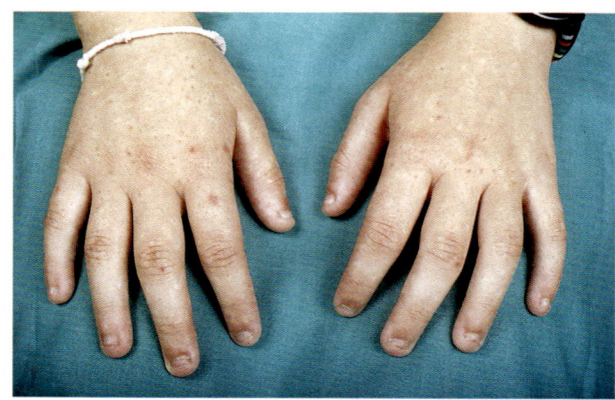

Figure 20.40

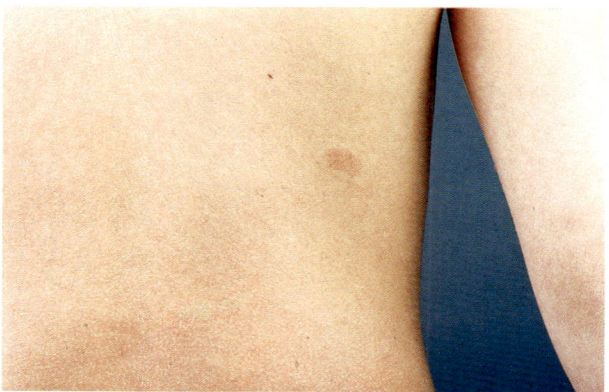

Figure 20.41

Course and prognosis

The disease is steady throughout life.

Laboratory findings

There are none specific.

Genetics and pathogenesis

The disorder is autosomal dominant.

Recent linkage studies allowed us to map the disease to chromosome 5q14, excluding linkage with endoglin and ALK1, the two known genes responsible for hemorrhagic telangiectasia on chromosomes 9 and 17, respectively. The linked region on 5q14 (locus CMC1) contains a gene encoding a protein expressed by endothelial cells during embryogenesis.

Follow-up and therapy

- Routine examination to exclude internal abnormalities
- Laser therapy for esthetic reasons

Differential diagnosis

- Syndromes with PWS and CNS involvement

REFERENCES

Brancati F, Valente EM, Tadini G, et al. Autosomal dominant hereditary benign telangiectasia maps to the CMC1 locus for capillary malformation on chromosome 5q14 [Letter]. J Med Genet 2003; 40: 349–53

Breugem CC, Alders M, Salieb-Beugelaar GB, et al. A locus for hereditary capillary malformations mapped on chromosome 5q. Hum Genet 2002; 110: 343–7

UNILATERAL NEVOID AND GENERALIZED 'ESSENTIAL' TELANGIECTASIA

Definition

Even if the partial form is by far better known to dermatologists, the same condition may present in diffuse and familial forms, and must be considered as the same clinical entity.

Epidemiology

This is a rare condition.

Age of onset

- Rarely at birth, usually visible within the second decade

Clinical findings

- Diffuse (Figures 20.42 and 20.43) or nevoid (Figures 20.44 and 20.45) superficial telangiectases
- Lesions are preferentially located on the upper part of the body
- Paradominant transmission is possible (Figures 20.46 and 20.47, same family)
- Mosaic forms may be represented by superficial pinpoint lesions (Figures 20.48 and 20.49) or small telangiectatic lesions surrounded by a

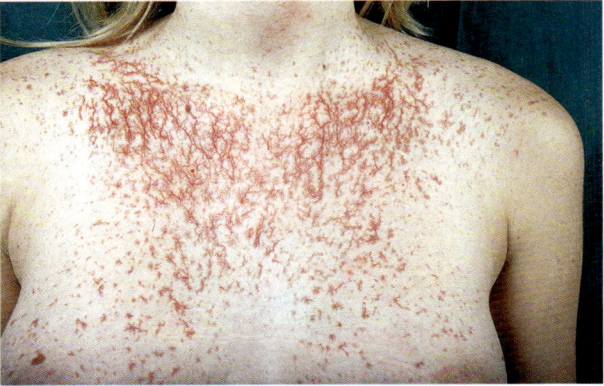

Figure 20.42

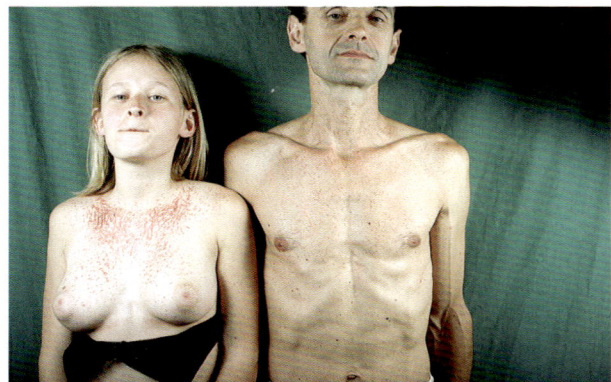

Figure 20.43

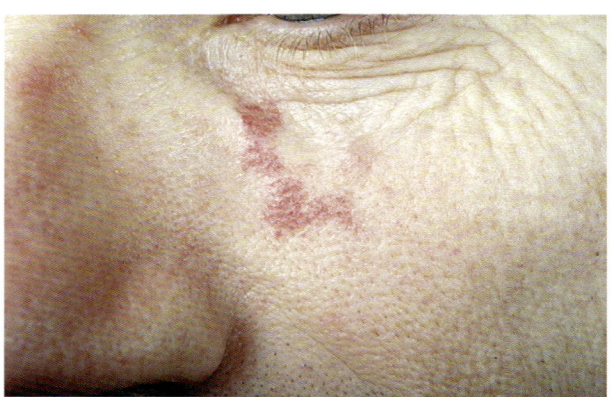

Figure 20.46

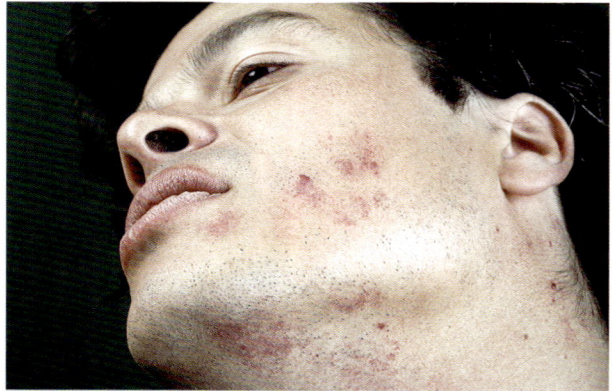

Figure 20.44

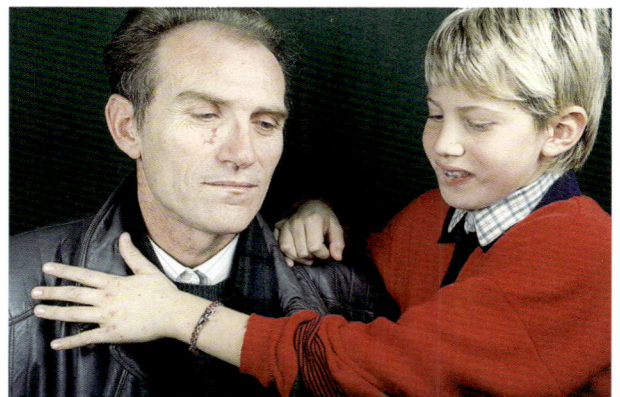

Figure 20.47

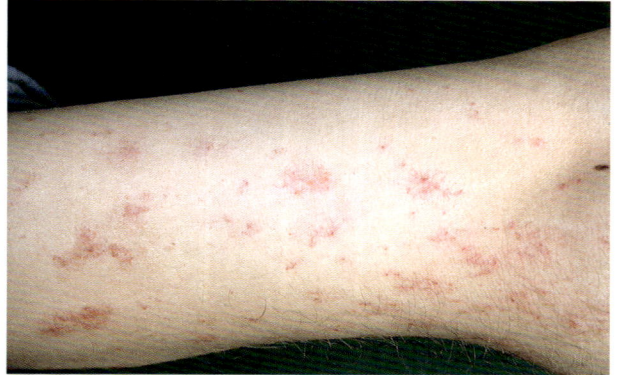

Figure 20.45

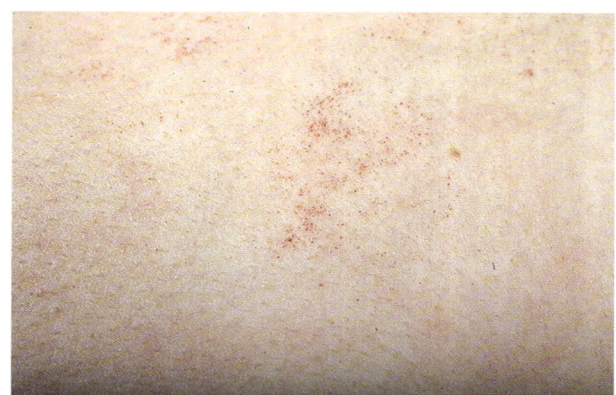

Figure 20.48

clear anemic halo (Figures 20.50–20.52), or 'spider nevi' arranged in a mosaic pattern (Figures 20.53 and 20.54)

Course and prognosis

Telangiectases are rarely seen at birth and may worsen with age.

Laboratory investigations

There are none specific.

Genetics and pathogenesis

- Autosomal dominant transmission is possible for the diffuse form (Figure 20.49)

Vascular disorders 317

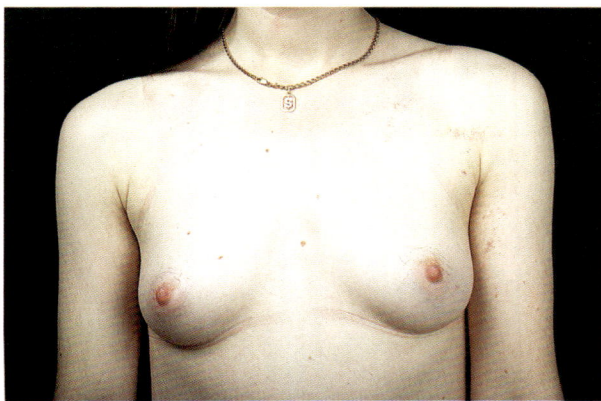

Figure 20.49

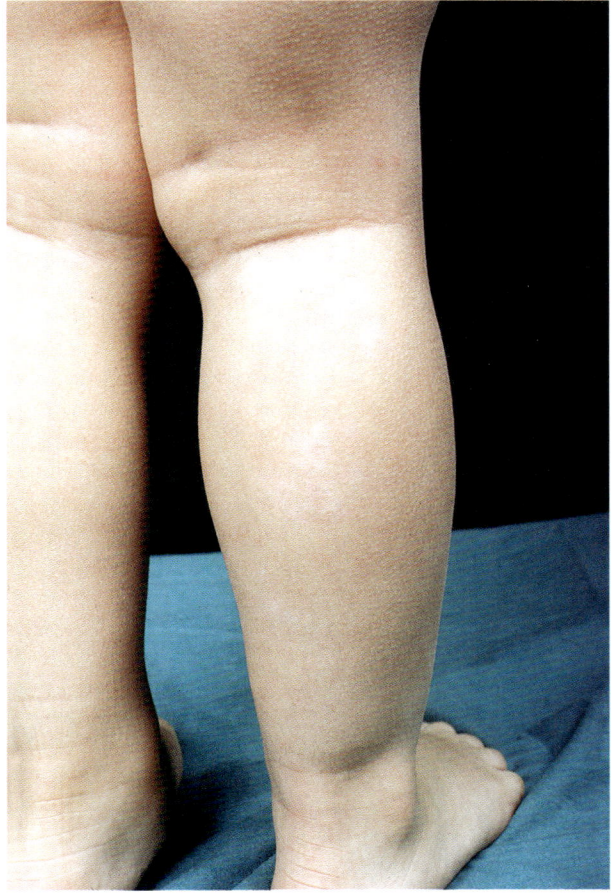

Figure 20.50

- Mosaic forms represent postzygotic mutations and may have paradominant transmission

Follow-up and therapy

- Laser therapy can be used if required

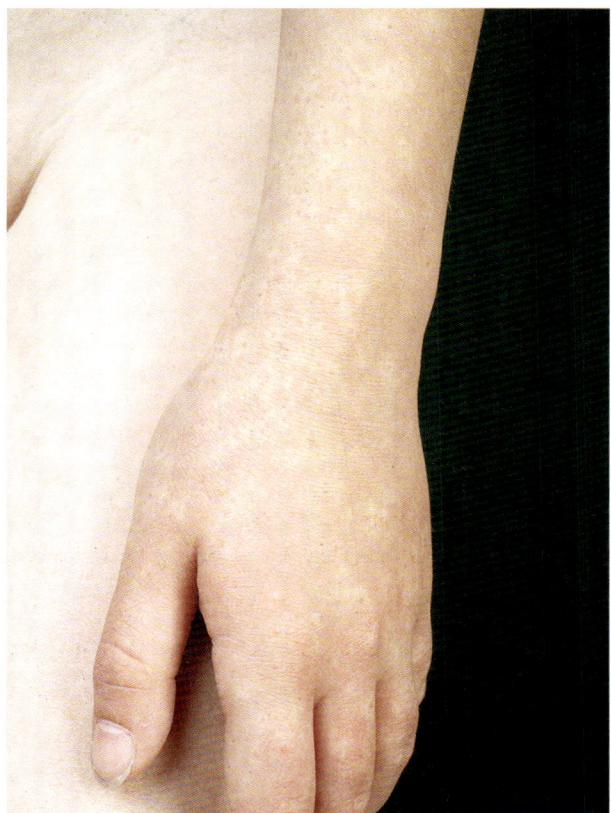

Figure 20.51

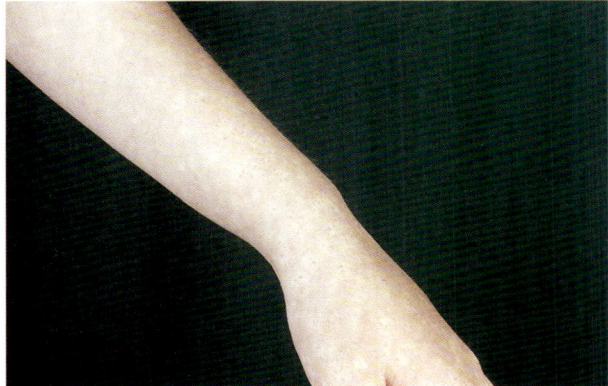

Figure 20.52

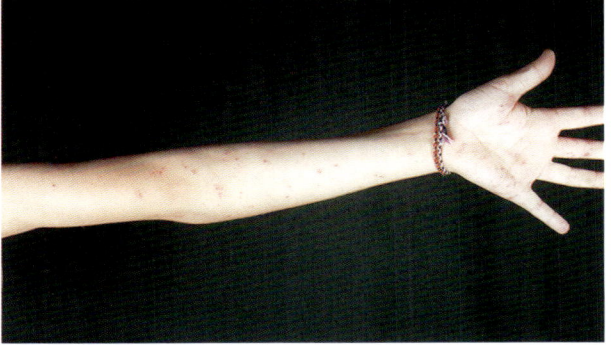

Figure 20.53

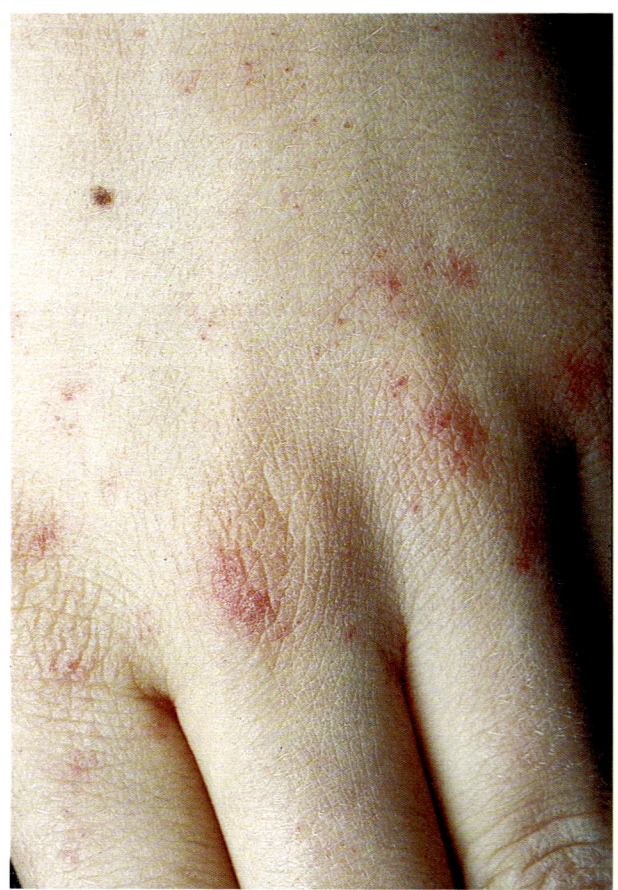

Figure 20.54

NEVUS ANEMICUS

Epidemiology

This is a very rare condition.

Age of onset

- At birth

Clinical findings

- Well circumscribed area of absence of visible vascularization (Figure 20.55, where peripheral erythema is due to rubbing)
- Visible in 'allelic twin-spots' together with PWS (Figure 20.56)
- Part of a subtype of phakomatosis pigmentovascularis (nevus anemicus and melanocytic nevus)

Course and prognosis

There are no modifications with age.

Differential diagnosis

- Syndromes with diffuse telangiectases (Rendu–Osler and ataxia–telangiectasia syndrome)

REFERENCE

Raff M, Bardach HG. Unilateral nevoid telangiectatic syndrome. Hautarzt 1982; 33: 148–51

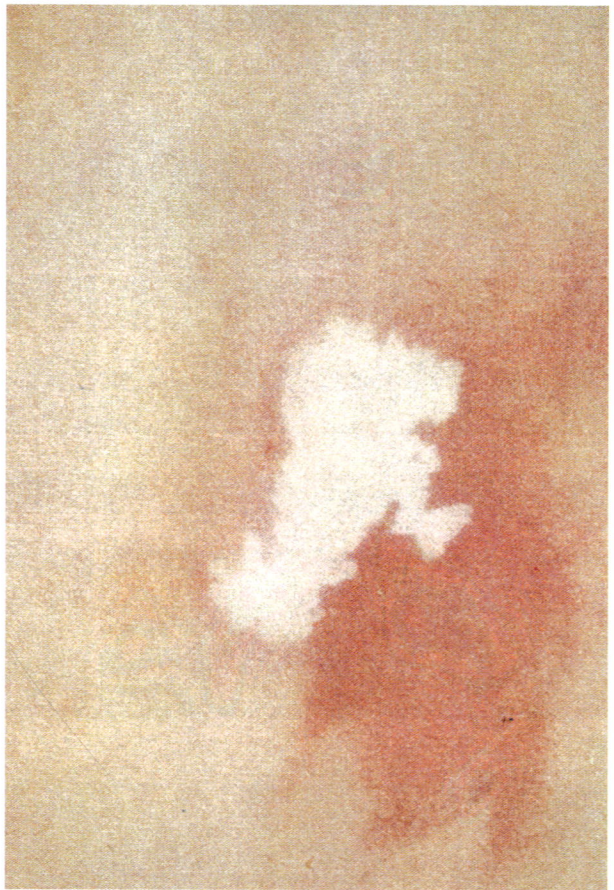

Figure 20.55

Vascular disorders

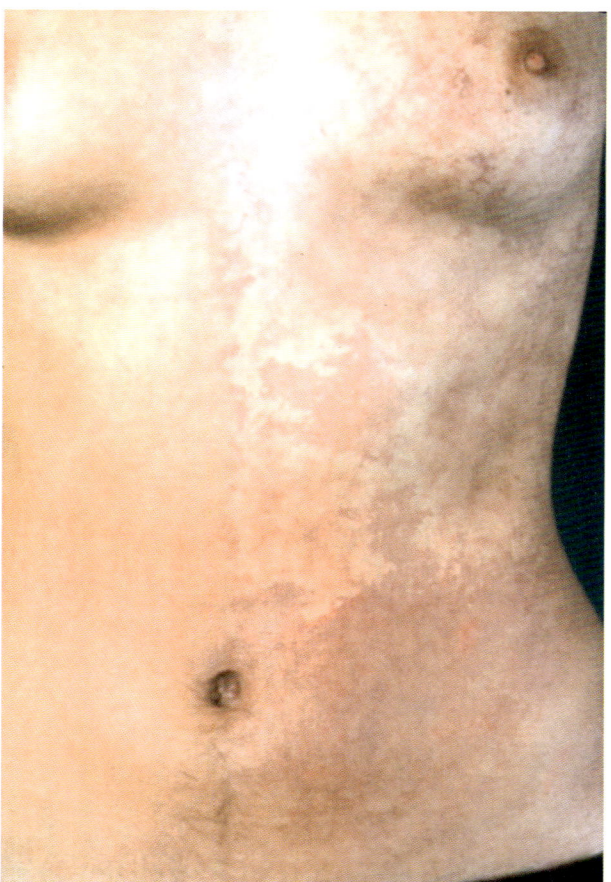

Figure 20.56

Genetics and pathogenesis

- Sporadic cases
- Seems to be the obvious negative counterpart of PWS, representing the homozygous conditions of doubled and absent expression, respectively, of a gene that modulates, at the embryologic level, the distribution of capillaries in the skin

Follow-up and therapy

- Camouflage can be applied if necessary

Differential diagnosis

- Hypopigmented nevus
- Vitiligo

REFERENCE

Ahkami RN, Schwartz RA. Nevus anemicus. Dermatology 1999; 98: 327–9

PHAKOMATOSIS PIGMENTOVASCULARIS

Epidemiology

This is a rare mosaic condition, with possibly a cluster in Japanese people.

Age of onset

- At birth, but often full-blown after some years of life

Clinical findings

Contemporaneous presence ('twin-spots' phenomenon) of port-wine stain (nevus flammeus) and melanocytic lesions, as follows:

- Speckled lentiginous nevus (Figure 20.57)
- Mongolian spots (Figure 20.58)
- Melanocytic nevus ('nevus pigmentosum') (Figure 20.59)
- Hypopigmented nevus (Figure 20.60)

Some reports also exist of a contemporaneous presence of nevus anemicus and melanocytic nevi, with or without concomitant and epidermal nevus.

Extracutaneous findings

There are no reports of relevant internal abnormalities among these patients.

Course and prognosis

- Disease stabilizes during infancy
- Some risk of malignant transformation for speckled lentiginous nevus

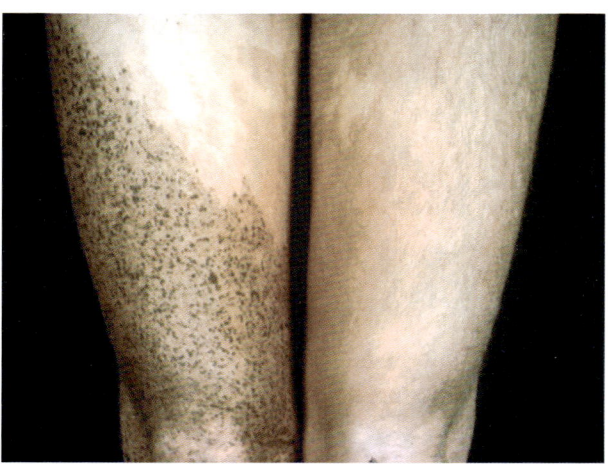

Figure 20.57

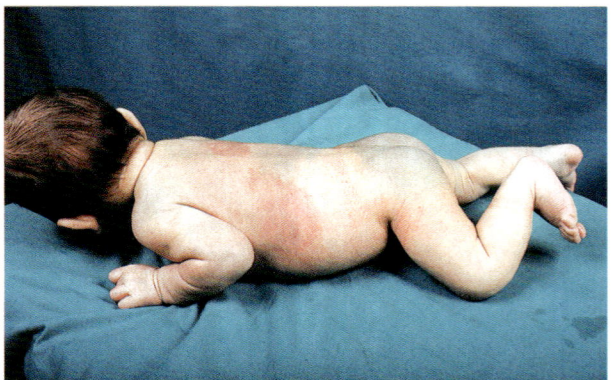

Figure 20.58

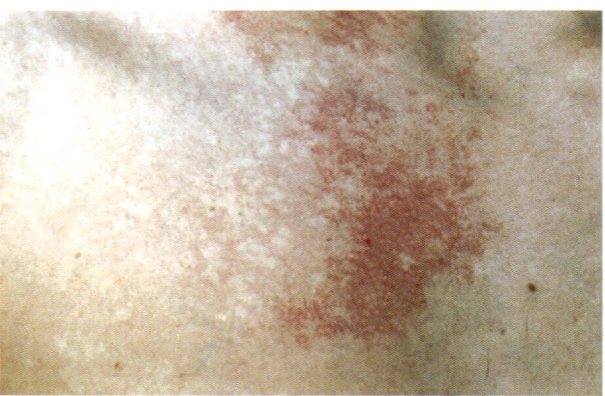

Figure 20.60

Genetics and pathogenesis

- Classic example of 'twin-spotting' phenomenon (see Chapter 25 'Cutaneous mosaicism')
- Sporadic cases, even if, theoretically, paradominant inheritance should be considered

Follow-up and therapy

- Laser and surgery for esthetic reasons
- UV protection for speckled lentiginous nevus to prevent risk of cancer

Differential diagnosis

- Phakomatosis pigmentokeratotica
- Syndromes with PWS

REFERENCES

Bielsa I, Paradelo C, Ribera M, Ferrandiz C. Generalized nevus spilus and nevus amemicus in patient with a primary lymphedema: a new type of phakomatosis pigmentovascularis? Pediatr Dermatol 1998; 15: 293–5

Di Landro A, Tadini GL, Marchesi L, Cainelli T. Phakomatosis pigmentovascualris: a new case with renal angiomas and some considerations about the classification. Pediatr Dermatol 1999; 16: 25–30

Van Gysel D, Oranje AP, Stroink H, Simonsz HJ. Phakomatosis pigmentovascularis. Pediatr Dermatol 1996; 13: 33–5

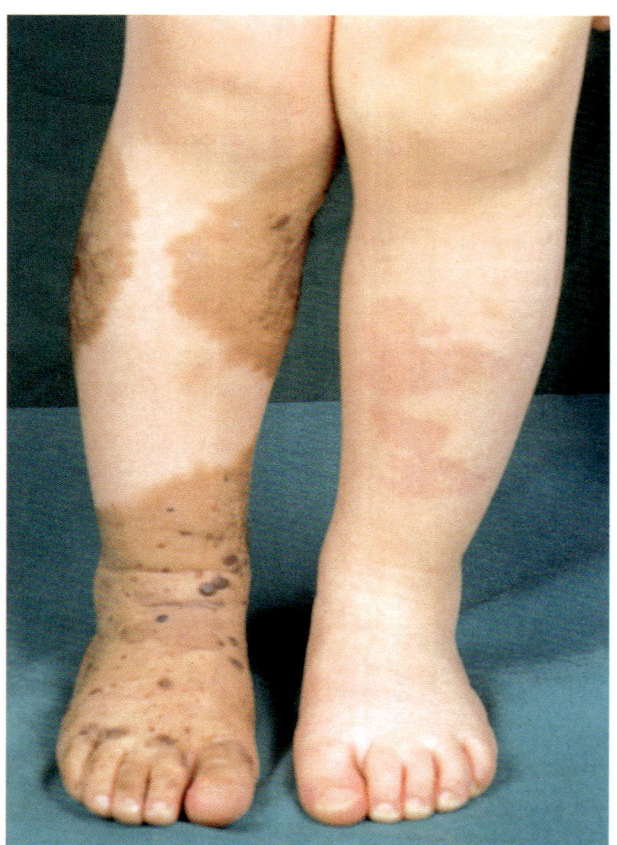

Figure 20.59

Laboratory findings

There are none specific.

LYMPHEDEMA

Synonyms

- Milroy's disease
- Milroy–Meige–Nonne disease
- Primary lymphedema

Age of onset

- Congenital (10%)
- Before the age of 35 (80%): lymphedema praecox
- After the age of 35 (10%): lymphedema tarda
- 70% of patients are female

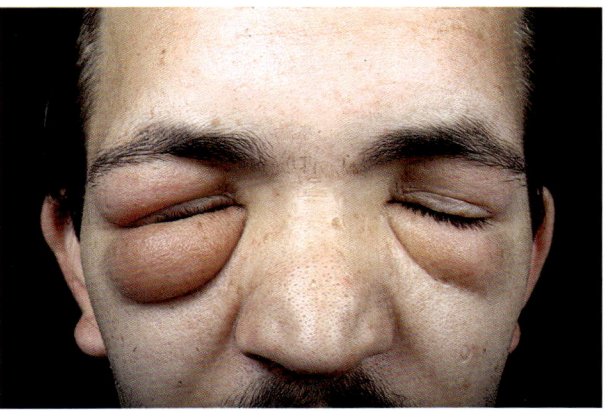

Figure 20.61

Clinical findings

In the early stages the edema is pitting and becomes firmer with the development of fibrosis; subsequently the skin increases in thickness and develops hyperkeratosis and a warty appearance.

The commonest localizations are the face (Figure 20.61), extremities (Figure 20.62) and genitalia; legs are involved in 80% of cases and in 70% only one extremity is involved initially.

Associations

- Hyper- or hypotrichosis
- Congenital malformations
- Yellow-nail syndrome
- Xanthomatous deposits

Course and complications

The disease is lifelong and usually progressive.

- Secondary infections (20%)
- Development of lymphangiosarcoma

Laboratory investigations and data

- Lymphangiography

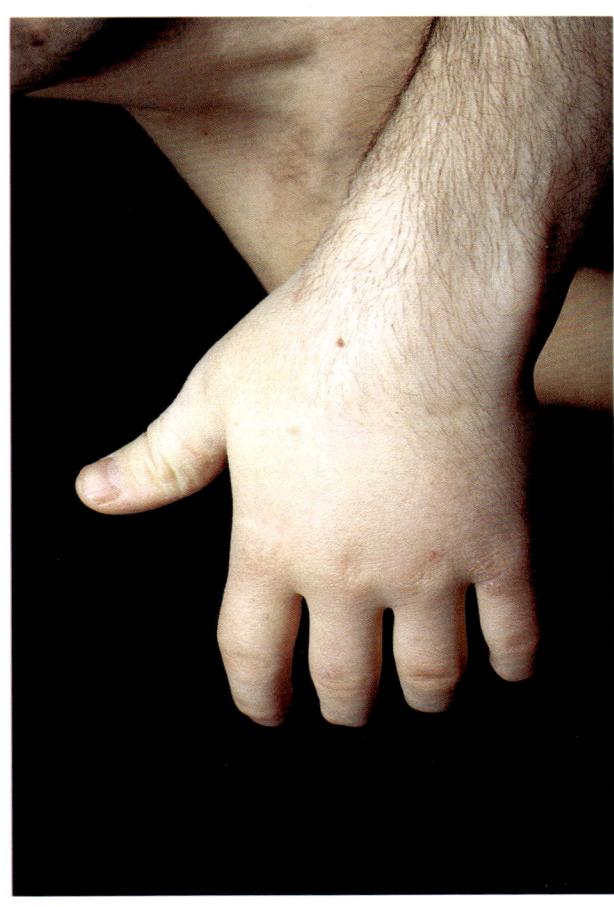

Figure 20.62

Genetics and pathogenesis

- Autosomal dominant inheritance
- Pathogenesis depends on aplasia/hypoplasia of lymphatics
- Vascular endothelial growth factor may be involved

Differential diagnosis

- Secondary lymphedema (infections, traumas, etc.)
- Idiopathic edema in women

- Secretan's syndrome
- Proteus syndrome
- Melkersson–Rosenthal syndrome

Follow-up and therapy

- Exercises to reduce venous pressure and drain lymphatic fluid
- Massage
- Compression
- Protection against infections

REFERENCES

Harwood CE, Mortimer PS. Causes and clinical manifestations of lymphatic failure. Clin Dermatol 1995; 13: 459–71

Offori TW, Platt CC, Stephens M, et al. Angiosarcoma in congenital hereditary lymphoedema (Milroy's disease): diagnostic beacons and a review of the literature. Clin Exp Dermatol 1993; 18: 174–7

Ruocco V, Schwartz RA, Ruocco E. Lymphedema: an immunologically vulnerable site for development of neoplasms. J Am Acad Dermatol 2002; 47: 124–7

GENERALIZED CYANOSIS, PHLEBECTASES AND SOFT SKIN SYNDROME

This is a previously undescribed syndrome characterized by a progressive reddish-blue hue of the entire skin, but especially of the extremities (arms, legs, neck and face), and abnormal soft skin, present in one large Italian pedigree through four generations.

Clinical findings

- Slowly progressive generalized cyanosis, starting within the first 2 years of life, involving the whole body surface with exacerbation on the face, neck arms and legs (Figures 20.63–68)
- Soft-touch skin, similar to that present in Ehlers–Danlos syndrome
- The color of the skin becomes progressively darker, reaching blue hues that readily disappear with pressure (Figures 20.64–20.66)

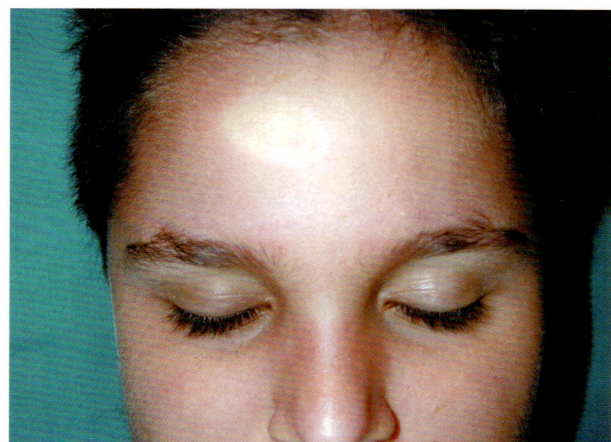

Figure 20.63

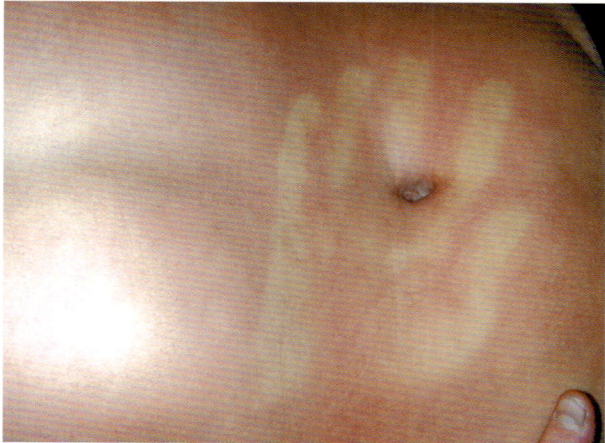

Figure 20.64

Vascular disorders   323

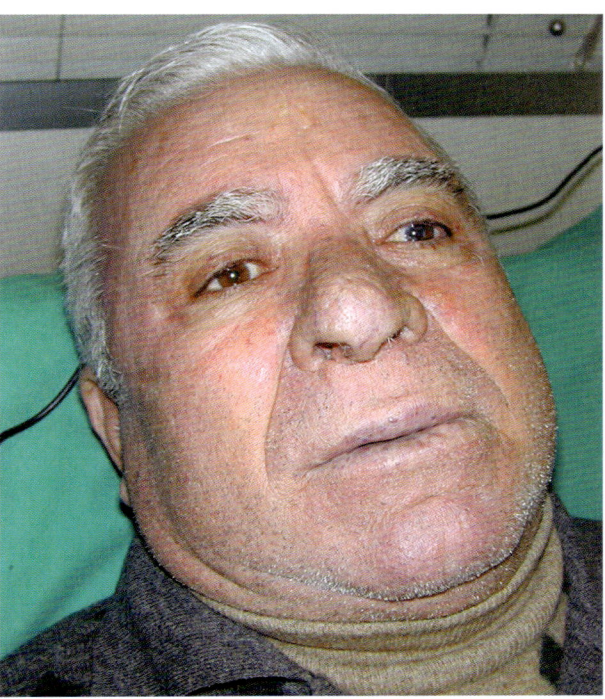

Figure 20.65

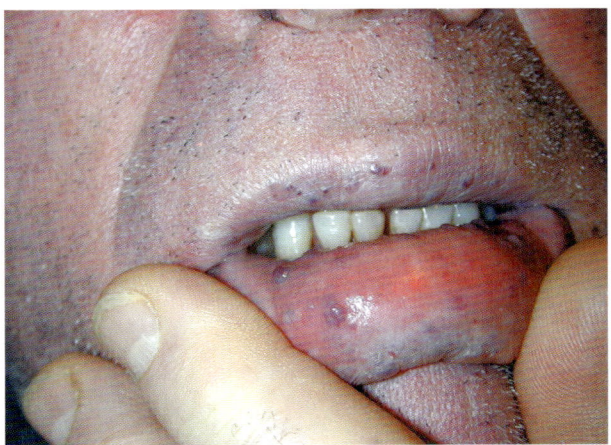

Figure 20.66

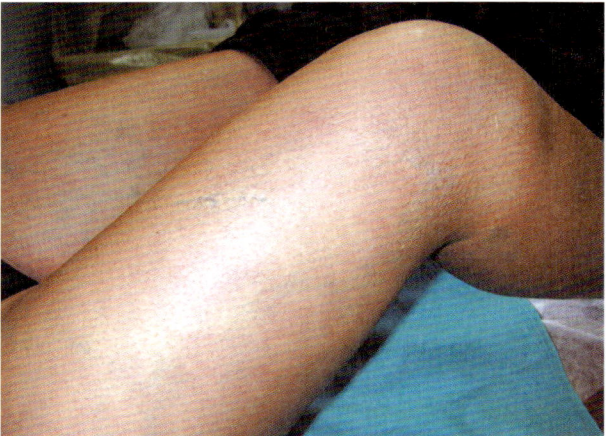

Figure 20.67

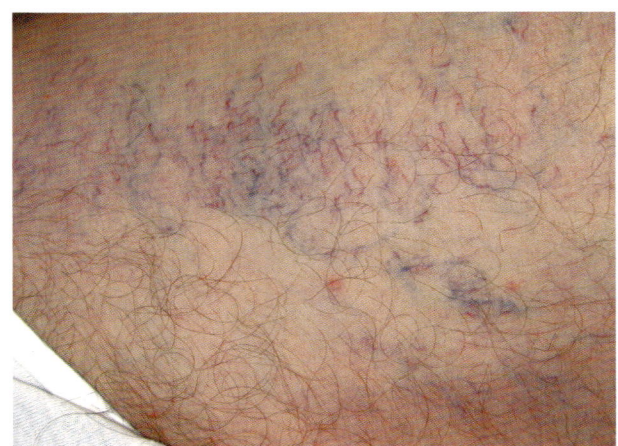

Figure 20.68

- Telangiectases and dilated venous blood vessels
- Adults present with phlebectases on lips and oral mucosa (20.66)
- In adulthood, lips may become hypertrophic

Extracutaneous findings

- In one patient hyponatremic episodes and hypertension
- Autoimmune thyroid diseases in thee out of ten patients
- No localizations of internal vascular anomalies can be found an Doppler ultrasonography

Course and prognosis

- The disease is slowly progressive with age, with worsening probably due to exposure to UV
- The disease seems to be not life-threatening

Laboratory investigations

- MRI and angio-MRI excludes internal vascular malformation
- Conventional histology shows abnormalities of elastic fibers

Genetics and pathogenesis

- The examination of the pedigree shows clearly that this syndrome is autosomal dominant
- The color of the skin indicates the capillarovenous origin of the cyanosis

Follow-up and therapy

- Photoprotection

Differential diagnosis

- Port-wine stains
- Sturge–Weber–Klippel–Trénaunay syndrome
- Louis–Bar syndrome
- Ehlers–Danlos IV

REFERENCE

Previously undescribed disease

GLOMUVENOUS MALFORMATION

Synonym

- Familial glomangiomas

Epidemiology

The disease is uncommon.

Age of onset

- Often present at birth

Clinical findings

- Multiple, red to purple-bluish nodular lesions preferentially located on the extremities (Figure 20.69)
- Lesions are painful and cannot be emptied using compression

Extracutaneous symptoms

- None

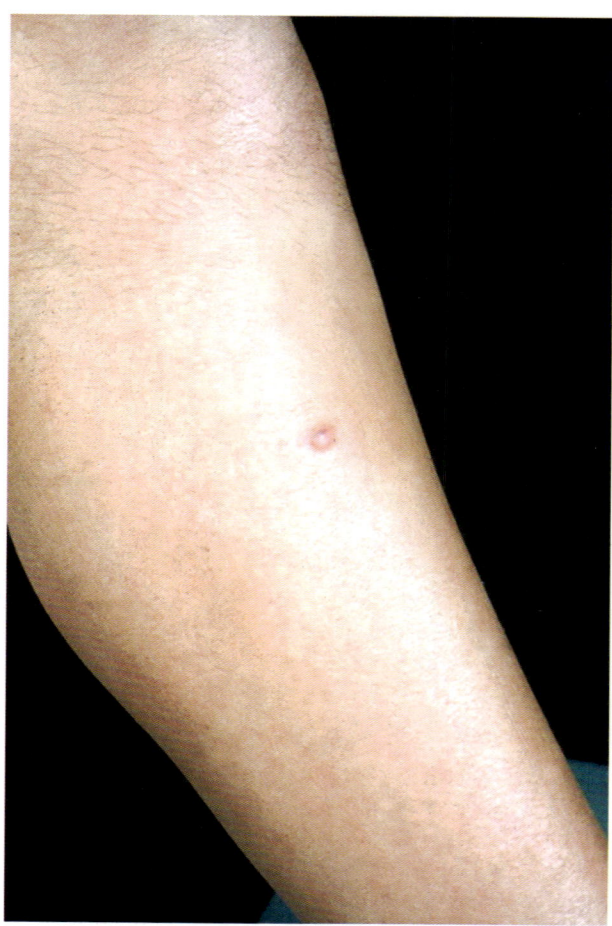

Figure 20.69

Course and prognosis

- Nodular lesions may merge into small plaques with cobblestone appearance and hyperkeratotic surface

Laboratory findings

- At histopathological examination, lesions involve cutis and subcutis

Genetics and pathogenesis

- The disease is autosomal dominant, with many sporadic cases
- The responsible gene is called GLMN (glomulin) located on chromosome 1
- One patient is reported to have paradominant (one germline and a 'second hit' somatic mutation) mode, with a complete localized loss of function of the involved gene. This finding may also explain the different extent of the disease even in patients belonging to the same pedigree

Follow-up and therapy

- Surgery or laser therapy

Differential diagnosis

- Blue rubber bleb nevus
- Subungual solitary glomus tumors
- Sporadic venous malformations
- Cutaneomucosal venous malformation
- Cutaneous and cerebral venous malformation syndrome due to mutation of KRIT 1 gene

REFERENCES

Arai T, Kasper JS, Skaar JR, et al. Targeted disruption of p185/Cul7 gene results in abnormal vascular morphogenesis. Proc Natl Acad Sci USA 2003; 100: 9855–60

Boon LM, Mulliken JB, Enjolras O, Vikkula M. Glomuvenous malformation (glomangioma) and venous malformation: distinct clinicopathologic and genetic entities. Arch Dermatol 2004; 140: 971–6

Brouillard P, Ghassibe M, Penington A, et al. Four common glomulin mutations cause two-thirds of glomuvenous malformations ('familial glomangiomas'): evidence for a founder effect. J Med Genet 2005; 42: e13

CHAPTER 21

Metabolic disease

PORPHYRIA CUTANEA TARDA AND HEPATOERYTHROPOIETIC PORPHYRIA

Epidemiology

Porphyria cutanea tarda (PCT) is frequent and often underestimated. Hepatoerythropoietic porphyria (HEP) is rare.

Age of onset

- Usually during the fourth decade of life
- In homozygous patients symptoms are visible within the first decade (HEP)

Clinical findings

In PCT, hyperfragility in sun-exposed areas leads to vesicobullous lesions after even minor trauma (dorsa of the hands, forearms, face and ears) (Figure 21.1)

- Blisters evolve in erosions, leaving milia and scarring (Figure 21.2)
- Malar and periorbital hypertrichosis is common, with facial hirsutism even in females (Figures 21.3 and 21.4)
- Hyperpigmentation of different degrees in sun-exposed areas occurs without photosensitivity
- In men, large and dark comedones may appear in malar areas (Figure 21.4)

In HEP, clinical manifestations are precocious and severe, with relevant ultraviolet (UV) light hypersensitivity, cutaneous fragility, bullae and erosions (Figure 21.5). During adulthood sclerodermiform changes, scarring, atrophy and scleromalacia lead to a clinical picture resembling Gunther's disease (Figures 21.6–21.8).

Extracutaneous symptoms

- Hepatic involvement, due to extragenetic factors such as alcohol abuse, hepatitis C virus (HCV) infection or estrogens

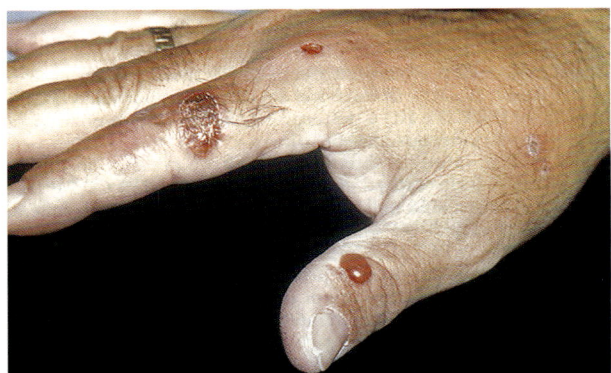

Figure 21.1

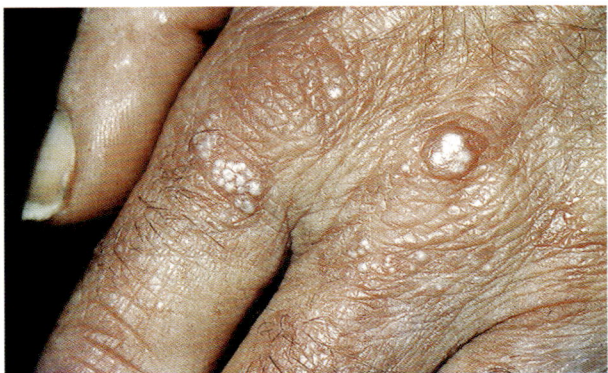

Figure 21.2

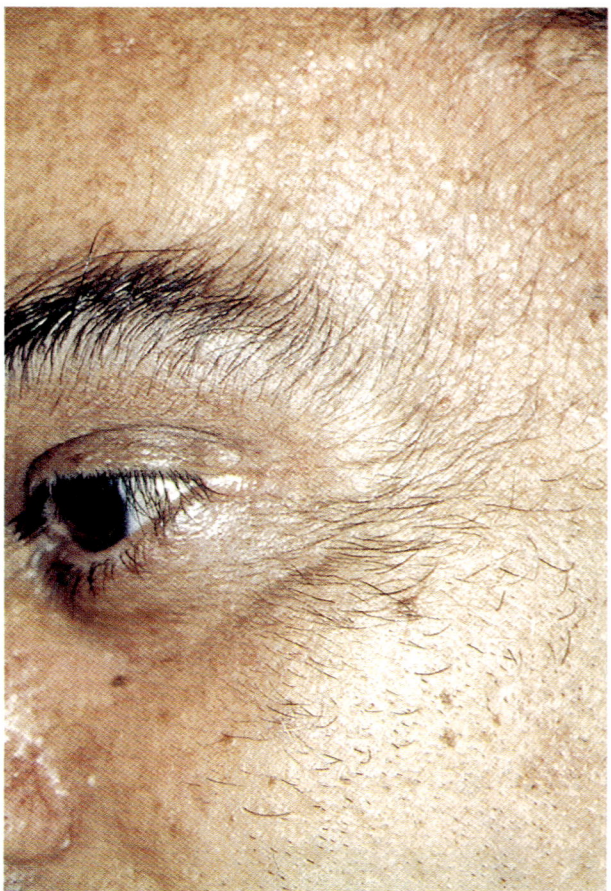

Figure 21.3

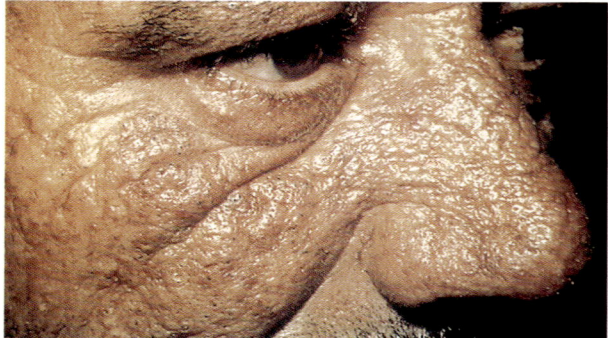

Figure 21.4

- Hypersideremia
- Glucose intolerance
- Human immunodeficiency virus (HIV) infection may trigger PCT

Course and complications

- Chronic actinic dermatosis with plicae on the face and cutis rhomboidalis nuchae
- Sclerodermatous changes in homozygous patients (Figure 21.7 and seleromelacia 21.8)
- Cutaneous calcinosis (Figure 21.9)

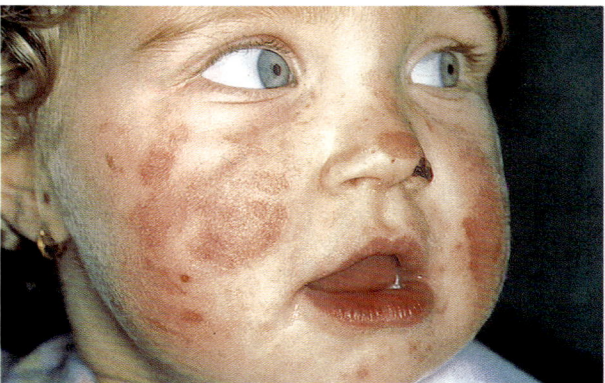

Figure 21.5

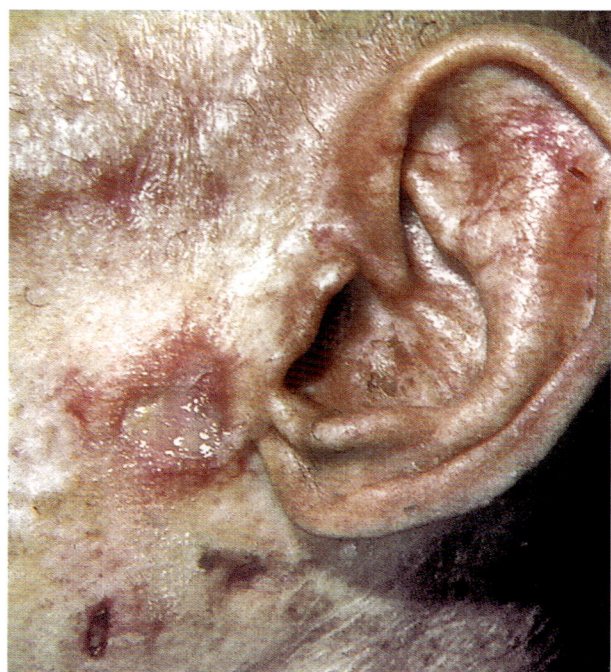

Figure 21.6

- Cicatricial alopecia (Figure 21.10)
- Hepatic cirrhosis and hepatocarcinomas

Laboratory findings

- Dark urine ('coca-cola like') with fluorescence
- Highly characteristic presence of isocoproporphyrin in the feces
- Hepatic metabolism is altered, with high levels of transaminase
- Sideremia is usually high (many patients are carriers of hemochromatosis gene defects)
- Hyperglycemia

Genetics and pathogenesis

PCT is due to genetic defects in the uroporphyrinogen decarboxylase gene (point mutations and deletions)

Metabolic disease 329

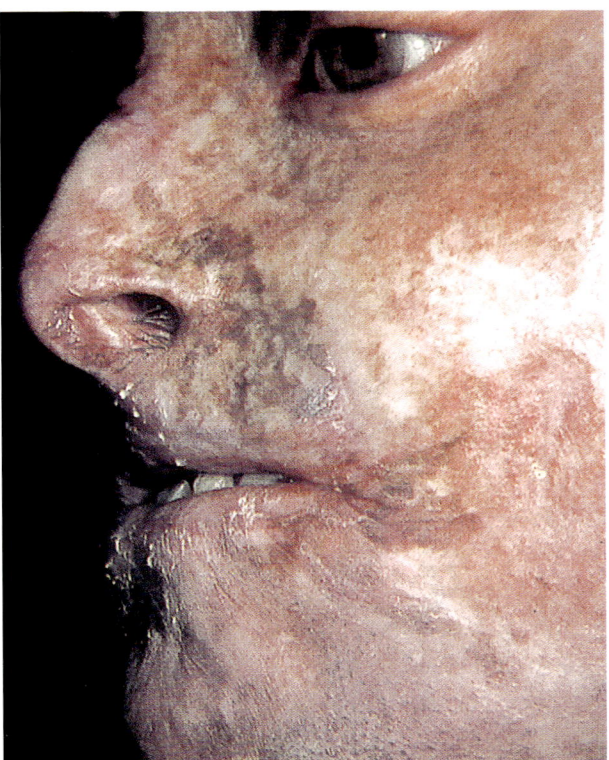

Figure 21.7

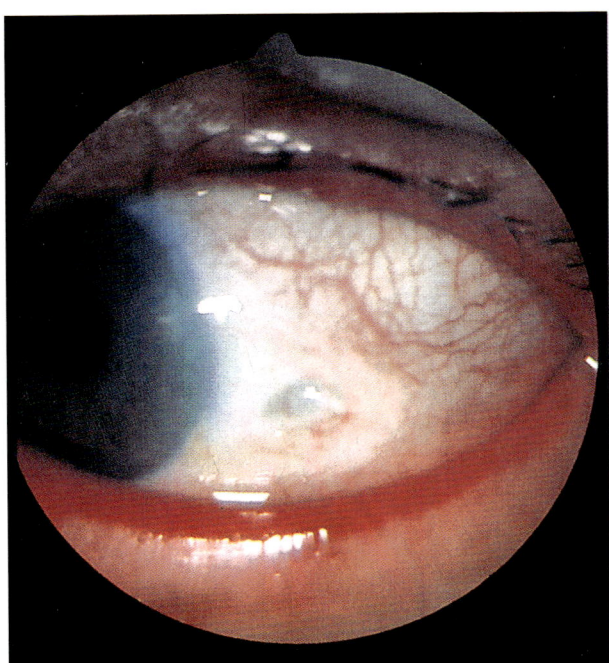

Figure 21.8

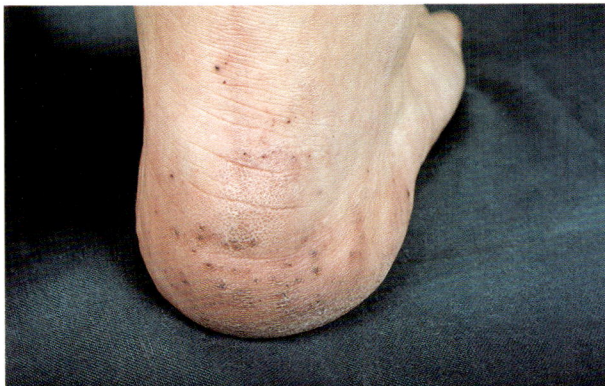

Figure 21.9

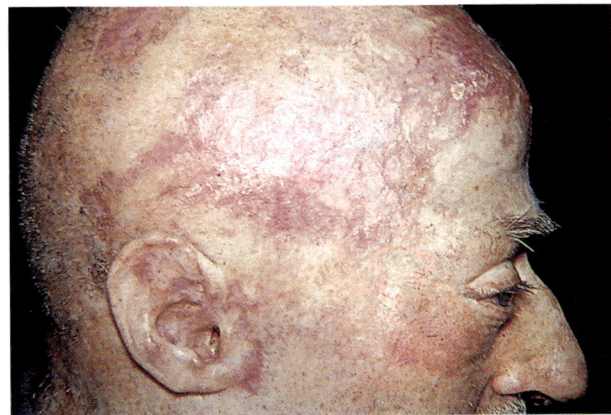

Figure 21.10

Follow-up and therapy

- Photoprotection!
- Phlebotomy (300–500 cm^3)
- Chloroquine (100 mg twice a week)
- Hepatology unit to manage liver disease progression

Differential diagnosis

- Remember that mixed porphyrias, such as variegated porphyria and hereditary coproporphyria, may have similar cutaneous lesions associated with abdominal acute pain
- Epidermolysis bullosa
- Kindler's disease
- Acquired PCT (HIV associated, drug associated, dialysis associated)

that decrease, but do not abolish, the activity of the enzyme.

HEP represents the rare double-heterozygous or homozygous form of the same genetic defect in which the activity of the enzyme is absent or greatly reduced.

REFERENCE

Ged C, Ozalla D, Herrero C, et al. Description of a new mutation in hepatoerythropoietic porphyria and prenatal exclusion of a homozygous fetus. Arch Dermatol 2002; 138: 957–60

ERYTHROPOIETIC PROTOPORPHYRIA

Epidemiology

This represents the more common pediatric porphyria. No data are available on prevalence and incidence.

Age of onset

- Usually within the first 4 years of life until adolescence

Cutaneous findings

- Acute photosensitivity with erythema, edema and rarely purpuric lesions after UV (natural and artificial light) exposure (face, hands and ears), with heat and burning sensations resulting in pruritus ('sunburnt face' with 'papillon' erythema sparing eyelids and philtrum) (Figures 21.11 and 21.12)
- Vesicobullous lesions after prolonged exposure, with fever and malaise
- Later in life there may be thickening of the skin of the face (Figure 21.13) and dorsa of the hands
- Fissurative radial lesions of the lips and face (Figure 21.14) are characteristic
- Cribriform scars are visible on the nose
- Cerebriform thickening of the pads (Figure 21.15)

Extracutaneous symptoms

- Hepatic involvement with rare fibrosis, and cirrhotic changes with acute hepatic failure and severe jaundice
- Cholestasis and gall-bladder stones in 10%
- Anemia in 20%
- Pseudogottous lesions of the hands in a small percentage of patients (Figure 21.15)
- Rarely, acute psychiatric symptoms

Course and prognosis

- The disease starts with aspecific signs of photophobia and mild photosensitivity and may be misdiagnosed for a long time
- Progressive worsening of skin signs is discussed above
- Liver insufficiency may lead to severe hepatic disease in 1–5% of patients

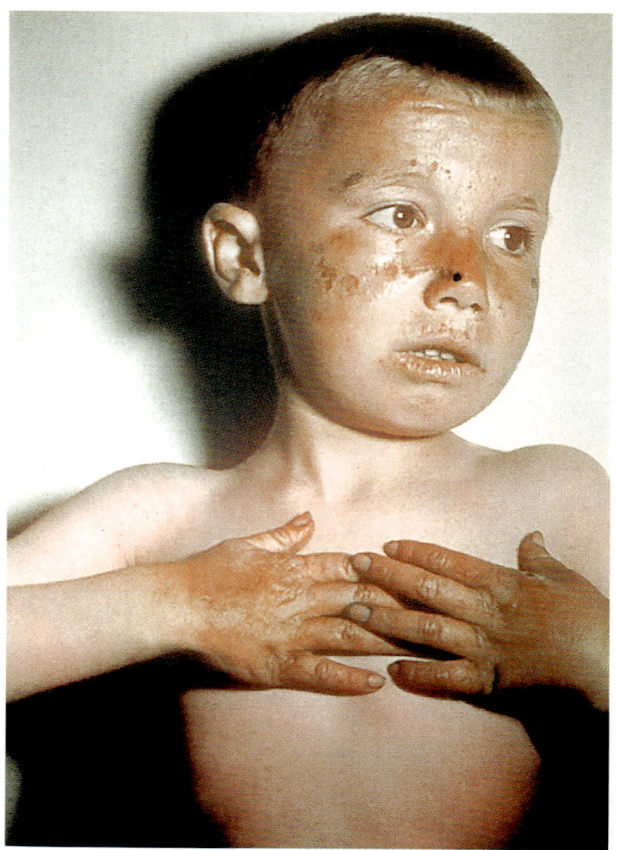

Figure 21.11

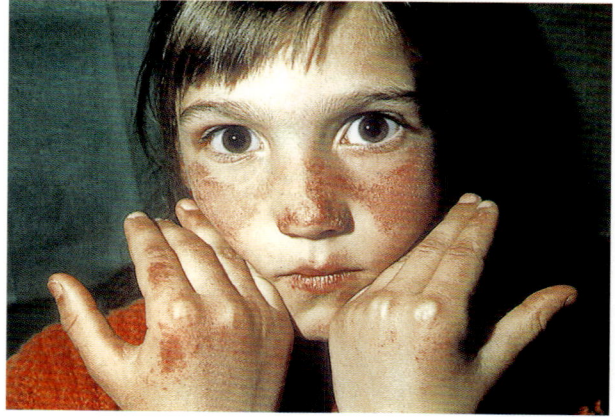

Figure 21.12

Laboratory findings

Urine porphyrins are normal but conversely higher in stool plasma and red blood series cells (protoporphyrins).

Genetics and pathogenesis

Mutations of the gene that synthesizes for the ferrochelatase enzyme are responsible for the disease.

Metabolic disease

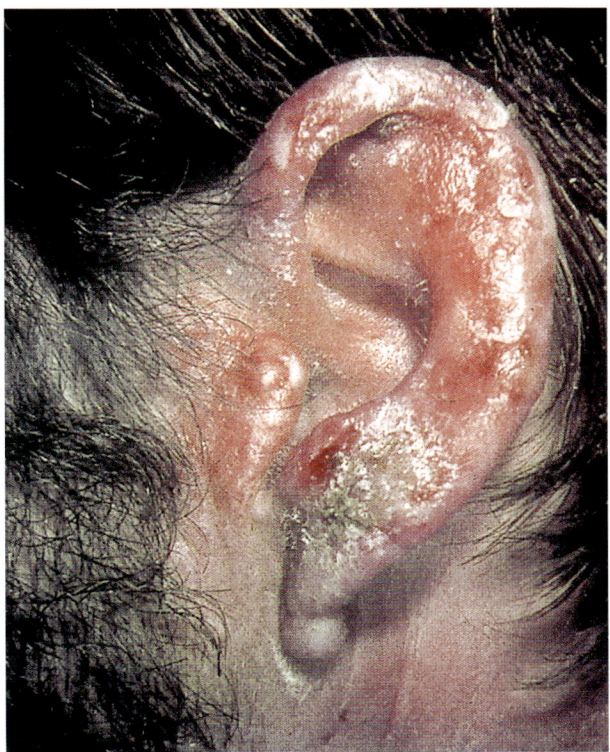

Figure 21.13

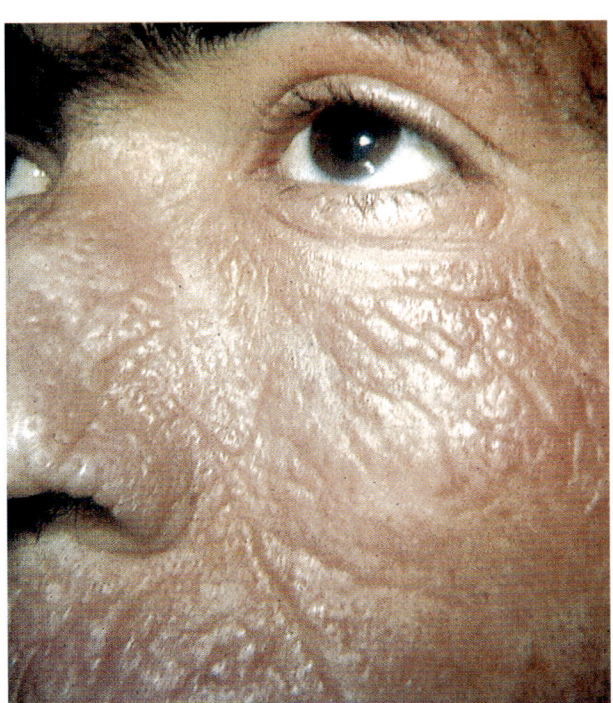

Figure 21.14

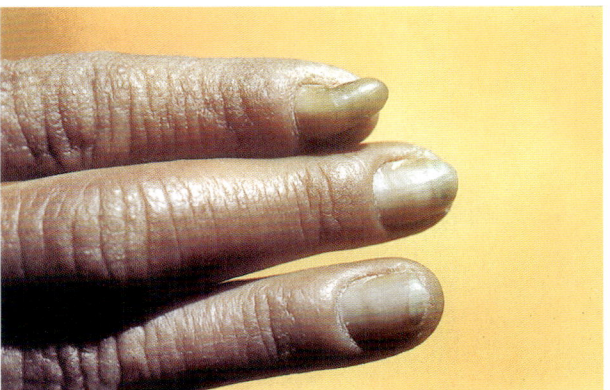

Figure 21.15

Follow-up and therapy

- Prevention of UV damage
- Hepatic function should be checked in all patients
- β-Carotenes to prevent UV damage
- Blood transfusions and plasmapheresis may be useful
- Drug therapy is controversial (bile salts, chelators)

Differential diagnosis

- Other porphyrias
- Kindler's disease
- Epidermolysis bullosa
- Polymorphous light eruption

REFERENCE

Wiman A, Floderus Y, Harper P. Novel mutations and phenotype effect of the splice site modulator IVS3-49C in nine Swedish families with erythropoietic protoporphyria. J Hum Genet 2003; 48: 70–6

ERYTHROPOIETIC PORPHYRIA

Synonym

- Gunther's disease

Epidemiology

This is a very rare disease; about 50 cases are reported in molecular biology studies.

Age of onset

- Rarely there are symptoms at birth
- Often signs are visible soon after first UV exposure

Clinical findings

- Extreme photosensitivity in sun-exposed areas (Figures 21.16 and 21.17)
- Erythema, vesicles, bullae and erosions on the face and hands (Figure 21.18)
- The skin of sun-exposed areas becomes progressively more severely affected, with ulcerations and scarring, severe loss of substance and amputations (nose, lips, fingers) (Figures 21.19 and 21.20)
- Hirsutism and sclerodermiform changes at involved sites
- Cutaneous calcinosis
- Nail dystrophy
- Scarring alopecia

Extracutaneous symptoms

- Teeth of both dentitions are grayish-red (erythrodontia) in color and are red-fluorescent under Wood's lamp (Figure 21.21)
- Recurrent conjunctivitis with scarring and pterygia formation is very common

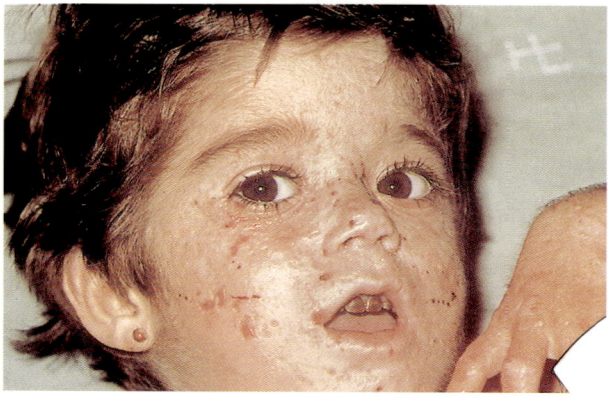

Figure 21.17

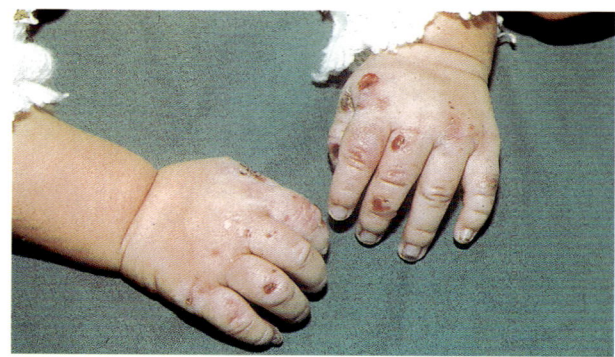

Figure 21.18

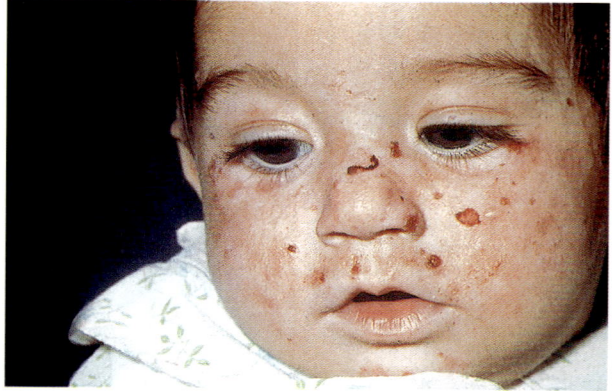

Figure 21.16

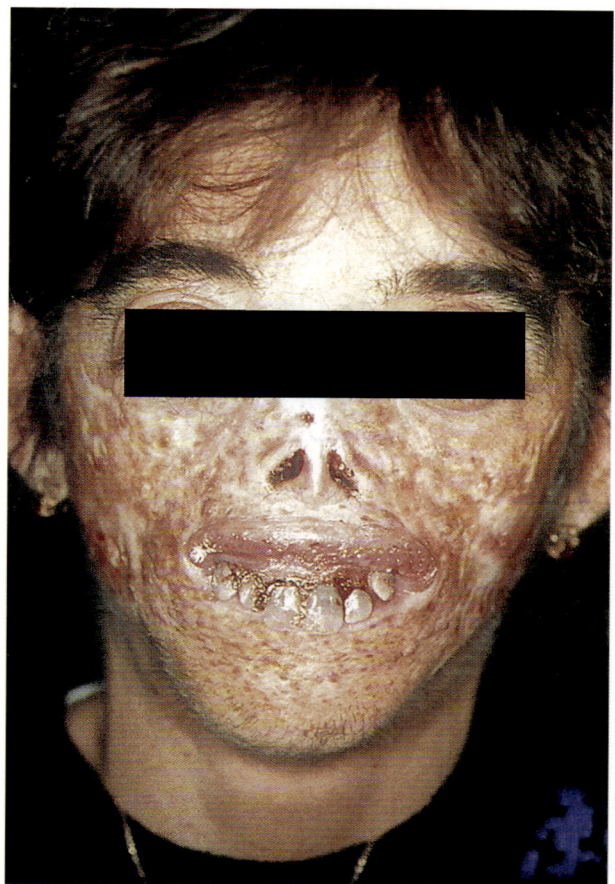

Figure 21.19

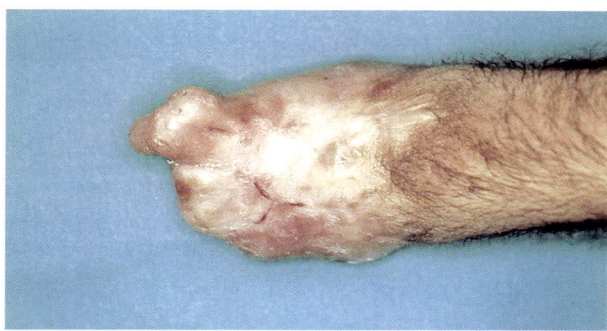

Figure 21.20

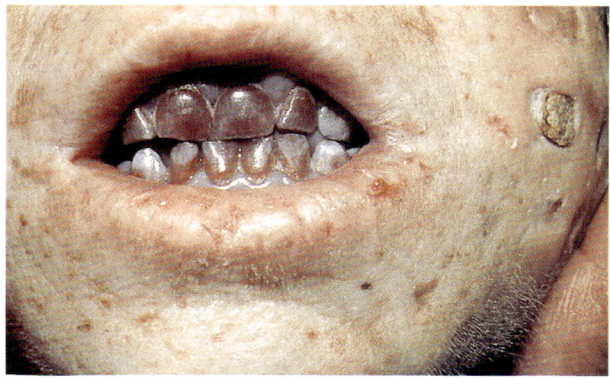

Figure 21.21

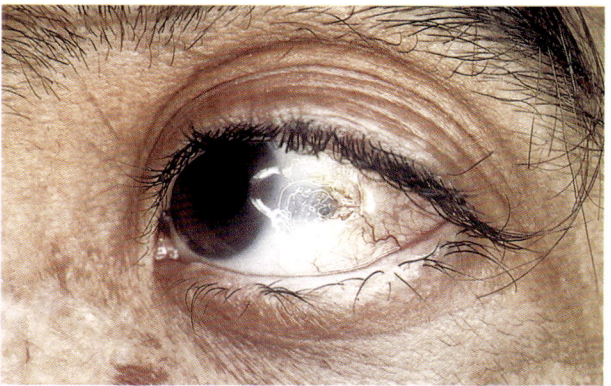

Figure 21.22

- Wood's lamp is useful to detect less severe cases
- Accumulation of type I isomers, especially in bone marrow, can be documented

Genetics and pathogenesis

Mutations in the gene encoding uroporphyrinogen III co-synthetase are responsible for the disease.

Follow-up and therapy

- Prevention of UV irradiation
- Trauma prevention, with tutor, parent and patient advice, to reduce mutilations
- Hydroxyurea and vegetal carbons to reduce porphyrin synthesis
- Biphosphonates to reduce osteolysis
- Bone-marrow transplant from compatible donor
- Genetic therapy is under experimentation

Differential diagnosis

- Polymorphous light eruption
- Epidermolysis bullosa (Hallopeau–Siemens dermolytic forms)
- Kindler's disease
- Scleroderma
- Maffucci's disease

REFERENCES

Arne JL, Depeyre C, Lesueur L. [Corneoscleral involvement in congenital erythropoietic porphyria. Gunther disease.] J Fr Ophthalmol 2003; 26: 498–502

Ged C, Megarbane H, Chouery E, et al. Congenital erythropoietic porphyria: report of a novel mutation with absence of clinical manifestations in a homozygous mutant sibling. J Invest Dermatol 2004; 123: 589–91

- Scleromalacia perforans is characteristic (Figure 21.22)
- Urine is dark and shows red fluorescence when exposed to UV light
- Deposition of pathologic porphyrins in red blood cells is highly characteristic, leading to hemolysis that can occur suddenly after UV exposure
- Anemia with jaundice and splenomegaly, hepatic involvement and renal failure
- Acro-osteolysis, osteoporosis and pathologic fractures due to deposition of porphyrins in osseous tissue

Course and complications

- Scars originate from bullous lesions, progressively worsen and lead to fibrosis, retractions and mutilations of the phalanges, nose tip, lips, eyelids and ears
- Face and hand mutilations are so severe in homozygous patients as to impede a normal social life
- Rarely, neoplastic changes in scarring areas
- Life span is reduced (renal and hepatic failure, acute hemolysis)

Laboratory findings

- Anemia, hepatic and renal functions are detected by routine tests

ACRODERMATITIS ENTEROPATHICA

Synonyms

- Brandt's syndrome
- Danbolt–Closs syndrome

Age of onset

- After weaning
- Infancy

Clinical findings

Skin and mucosal lesions (Figures 21.23–21.25)

- Crops of vesicles and pustules evolving in erythematous psoriasiform plaques involving periorificial areas, distal extremities and scalp. Distribution is symmetrical
- Alopecia of scalp, eyebrows and eyelashes
- Nail dystrophy and paronychia
- Stomatitis, glossitis, perlèche

Extracutaneous symptoms

- Severe and persistent diarrhea
- Failure to thrive and retardation of growth
- Apathy, irritability, mental retardation
- Blepharitis, conjunctivitis, photophobia

Complications

There can be secondary infection by bacteria and *Candida* species.

Course

The disease is persistent, with periods of remission and exacerbation.

Laboratory findings

- Low serum zinc level (less than 50 mg/dl)
- Low serum alkaline phosphatase levels
- Histopathologic features: marked ballooning of keratinocytes in the upper part of the epidermis, hypogranulosis and parakeratosis

Genetics and pathogenesis

- Autosomal recessive disease
- Mutations in the gene called SLC39A4 underlie the disease, affecting transport activity and zinc-responsive trafficking of zinc-binding proteins
- Genetic deficiency of zinc-binding ligands induces a deficit in zinc absorption when bovine milk is introduced and is responsible for low serum zinc level and typical phenotype
- Zinc is an indispensable constituent of over 200 metalloenzymes

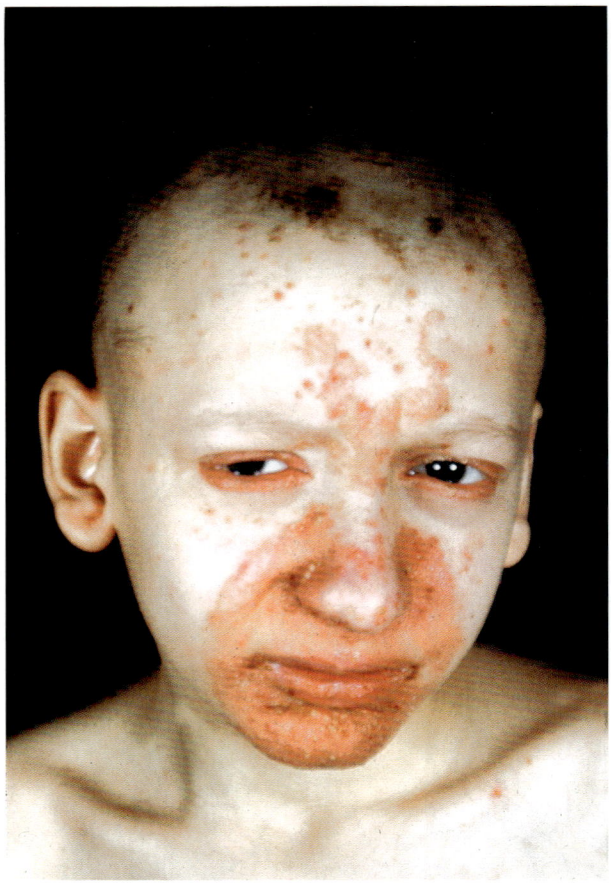

Figure 21.23

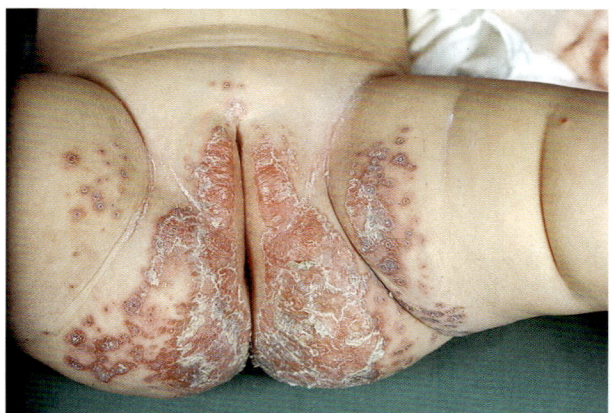

Figure 21.24

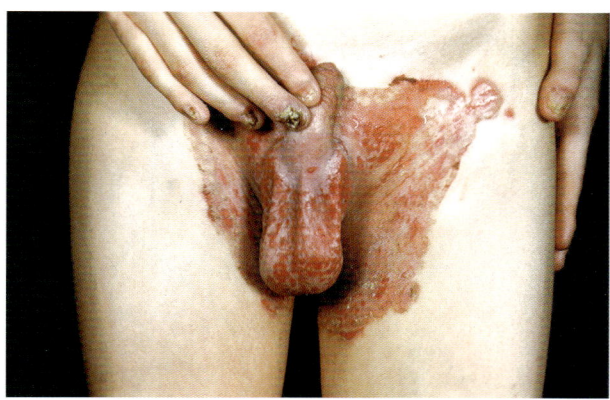

Figure 21.25

Differential diagnosis

- Widespread candidiasis
- Epidermolysis bullosa
- Glucagonoma syndrome
- Acquired zinc deficiencies

Follow-up and therapy

- Periodic measurements of zinc serum level to avoid hyperzincaemia
- Zinc sulfate or gluconate 5 mg/kg/day indefinitely
- Oral zinc supplementation induces a dramatic cessation of signs and symptoms within a few days and a normal life without sequelae
- Exacerbations during pregnancy

REFERENCES

Ben-Asher E, Lancet D. NIPBL gene responsible for Cornelia de Lange syndrome, a severe developmental disorder. Isr Med Assoc J 2004; 6: 571–2.

Kury S, Dreno B, Bezieau S, et al. Identification of SLC39A4, a gene involved in acrodermatitis enteropathica. Nature Genet 2002; 31: 239–40. Epub 2002 Jun 17

Kury S, Kharfi M, Kamoun R, et al. Mutation spectrum of human SLC39A4 in a panel of patients with acrodermatitis enteropathica. Hum Mutat 2003 Oct; 22: 337–8

Wang F, Kim BE, Dufner-Beattie JV Acrodermatitis enteropathica mutations affect transport activity, localization and zinc-responsive trafficking of the mouse ZIP4 zinc transporter. Hum Mol Genet 2004; 13: 563–71. Epub 2004 Jan 06

FABRY'S DISEASE

Synonyms

- Angiokeratoma corporis diffusum
- Fabry–Anderson disease

Epidemiology

Estimated prevalence 1 : 20 000 to 1 : 40 000 in Europe.

Age of onset

- First decade

Clinical findings

- Cutaneous lesions start as pointed erythematous macules that become progressively dark red or purple-blackish and larger papules scattered especially in the central body areas but also, less frequently, at other body sites (Figures 21.26 and 21.27)
- Slight hyperkeratosis gives the rough pattern to these lesions ('angio' + 'keratomas')
- Oral mucosa is involved (i.e. base of the tongue)
- Sometimes distal edema prior to renal involvement is described
- Alterations of peripheral nervous autonomic system can cause imbalance of thermoregulatory and vasomotor functions
- Presence of mosaic pattern distribution of angiokeratomas is visible in female carriers (buttocks, thighs and abdomen, rarely arms) (Figure 21.8)

Extracutaneous symptoms

- Dysesthesias and burning pain in hands and feet are often the first sign of the disease during the first decade of life and may precede cutaneous signs
- Episodes may be short- or long-lasting and may be associated with fever ('Fabry crises')
- Abdominal colic pain is common
- Headaches, migraine, vertigo and central hearing loss
- Secondary cerebrovascular thrombotic accidents
- Corneal opacities with a circular pattern; retinal angiomatous abnormalities
- Renal involvement is highly characteristic and severe
- Cardiac involvement, both valvular and conduction

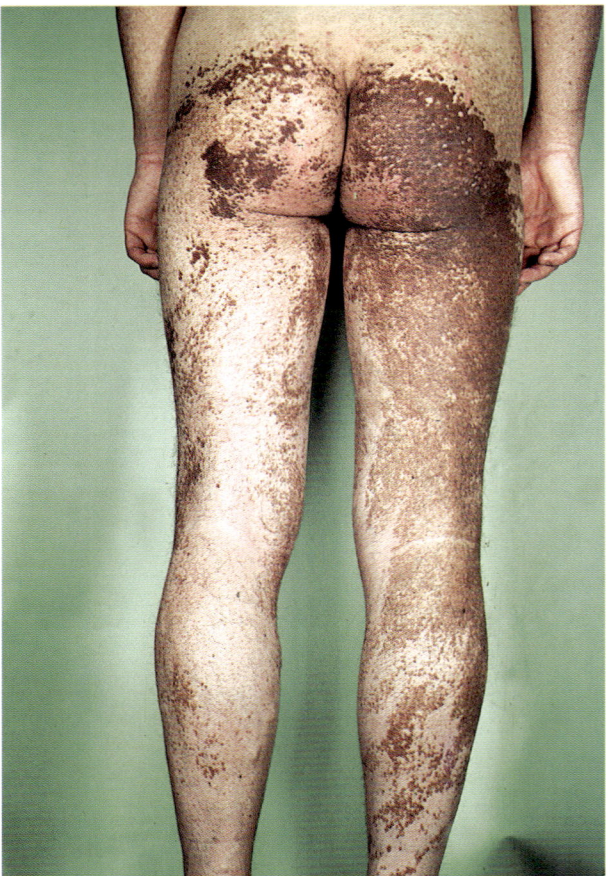

Figure 21.26

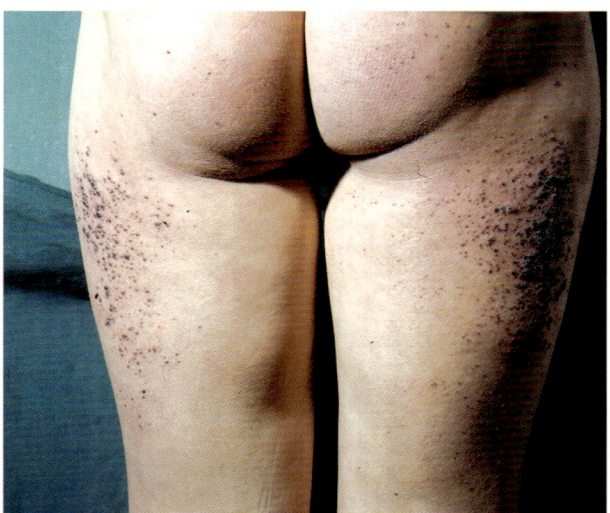

Figure 21.27

Course and complications

- Female carriers may show all the symptoms to an extent
- The disease is progressive and renal involvement is the major cause of death owing to untreatable renal failure

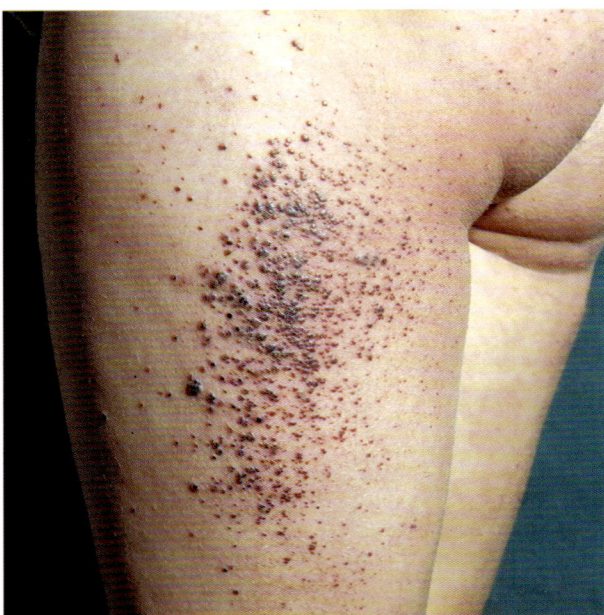

Figure 21.28

- Strokes and myocardial infarction are the second cause of premature death
- Life expectancy for males is the fourth decade

Laboratory investigations

- On electron microscopy examination of the skin, electron-dense bodies are visible in the cytoplasm of keratinocytes
- Enzyme assay can detect female carriers without cutaneous signs

Genetics and pathogenesis

- X-linked recessive
- Mosaic form is frequent in our experience; particular attention may be paid to genetic counseling in these cases
- The genetic defect is related to the gene that encodes α-galactosidase A
- Mutations cause storage of sphingolipids in almost all cells and are causative for the entire clinical spectrum of the disease
- The severity of the phenotype is related to the residual α-galactosidase A activity in each individual

Differential diagnosis

- Fucosidosis
- Gangliosidoses

- Galactosialidosis
- Porokeratosis of Mibelli
- Fordyce angiokeratomas
- Rendu–Osler syndrome
- Acute intermittent porphyria

Follow-up and therapy

The nephrologist has a pivotal role in the management of renal failure; transplantation gives controversial results in male patients.

Infusions of α-galactosidase have been introduced to treat Fabry's patients.

High doses of pure antidolorific agents may be helpful to reduce the painful paresthesias.

REFERENCES

Hopkin RJ, Bissier J, Grabowski GA. Comparative evaluation of alpha-galactosidase A infusions for treatment of Fabry disease. Genet Med 2003; 5: 144–53

Morrone A, Cavicchi C, Bardelli T, et al. Fabry disease: molecular studies in Italian patients and X inactivation analysis in manifesting carriers. J Med Genet 2003; 40: e103

Yasuda M, Shabbeer J, Osawa M, Desnick RJ. Fabry disease: novel alpha-galactosidase A 3'-terminal mutations result in multiple transcripts due to aberrant 3'-end formation. Am J Hum Genet 2003; 73: 162–73

SEA-BLUE HISTIOCYTOSIS

Age of onset

- First or second decade of life

Clinical findings

Cutaneous manifestations (present in about 30% of patients)

- Maculonodular lesions scattered on the face, trunk, hands and feet (Figure 21.29)
- The prominent cutaneous features consist of eyelid infiltration and facial waxy plaques resulting in a puffy appearance (Figures 21.30 and 21.31)

Extracutaneous manifestations

- Hepatosplenomegaly
- Lymphadenopathies
- Hemorrhagic diathesis

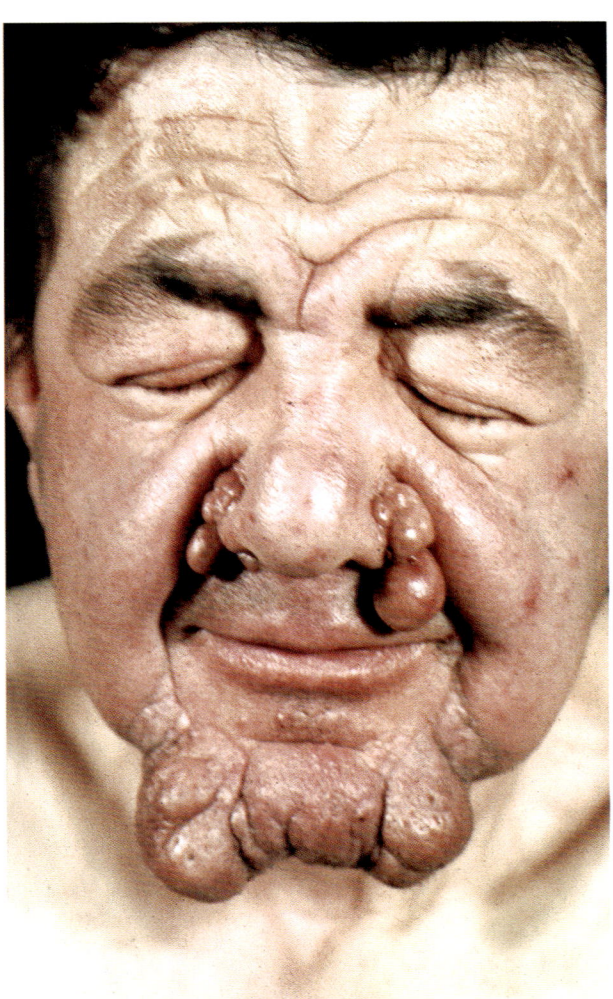

Figure 21.29

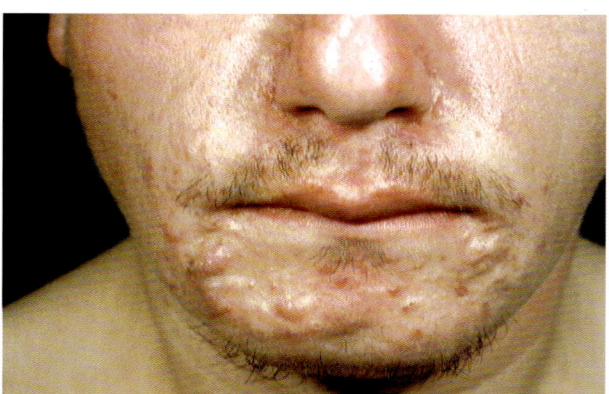

Figure 21.30

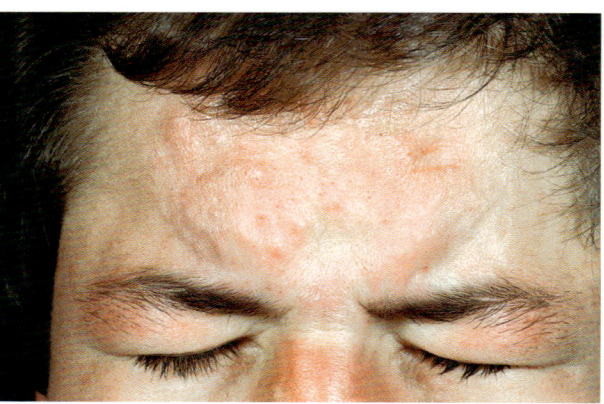

Figure 21.31

- Lung infiltrate
- Nervous system involvement
- Thrombocytopenia

Course

The disease is progressive. Death is due to pulmonary or hepatic failure.

Laboratory investigations and data

Histopathologic findings include proliferation of large macrophages whose cytoplasm is filled with granules staining blue or blue-green with Giemsa.

Genetics and pathogenesis

- Autosomal recessive inheritance

- The granules of sea-blue histiocytes are constituted of a glycophospholipid representing the product of a peculiar storage process

Differential diagnosis

- Reticulohistiocytosis
- Nieman–Pick disease

Therapy

There is no treatment.

REFERENCE

Zina AM, Bundino S. Familial sea-blue histiocytosis with cutaneous involvement. A case report with ultrastructural findings. Br J Dermatol 1983; 108: 355–61

CEREBROTENDINOUS XANTHOMATOSIS

Synonym

- Cholestanolysis

Epidemiology

There are no data available in the literature. We have personally observed at least ten cases in a 25-year survey.

Age of onset

- During late childhood or even later in some pedigrees

Clinical findings

- Yellowish-orange or pink papules, nodules and plaques, especially on the extensor surfaces (knees, elbows, dorsa of hands) (Figures 21.1–21.5)
- Peculiar lesions over the tendons (Figure 21.6)
- Xanthelasmas

Extracutaneous findings

- Atherosclerosis in all regions, leading to:
  - angina and myocardial infarction
  - central nervous system (CNS) involvement with progressive mental retardation, ataxia and atrophy due to extensive demyelinization
  - early-onset cataracts
  - ovarian abnormalities
- Personal observation of xanthomatosis with biliary atresia and cirrhosis

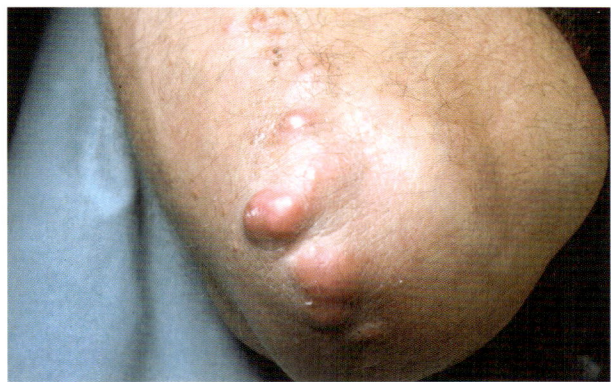

Figure 21.33

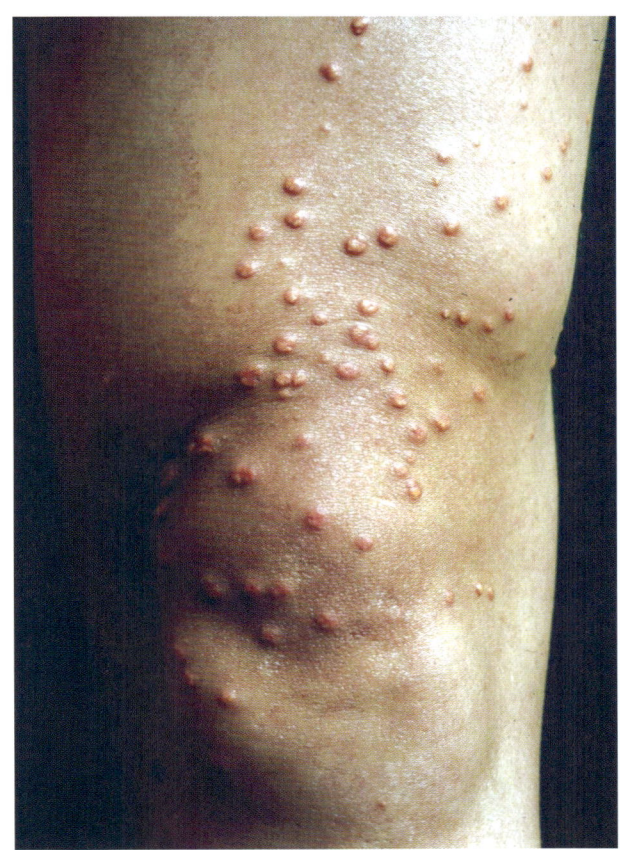

Figure 21.34

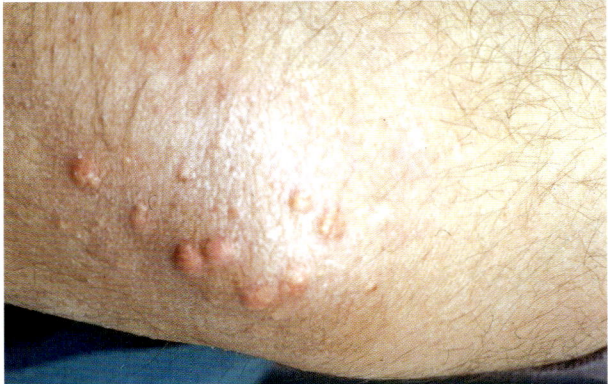

Figure 21.32

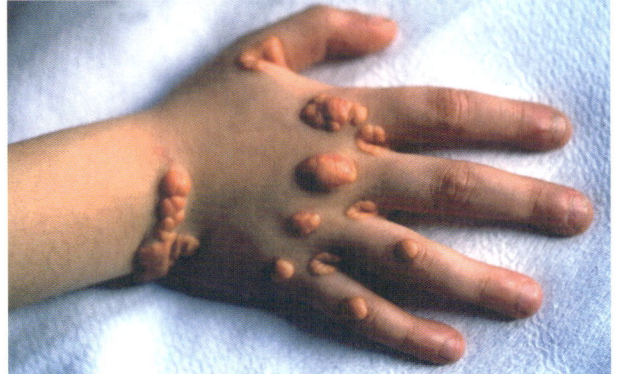

Figure 21.35

340 Atlas of Genodermatoses

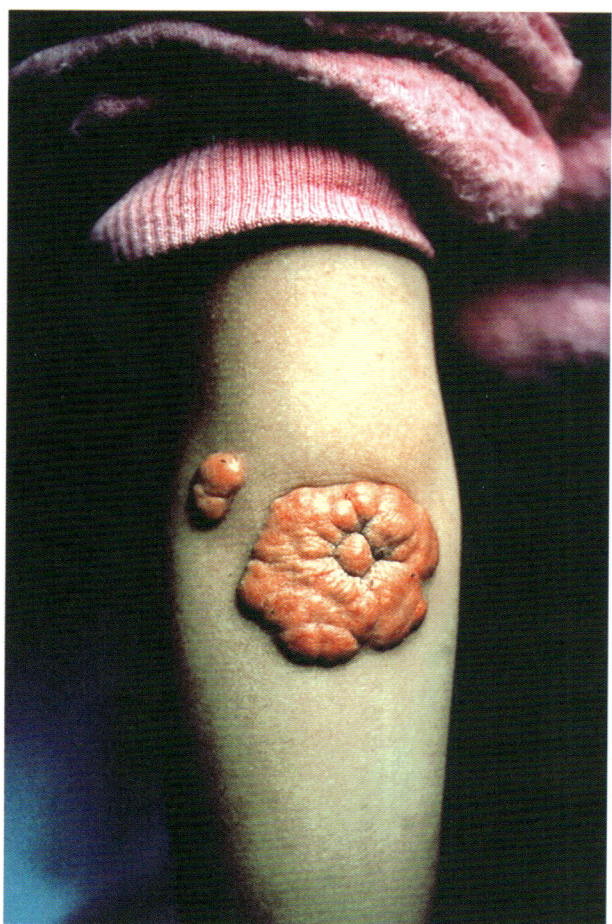

Figure 21.36

Figure 21.37

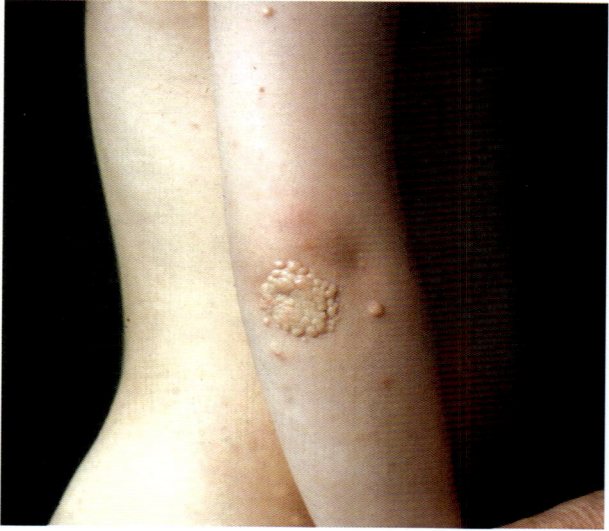

Figure 21.38

Course and prognosis

The life span is reduced. The major causes of premature death are myocardial infarction and stroke.

Laboratory findings

- Large and light histiocytes with crystals of cholestanol in the dermis upon electron microscopic examination

Genetics and pathogenesis

The disease is autosomal recessive. Mutations have been established in the CYP27 gene encoding a sterol 27-hydroxylase enzyme.

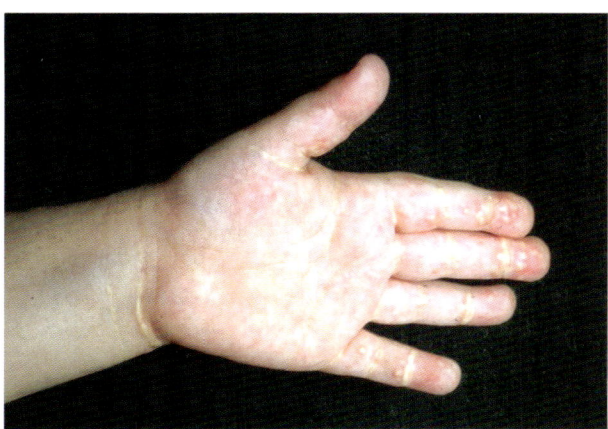

Figure 21.39

Follow-up and therapy

- Cardiologic and neurologic examinations are mandatory, in order to prevent major events
- A few trials with biliary acid are reported
- Statins may be helpful

Differential diagnosis

- Familial hyperlipoproteinemias

REFERENCES

Bartholdi D, Zumsteg D, Verrips A, et al. Spinal phenotype of cerebrotendinous xanthomatosis – a pitfall in the diagnosis of multiple sclerosis. J Neurol 2004; 251: 105–7

Federico A, Dotti MT. Cerebrotendinous xanthomatosis: clinical manifestations, diagnosis criteria, pathogenesis, and therapy. J Child Neurol 2003; 18: 633–8

Mak CM, Lam KS, Tan KC, et al. Cerebrotendinous xanthomatosis in a Hong Kong Chinese kinship with a novel splicing site mutation IVS6-1G>T in the sterol 27-hydroxylase gene. Mol Genet Metab 2004; 81: 144–6

PROLIDASE DEFICIENCY

Epidemiology

- About 50 patients reported worldwide

Age of onset

- During infancy or adolescence

Clinical findings

- Purpuric rashes
- Chronic infiltrated eczematous-like dermatitis
- Recurrent ulcers (legs) (Figures 21.40–21.42)

Extracutaneous symptoms

- Recurrent infections and hyperimmunoglobulin E
- Psychomotor retardation
- Joint laxity

Course and prognosis

- The disease is progressive if untreated
- Many patients may be paucisymptomatic

Laboratory findings

- Enzymatic test on erythrocytes or cultured fibroblasts reveal low or absent prolidase levels

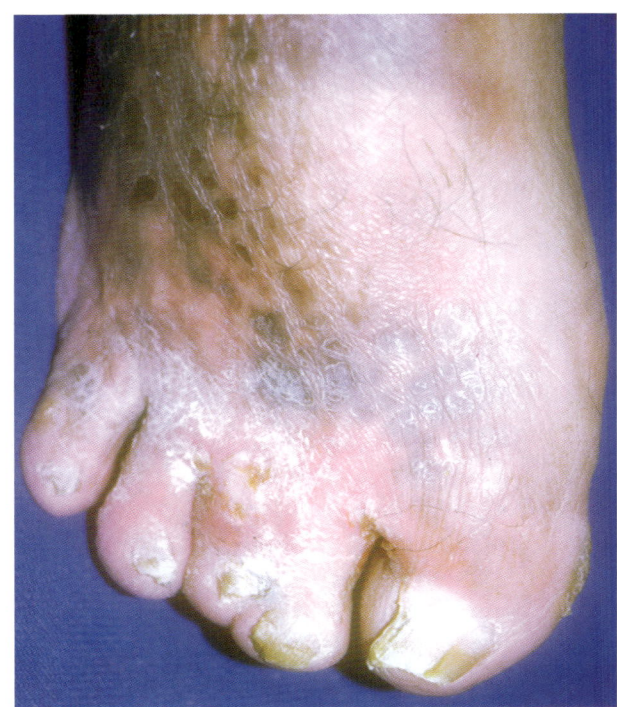

Figure 21.40

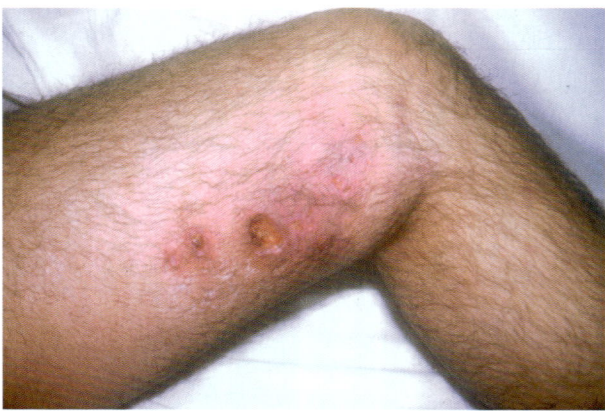

Figure 21.41

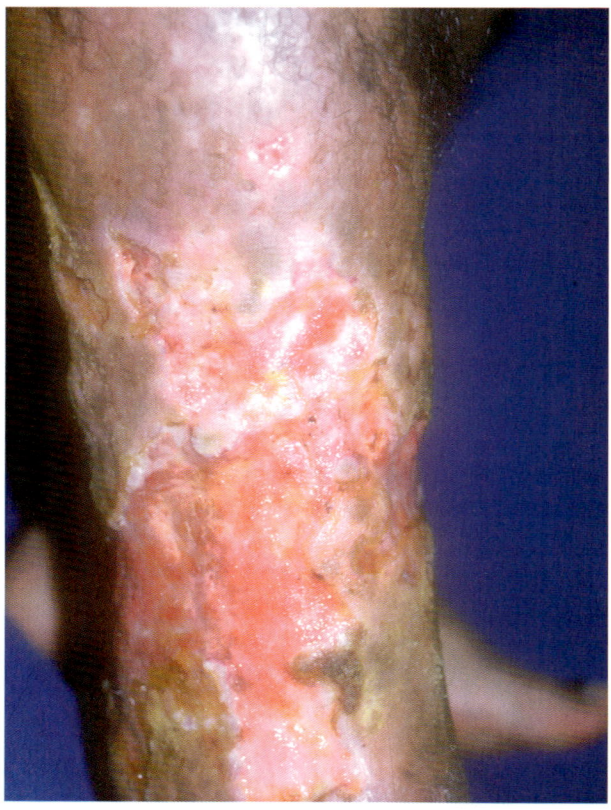

Figure 21.42

- Urinary secretion of imidopeptides
- Mitochondrial abnormalities are easily detectable using electron microscopy

Genetics and pathogenesis

- The disease is autosomal recessive
- The prolidase gene code for an ubiquitous dipeptidase involved in the latter stage of degradation of endogenous and dietary proteins, especially collagen catabolism
- Prolidase deficiency causes the activation of a necrosis-like cellular death that is responsible for cutaneous lesions

Follow-up and therapy

- Oral supplementation with proline, vitamin C and manganese may be useful
- Topical proline and glycine have been tested for topical application
- Apheresis exchange
- Topical antiseptics and antibiotics
- Heterologous grafts

Differential diagnosis

- Infectious diseases causing leg ulcerations
- Diabetes

REFERENCE

Forlino A, Lupi A, Vaghi P, et al. Mutation analysis of five new patients affected by prolidase deficiency: the lack of enzyme activity causes necrosis-like cell death in cultured fibroblasts. Hum Genet 2002; 111: 314–22

METHYLMALONIC ACIDURIA

Epidemiology

- Classical isolated methylmalonic aciduria is a rare disease, occurring in 1: 50 000–1: 80 000 newborns

Age of onset

- At birth until late childhood

Clinical findings

- Great heterogeneity of clinical presentation
- Large eroded areas in the periorificial areas (Figures 21.43 and 21.44) in neonatal period
- Ichthiotic skin during childhood and in adults
- Skin may be normal in milder cases

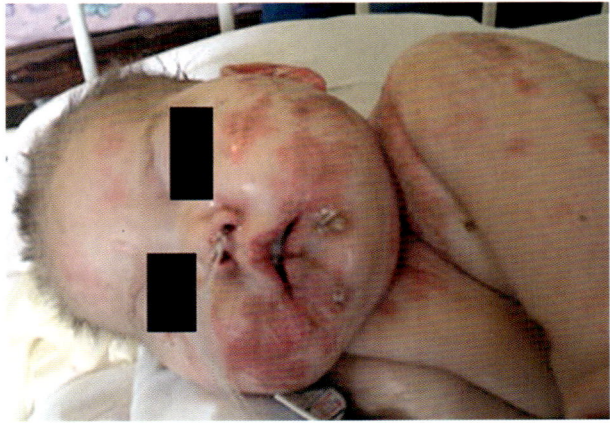

Figure 21.43

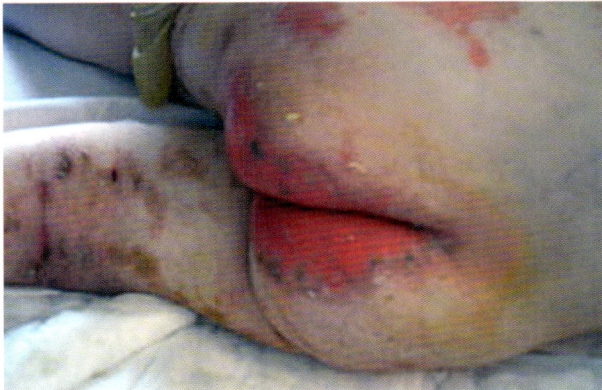

Figure 21.44

Extracutaneous findings

- Chronic renal failure
- Neurological abnormalities:
  - extrapyramidal movement disorder caused by progressive destruction of basal ganglia
  - myoclonic convulsions and hypsarrythmia
  - psychomotor retardation

Course and prognosis

- The disease may be silent and diagnosed during screening
- Even in milder cases there is frequent worsening during intercurrent illnesses with psoriasiform eruption
- Severe and recurrent staphylococcal infections

Laboratory findings

- Urine gas chromatography is useful to detect methylmalonate
- Enzyme activity in cultured fibroblasts or amniotic cells is considerably low

Genetics and pathogenesis

At least six genes can cause this relatively rare metabolic disease.

The involved pathways are mainly the transformation of methylmalonyl-CoA to succinyl-CoA (methylmalonyl-CoA mutase: mut0 (total absence) or mut– (partial activity) of the adenosyl cobalamin (cblA and cblB patients) pathway that is relevant at the same level of transformation.

The rarest cases are defined as cblC and cblD which cause the methylmalonic aciduria syndrome with homocystinuria.

This genetic heterogeneity explains the different phenotype of these patients.

Follow-up and therapy

- Detection of silent or milder familial cases
- Specially formulated protein diet
- Vitamin B_{12} and carnitine supplementation
- Emergency treatment during intercurrent illnesses and infections

Differential diagnosis

- Acrodermatitis enterpathica

REFERENCES

Horster F, Hoffmann GF. Pathophysiology, diagnosis, and treatment of methylmalonic aciduria – recent advances and new challenges. Pediatr Nephrol 2004; 19: 1071–4 [Review]

Martinez MA, Rincon A, Desviat LR, et al. Genetic analysis of three genes causing isolated methylmalonic acidemia: identification of 21 novel allelic variants. Mol Genet Metab 2005; 84: 317–25

CHAPTER 22

Immunodeficiency disorders

OMENN'S SYNDROME

Synonym

- Familial reticuloendotheliosis with eosinophilia

Age of onset

- Shortly after birth or early infancy (first–second month of life)

Clinical findings

Skin manifestations

- Erythematous pruritic rash evolving into an infiltrated, exfoliative and exudative erythroderma: first symptom of the disease (Figures 22.1–22.3)
- Diffuse alopecia on the scalp and eyebrows (Figure 22.4)

Extracutaneous manifestations

- Hepatosplenomegaly (88%)
- Lymphadenopathy (80%)
- Recurrent infections (72%)
- Chronic diarrhea
- Failure to thrive

Course and prognosis

Rapid death can occur from severe recurrent infections if untreated.

Laboratory findings

- High serum immunoglobulin E (IgE) level (91%)
- Eosinophilia (55%)
- B-cell count decreased
- T-cell count increased

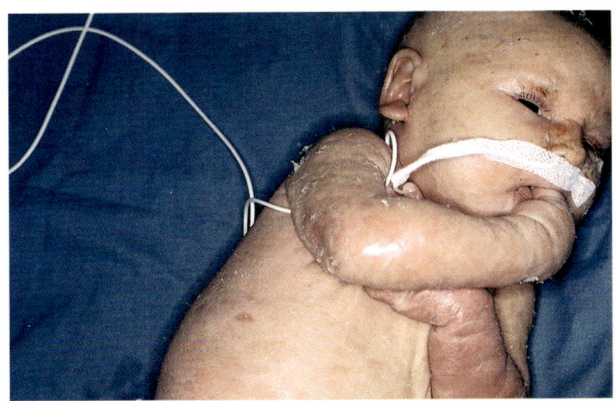

Figure 22.1

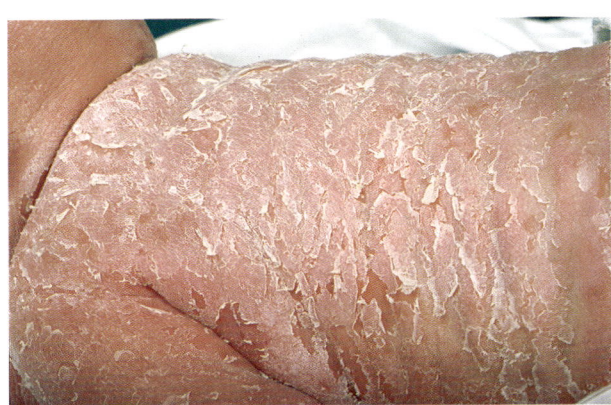

Figure 22.2

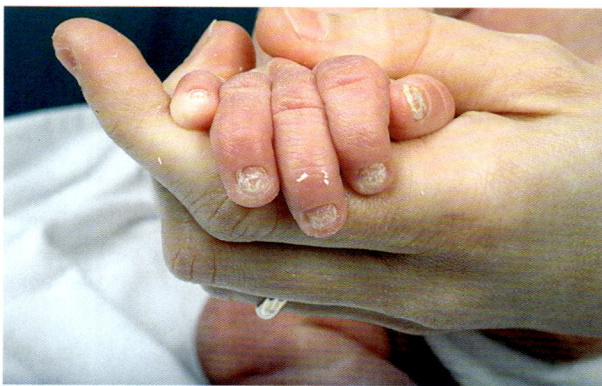

Figure 22.3

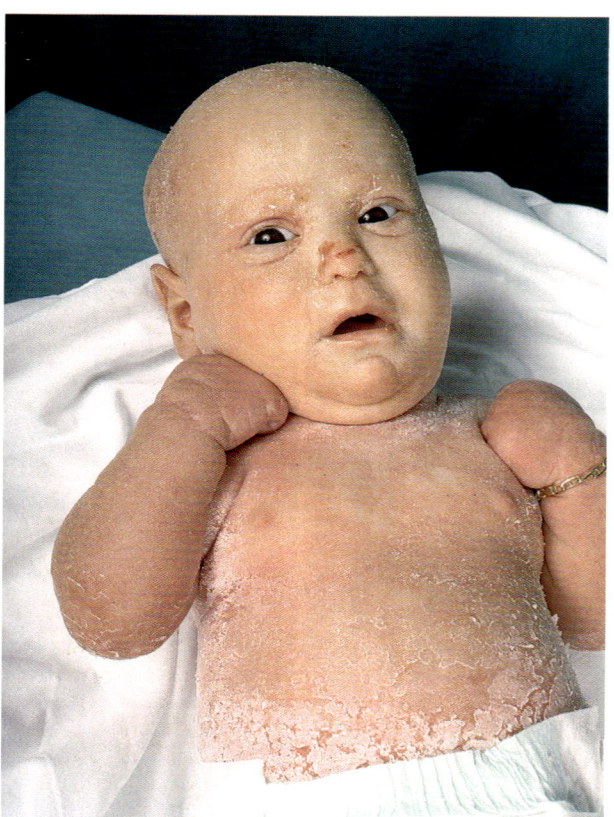

Figure 22.4

- Hypogammaglobulinemia
- Histopathologic findings: lymphohistiocytic and eosinophilic infiltration of superficial dermis and lymph nodes

Genetics and pathogenesis

- Autosomal recessive inheritance
- Severe combined immunodeficiency due to identical mutations in RAG1 or RAG2 genes leading to defective V(D)J recombinase activity

Differential diagnosis

- Netherton syndrome
- Graft versus host disease
- Leiner's syndrome

Follow-up and therapy

The mortality (still very high at 46%) may be reduced when diagnosis is established early and treatment initiated rapidly.

- Supportive therapy for diarrhea, electrolyte imbalance and infections
- Allogenic bone marrow transplantation
- Cord blood stem cell transplantation

REFERENCES

Aleman K, Noordzij JG, de Grost R, et al. Reviewing Omenn syndrome. Eur J Pediatr 2001; 160: 718–25

Pruszkowski A, Bodemer C, Fraitag S, et al. Neonatal and infantile erythrodermas. A retrospective study of 51 patients. Arch Dermatol 2000; 136: 875–80

Santagata S, Villa A, Sobacchi C, et al. The genetic and biochemical basis of Omenn syndrome. Immunol Rev 2000; 178: 64–74

HYPER IgE SYNDROME

Synonyms

- Hyperimmunoglobulinemia E syndrome
- Job's syndrome
- Staphylococcal abscess syndrome

Age of onset

- Early infancy

Clinical findings

Cutaneous manifestations

- Atopic-like dermatitis mainly localized on the scalp and flexures (Figure 22.5)
- Recurrent skin infections, including impetigo, furunculosis, paronychia, cellulitis and characteristic abscesses (cold abscesses) (Figure 22.6), warts (Figure 22.7), without warmth, tenderness or erythema occurring mainly on the head and neck
- Mucocutaneous candidiasis

Extracutaneous manifestations

- Recurrent pulmonary bacterial abscesses and pneumonia due to *Staphylococcus aureus* and *Haemophilus influenzae* resulting in pneumatoceles and empyemas
- Distinctive progressive coarsening of the facial features, including facial asymmetry, prominent forehead, broad nasal bridge, deep-set eyes
- Occasionally dental abnormalities, bone fractures, scoliosis, hyperextensible joints
- Lymphomas

Course and prognosis

In case of prompt diagnosis and treatment the disease may have a chronic course, but death may occur early owing to deep infections.

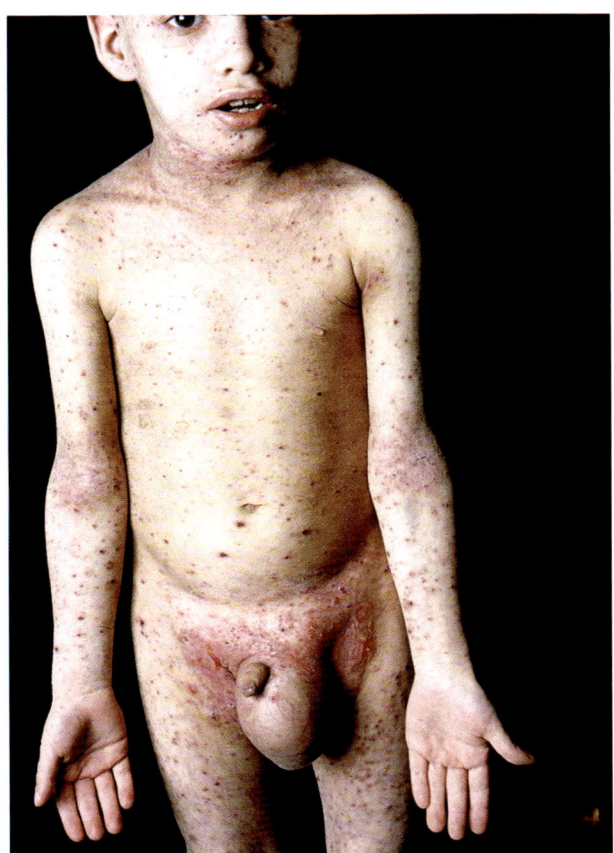

Figure 22.5

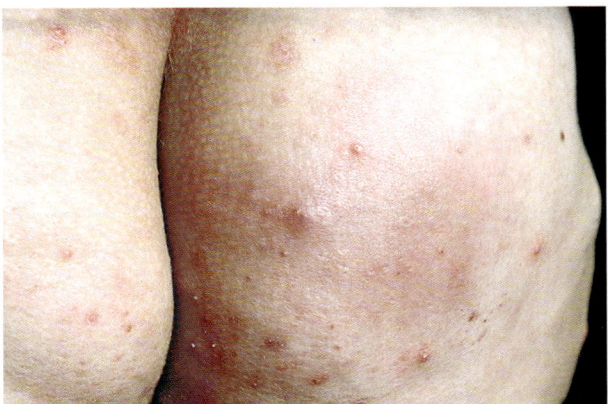

Figure 22.6

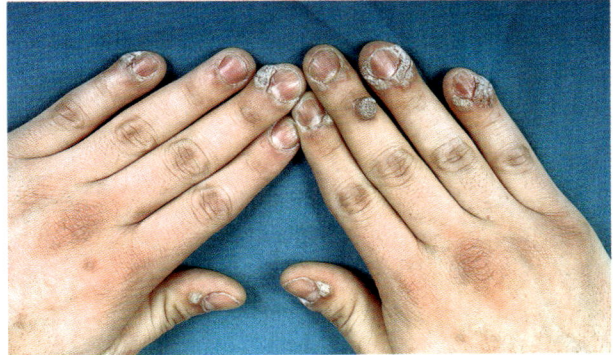

Figure 22.7

Laboratory investigations and data

- Elevated serum IgE levels
- Blood eosinophilia
- Abnormal neutrophil chemotaxis
- Defect of T-cell mediated immunity
- Radiography of bones and lungs
- Bacterial cultures

Genetics and pathogenesis

- Autosomal dominant inheritance; many sporadic cases
- Gene locus unknown
- Cytokine and chemokine dysregulation plays an important role in susceptibility to infections

Differential diagnosis

- Severe forms of atopic dermatitis
- Wiskott–Aldrich syndrome

Follow-up and therapy

Patients must be closely followed for infections and association with malignancies.

- Antibiotics
- Intravenous human immunoglobulins
- Cimetidine or ranitidine to induce an improvement in recurrent infections
- Incision and drainage of abscesses
- Bone marrow transplantation does not correct the syndrome

REFERENCES

Garraud O, Mollis SN, Holland SM, et al. Regulation of immunoglobulin production in hyper IgE syndrome. J Allergy Clin Immunol 1999; 103: 333–40

Grimbacher B, Holland SM, Gallin JI, et al. Hyper IgE syndrome with recurrent infections. An autosomal dominant multisystem disorder. N Engl J Med 1999; 340: 692–702

Shemer A, Weiss G, Confins Y, et al. The hyper IgE syndrome. Two cases and review of the literature. Int J Dermatol 2001; 40: 622–8

C1Q ESTERASE INHIBITOR DEFICIENCY

Synonym

- Hereditary angioedema

Epidemiology

No data are available in the literature. Many cases are underestimated as simply chronic urticaria.

Age of onset

- Usually within the first decade

Clinical findings

- Recurrent swelling of mucosae and skin, especially lips, face and hands (Figure 22.8)
- Episodes heal spontaneously in hours or days
- Erythema marginatum in a minority of patients (that may herald the edema)

Extracutaneous findings

- Severe involvement of oral mucosa and upper respiratory tract is common
- Gastrointestinal symptoms (diarrhea and colic pain)
- Autoimmune disorders such as lupus erythematosus and glomerulonephritis are reported

Course and prognosis

The disease persists throughout life. Episodes may be caused by emotional and thermal stress or intercurrent diseases. Severe episodes characterized by laryngeal involvement may be life-threatening if not promptly cured.

Laboratory findings

- Low levels of C1 esterase inhibitor
- Skin biopsies give aspecific results

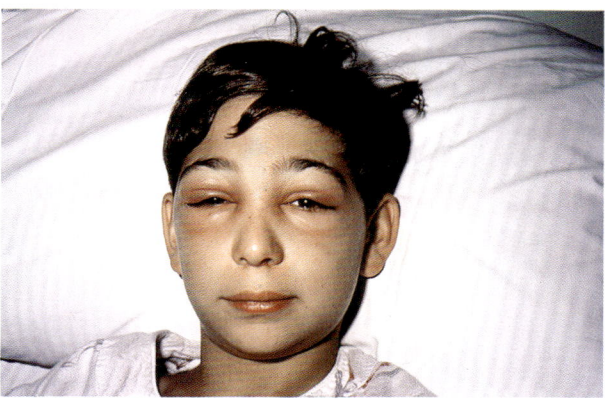

Figure 22.8

Genetics and pathogenesis

- Autosomal dominant disease
- Mutations in the C1q esterase inhibitor gene

Follow-up and therapy

- Prompt rescue for severe laryngeal episodes
- Detection of affected relatives
- Anabolic steroid treatment

Differential diagnosis

- Common urticaria
- Autoimmune skin diseases
- Common hypersensitivity and allergic episodes

REFERENCES

Bork K, Hardt J, Schicketanz KH, Ressel N. Clinical studies of sudden upper airway obstruction in patients with hereditary angioedema due to C1 esterase inhibitor deficiency. Arch Intern Med 2003; 163: 1229–35

Cumming SA, Halsall DJ, Ewan PW, Lomas DA. The effect of sequence variations within the coding region of the C1 inhibitor gene on disease expression and protein function in families with hereditary angio-oedema. J Med Genet 2003; 40: e114

Pappalardo E, Zinglae LC, Cicardi M. Increased expression of C1 inhibitor mRNA in patients with herediary angioedema treated with Danazol. Immunol Lett 2003; 86: 271–6

CHEDIAK–HIGASHI SYNDROME

Epidemiology

This is a very rare disorder; no further data are available.

Age of onset

- At birth

Skin findings

- Skin is lighter than expected for racial background; there is a sort of pigmentary 'dilution', especially on the central face (Figure 22.9, in a native Central-American boy)
- Silvery hair
- Freckles

Extracutaneous symptoms

- Proneness to bacterial infections
- Visual disturbances
- Lymphoproliferative diseases
- Pancytopenia
- Recurrent fevers
- Progressive neuropathy (impaired walking and dysesthesia)
- Rarely, mental retardation

Course and prognosis

The disease is often fatal by the 10th year of life.

Laboratory findings

Upon ultrastructural examination giant, dense granules in leukocytes, fibroblasts and giant melanosomes in melanocytes may be found.

Genetics and pathogenesis

- The disease is autosomal recessive
- The causative gene is LYST
- Chediak–Higashi syndrome is a vesicular trafficking disease causing abnormal transfer of proteins in white blood cells, melanocytes, retina

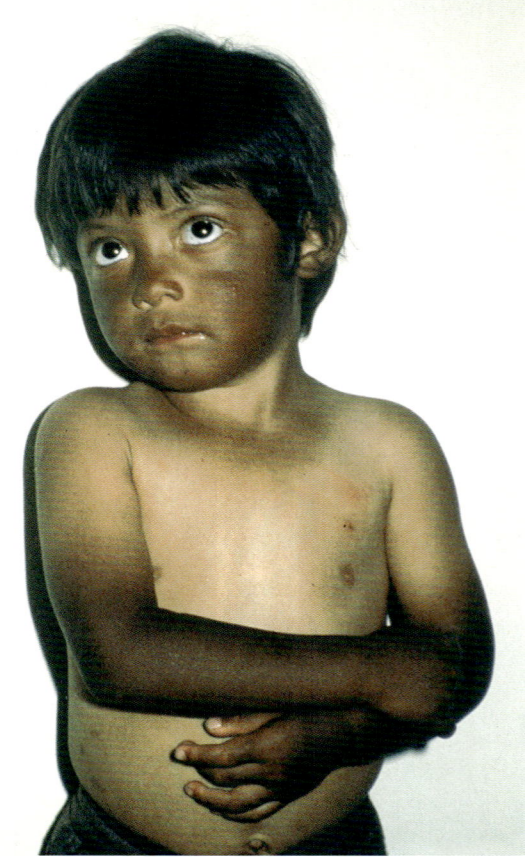

Figure 22.9

Follow-up and therapy

- Hematological assessment to prevent cytopenia and neoplasia
- Ophthalmological examination
- Antibiotics for recurrent infections

Differential diagnosis

- Elejalde's syndrome
- Griscelli's syndrome
- Hermansky–Pudlak syndrome

REFERENCES

Masui N, Nishikawa T, Takagi Y, et al. The rat lysosmal trafficking regulator (Lyst) gene is mapped on the telomeric region of chromosome 17. Exp Anim 2003; 52: 89–91

Mori M, Yamasaki K, Nakanishi S, et al. A new beige mutant rat ACI/N-Lystbg-Kyo. Exp Anim 2003; 52: 31–6

Mottonen M, Lanning M, Baumann P, et al. Chediak-Higashi syndrome: four cases from Northern Finland. Acta Pediatr 2003; 92: 1047–51

Scheinfeld NS. Syndromic albinism: a review of genetics and phenotypes. Dermatol Online J 2003; 9: 5. Review

Stein SM, Dale DC. Molecular basis and therapy of disorders associated with chronic neutopenia. Curr Allergy Asthma Rep 2003; 3: 385–8

Tomita Y, Suzuki T. Genetics of pigmentary disorders. Am J Med Genet 2004; 15: 131C: 75–81. PMID: 15452859

CHAPTER 23

Complex malformative syndromes with distinctive cutaneous signs

RUBINSTEIN–TAYBI SYNDROME

Synonyms

- Broad thumb–great toe syndrome
- Rubinstein syndrome

Age of onset

- Birth to first months of life; fully visible phenotype during childhood

Epidemiology

An estimated birth prevalence of 1 : 125 000 is reported in the literature.

Clinical findings

Cutaneous manifestations

- Hypertrichosis of the arms and back (75%) (Figure 23.1)
- Capillary hemangiomas on forehead, nape and lumbar region (60%)
- Simian crease and abnormal dermatoglyphics (50%) (Figure 23.2)
- Increased tendency to form keloids (5–22%) (Figure 23.3)
- Supernumerary nipples (16%)
- Racquet nails
- Thick and highly arched eyebrows
- Unusually long eyelashes

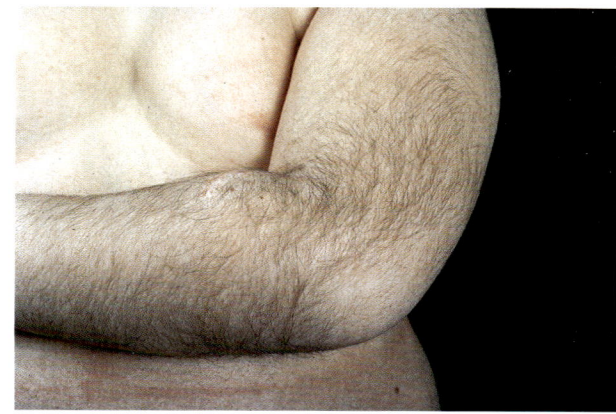

Figure 23.1

- Atopy, keratosis pilaris, ulerythema ophryogenes
- Piebaldism
- Multiple pilomatricomas (Figure 23.3)
- Epidermal nevi and nevus flammeus in 20% of patients

Extracutaneous manifestations

- Characteristic broad thumbs and great toes (Figure 23.2)
- Broad terminal phalanges in the other fingers (Figure 23.2)
- Clinodactyly of the fourth toe and of the fourth and fifth fingers
- Distinctive facies consisting of microcephaly, prominent forehead, beaked nose with nasal septum below alae, deformed ears, high arched palate, irregular and crowded teeth (Figure 23.4)

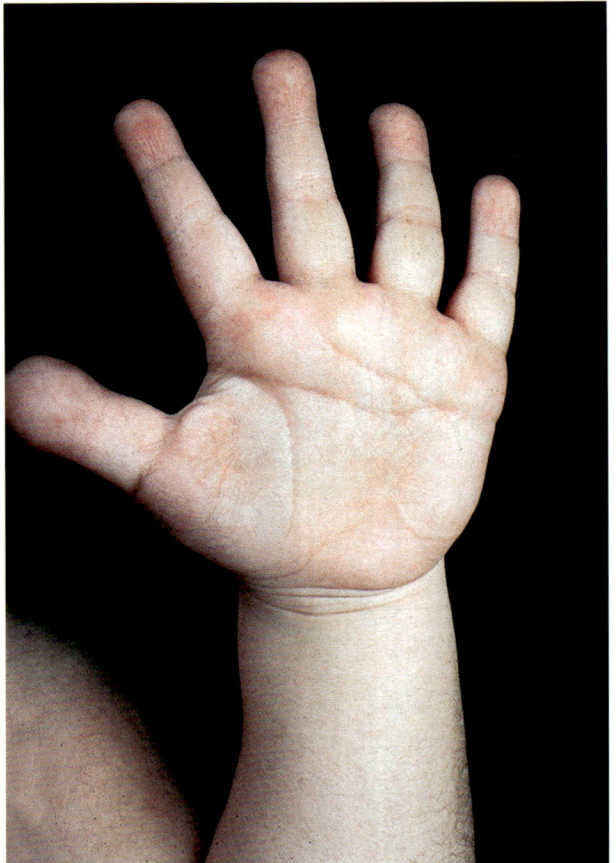

Figure 23.2

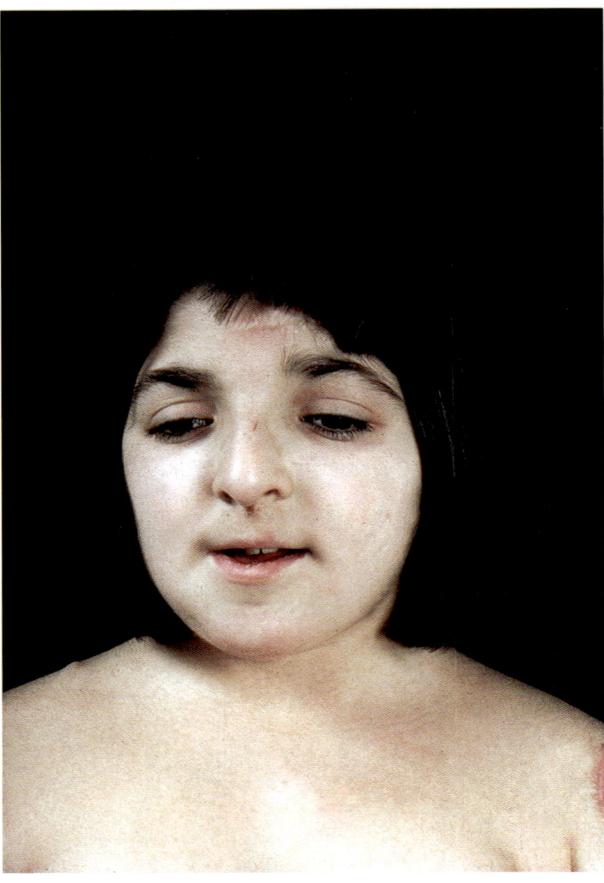

Figure 23.4

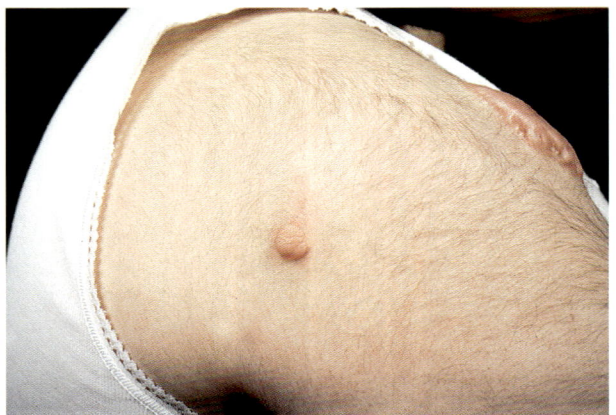

Figure 23.3

- Ocular abnormalities including strabismus, cataract, blepharoptosis; hearing loss
- Short stature with bony abnormalities of ribs, vertebrae and sternum; obesity
- Cryptorchidism

- Cardiac abnormalities; septa; heart defects (30%)
- Severe mental and motor retardation
- Report of increased incidence of polyhydramnios during pregnancy
- Increased tumor risk

Complications

There can be frequent infections.

Course

The disease is lifelong. Life expectancy is reduced, related to the severity of internal organ malformations.

Laboratory investigations and data

- Complete radiographic studies of bones
- Electrocardiography (ECG) and electroencephalography (EEG)

Genetics and pathogenesis

- Possible autosomal dominant and autosomal recessive inheritance, but most cases sporadic
- Gene locus: 16p13.3
- Disease seems to be caused by mutations in the transcriptional coactivator cyclic adenosine monophosphate (AMP) response element *binding protein* (CREB) axiel (CBP acetyltransferase)

Differential diagnosis

- Apert's syndrome
- Patau's syndrome
- Trisomy 13 syndrome
- Cornelia de Lange syndrome

Follow-up and therapy

Increased mortality at young age is secondary to cardiac failure, and secondary infections need periodic screening.

- Referral to symptom-specific specialists

REFERENCES

Lacombe D, Saura R, Taine L, et al. Confirmation of assignement of a locus for Rubinstein–Taybi syndrome gene to 16p13.3. Ann J Med Genet 1992; 44: 126–8

Petrij F, Giles RH, Danwerse HG, et al. Rubinstein–Taybi syndrome caused by mutations in transcriptional coactivator CBP. Nature (London) 1995; 376: 348–51

Selmanowitz VJ, Stiller MJ. Rubinstein–Taybi syndrome. Cutaneous manifestations and colossal keloids. Arch Dermatol 1981; 117: 504–6

CORNELIA DE LANGE SYNDROME

Synonyms

- Brachmann–de Lange syndrome
- de Lange syndrome

Epidemiology

- Over 400 cases are described
- Estimated birth prevalence in USA is 1 : 10 000 and population prevalence in a Danish study is calculated to be 0.6 : 100 000

Age of onset

- At birth

Clinical findings

Diffuse hirsutism, with long, thin and whorled hair over shoulders, elbows, thighs and lumbar areas

- Characteristic facies (Figure 23.5) with:
  - Microbrachycephaly
  - Synophris and low hairline
  - Hypertelorism
  - Small nose with anteverted nostrils
  - Thin lips and micrognathia
  - Low-set and deformed external ears with lanugo
- Livedo reticularis in over half of patients
- Dermatoglyphic abnormalities
- Nipples may be hypoplastic

Extracutaneous symptoms

- Severe postnatal growth in almost all patients with swallowing disturbances
- Severe mental retardation is a hallmark of this disease
- Micromelia and phocomelia
- Hands are usually small and with different finger abnormalities (Figure 23.6)
- Cryptorchidism and hypospadias (in over 70% of patients)
- 'Growling' cry and later hoarse dysphony
- Cleft palate in 20% of patients and hearing loss
- Late eruption and widely spaced teeth are characteristic
- Congenital heart defects and diaphragmatic hernia in 20%

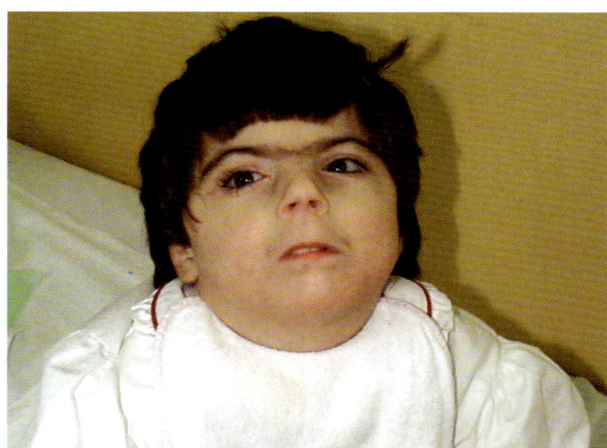

Figure 23.5

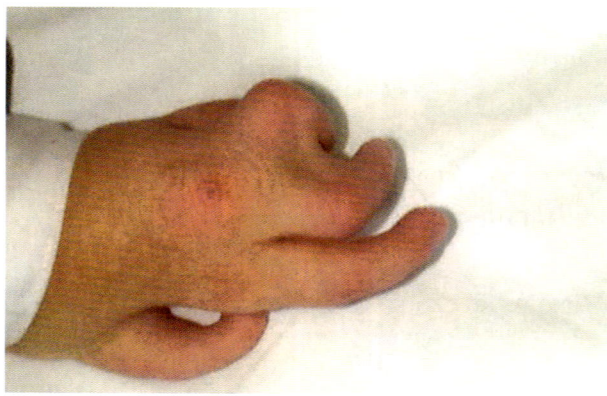

Figure 23.6

- Intestinal malrotation, annular pancreas and renal abnormalities in 10–20% of patients

Course and complications

- Life expectancy is reduced (20–30 years)
- Cardiopathy and pneumonitis 'ab ingestis' are major causes of death

Genetics and pathogenesis

- Sporadic
- Many pedigrees with vertical transmission have been reported
- NIPBL gene is responsible for Cornelia de Lange syndrome

Laboratory findings

Second-level ultrasonography during pregnancy may reveal some of the reported anomalies.

Differential diagnosis

- Duplication (3q) syndrome
- Coffin–Syris syndrome

Follow-up and therapy

A multidisciplinary approach is needed in order to manage all the eventual multiorgan disturbances.

REFERENCES

Ben–Asher E, Lancet D. NIPBL gene responsible for Cornelia de Lange syndrome, a severe developmental disorder. Isr Med Assoc J 2004; 6: 571–2

Dorsett D. Adherin: key to the cohesin ring and cornelia de Lange syndrome. Curr Biol 2004; 14: R834–6

Gilgenkrantz S. [Cornelia de Lange syndrome] Med Sci (Paris) 2004; 20: 954–6. [French]

COHEN'S SYNDROME

Epidemiology

- Over 100 cases have been described

Age of onset

- At birth

Clinical findings

In two unrelated patients of personal observation, we found diffuse hyperpigmented lesions along the Blaschko lines (Figures 23.7–23.9).

Extracutaneous findings

- Facies with downslanted palpebral fissures, open mouth with prominent upper central incisors, maxillary hypoplasia (Figure 23.10)
- Early-onset obesity (Figures 23.7 and 23.8)
- Narrow hands and feet
- Long and thin fingers
- Myopia and strabismus in 50% of patients, retinal pigmentary anomalies in 70%
- Heart defects in 10%
- Usually medium to severe mental retardation with 'party behavior'

Course and prognosis

Mental retardation may progress with age, as well as retinal defects that do not lead to blindness.

Laboratory findings

- In our two patients cytological examination of normal and hyperpigmented demonstrated diploidy for the former and triploidy for the latter
- Hyperhyaluronicaciduria has been reported
- Asymptomatic neutropenia

Genetics and pathogenesis

Inheritance is autosomal recessive.

Cohen's syndrome is related to mutations in COH1 gene, coding for a transmembrane protein with a role

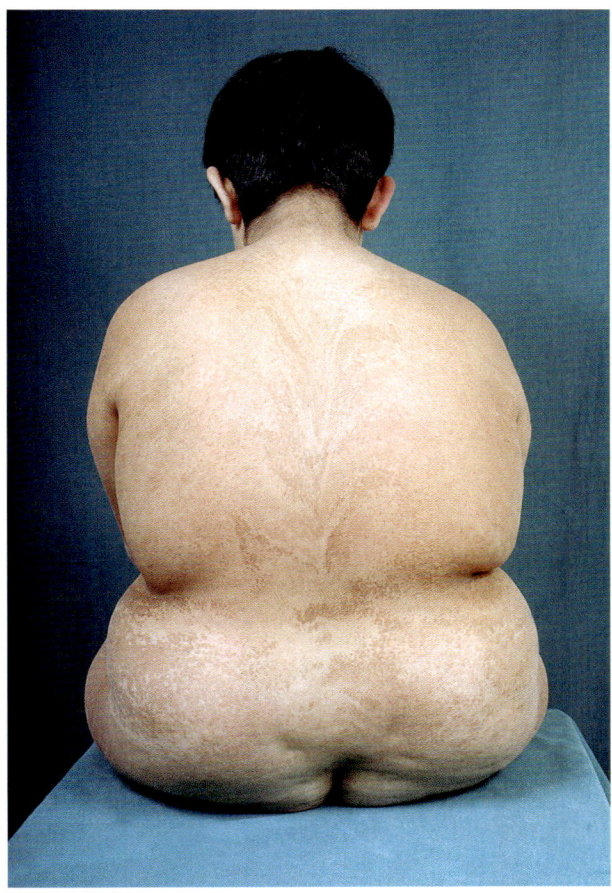

Figure 23.8

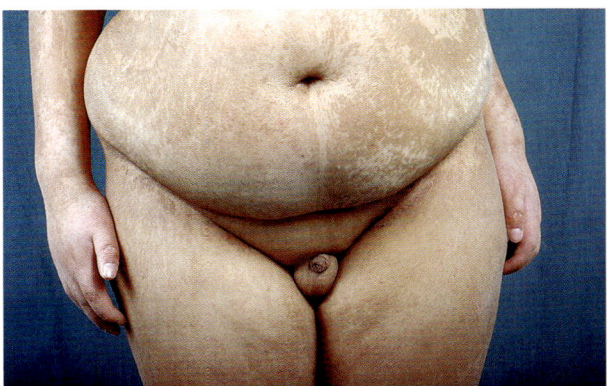

Figure 23.7

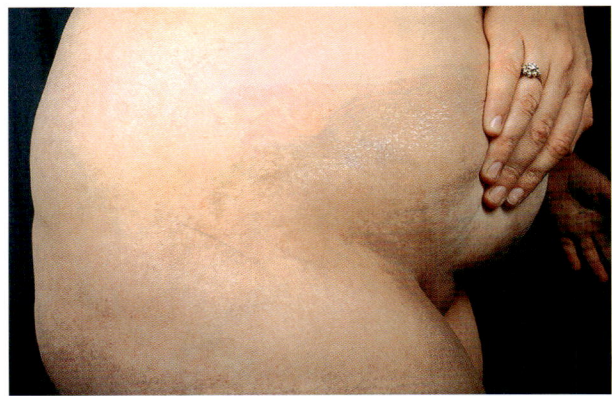

Figure 23.9

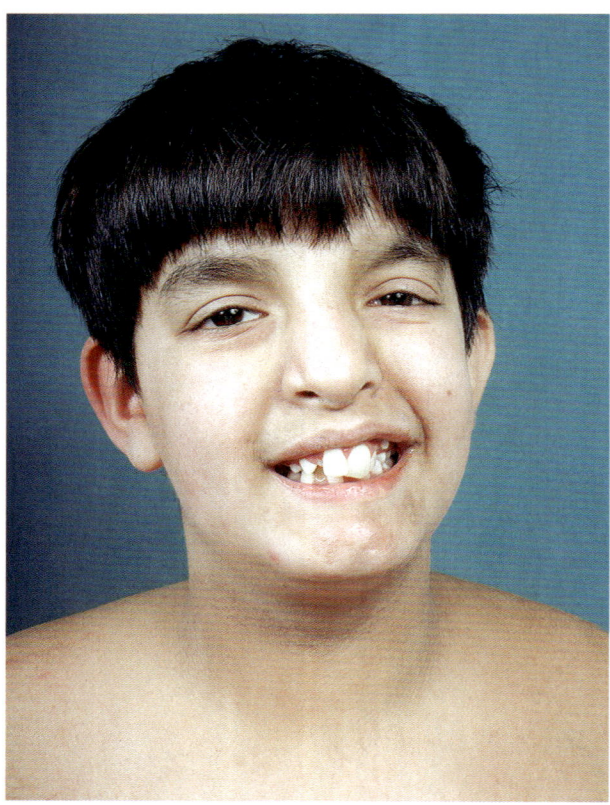

Figure 23.10

in vesicle-mediated sorting and intracellular proteins transfer.

Follow-up and therapy

- Dietary regimen
- Orthodontic management
- Cardiac echotomography for early detection of cardiac anomalies
- Correction of ocular defects
- Psychological assessment

Differential diagnosis

- Prader–Willi syndrome (obesity)

REFERENCES

Falk MJ, Feiler HS, Neilson DE, et al. Cohen syndrome in the Ohio Amish. Am J Med Genet A 2004; 128: 23–8

Kondo I, Shimizu A, Asakawa S, et al. COH1 analysis and linkage study in two Japanese families with Cohen syndrome. Clin Genet 2005; 67: 270–2

Mrugacz M, Sredzinska-Kita D, Bakunowicz-Lazarczyk A. Pediatric opthalmologic findings of Cohen syndrome in twins. J Pediatr Opthalmol Strabismus 2005; 42: 54–6

BRANCHIO-OCULOFACIAL SYNDROME

Synonym

- BOF syndrome

Epidemiology

A review of 43 cases was published in 1995.

Age of onset

- At birth

Clinical findings

- Laterocervical areas of erythematous and scaly skin (psoriasiform aspect) over the sternocleidomastoid muscles (bilateral) (100% of patients) (Figures 23.11 and 23.12). These areas are referred to by some authors as aplasia cutis congenita, but the concept is not true, even if areas of true aplasia cutis congenita are described in fewer than 10% of patients
- Early canities and sebaceous scalp cysts
- Pinnae are low and posteriorly placed (Figures 23.13 and 23.14) in almost all cases and may have

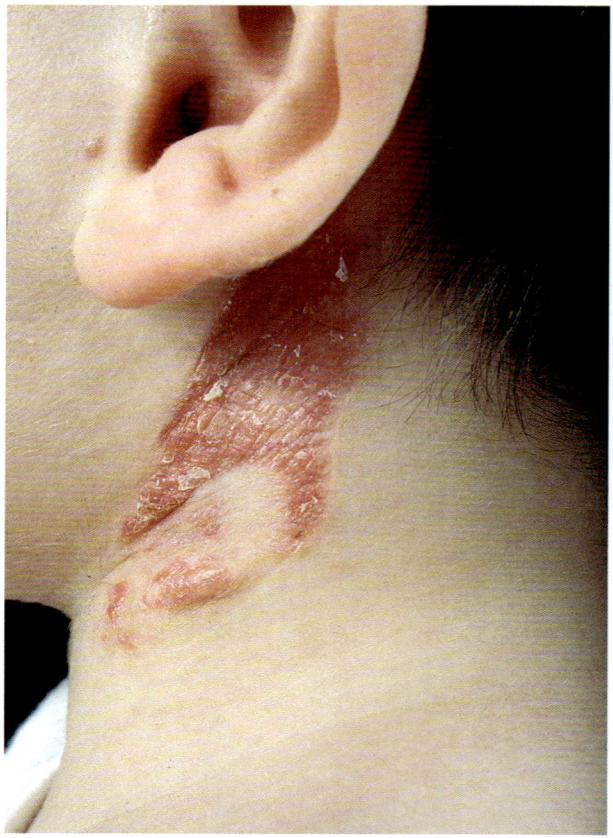

Figure 23.11

minor malformation of helix, antihelix and lobules; accessory tragi in 20% of patients

Extracutaneous symptoms

- Facies with hypertelorism, broad nose, short and prominent philtrum and upper lips with or without pseudocleft and cleft lips (and palate) and micrognathia (Figures 23.13 and 23.14)
- Loss of punctae is common, with absent or rudimentary nasolacrimal ducts (> 70%)
- Strabismus, cataracts, myopia, colobomas, microphthalmia and anophthalmia in some cases
- Clinodactyly of the fifth finger (20%)
- Anomalies of eustachian tubes
- Renal cystic disease in a subset of patients
- Mental retardation of various degrees in a third of patients
- Conductive hearing loss
- Susceptibility to dental caries

Course and complications

The main issues are represented by recurrent infections due to rudimentary nasolacrimal ducts, leading to severe conjunctivitis, otitis media and externa, rhinitis and ozena. These infections may lead to permanent defects such as hearing loss or impairment of vision.

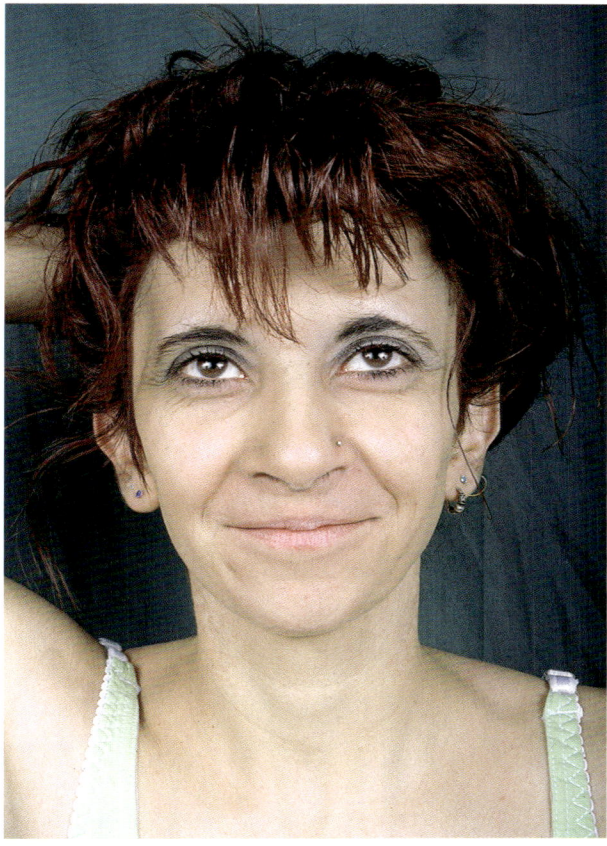

Figure 23.13

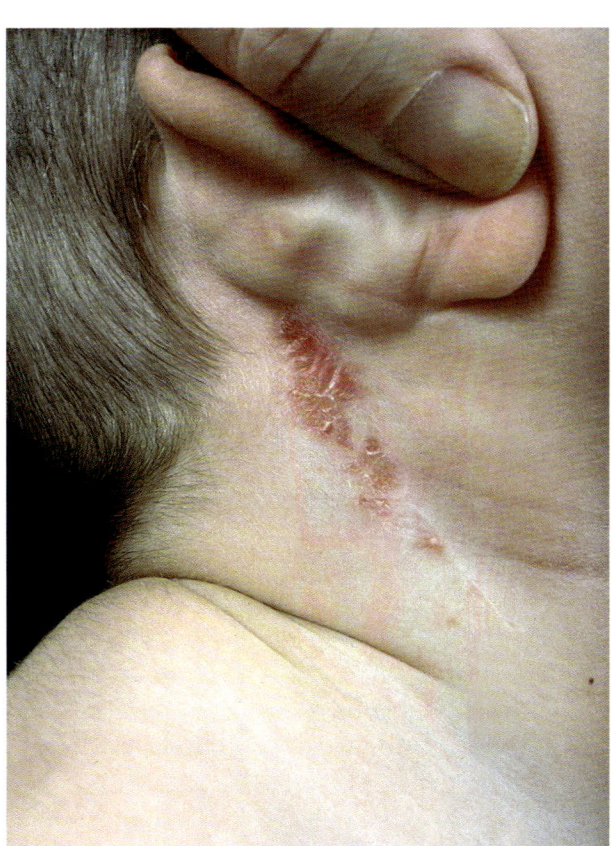

Figure 23.12

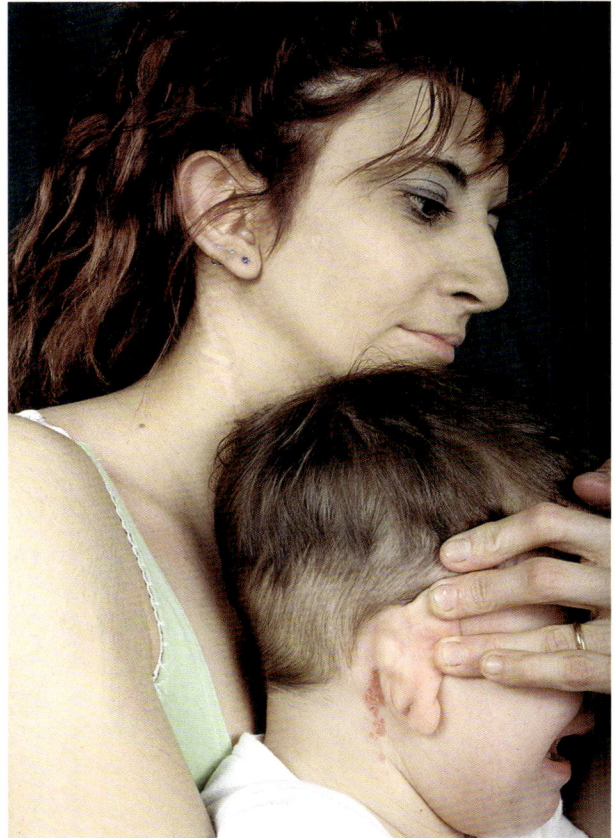

Figure 23.14

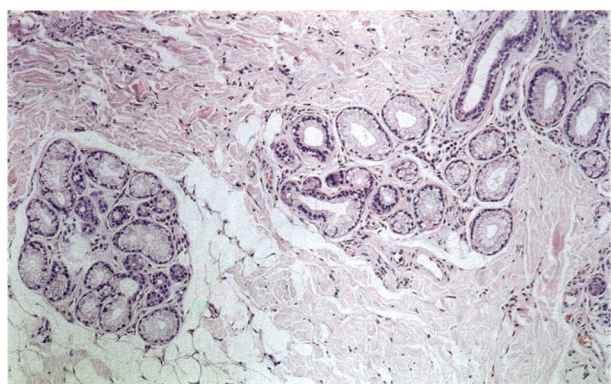

Figure 23.15

Laboratory findings

Histology of the infiltrated laterocervical skin may reveal ectopic thymus, mucous glands of the third branchial arch and ectopic salivary glands (Figure 23.15).

Genetics and pathogenesis

The disease is autosomal dominant, and is part of the chapter of orofacial clefting syndromes representing defects of closure of the embryonic branchial arches.

The gene does not map to the locus of branchio-otorenal (BOR) disease, EYA1.

Follow-up and therapy

- Surgery for nasolacrimal duct defect and eventual cleft lip and palate
- Surgery for ectopic hamartomatous laterocervical areas, mainly for esthetic reasons
- Control of recurrent infections of ears and conjunctiva by antibiotics
- Assessment for renal defects (ultrasonography)
- Neurological evaluation for mental retardation

Differential diagnosis

- Branchio-otorenal disease
- Other cleft lip and palate syndromes
- Rapp–Hodgkin–AEC complex (p63 disease)

REFERENCES

Drut R, Galliani C. Thymic tissue in the skin: a clue to the diagnosis of the branchio-oculo-facial syndrome: report of two cases. Int J Surg Pathol 2003; 11: 25–8

Lin AE, Semina EV, Daack-Hirsch S, et al. Exclusion of the branchio-oto-renal syndrome locus (EYA1) from patients with branchio-oculo-facial syndrome. Am J Med Genet 2000; 91: 387–90

BARBER–SAY SYNDROME

Synonym

- Unusual face, atrophic skin, hirsutism syndrome

Epidemiology

Fewer than ten cases have been described.

Age of onset

- At birth

Clinical findings

- Hypertrichosis (forehead, neck and back) (Figure 23.16)
- Atrophy and laxity of the skin
- Abnormal fingerprints

Extracutaneous symptoms

- Unusual face with (Figures 23.17 and 23.18):
    - Severe hypertelorism and mongolian shape
    - Shallow orbits and partial ablepharon
    - Ectropion and strabismus
    - Bulbous nose tip and prominent alae
    - Thin lips and macrostomia
    - Abnormal pinnae
- Absent or hypoplastic nipples and mammary glands
- Growth retardation
- Mild to severe mental retardation
- Cryptorchidism

Course and complication

Ectropion may cause corneal opacities.

Laboratory findings

There are none particular.

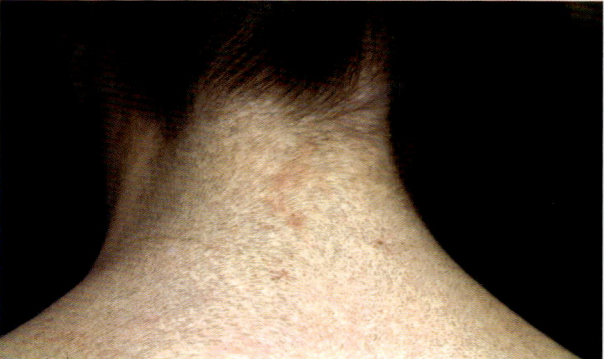

Figure 23.16

Genetics and pathogenesis

- Sporadic cases and autosomal dominant inheritance
- Gene locus unknown

Follow-up and therapy

- Ophthalmological therapy for ectropion

Differential diagnosis

- Ablepharon–macrostomy syndrome

REFERENCES

Dimulos MB, Pagon RA. Autosomal dominant inheritance of Barber–Say syndrome. Am J Med Genet 1999; 86: 54–6

Pellegrino JE, Schur RE, Boghosian-Sell L, et al. Ablepharon macrostomia syndrome with associated cutis laxa: possible localization to 18q. Hum Genet 1996; 97: 532–6

Sod R, Izbizky G, Cohen-Salama M. Macrostomia, hypertelorism, atrophic skin, severe hypertrichosis without ectropion: milder form of Barber–Say syndrome. Am J Med Genet 1997; 73: 366–7

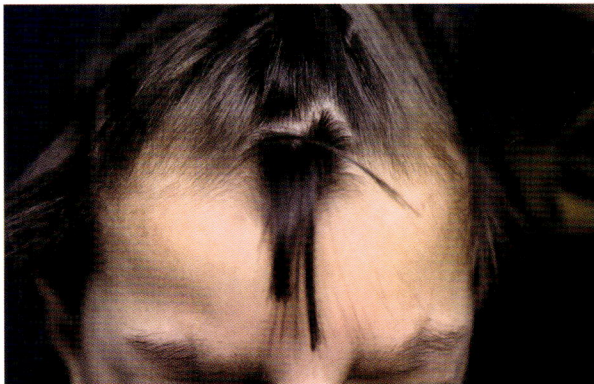

Figure 23.17

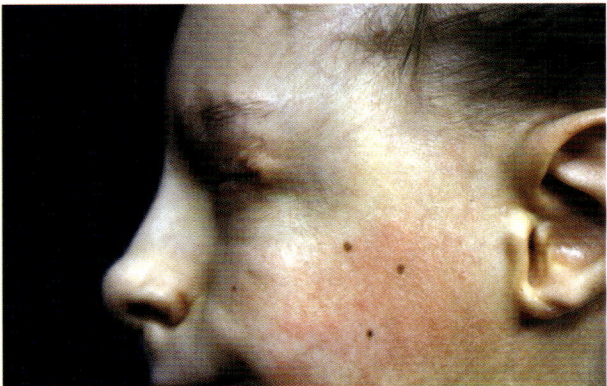

Figure 23.18

TURNER'S SYNDROME

Synonym

- XO syndrome

Epidemiology

The prevalence is 1 : 2500 female births.

Age of onset

- At birth

Clinical findings

- Webbed neck (pterygium colli) with redundant skin at birth (Figure 23.19)
- Dystrophic nails
- Low posterior nuchal hairline (Figure 23.20)
- Hirsutism
- Peripheral lymphedema at birth
- Thickening of central areas of palms, soles and dermatoglyphic abnormalities
- Multiple pigmented nevi in two-thirds of patients (Figure 23.21)

Extracutaneous symptoms

- Short stature (130–145 cm)
- Gonadal dysgenesis

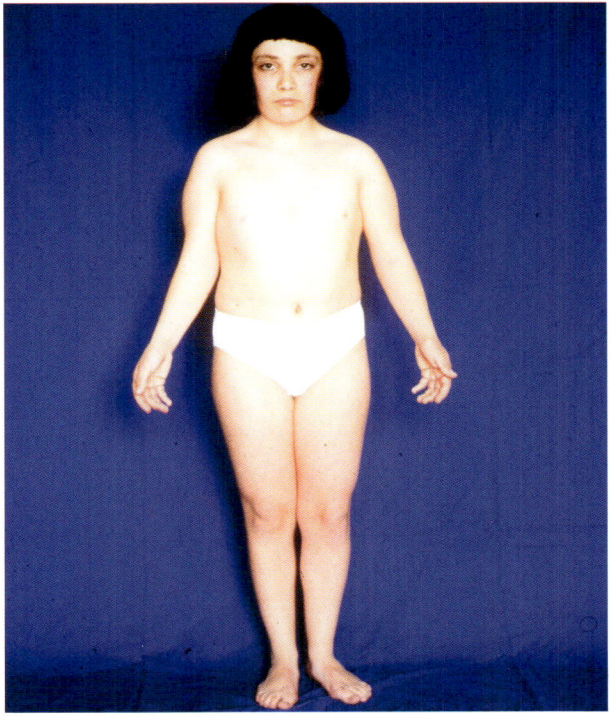

Figure 23.19

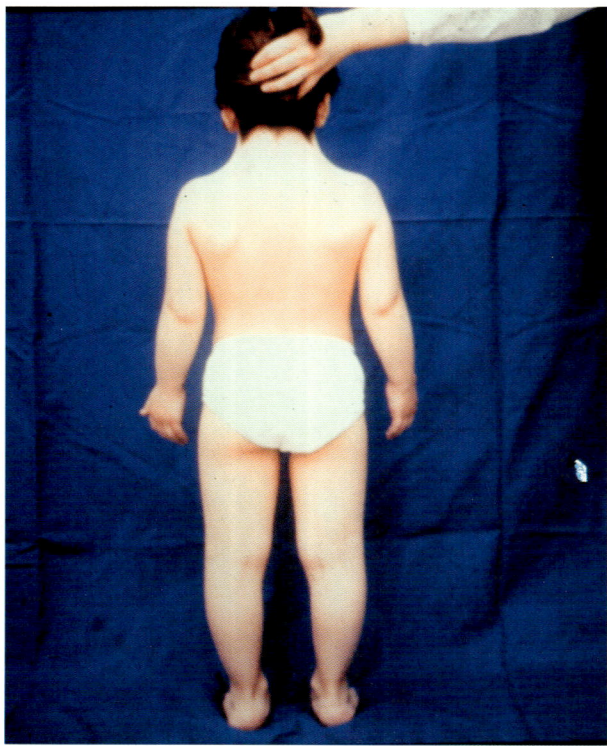

Figure 23.20

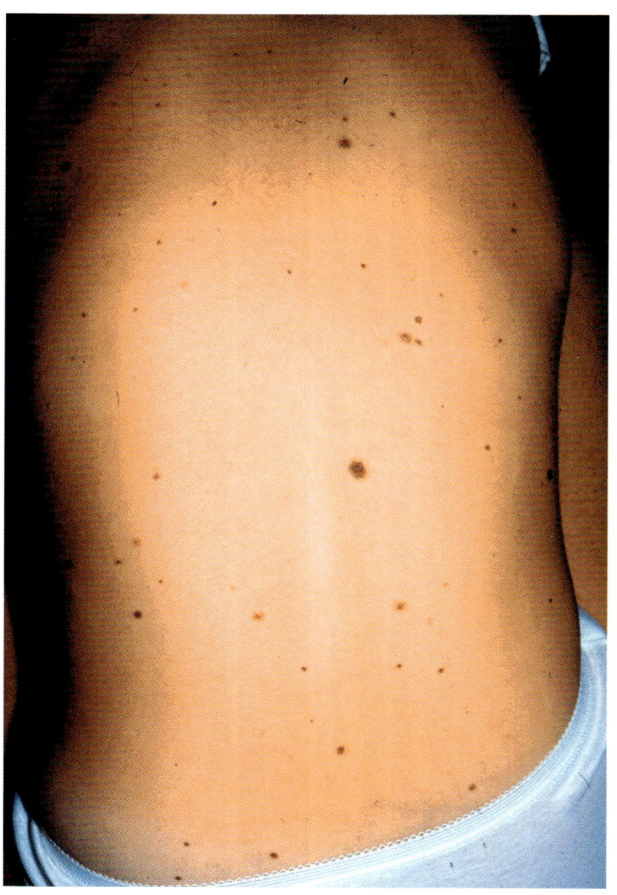

Figure 23.21

- Broad chest
- Coarctation of the aorta (15%)
- Renal abnormalities ('horseshoe kidney') in 40%
- Cubitus valgus, short metacarpals and metatarsals
- Mild mental retardation and learning disabilities (30%)
- Visual and auditory problems (30–40%)

Course and prognosis

- Peripheral lymphedema resolves during the third year
- Life expectancy is normal and linked to cardiac and renal diseases
- Increased risk of gonadoblastoma and extragonadal neoplasia

Laboratory findings

Estrogen levels are low.

Genetics and pathogenesis

- 45XO in half of patients
- Isochromosome X in 12–20%
- Mosaicism in 30–40%: 45,X–46,XX, 45,X–46,XY, 45,X–47,XXX and other rarest

Follow-up and therapy

- Surgical approach for renal and cardiac diseases
- Plastic surgery for neck abnormalities

Differential diagnosis

- Multiple pterygium syndrome
- Noonan's syndrome

REFERENCES

Kawakami Y, Oyama N, Kishimoto K, et al. A case of generalized pustular psoriasis associated with Turner syndrome. J Dermatol 2004; 31: 16–20

Longui CA, Rocha MN, Martinho LC, et al. Molecular detection of XO – Turner syndrome. Genet Mol Res 2002; 1: 266–70

Wallerstein R, Musen E, McCarrier J, et al. Turner syndrome phenotype with 47,XXX karyotype: further investigation warranted? Am J Med Genet 2004; 125: 106–7

PALLISTER–KILLIAN SYNDROME

Synonyms

- Mosaic tetrasomy 12p
- Isochromosome 12p syndrome

Epidemiology

The disease was described by Pallister in 1977; there are at least 50 studies and reports in the literature.

Age of onset

- At birth

Clinical findings

- Hyperpigmented streaks along the lines of Blaschko (Figures 23.22 and 23.23), reflecting mosaic conditions
- Hypopigmented lesions have also been reported
- Hypotrichosis of frontal and temporal areas (Figure 23.24)

Extracutaneous symptoms

- Facies with coarse face, high forehead, hypotrichosis, ptosis, flat nasal bridge with anteverted nostrils, downturned mouth, thin upper lip (Figure 23.24)
- Usually severe mental retardation
- Seizures
- Cardiovascular anomalies in 25% of patients
- Diaphragmatic hernia and anal abnormalities
- Supernumerary nipples

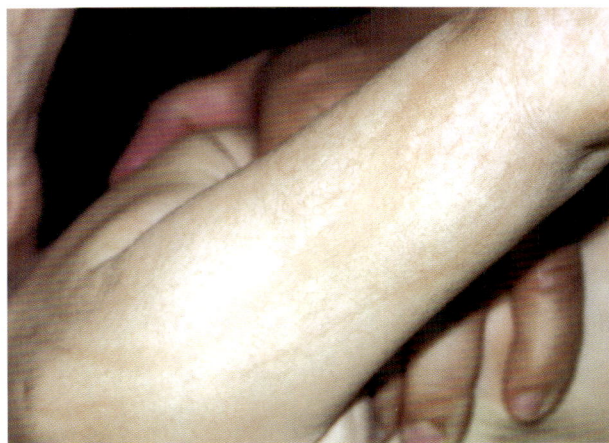

Figure 23.23

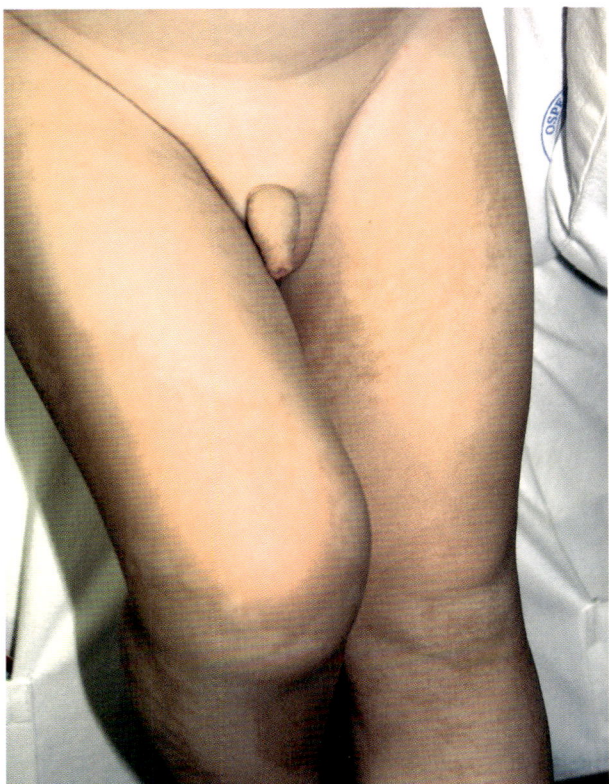

Figure 23.22

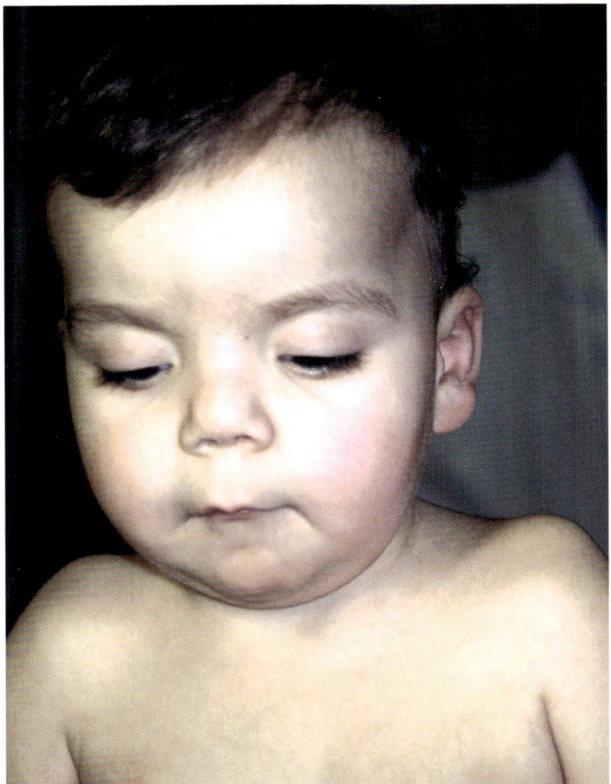

Figure 23.24

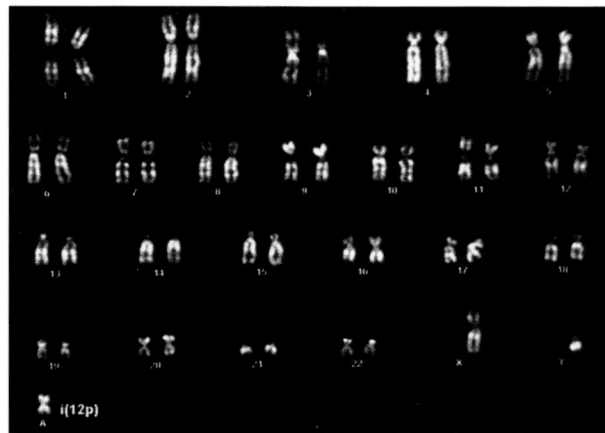

Figure 23.25

- Generalized hypotonia
- Short limbs, fingers and thumbs with retarded bone age

Course and prognosis

- This syndrome may be lethal at neonatal age (asphyxia) or in infancy
- Adults have severe mental retardation and epilepsy
- Skin signs are steady

Laboratory findings

- Tetrasomy 12p and mosaic conditions may be revealed by fibroblast cultures (Figure 23.25)
- Magnetic resonance imaging (MRI) may reveal arachnoid cysts and other anomalies of the central nervous system (CNS)

Genetics and pathogenesis

- Maternal age is a factor in the pathogenesis
- Tetrasomy 12p itself explains the malformations
- Mosaic conditions are frequent and explain the relative phenotypic differences

Follow-up and therapy

- Neurologic consultations
- Anticonvulsant drugs
- Psychologic support for patients and families
- Physiotherapy

Differential diagnosis

- Incontinentia pigmenti
- Fryns' syndrome
- Other linear hyperpigmentations with or without CNS involvement

REFERENCES

Chiesa J, Hoffet M, Rousseau O, et al. Pallister–Killian syndrome [i(12p)]: first pre-natal diagnosis using cordocentesis in the second trimester confirmed by in situ hybridization. Clin Genet 1998; 54: 294–302

Cormier-Daire V, Le Merrer M, Gigarel N, et al. Prezygotic origin of the isochromosome 12p in Pallister–Killian syndrome. Am J Med Genet 1997; 69: 166–8

Takakuwa K, Hataya I, Arakawa M, et al. A case of mosaic tetrasomy 12p (Pallister–Killian syndrome) diagnosed prenatally: comparison of chromosome analyses of various cells obtained from the patient. Am J Perinatol 1997; 14: 641–3

ENCEPHALOCRANIOCUTANEOUS LIPOMATOSIS

Age of onset

- At birth

Clinical findings

Cutaneous manifestations

- Cutaneous lipomatous nevi mostly confined to the scalp, often with unilateral localization
- Nevus psiloliparus is the name used by Happle to define this particular nevus (from the Greek psilos = hairless and liparos = formed by adipose tissue)
- Areas of alopecia frequently corresponding to underlying soft tumors (Figures 23.26 and 23.27)
- Papular or polypoid cutaneous lesions mostly involving the face (Figure 23.28)

Extracutaneous manifestations

- Ocular lesions: desmoid tumors of the scleral limb, dislocation of lens capsule, clouding of the cornea (Figure 23.29)
- Cerebral alteration (normally ipsilateral to the main cutaneous lesions): constant ventricular dilatation, monolateral cerebral atrophy, arachnoid cysts, pontocerebellar and paramedullary lipomas, porencephaly
- Neuromuscular retardation, monolateral spasticity, mental retardation, seizures

Course and prognosis

- Cutaneous and ocular lesions are stable
- Prognosis is strictly dependent on central nervous system involvement
- Usually, mental retardation and motor underdevelopment
- Neurologic symptoms not related to the extent of anatomic damage

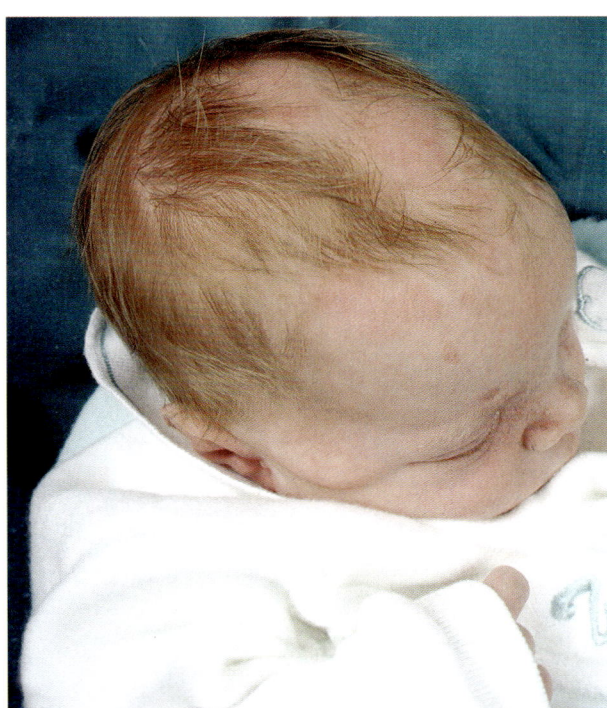

Figure 23.27

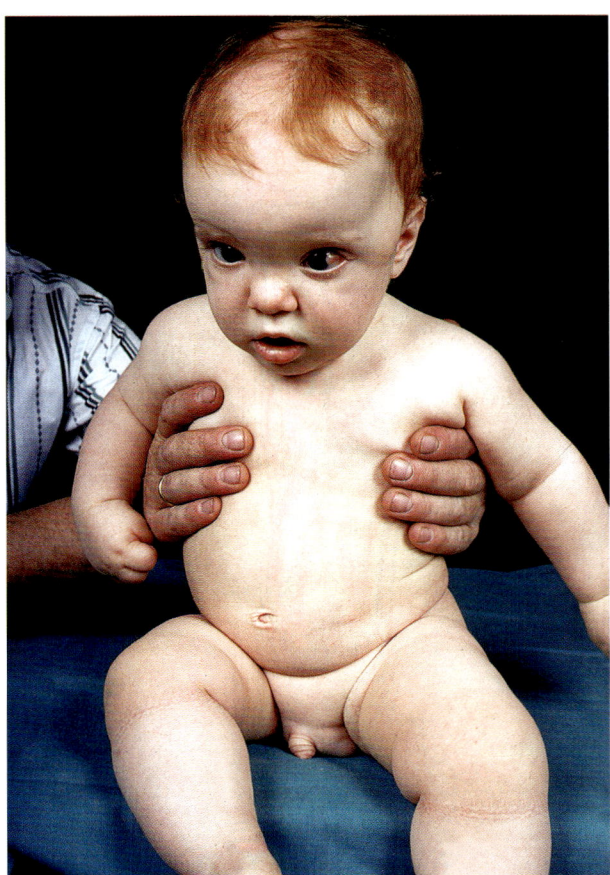

Figure 23.26

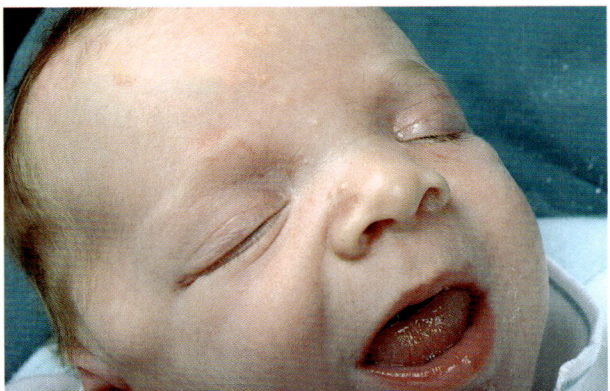

Figure 23.28

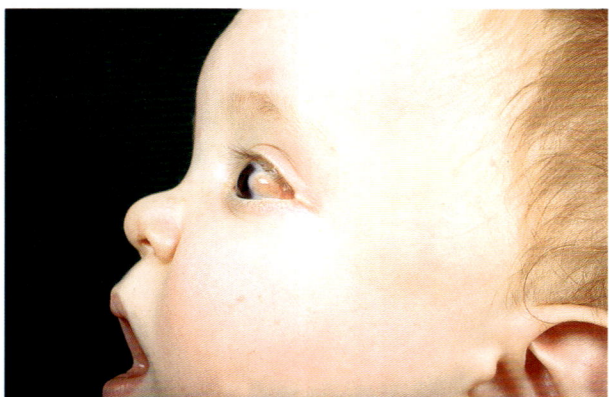

Figure 23.29

Laboratory examinations

- Histopathologic findings of cutaneous lesions: lipoma or fibrolipoma
- Ultrasonography, computerized tomographic scan, magnetic resonance imaging of the cranium
- Electroencephalography for seizures

Genetics and pathogenesis

- Sporadic
- Lethal autosomal dominant mutation, surviving by mosaicism

Differential diagnosis

- Proteus syndrome
- Epidermal nevus syndrome (Schimmelpenning's syndrome)

Follow-up and therapy

- Symptomatic neurologic drugs
- Surgical excision of cutaneous and ocular lipomas

REFERENCES

Grimalt R, Ermacora E, Mistura L, et al. Encephalocraniocutaneous lipomatosis: case report and review of the literature. Pediatr Dermatol 1993; 10: 164–8

Happle R. Lethal genes surviving by mosaicism: a possible explanation for sporadic birth defects involving the skin. J Am Acad Dermatol 1987; 16: 899–906

Nosti-Martinez D, del Castillo V, Duran C, et al. Encephalocraniocutaneous lipomatosis: an uncommon neurocutaneous syndrome. J Am Acad Dermatol 1995; 32: 387–9

GAPO SYNDROME

Synonym

- **G**rowth retardation, **A**lopecia, **P**seudoanodontia, **O**ptic atrophy

Epidemiology

Twenty-two cases are reported.

Age of onset

- Skin signs may be visible after the first 2 years of life
- Cranial anomalies at birth

Clinical findings

- Scalp and body hair is present at birth but is invariably lost during the first years of life (Figure 23.30)
- Eyelashes and eyebrows are involved
- Face wrinkles and visible dilated scalp veins

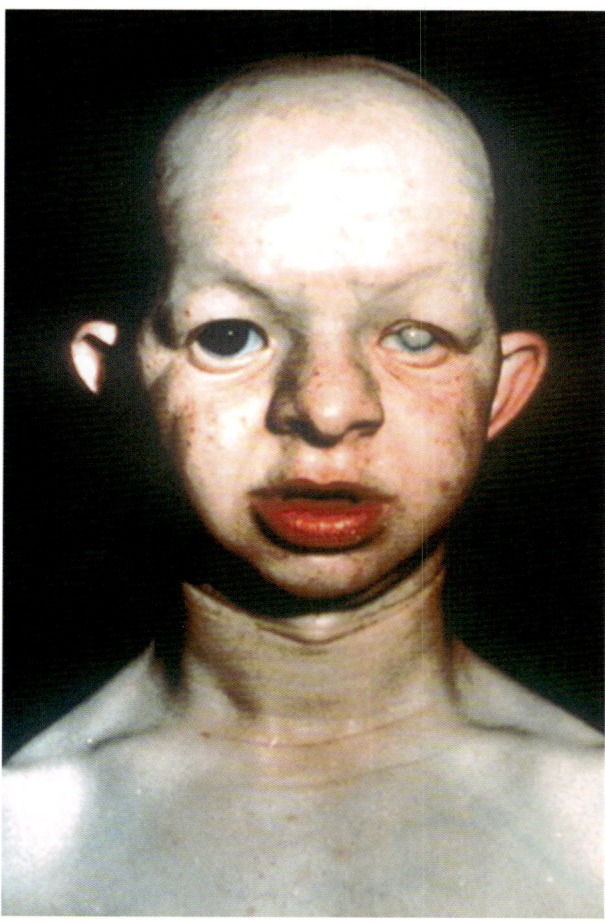

Figure 23.30

Extracutaneous manifestations

- Facies with frontal bossing, high forehead, midfacial hypoplasia, broad nose with anteverted nostrils, large mouth with thick lips and large ears, creating a comprehensive elderly appearance
- Edentulous jaws (Figure 23.31) with radiography showing an overcrowded mouth for the contemporaneous presence of two unerupted dentitions (pseudoanodontia)
- Optic nerve atrophy (30%) due to glaucoma and keratoconus (Figure 23.30)
- Umbilical hernia (90%)
- Reduced body length with retarded bone age and 'muscular appearance'
- Renal abnormalities

Course and prognosis

- Scalp and body hair is rapidly lost during infancy
- Ophthalmological abnormalities lead to severely impaired vision
- Expected life span is reduced

Laboratory findings

Biopsies demonstrate the deposition of an anomalous hyaline substance and fibrosis.

Genetics and pathogenesis

The disease is autosomal recessive (consanguinity), due to an unkown defect.

Follow-up and therapy

- Maxillofacial and ophthalmological survey

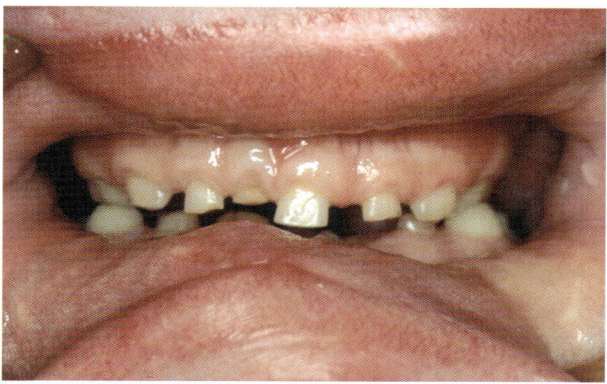

Figure 23.31

Differential diagnosis

- Hutchinson–Gilford progeria syndrome

REFERENCES

Bacon W, Hall RK, Roset JP, et al. GAPO syndrome: a new case of this rare syndrome and a review of the relative importance of different phenotypic features in diagnosis. J Craniofac Genet Dev Biol 1999; 19: 189–200. Review

Baxova A, Kozlowski K, Obersztyn E, Zeman J. GAPO syndrome (radiographic clues to early diagnosis). Radiol Med (Torino) 1997; 93: 289–91

Ilker SS, Ozturk F, Kurt E, et al. Ophthalmic findings in GAPO syndrome. Jpn J Ophthalmol 1999; 43: 48–52

Mullaney PB, Jacquemin C, al-Rashed W, Smith W. Growth retardation, alopecia, pseudoanodontia, and optic atrophy (GAPO syndrome) with congenital glaucoma. Arch Ophthalmol 1997; 115: 940–1

Orbak Z, Orbak R, Ozkan B, Okten A. GAPO syndrome: first patients with partially empty sella. J Pediatr Endocrinol Metab 2002; 15: 865–8

CHAPTER 24

Genodermatoses related to malignancy

NEVOID BASAL CELL CARCINOMA SYNDROME

Synonyms

- Gorlin syndrome
- Basal cell nevus syndrome

Age of onset

- From birth to childhood

Clinical findings

- Multiple basal cell carcinomas appearing as smooth, flesh-colored to red-brown papules distributed mainly on the face, neck, back and chest (90%) (Figures 24.1–24.4)
- Palmar and plantar pits 2–3 mm in diameter in 65–80% of patients (Figure 24.5)
- Facial milia and epidermal cysts on the limbs and trunk (~50%) (Figure 24.6)
- Occasionally acrochordons (Figure 24.7)

Extracutaneous manifestations

- Odontogenic cysts of the jaw in about 80% of patients: multiple, often symptomatic, causing marked tooth displacement
- Calcification of falx cerebri in about 85% of patients
- Musculoskeletal abnormalities: enlarged occipito-frontal circumference (80%), frontal bossing (65%), fused or bifid ribs (50%), spina bifida occulta of cervical or thoracic vertebrae (60%), kyphoscoliosis (30%), scapular deformity (30%), brachymetacarpalism (15–45%), cleft palate (5%), polydactyly (4%)

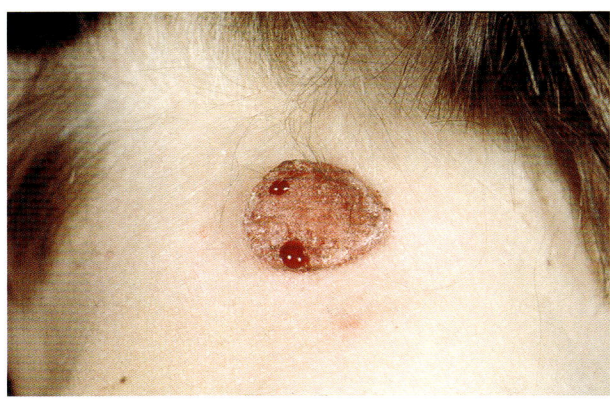

Figure 24.1

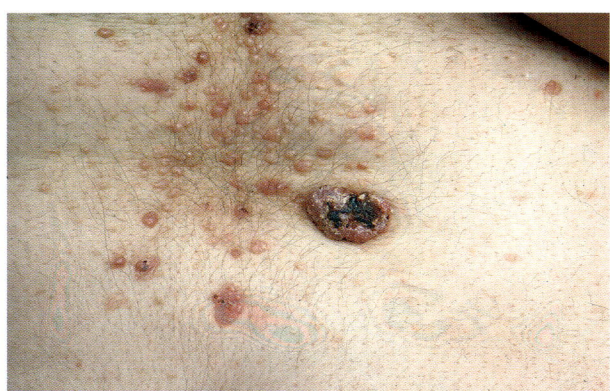

Figure 24.2

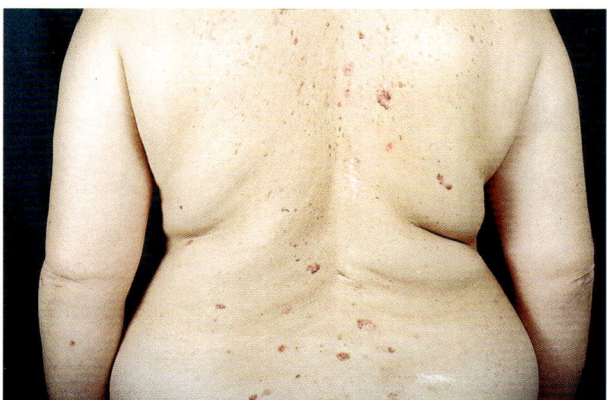

Figure 24.3

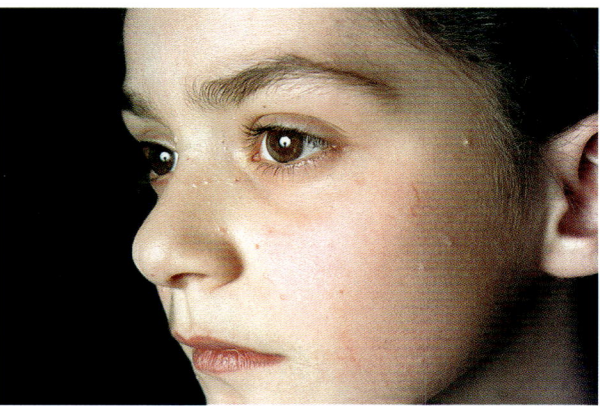

Figure 24.6

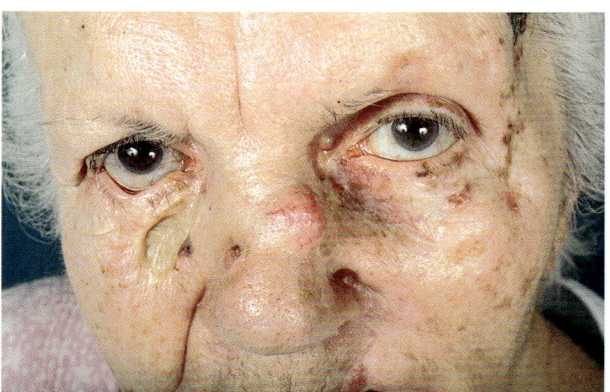

Figure 24.4

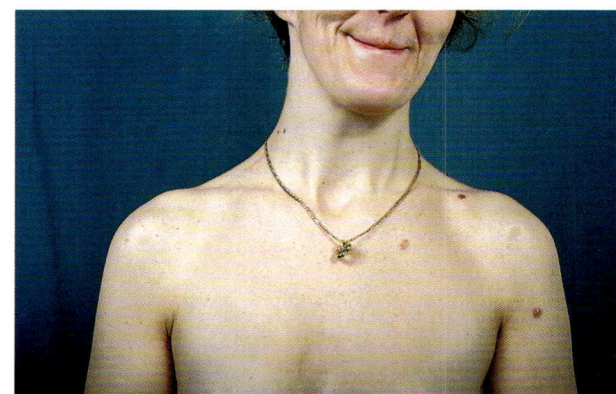

Figure 24.7

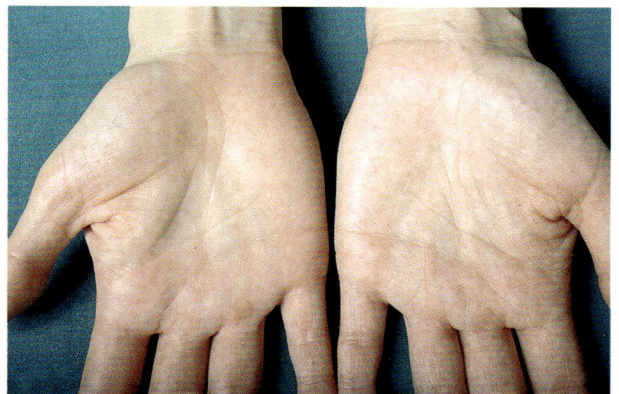

Figure 24.5

- Eye anomalies in 10–25% of patients: cataract, strabismus, colobomas of iris, choroid or optic nerve, hypertelorism
- Hypogonadism in 5–10% of male patients

- Kidney anomalies (5%): horseshoe kidney, unilateral renal agenesis
- Occasionally, mental retardation and seizures due to cerebellar medulloblastoma in 3–5% that may be the first manifestation of the disease
- Ovarian fibroma in about 15%
- Cardiac fibroma (3%)
- Mesenteric cysts
- Fetal rhabdomyoma, fibrosarcoma, leiomyomas

Course and prognosis

- Basal cell carcinomas may increase in number and become aggressive after puberty
- Odontogenic cysts occur frequently before basal cell carcinomas and may easily recur after removal
- Musculoskeletal abnormalities may be congenital and medulloblastoma may occasionally be the first manifestation

Laboratory investigations

- Histopathologic findings: typical aspect of basal cell carcinoma or rarely of infundibulocystic basal cell carcinoma
- Skeletal radiography
- Total body magnetic resonance imaging

Genetics and pathogenesis

- Autosomal dominant inheritance
- The responsible gene, the PTCH gene, is mapped to chromosome 9q22.3–q31
- The PTCH gene is a tumor suppressor gene and patients with mutations in this gene have a predisposition not only for multiple basal cell carcinomas but also for other tumors and skeletal abnormalities

Differential diagnosis

- Bazex syndrome
- Other cancer-related genodermatoses

Follow-up and therapy

- Close surveillance is mandatory, with periodic radiography and nuclear magnetic resonance examinations
- It is necessary to avoid sun exposure and radiotherapy
- Basal cell carcinomas: topical 5-fluorouracil or imiquimod cream, surgical excision, electrodesiccation, CO_2 laser, photodynamic therapy, oral retinoids
- Odontogenic cysts: surgical excision

REFERENCES

Boutet N, Bignon YJ, Drouin-Garraud V, et al. Spectrum of PTCH1 mutations in French patients with Gorlin syndrome. J Invest Dermatol 2003; 121: 478–81

Chiritesen E, Maloney ME. Acrochordons as a presenting sign of nevoid basal cell carcinoma syndrome. J Am Acad Dermatol 2001; 44: 789–94

Cohen MM Jr. Craniofacial anomalies: clinical and molecular perspectives. Ann Acad Med Singapore 2003; 32: 244–51

Gorlin RJ. Nevoid basal cell carcinoma syndrome. Dermatol Clin 1995; 13: 113–25

Olivieri C, Maraschio P, Caselli D, et al. Intersitial deletion of chromosome 9, int del(9)(9q22.31.2), including the genes causing multiple basal cell nevus syndrome and Robinow/brachydactyly 1 syndrome. Eur J Pediatr 2003; 162: 100–3

MUIR–TORRE SYNDROME

Synonym

- Torre syndrome

Age of onset

- Fourth or fifth decade of life

Clinical findings

Skin lesions

- Sebaceous gland tumors (hyperplasias, adenomas, carcinomas) presenting as yellow papules or nodules located mainly on the face (Figures 24.8–24.10)
- Keratoacanthomas (one or more) spontaneously involuting as associated cutaneous finding (23%)

Extracutaneous features

- Colorectal cancers (53%)
- Colon polyps
- Genitourinary neoplasms (25%)
- Breast and lung tumors
- Hematologic malignancies

Course and prognosis

Visceral malignancies, usually of low grade, may precede the appearance of sebaceous tumors in 60%.

Laboratory findings

- Skin and colon biopsies
- Colonoscopy
- Carcinoembryonic antigen
- Stool examination for occult blood
- Chest radiography

Genetics and pathogenesis

- Autosomal dominant disease with variable degree of penetrance; few sporadic cases
- Germline mutation in the mismatch DNA-repair gene $hMSH_2$, located on chromosome 2p

Differential diagnosis

- Cowden's syndrome
- Gardner's syndrome
- Gorlin syndrome

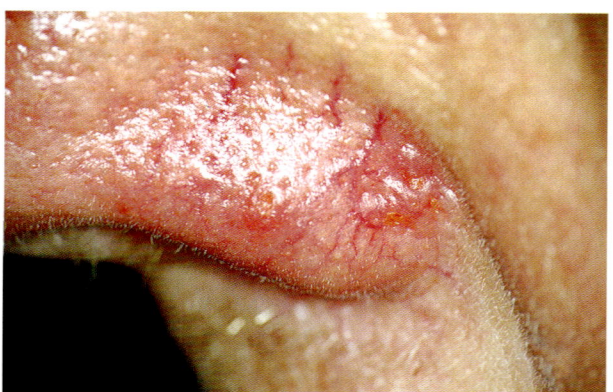

Figure 24.8

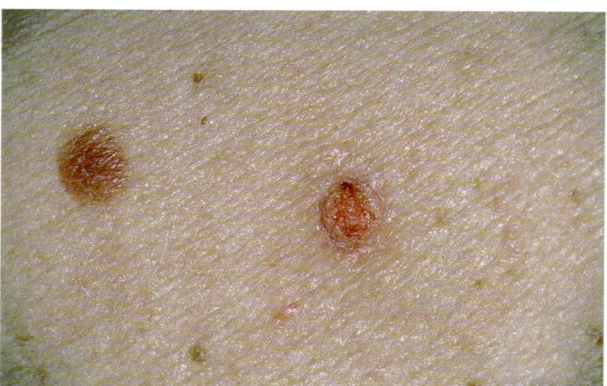

Figure 24.10

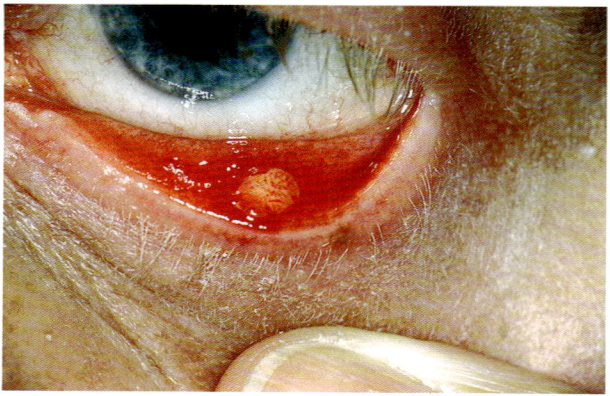

Figure 24.9

- Multiple self-healing keratoacanthomas
- Tuberous sclerosis

Follow-up and therapy

- Periodic accurate screening for visceral tumors
- Evaluation for internal malignancy in asymptomatic relatives
- Treatment of skin tumors surgically or with CO_2 laser
- Prevention may be tried with oral retinoids
- Surgery for bowel neoplasms

REFERENCES

Cohen PR, Kohn SR, Davis DA, et al. Muir Torre syndrome. Dermatol Clin 1995; 13: 79–89

Esche C, Kruse R, Lamberti C, et al. Muir Torre syndrome: clinical features and molecular genetic analysis. Br J Dermatol 1997; 136: 913–17

Kruse R, Rutten A, Schweiger N, et al. Frequency of microsatellite instability in unselected sebaceous gland neoplasias and hyperplasias. J Invest Dermatol 2003; 120: 858–64

Machin P, Catasus L, Pons C, et al. Microsatellite instability and immunostaining for MSH-2 and MLH-1 in cutaneous and internal tumors from patients with the Muir–Torre syndrome. J Cutan Pathol 2002; 29: 415–20

Popnikolov NK, Gatalica Z, Colome-Grimmer MI, Sanchez RL. Loss of mismatch repair proteins in sebaceous gland tumors. J Cutan Pathol 2003; 30: 178–84

COWDEN'S SYNDROME

Synonym

- Multiple hamartoma syndrome

Age of onset

- Usually third to fourth decade of life

Clinical findings

- Facial papules (83%): yellow or flesh colored, flat topped papules, 1–4 mm in diameter sometimes with a central keratin-plugged opening, generally concentrated around the orifices (Figures 24.11 and 24.12)
- Oral mucosal papillomatosis (83%): smooth-surfaced rose-red papules located primarily on the gingival, labial and palatal surfaces. Coalescence of the lesions gives a cobblestone appearance (Figure 24.13)
- Acral keratoses (63%): flesh-colored, smooth or rough-surfaced papules, 1–4 mm in diameter, located mainly on the dorsa of the hands and feet (Figures 24.14 and 24.15)
- Palmoplantar keratoses (42%): hard translucent punctate papules on the palms and soles (Figure 24.16)
- Scrotal tongue (17%)
- Cutaneous lipomas (39%), hemangiomas (21%), neuromas (10%)

Extracutaneous findings

- Thyroid gland lesions (67%): goiter, adenomas, follicular adenocarcinomas
- Breast lesions (76% of female patients): fibrocystic disease, ductal adenocarcinoma (25%)
- Gastrointestinal lesions (40%): polyposis
- Genitourinary tract lesions (55% of female patients): ovarian cysts, leiomyomas, menstrual irregularities
- Skeletal lesions (37%): macrocephaly, adenoid facies, high arched palate, kyphosis
- Eye lesions (13%): myopia, photophobia, angioid streaks
- Nervous system lesions (19%): low intelligence, disturbances of coordination, electroencephalographic abnormalities

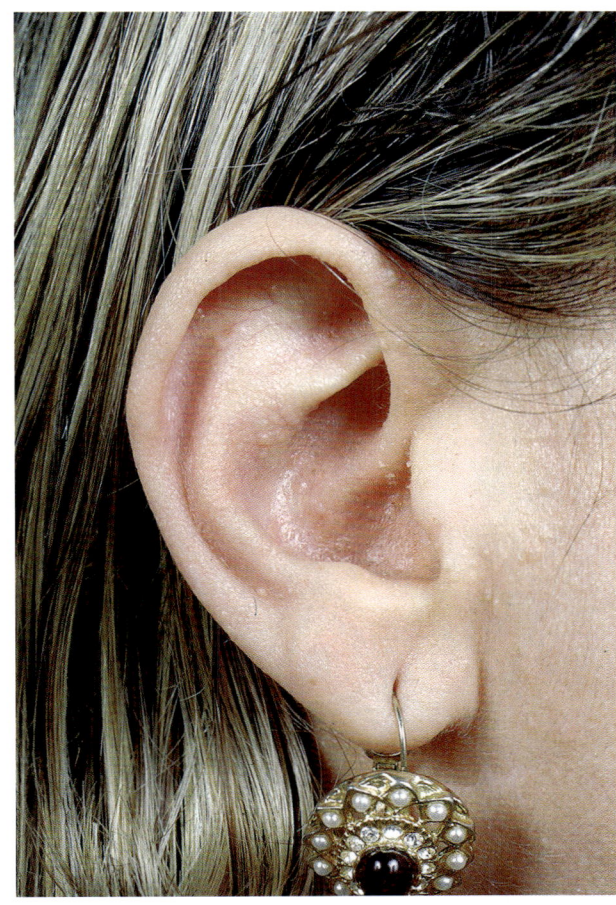

Figure 24.12

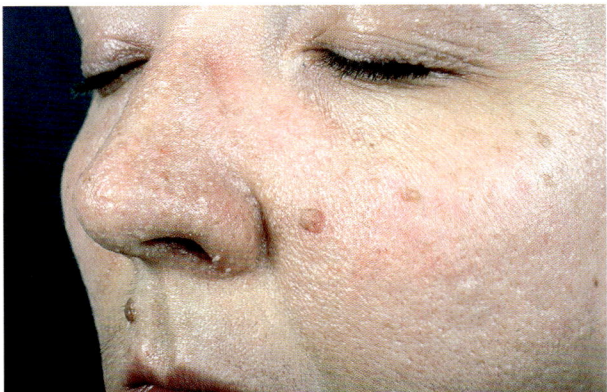

Figure 24.11

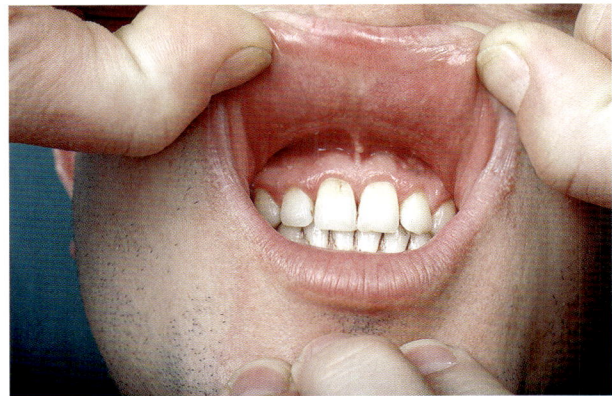

Figure 24.13

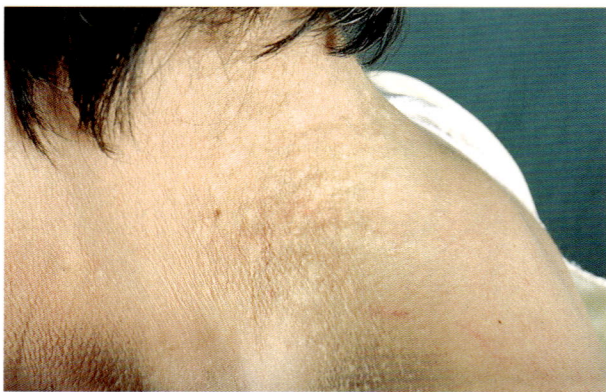

Figure 24.14

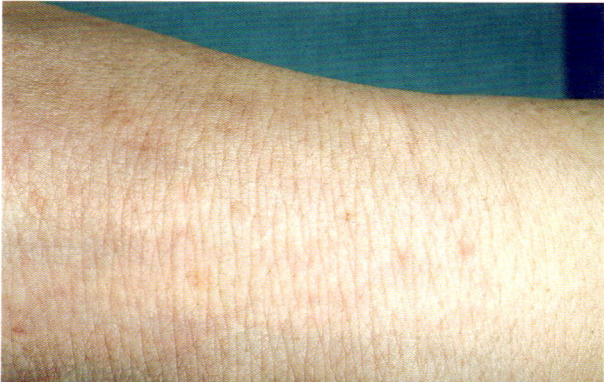

Figure 24.15

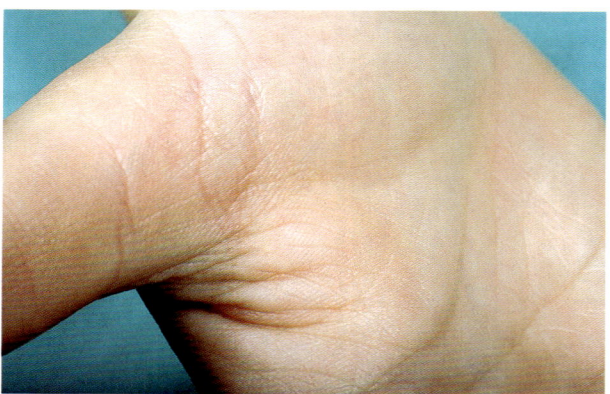

Figure 24.16

Course and progression

- Facial, oral and acral lesions usually precede the development of extracutaneous manifestations
- Normal life span in the absence of malignancies

Laboratory examinations

- Histopathologic findings of skin and mucosal lesions: facial lesions, trichilemmomas; oral and acral lesions, papillomas

- Thyroid test and scan
- Mammography
- Radiography of bones
- Electroencephalogram
- Gastro- and colonoscopy

Genetics and pathogenesis

- Autosomal dominant disease
- Germline mutations of the tumor suppressor gene PTEN (phosphatase and tensin homolog) on chromosome 10q23. Mutations are located mainly on exons 5, 6, 7, and 8
- Bannayan–Riley–Ruvalcaba syndrome, characterized by macrocephaly, intestinal polyposis, lipomas, pigmented macules of glans penis and mental retardation, is due to mutation on PTEN gene and considered allelic to Cowden syndrome

Differential diagnosis

- Gorlin syndrome
- Tuberous sclerosis
- Lipoid proteinosis
- Muir–Torre disease
- Darier's disease

Follow-up and therapy

- Accurate, periodic control by gynecologists and gastroenterologists
- 52% of women and 23% of men develop cancer
- Breast cancer develops in 36–50% of female patients
- Prophylactic mastectomy
- Excision of hamartomas and neoplasias
- Dermabrasion, CO_2 laser and systemic retinoids for skin and mucosal lesions

REFERENCES

Eng C. PTEN: one gene, many syndromes. Hum Mutat 2003; 22: 183–98

Schaller J, Rohwedder A, Burgdorf WH, et al. Identification of human papillomavirus DNA in cutaneous lesions of Cowden syndrome. Dermatology 2003; 207: 134–40

Zhou XP, Waite KA, Pilarski R, et al. Germline PTEN promoter mutations and deletions in Cowden/Bannayan–Riley–Ruvalcaba syndrome result in aberrant PTEN protein and dysregulation of the phosphoinsitol-3-kinase/AKT pathway. Am J Hum Genet 2003; 73: 404–11

GARDNER SYNDROME

Age of onset

- Childhood and adolescence for skin and bone lesions
- Adulthood for gastrointestinal lesions

Clinical findings

- Multiple epidermal cysts in 50–65% of patients mainly localized on the face, scalp and extremities (Figures 24.17–24.19)

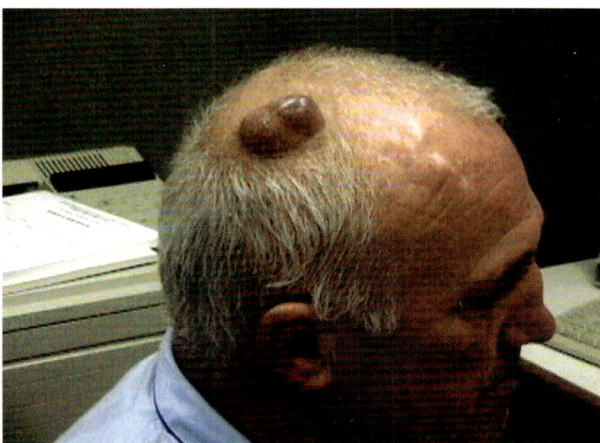

Figure 24.17

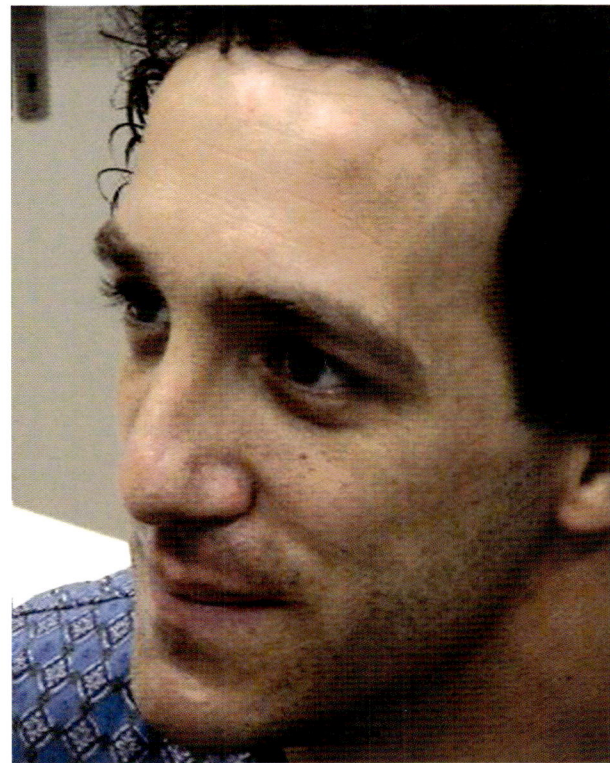

Figure 24.18

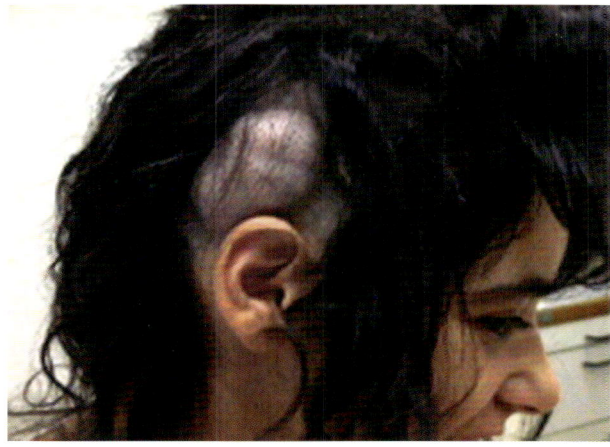

Figure 24.19

- Desmoid tumors presenting as poorly defined, deep lesions within the soft tissue of the anterior abdominal wall triggered by trauma
- Less frequently, fibromas, lipomas, leiomyomas, neurofibromas

Extracutaneous findings

- Multiple gastrointestinal polyps with high predisposition to malignant adenocarcinoma, more frequently localized on the colon and rectum in 100% of patients
- Osteomas in more than 50% of patients, mostly involving the mandible and the skull
- Multifocal pigmented lesion of the ocular fundus in about 80% of patients: an early and important marker of the disease
- Dental abnormalities (~ 18%), including congenitally absent teeth, odontomas, rudimentary and supernumerary teeth, multiple caries
- Adenocarcinoma of the colon in almost 100% of patients
- Periampullary carcinoma (~ 12%)
- Less frequently thyroid ovarian and pancreatic carcinoma, hepatoblastoma, medulloblastoma, glioblastoma, craniopharyngioma, osteosarcoma, liposarcoma

Course and prognosis

- Ocular lesions are congenital or present shortly after birth
- Skin and bone lesions precede colonic polyposis and may increase in number and size with age
- Average age for diagnosis of colon cancer is 40 years

Laboratory investigations and data

- Endoscopy, colonoscopy and radiologic evaluation of the gastrointestinal tract
- Radiologic evaluation of bones
- Fundoscopic evaluation
- Fecal occult blood studies
- Histologic findings of epidermoid cyst: keratin-filled cystic cavity within the dermis lined by a well of stratified squamous epithelium containing granular layer, sometimes with focal pilomatricoma-like changes

Genetics and pathogenesis

- Autosomal dominant inheritance
- Gene locus location in an area on the long arm of chromosome 5 (5q21) and referred to as the adenomatous polyposis coli locus (APC)

Differential diagnosis

- Epidermoid cysts
- Familial adenomatous polyposis: without skin and bone lesions
- Turcot's syndrome: characterized by colonic polyposis, café-au-lait spots and malignant tumors of the central nervous system

Follow-up and therapy

- Regular screening of the gastrointestinal tract is mandatory
- Careful examination of relatives
- Molecular genetics screening in all the pedigrees
- Surgical excision of cysts and osteomas
- Endoscopic excision of polyps
- Prophylactic colectomy

REFERENCES

Pernciara C. Gardner's syndrome. Dermatol Clin 1995; 13: 51–6

Tsao H. Update on familial cancer syndromes and the skin. J Am Acad Dermatol 2000; 42: 939–69

Williams SC, Peller PJ. Gardner's syndrome: case report and discussion on the manifestations of the disorder. Clin Nucl Med 1994; 19: 668–70

BLOOM'S SYNDROME

Synonym

- Congenital telangiectatic erythema

Age of onset

- During the first or second summer of life

Clinical findings

- Sun-sensitive erythematous telangiectatic patches on the face distributed in a butterfly configuration, resembling lupus erythematosus (main feature) (Figure 24.20)
- Occasionally, erythematous lesions on the forearms and dorsa of the hands
- Patchy areas of hyperpigmentation and hypopigmentation on the trunk and extremities (in about 50%)
- Blistering and crusting of the lips
- Conjunctivitis and loss of eyelashes
- Café-au-lait spots

Extracutaneous findings

- Stunted growth: small body size with normal proportions and without identifiable endocrine dysfunctions (main feature)
- Characteristic facies due to dolichocephaly, small narrow face, nasal prominence
- Skeletal malformations such as clinodactyly and syndactyly
- Characteristic high-pitched voice
- Testicular atrophy
- Variable degree of vomiting and diarrhea
- Diabetes mellitus
- Mental retardation
- Immunodeficiency

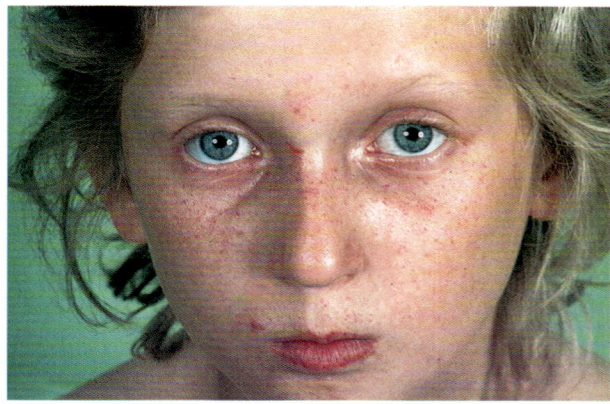

Figure 24.20

Complications

- Predisposition to cancer (a quarter of patients): leukemia, lymphoid tumors, carcinomas
- Increased occurrence of respiratory and gastrointestinal infections

Course and prognosis

The intensity of facial erythema and of the sun sensitivity diminishes with age, but there is an incidence of early death from cancers or infections (mean life span is 18 years).

Laboratory investigations

- Chromosomal studies showing high frequency of sister chromatid exchanges and quadriradial configurations in cultured lymphocytes: diagnostic for the disease
- Increased sensitivity to ultraviolet light
- Immunoglobulin deficiency of at least one class: IgG, IgM or IgA
- Complete blood count and bone marrow examination

Genetics and pathogenesis

- Autosomal recessive disease
- Gene for α helicase (DNA-repair) is mutated in these patients

Differential diagnosis

- Ataxia telangiectasia syndrome
- Rothmund Thomson syndrome
- Cockayne's syndrome
- Dyskeratosis congenita
- Xeroderma pigmentosum
- Kindler syndrome
- Porphyrias

Follow-up and therapy

- Continuous screening of these patients for increased occurrence of malignancies and severe infections is mandatory
- Prenatal diagnosis is possible by detection of a high number of sister chromatid exchanges in amniotic fluid cells and from molecular genetics data
- Sun protection
- Bone marrow replacement
- Antibiotics
- Specific therapy for associated neoplasms

REFERENCES

Boda KN, Bodemer C. Photosensibilité chez l'enfant. Ann Dermatol Venereol 2002; 129: 244–50

Charames GS, Bapat B. Genomic instability and cancer. Curr Mol Med 2003; 3: 589–96

German J. Bloom's syndrome. Dermatol Clin 1995; 13: 7–18

Gretzula JC, Herva D, Weber PJ. Bloom's syndrome. J Am Acad Dermatol 1987; 17: 479–88

Rassool FV, North PS, Mufti GJ, Hickson ID. Constitutive DNA damage is linked to DNA replication abnormalities in Bloom's syndrome cells. Oncogene 2003; 22: 8749–57

Wu L, Hickson ID. The Bloom's syndrome helicase suppresses crossing over during homologous recombination. Nature (London) 2003; 426: 870–4

HOWEL–EVANS SYNDROME

Synonym

- Tylosis and esophageal carcinoma

Epidemiology

The syndrome is rare. No further data are available.

Age of onset

- Later than in other palmoplantar keratodermas (PPK), usually after the first decade

Clinical findings

- Blotchy plantar hyperkeratosis, especially in pressure areas (Figure 24.21), with or without underlying erythema
- Palmar involvement is much less severe
- Skin may be dry, with follicular hyperkeratosis
- Onychodystrophy and leukoplakia are possible

Extracutaneous findings

Esophageal carcinoma of the lower two-thirds of the esophagus is found in almost all affected subjects (>90%).

Course and prognosis

Esophageal neoplasms occur almost invariably in the affected subject within the fourth–fifth decades.

Laboratory investigations

Aspecific data owing to the presence of esophageal carcinomas may be present.

Genetics and pathogenesis

- Autosomal dominant
- The gene is unknown and is located in a minimal region (42.5kb) of chromosome 17q25

Follow-up and therapy

- Any PPK of unclear diagnosis must be assessed for even minimal signs of dysphagia

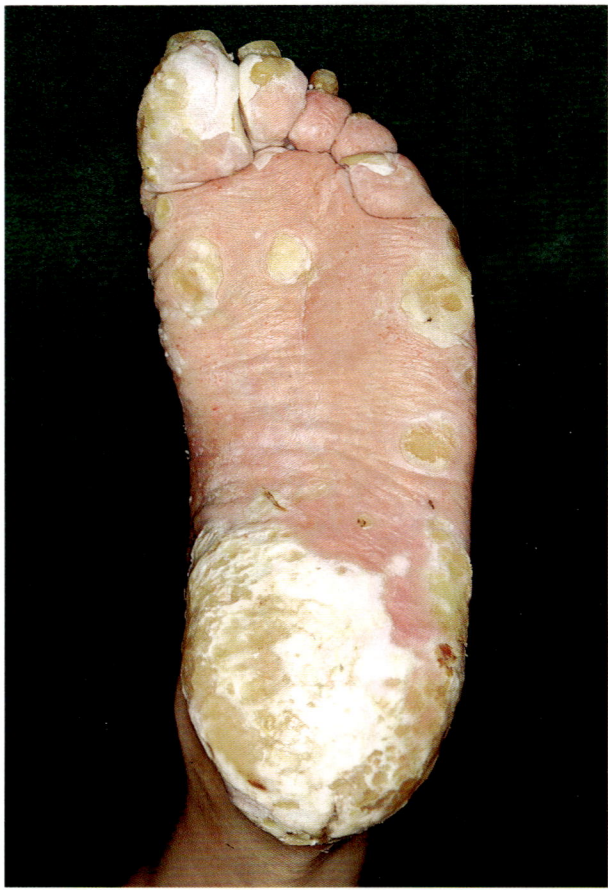

Figure 24.21

- Surgery for neoplasms
- Usual keratolytic agents for PPK
- Endoscopy in the relatives of patients

Differential diagnosis

It is very difficult to discriminate the PPK of Howel–Evans syndrome from many other non-syndromic palmoplantar keratodermas.

The late onset and the predominant plantar involvement may be useful to detect carriers before the occurrence of dysphagia and neoplastic stenosis.

REFERENCE

Bethke G, Kolde G, Bethke G, Reichart PA. [Focal palmo-plantar and oral mucosa hyperkeratosis syndrome.] Mund Kiefer Gesichtschir 2001; 5: 202–5

MULTIPLE ENDOCRINE NEOPLASIA SYNDROME, TYPE 2B

Synonym

- MEN 2B syndrome

Epidemiology

More than 150 cases are described, but it may be that numerous familial cases have been misdiagnosed.

Clinical findings

- Hyperpigmentation of entire skin is reported, rarely perioral lentiginosis
- Enlarged, swollen and often nodular lips (Figures 24.22 and 24.23)
- Occasionally, hypertrichosis and synophris (Figures 24.22 and 24.23)
- Multiple plexiform neuromata in oral mucosa (lips and internal cheeks) and tongue

Extracutaneous symptoms

- Peculiar facies, elongated in shape, with hypertelorism, synophris, broad nose, enlarged lips and occasionally tarsal hypertrophy (Figure 24.23)
- Medullary carcinoma of the thyroid ('C' cells) (90%)
- Pheochromocytoma (50–90%)
- Megacolon (30–50%), diverticulosis and diarrhea
- Asthenic–marfanoid habitus with muscular hypotrophy
- Pubertal delay
- Neuromas are present in the upper and lower respiratory tract
- White, medullated corneal nerve fibers are visible under slit-lamp examination (>50%)

Laboratory findings

- Urinary catecholamines are higher than normal
- Aspecific cancer-related data (FT3-FT4, TSH)

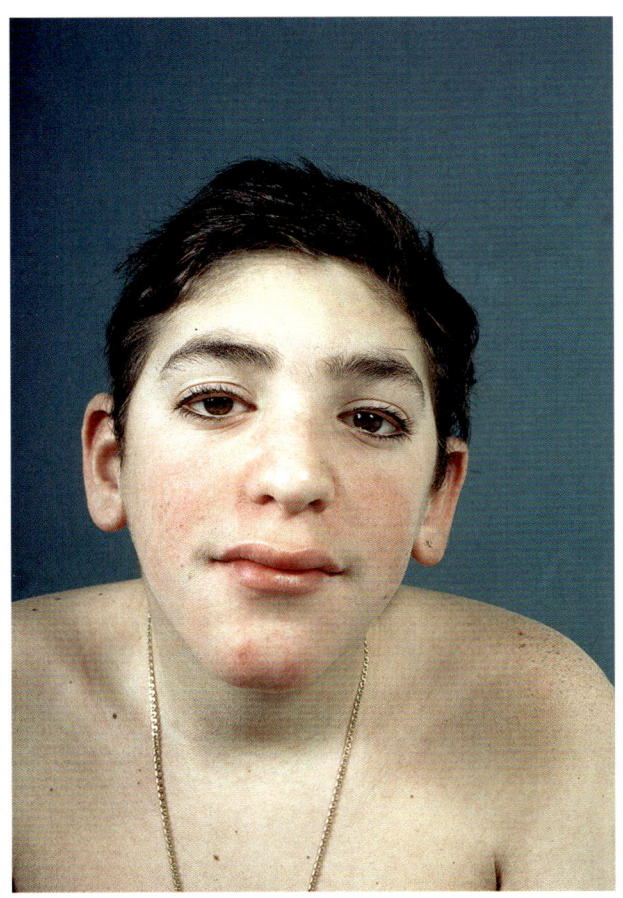

Figure 24.22

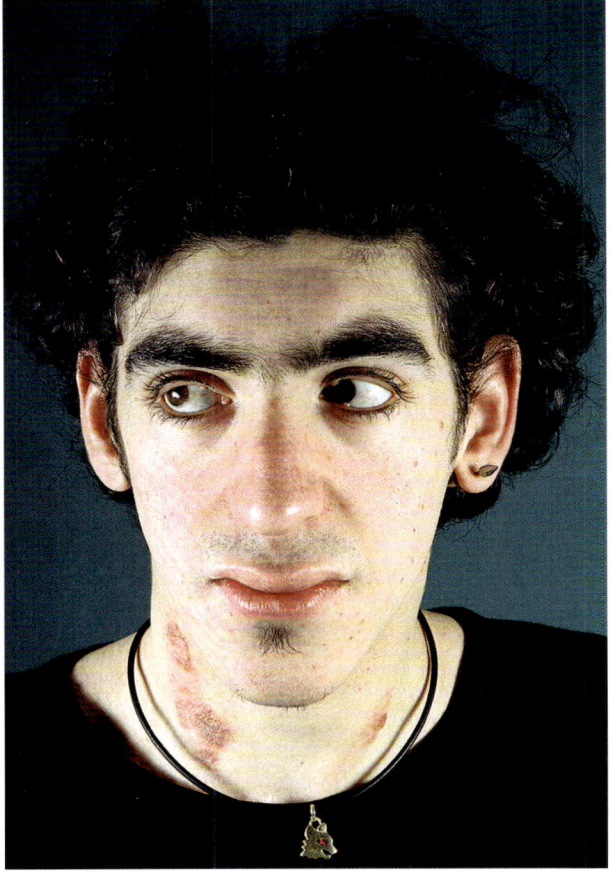

Figure 24.23

Course and complications

Medullary carcinoma of the thyroid metastatizes early and frequently and is the more likely cause of death in these patients (in a published series the average age at death from metastatic medullary thyroid carcinoma was 21 years).

Genetics and pathogenesis

- The disease is inherited in an autosomal dominant fashion with high penetrance and variable expression
- Half of patients are sporadic cases
- Missense mutations in the receptor tyrosine kinase of the *ret* proto-oncogene cause MEN 2B (95% are in the 'hot-spot' of M918T substitution and others are A883F). These mutations cause hyperplasia and neoplasia of cells derived from the neural crest and the related findings of MEN 2B

Follow-up and therapy

- Medullary carcinoma may be present in early childhood
- Preventive ablation is mandatory in known familial cases
- Surgery for pheochromocytoma
- Medical therapy for pheochromocytoma-related symptoms

Differential diagnosis

- MEN 2A (with cutaneous amyloidosis)
- Neurofibromatosis
- Cowden's syndrome
- Marfan's syndrome
- Hirschsprung's disease
- Melkersson–Rosenthal syndrome
- Multiple systematized neuromata of the skin and mucosa

REFERENCES

Hennige AM, Lammers R, Arit D, et al. Ret oncogene signal transduction via a IRS-2/PI 3-kinase/PKB and a SHC.Grb-2 dependent pathway: possible implication for transforming activity in NIH3T3 cells. Mol Cell Endocrinol 2000; 167: 69–76

Watanabe T, Ichihara M, Hashimoto M, et al. Characterization of gene expression induced by RET with MEN2A or MEN2B mutation. Am J Pathol 2002; 161: 249–56

PEUTZ–JEGHERS SYNDROME

Synonym

- Intestinal polyposis (generalized) type II

Epidemiology

No specific data are available.

Age of onset

- Early childhood

Clinical findings

- Dark-pigmented pinpoint macules on the lips, perioral and facial areas (Figure 24.24), less frequently on hands (fingertips) (Figure 24.25) and other areas (genital and perianal) and soles (Figure 24.26)

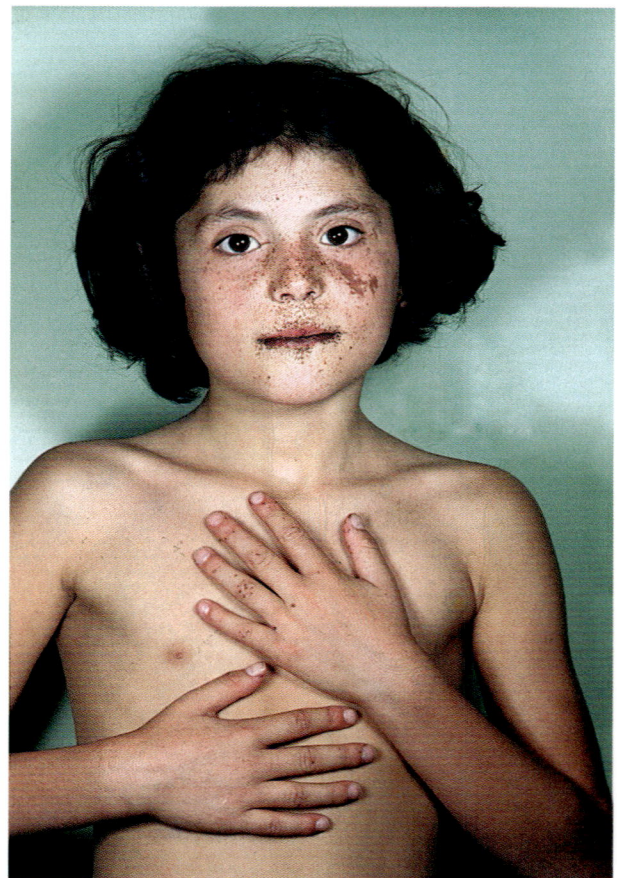

Figure 24.24

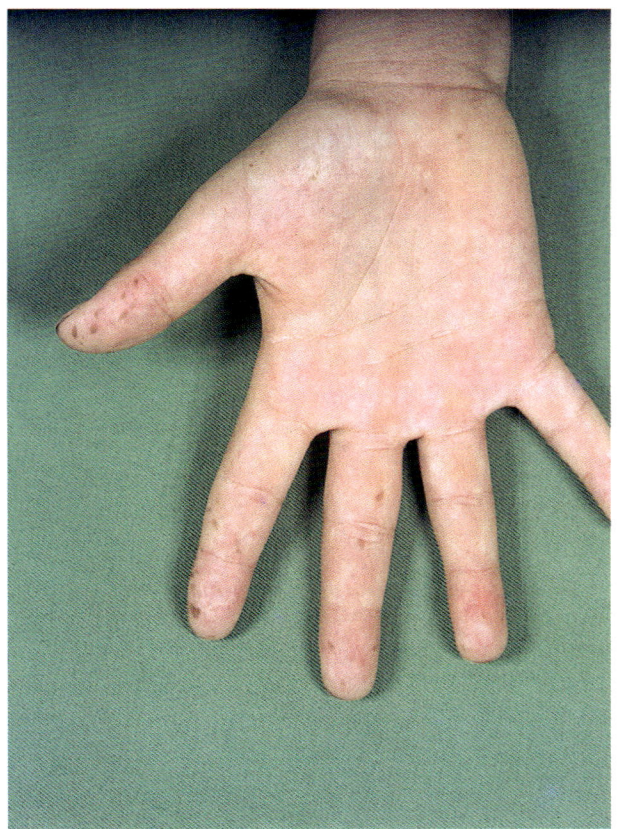

Figure 24.25

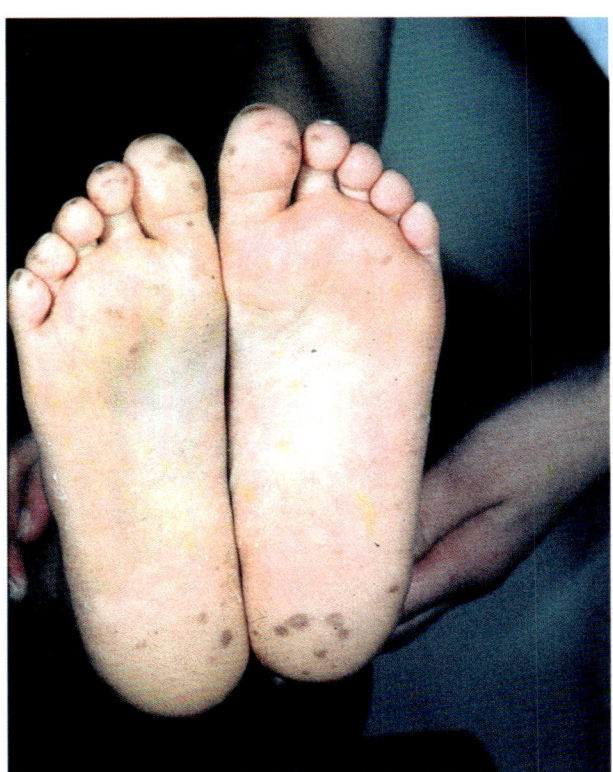

Figure 24.26

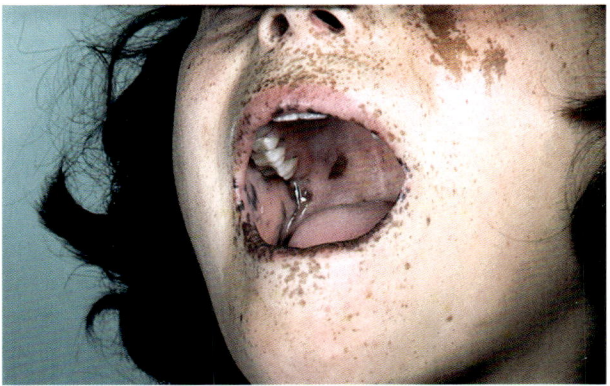

Figure 24.27

- Oral mucosal dark brown macular lesions may be large and highly characteristic (Figure 24.27)
- Rarely, telangiectases are visible on oral mucosa and pigmented lesions reach eyelids and conjunctiva

Extracutaneous symptoms

- Generalized eruption of hamartomatous polyps associated with abdominal colic pain, bleeding, intussusception and early-onset rectal prolapse
- High susceptibility to cancer (breast, uterus, ovary and testes, pancreas)
- Early onset of puberty

Course and complications

- Pigmentation of lips tends to fade at puberty
- Malignant transformation of polyps in gastrointestinal tract is relatively common (20–40%)
- Secondary anemia due to intestinal bleeding

Genetics and pathogenesis

- Autosomal dominant inheritance and high penetrance, with a third of cases representing new germline mutations
- Due to a gene called STRK11/LKB1 (a serine–threonine kinase), that encodes a tumor suppressor gene
- As occurs in other syndromes with hamartomata development (NF1 and STC), loss of heterozygosity (postzygotic) has been shown

Differential diagnosis

- LEOPARD syndrome (see Chapter 19 for definition)
- Carney's complex
- Cronkhite–Canada syndrome
- Laugier–Hunziker syndrome (acquired oral mucosa pigmentation)

Follow-up and therapy

- Endoscopy and ultrasonography are mandatory in order to prevent any malignant or proliferative transformation of intestinal and ovarian hamartomata
- Surgical excision of premalignancies and cancer if advised

REFERENCES

Eng C. Constipation, polyps, or cancer? Let PTEN predict your future. Am J Med Genet 2003; 122A: 315–22

Qunungo S, Haldar S, Basu A. Restoration of silenced Peutz–Jeghers syndrome gene, LKB1, induces apoptosis in pancreatic carcinoma cells. Neoplasia 2003; 5: 367–74

Zanoni EC, Averbach M, Borges JL, et al. Laparoscopic treatment of intestinal intussusception in the Peutz–Jeghers syndrome: case report and review of the literature. Surg Laparpsc Endosc Percutan Tech 2003; 13: 280–2

BIRT–HOGG–DUBÉ SYNDROME

Synonym

- Multiple fibrofolliculomas, trichodiscomas and acrochordons

Epidemiology

This is a very rare disease. No data are available.

Age of onset

- In early adulthood

Clinical findings

- Perifollicular fibromas, acrochordons and trichodiscomas on the face, neck and trunk (Figures 24.28–24.30)

Extracutaneous signs

- Intestinal polyposis
- Colonic cancer in a few pedigrees

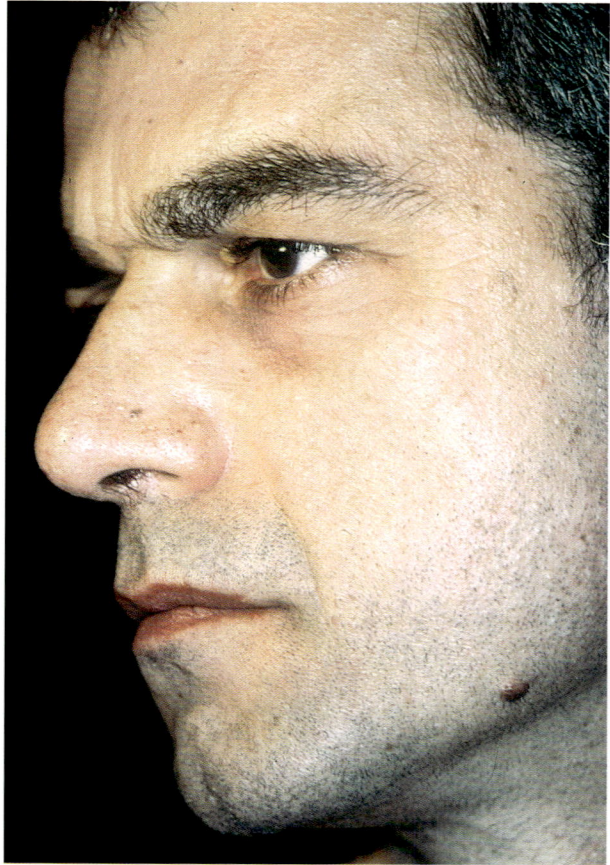

Figure 24.28

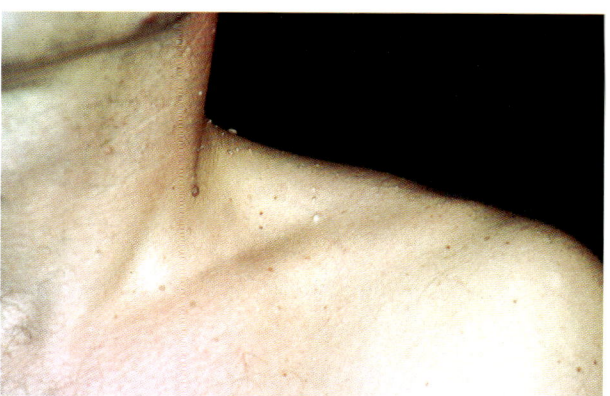

Figure 24.29

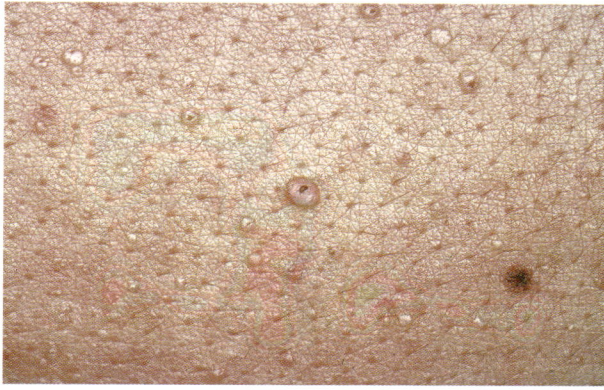

Figure 24.30

Course and prognosis

The cutaneous lesions progressively increase in number and size.

Laboratory findings

Radiography examinations of the colon may reveal polyposis and malignancies.

Genetics and pathogenesis

The disease is due to a mutation in an oncogene suppressor gene called BHD1. Mutations cause a loss of proliferation control and susceptibility to hyperproliferation and neoplastic transformation.

Follow-up and therapy

Once diagnosed, patients must be investigated for colon disease.

Differential diagnosis

- Cowden's syndrome
- Muir–Torre syndrome
- Gardner syndrome

REFERENCES

Khoo SK, Kahnoski K, Sugimura J, et al. Inactivation of BDH in sporadic renal tumors. Cancer Res 2003; 63: 4583–7

Musse L. Birt–Hogg–Dube syndrome. Dermatol Nurs 2003; 15: 178

Shin JH, Shin YK, Ku JL, et al. Mutations of the Birt–Hogg–Dube (BHD) gene in sporadic colorectal carcinomas and colorectal carcinoma cell lines with microsatellite instability. J Med Genet 2003; 40: 364–7

CARNEY'S COMPLEX

Synonyms

- NAME (nevi, atrial myxoma, myxomatous neurofibromata, ephelids)
- LAMB (lentigines, atrial myxoma, myxoid tumors, blue nevi)

Age of onset

- Early childhood to adolescence

Clinical findings

- Macules (bluish to brown ephelids), especially on the face, neck and, characteristically, on the lips (Figure 24.31)
- Intermingled blue nevi
- Brownish discoloration of major folds (Figures 24.32 and 24.33)
- Myxoid tumors (Figure 24.34)
- Pigmentation of conjunctiva

Extracutaneous findings

- Cardiac myxoma
- Adrenocortical hypertrophy
- Sertoli cell tumors
- Hypophyseal tumors
- Mammary precancerous dysplasias

Course and complications

- Mammary neoplasia can occur
- Strokes can develop from cardiac emboli due to atrial myxomas

Laboratory findings

There are none specific.

Genetics and pathogenesis

- Autosomal dominant
- Mutations of PRKAR1A gene, coding for protein kinase A, are responsible for the disease

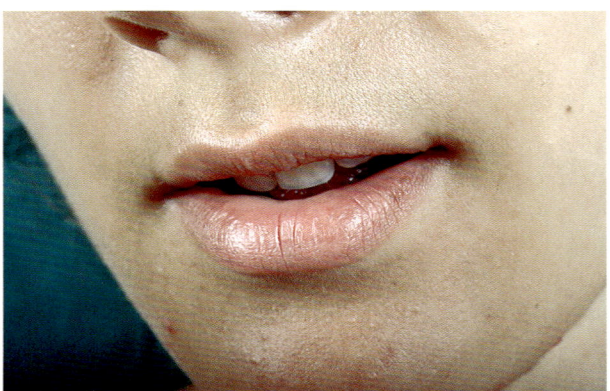

Figure 24.31

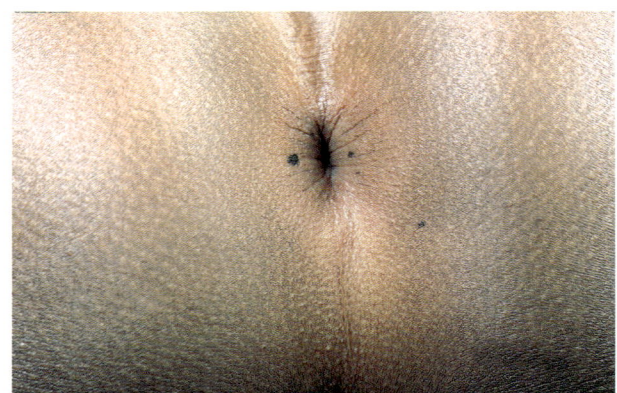

Figure 24.33

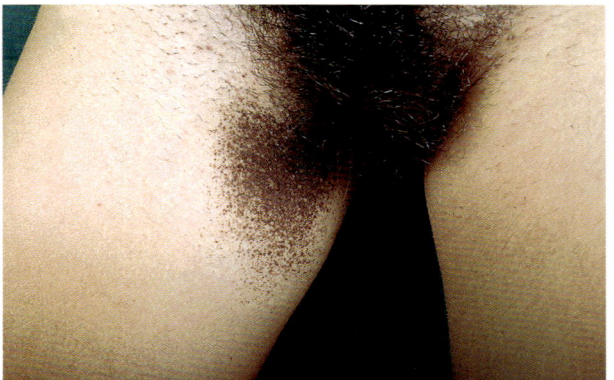

Figure 24.32

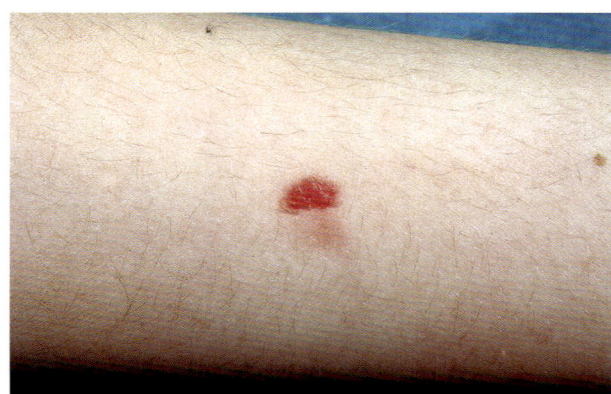

Figure 24.34

Differential diagnosis

- LEOPARD syndrome
- Xeroderma pigmentosum
- Lentiginoses
- Peutz–Jeghers syndrome

Follow-up and therapy

- Prevention of strokes
- Surgery for atrial and intracardiac myxoma when necessary
- Plastic surgery for skin myxomata

REFERENCES

Robinson-White A, Hundley TR, Shiferaw M, et al. Protein kinase-A activity in PRKAR1A-mutant cells, and regulation of mitogen-activated protein kinases ERK1/2. Hum Mol Genet 2003; 12: 1475–84

Skamrov AV, Feoktistova ES, Khaspekov GL, et al. [PRKAR1A gene mutations in two patients with carney complex.] Kardiologiia 2003; 43: 77–82

Stergiopoulos SG, Stratakis CA. Human tumors associated with Carney complex and germline PRKAR1A mutations: a protein kinase A disease! FEBS Lett 2003; 546: 59–64

BAZEX–DUPRÉ–CHRISTOL SYNDROME

Synonyms

- Bazex's syndrome
- Follicular atrophoderma and basal cell carcinoma

Age of onset

- At birth

Clinical findings

- Follicular atrophoderma most frequently localized on the dorsa of the hands and feet, on the face and on the extensor surface of the elbows and knees (Figures 24.35)
- 'Spiny' hyperkeratosis (Figure 25.36)
- Basal cell carcinoma (~50%) mostly localized on the face
- Hypotrichosis with pili torti and trichorrhexis nodosa
- Milia on the face ('ulerythema ophryogenes') and upper trunk
- Atopy
- Rarely, hypohidrosis is reported

Extracutaneous findings

- Neuropsychic disorders
- Scrotal tongue

Course and prognosis

- Follicular atrophoderma at birth or in early infancy
- Hypotrichosis at birth and steady throughout life
- Basal cell carcinomas starting in the second and third decades of life

Laboratory investigations

- Histopathologic findings: follicular atrophoderma: depression in the epidermis with clusters of basaloid cells in the superficial dermis; nevoid basal cell proliferations
- Microscopic examination of the hair shows rudimentary hair shaft

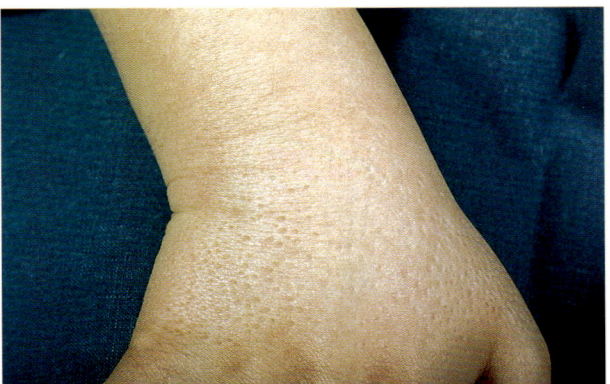

Figure 24.35

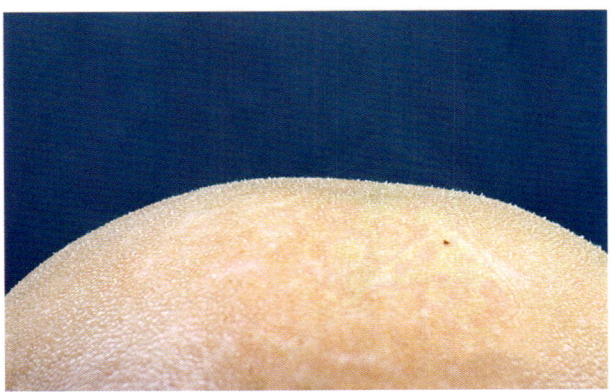

Figure 24.36

Genetics and pathogenesis

- X-linked dominant inheritance
- Gene locus on the distal part of the long arm of the X chromosome in the Xq24–Xq27.1 region
- Primary defect unknown

Differential diagnosis

- IFAP syndrome
- Basal cell carcinoma syndrome
- Rombo syndrome
- Chondrodysplasia punctata
- Isolated atrophodermas (Moulin)
- Oley's syndrome: congenital hypotrichosis, milia with spontaneous regression during adolescence, is merely a variant of Bazex–Dupré–Christol syndrome

Follow-up and therapy

The disease is a genodermatosis with malignant potential, requiring regular screening.

- Topical retinoids and imiquimod
- Oral retinoids
- Surgical, cryosurgical, CO_2 laser treatments

REFERENCES

Andreani V, Richard M, Folchetti G, et al. [Congenital hypotrichosis and milia with spontaneous regression during adolescence or Oley syndrome: a variant of Bazex–Dupre–Christol syndrome.] Ann Dermatol Venereol 2000; 127: 285–8

Goetey M, Geerts ML, Kint A, et al. The Bazex–Dupré–Christol syndrome. Arch Dermatol 1994; 130: 337–42

Inoue Y, Ono T, Kayashima K, Johno M. Hereditary perioral pigmented follicular atrophoderma associated with milia and epidermoid cysts. Br J Dermatol 1998; 139: 713–18

Moreau-Cabasiot A, Bonafé JL, Hachich N, et al. Atrophodermie folliculaire, proliférations baso-cellulaires et hypotrichose (syndrome de Bazex, Dupré, Christol). Etude de deux familles. Ann Dermatol Venereol 1994; 121: 297–301

Vabres P, Lacombe D, Ralinowitz LG, et al. The gene for Bazex–Dupré–Christol syndrome maps to chromosome Xq. J Invest Dermatol 1995; 105: 87–91

EPIDERMODYSPLASIA VERRUCIFORMIS

Synonym

- Lewandowsky–Lutz disease

Age of onset

- 4–8 years

Clinical findings

The disease is limited to the skin (Figures 24.37–24.40)

- Plane warts lesions on the face and neck
- Papillomatous–vegetant lesions and seborrheic wart-like lesions elsewhere on the body
- Microinvasive and invasive squamous cell carcinomas (25/50%), usually beginning in the fourth decade of life, especially in sun-exposed areas

Course and prognosis

The disease is lifelong.

Laboratory findings

There is decreased cell-mediated immunity, specifically delayed-type hypersensitivity towards epidermodysplasia verruciformis human papilloma viruses (EV HPVs).

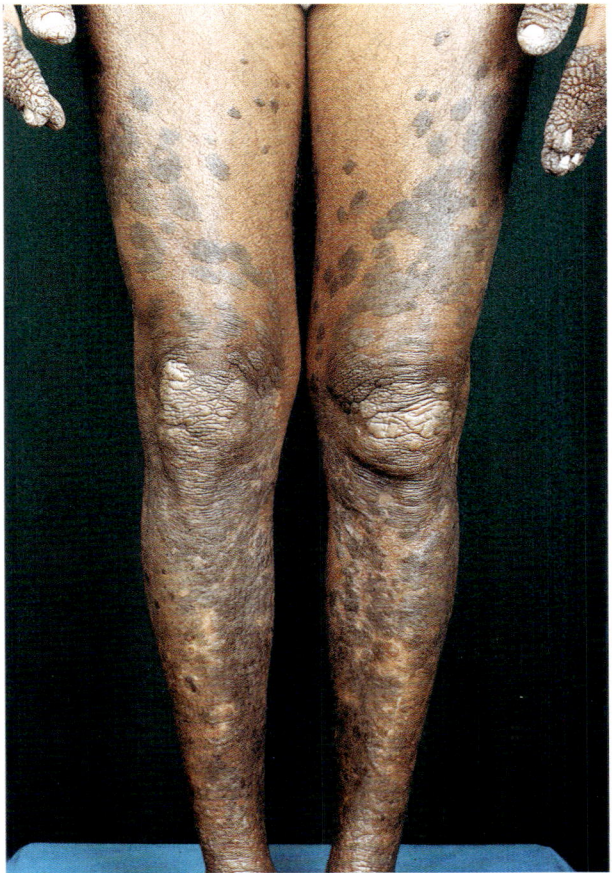

Figure 24.38

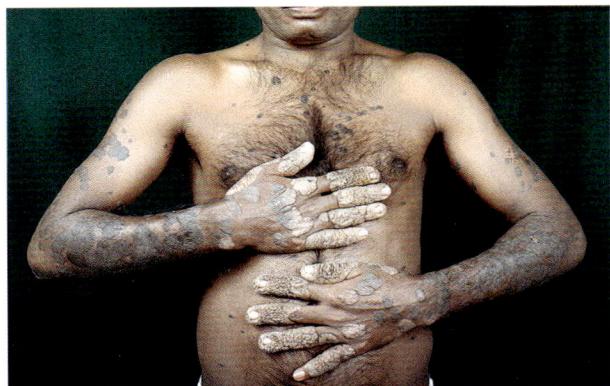

Figure 24.37

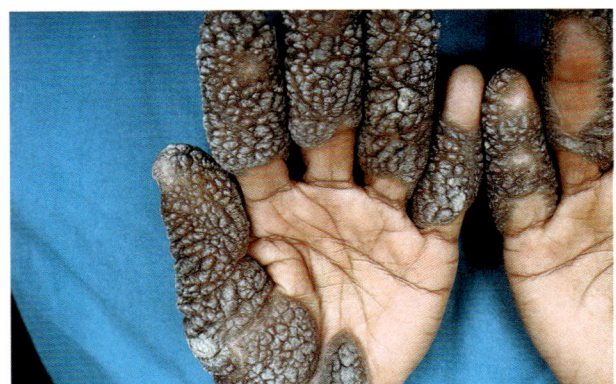

Figure 24.39

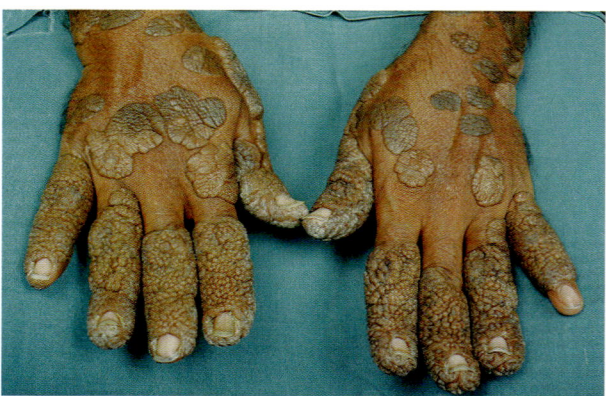

Figure 24.40

Genetics and pathogenesis

- Autosomal recessive and occasionally X-linked mode of inheritance; many sporadic cases
- Gene locus: chromosome arm 17q + e2
- Inherited immunosuppression with susceptibility to many HPV strains (5, 8, 14, 20)
- A dysfunction of the p53 gene is likely to play a part in EV carcinogenesis either due to ultraviolet B radiation (UVB)-induced p53 mutations or involving other mutagens
- In EV cancer HPV5 is a predominant type, and this virus and HPV8 are found in more than 90% of EV cancers

Follow-up and therapy

Cancers are locally destructive and the metastatic potential is low, but continuous observation is necessary.

- Oral retinoids alone or in combination with interferon α_2
- Surgery when mandatory

REFERENCES

Majewski S, Jablonska S. Do epidermodysplasia verruciformis human papilloma viruses contribute to malignant and benign epidermal proliferations? Arch Dermatol 2002; 138: 649–54

Majewski S, Jablonska S. Epidermodysplasia verruciformis as a model of human papillomavirus-induced genetic cancer of the skin. Arch Dermatol 1995; 131: 1312–18

Padlewska K, Ramon N, Cassonnet P, et al. Mutation and abnormal expression of the p53 gene in the viral carcinogenesis of epidermodysplasia verruciformis. J Invest Dermatol 2001; 117: 935–42

BROOKE–SPIEGLER SYNDROME

Synonym

- Multiple trichoepitheliomas and multiple cylindromas

Age of onset

- Late childhood (milia) to second decade of life (tumors)

Clinical findings

- Within a given family some members may have cylindromas mainly located on the scalp and trunk (Figures 24.41 and 24.42), whereas others may have trichoepitheliomas (Figure 24.43) mainly located on the face, or both
- Spiradenomas
- Milia and follicular cysts (Figure 24.44)

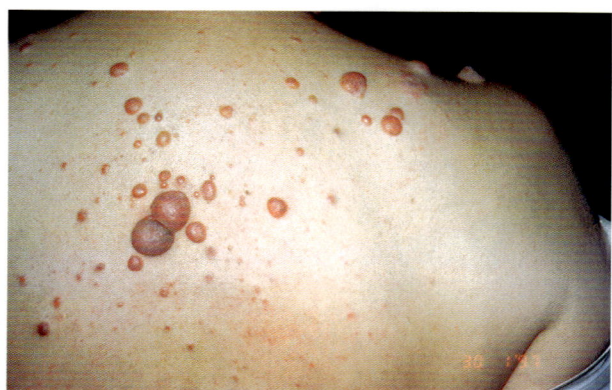

Figure 24.41

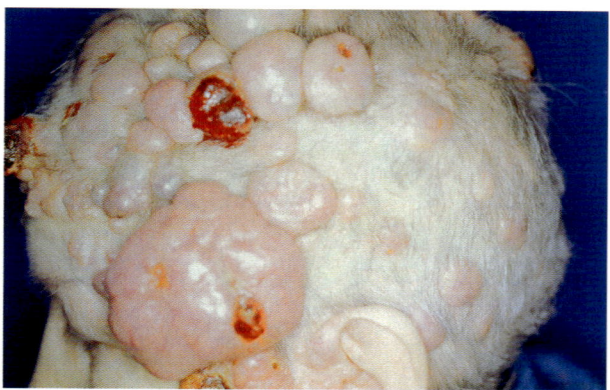

Figure 24.42

Genodermatoses related to malignancy

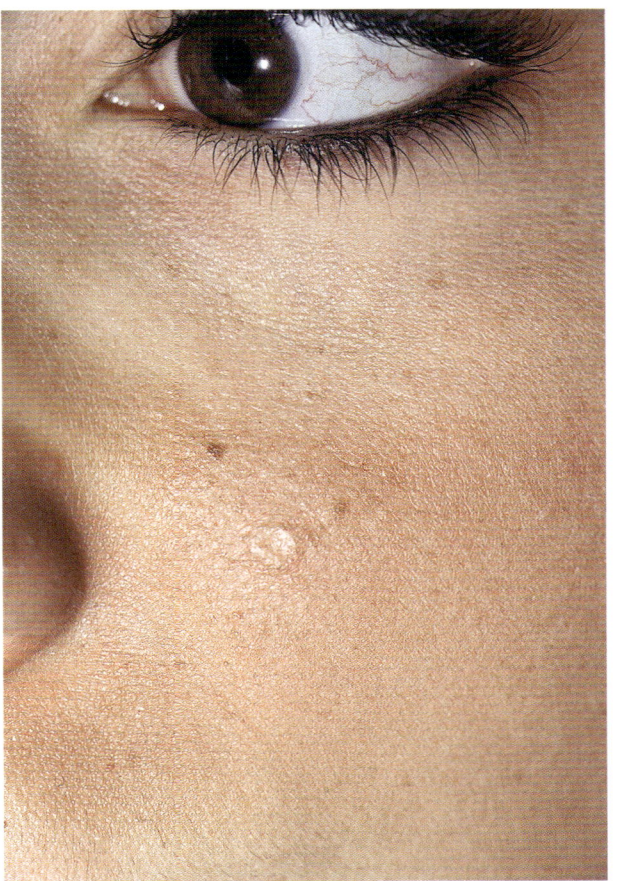

Figure 24.43

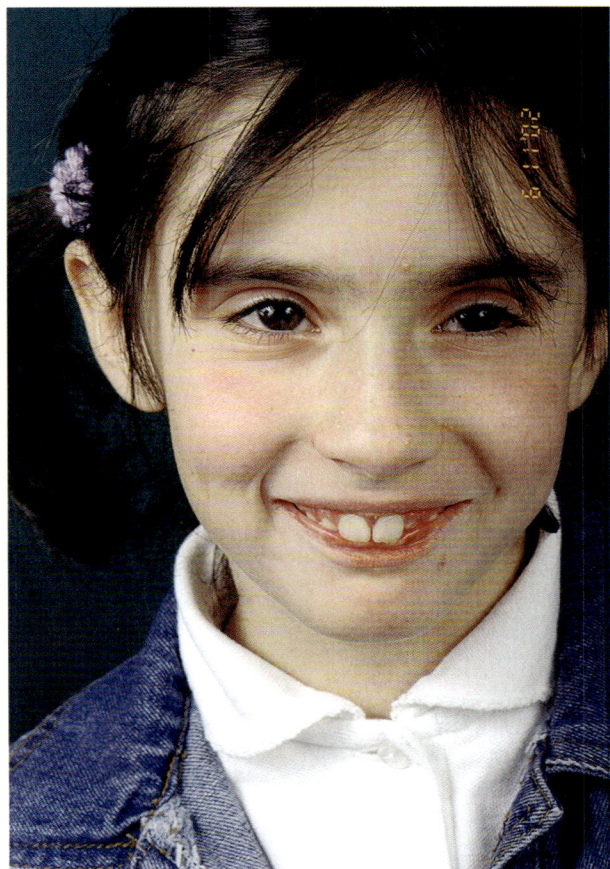

Figure 24.44

Course and prognosis

The disease is lifelong. Lesions may become multiple, disfiguring and of huge dimensions. The prognosis is related to the course of the neoplasia.

Laboratory investigations and data

Histopathologic findings include co-occurrence of typical lesions of cylindromas, trichoepitheliomas and rarely spiradenomas.

Genetics and pathogenesis

- Autosomal dominant inheritance
- Frameshift mutation in the CYLD gene located on chromosome 16q21–23. The reasons for different expression patterns of the same genetic may be related to the type and location of the mutation in the gene

Differential diagnosis

- Tuberous sclerosis
- Cowden's syndrome
- Gardner syndrome

Therapy

- Surgical excision
- CO_2 laser
- Recurrences are frequent

REFERENCES

Gutierrez PP, Eggermann T, Holler D, et al. Phenotype diversity in familial cylindromatosis: a frameshift mutation in the tumor suppressor gene CYLD underlies different tumors of skin appendages. J Invest Dermatol 2002; 119: 527–31

Szepietowoki JC, Wasik F, Srylejko-Machaj G, et al. Brooke–Spiegler syndrome. J Eur Acad Dermatol Venereol 2001; 15: 346–9

PROGRESSIVE MUCINOUS HISTIOCYTOSIS

Age of onset

- In infancy or childhood

Clinical findings

- Asymptomatic eruption of numerous skin-colored or red nodules, 2–15 mm in diameter scattered over the entire body. The lesions do not tend to ulcerate or to merge into plaques. Absence of mucous membrane and visceral involvement (Figures 24.45–24.48)
- Good general health

Course

The number of lesions increases gradually during life (several hundreds), and there is no spontaneous resolution.

Laboratory investigations and data

Histopatologic findings include infiltrate constituted of spindle-shaped or oval histiocytes (S100-negative and CD68- and factor XIII positive) with dermal deposition of mucinous material.

Genetics and pathogenesis

- Autosomal dominant inheritance
- Non-Langerhans' cell histiocytosis

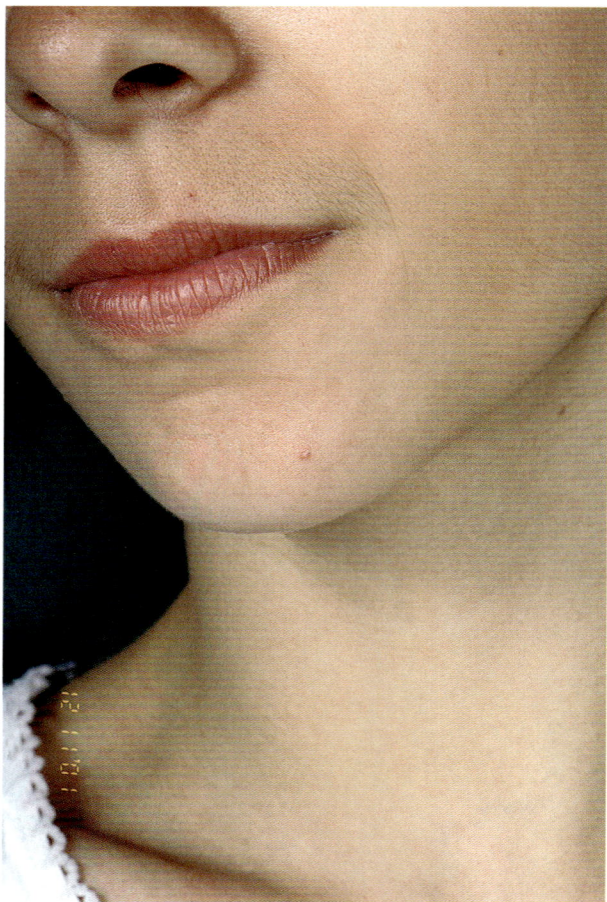

Figure 24.46

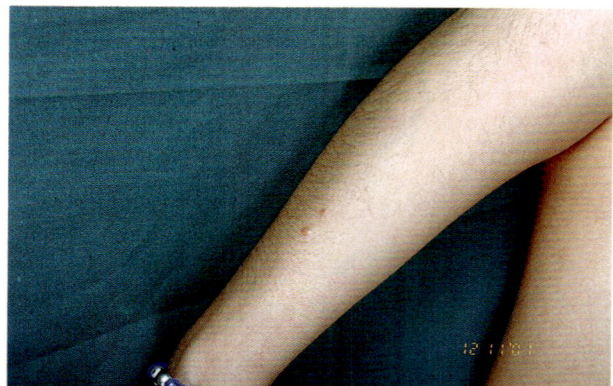

Figure 24.47

Differential diagnosis

- Other non-Langerhans' cell histiocytosis

Therapy

No treatment is helpful.

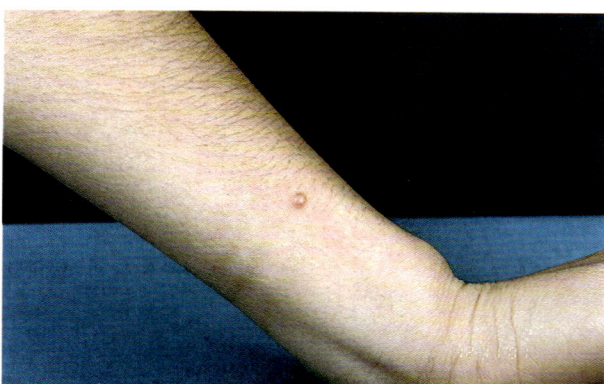

Figure 24.45

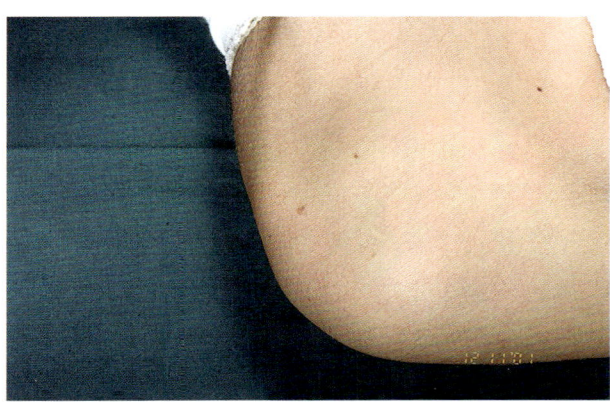

Figure 24.48

REFERENCES

Bork K, Hoede N. Hereditary progressive mucinous histiocytosis in women. Arch Dermatol 1988; 124: 1225–9

Bork K. Hereditary progressive mucinous histiocytosis: immunohistochemical and ultrastructural studies in an additional family. Arch Dermatol 1994; 130: 1300–1304

Schröder K, Hartmannoperger V, Schmuth M, et al. Hereditary progressive mucinous histiocytosis. J Am Acad Dermatol 1996; 35: 298–303

DEGOS' DISEASE

Synonym

- Familial atrophic papulosis

Age of onset

- Second decade of life

Clinical findings

- Slow appearance of asymptomatic pink to red papules that gradually develop umbilicated centers which progress into atrophic, porcelain white lesions with a sharply defined erythematous edge (Figures 24.49–24.51)
- The number of the lesions is variable (from a few to more than 100), mainly located on the trunk (Figure 24.50)

Extracutaneous manifestations

Intestinal (cramps, vomit, acute crisis), neurological and renal symptoms are found in about 50% of cases.

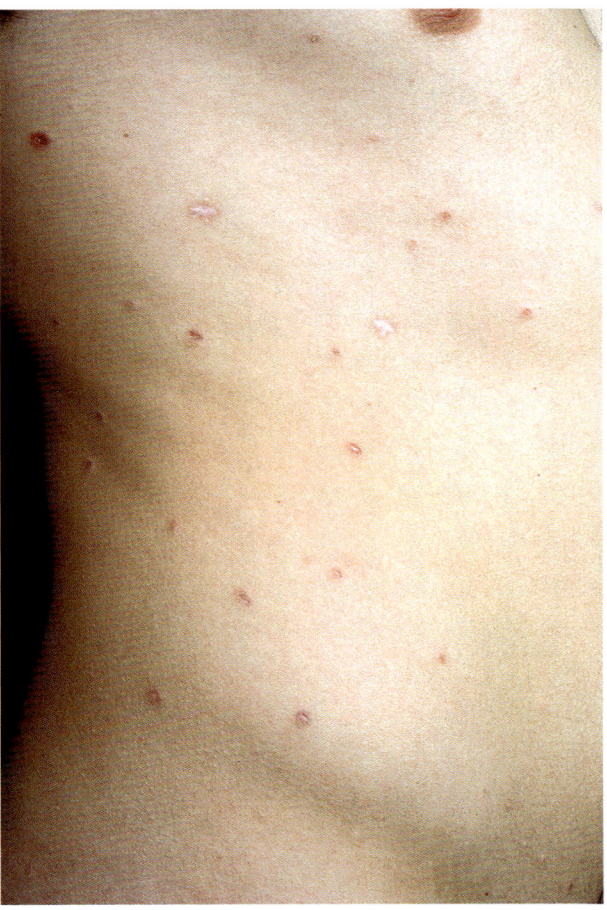

Figure 24.49

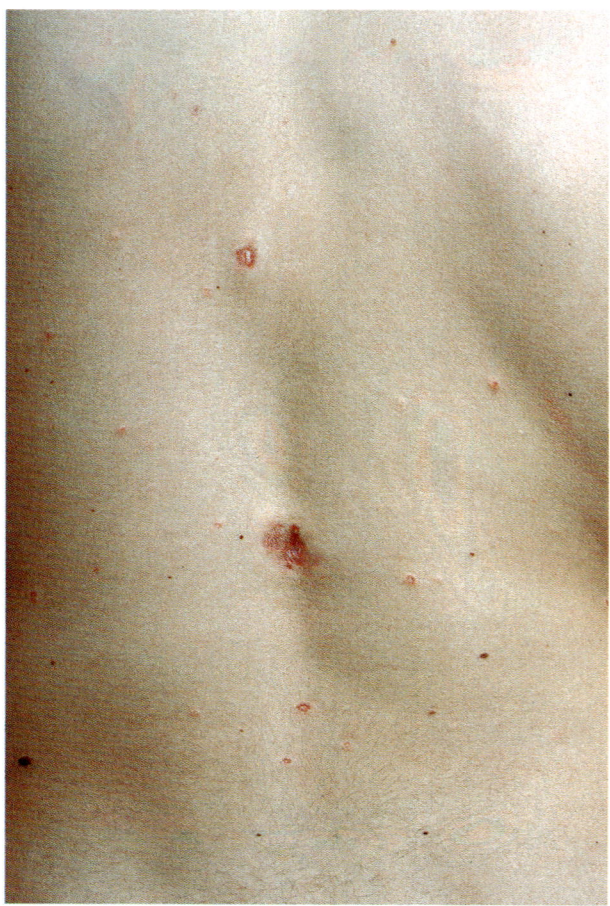

Figure 24.50

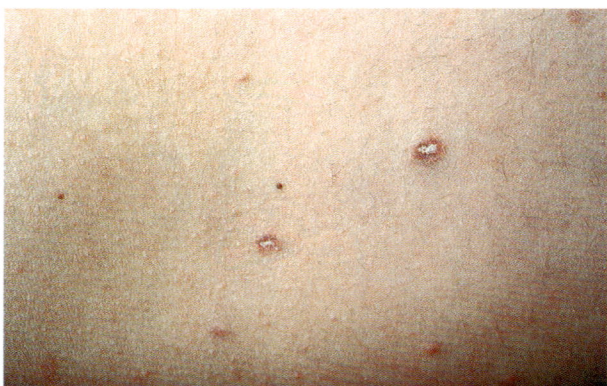

Figure 24.51

Course and complications

- Intestinal hemorrhage, perforation, peritonitis
- The lesions may continue to appear for several years
- Two forms may be recognized: a malignant form (~90%) with fatal evolution and a benign form (~10%) with only cutaneous lesions

Laboratory investigations and data

- Histopathological findings: endothelial proliferation in the deep dermal vessels and often partial or complete obstruction by a thrombus
- Complete blood tests
- Enteroscopy

Genetics and pathogenesis

- Autosomal dominant inheritance, but most cases are sporadic
- Controversial pathogenesis; infective, immunologically mediated

Differential diagnosis

- Lupus erythematosus
- Necrotic vasculitis

Follow-up therapy

- Accurate for a long period

There are no effective treatments. Anticoagulants and fibrinolytic drugs may occasionally be useful.

REFERENCES

Farrel AM, Moss J, Costello C, et al. Benign cutaneous Degos' disease. Br J Dermatol 1998; 139: 708–12

Kisch LS, Bruynzeel DP. Six cases of malignant atrophic papulosis (Degos' disease) occurring in one family. Br J Dermatol 1984; 111: 469–71

Powell J, Bordea C, Wojnarowska F, et al. Benign familial Degos disease worsening during immunosuppression. Br J Dermatol 1999; 141: 524–7

ROMBO SYNDROME

Epidemiology

Three families are reported.

Age of onset

- From 6–7 years of age

Clinical findings

- Pearly, milia-like papules and atrophoderma vermiculatum on the face (especially upper part) and more scattered on the neck and trunk, giving the skin a 'grainy' appearance (24.52 and 24.53)
- Diffuse hypotrichosis
- Cyanosis of lips, hands and feet
- Trichoepitheliomas
- Tendency to form basal cell carcinomas (24.53)

Extracutaneous findings

- None reported

Course and prognosis

- Gradually the skin become coarse with age and basal cell carcinomas become visible around the age of 30
- Cyanosis remains located to acral regions, without any detectable vascular abnormalities in large vessels
- Telangiectases are visible in older patients

Laboratory investigations

- Biopsies reveal irregularly distributed and atrophic hair follicles with keratotic plugging and, in the upper dermis, milia are visible as well as small dilated vessels
- Elastic fibers are thin and irregularly distributed

Genetics and pathogenesis

- The disease is autosomal dominant
- The propensity to form basal cell carcinomas in sun-exposed areas, together with the acrocyanosis strongly supports the hypothesis of a further syndrome with impaired DNA-repair cascade

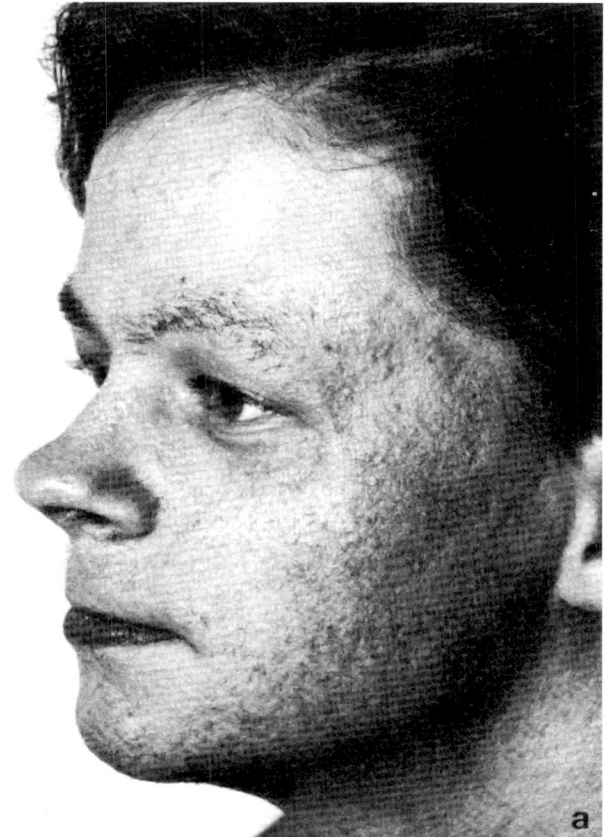

Figure 24.52

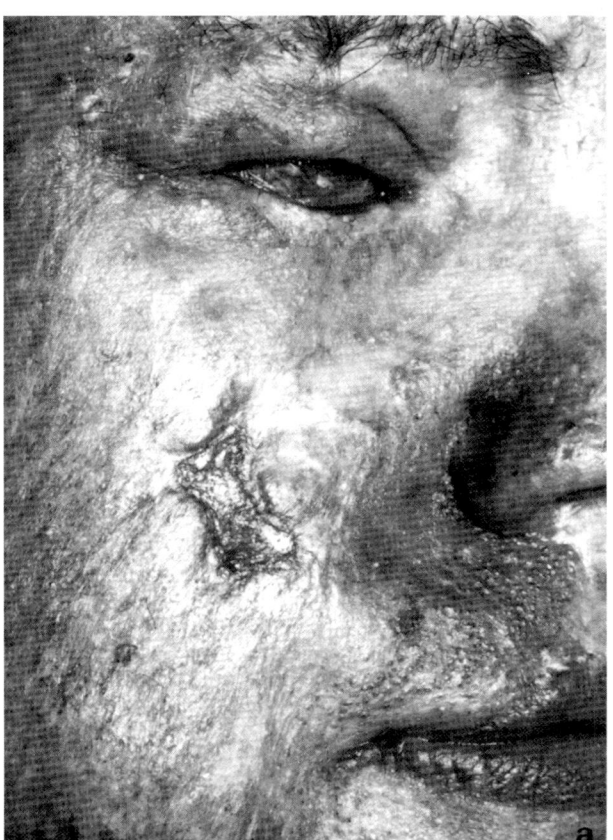

Figure 24.53

Follow-up and therapy

- Given the absence of internal diseases, periodic dermatological evaluation in order to prevent the formation of basal cell carcinomas
- Surgery for cutaneous neoplasms
- Protection from UV-radiations

Differential diagnosis

- Xeroderma pigmentosum
- Kindler's syndrome
- Cyanosis and soft skin syndrome
- Basex syndrome
- Cowden syndrome

REFERENCE

van Steensel MA, Jaspers NG, Steijlen PM. A case of Rombo syndrome. Br J Dermatol 2001; 144: 1215–18. Erratum in: Br J Dermatol 2002; 146: 715

CHAPTER 25

Cutaneous mosaicism

Definition

A mosaic is formed by two or more genetically different populations of cells originating from a single 'healthy' wild-type zygote. It is developed from an early-stage embryonic mutation, called 'somatic'. Mosaics are well known in biology, especially in plants and fruits and animals (insects, e.g. *Drosophila* species) but, in contrast, in humans they represent recent knowledge and even more recent understanding. From 1983 onward, many molecular biology studies have attempted to explain the pathogenesis of this phenomenon.

Pattern of clinical presentation of mosaicism

Mosaics are visible on the skin following the distribution visible in Figure 25.1. There are at least five patterns of distribution.

Lines of Blaschko

The lines of Blaschko represent the ideal lines of growth for the embryonic populations of keratinocytes. They follow a well-known pattern originating from the early posterior–anterior growth that is completed by longitudinal elongation of the embryo (V-shaped or 'fountain pattern' on the posterior midline) (Figure 25.1: diffuse epidermal nevus, Figure 25.2: hyperpigmented streaks in Cohen's syndrome with dyploidia–triploidia) and by visceral

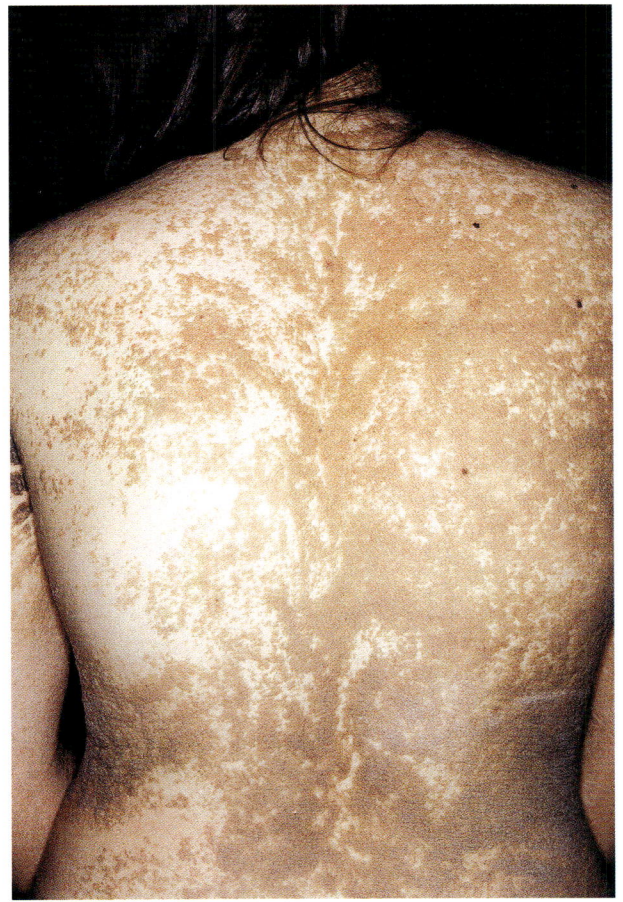

Figure 25.1

growth at different times of embryonic development (the S-shaped or wave-like figure on the lateral aspect of the thorax and abdomen) (Figure 25.3: diffuse epidermal nevus).

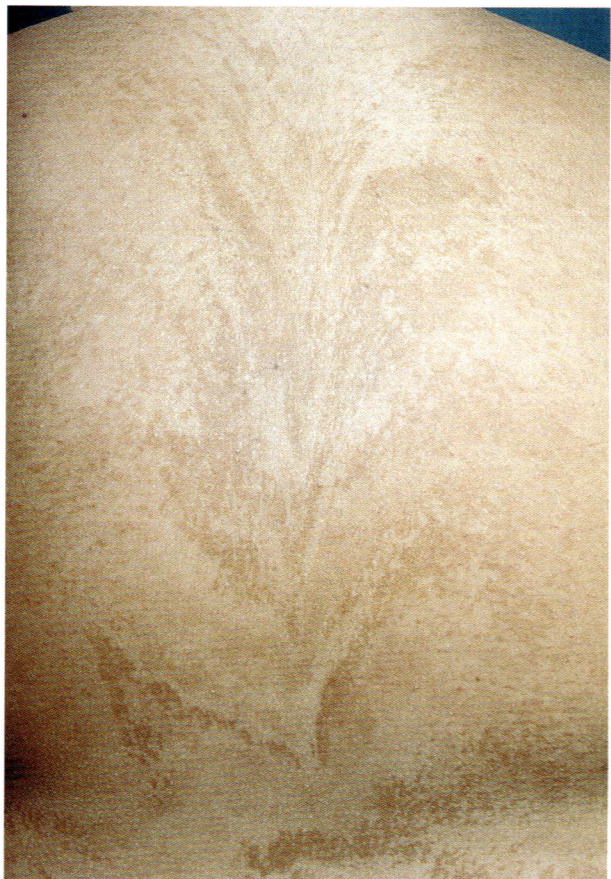

Figure 25.2

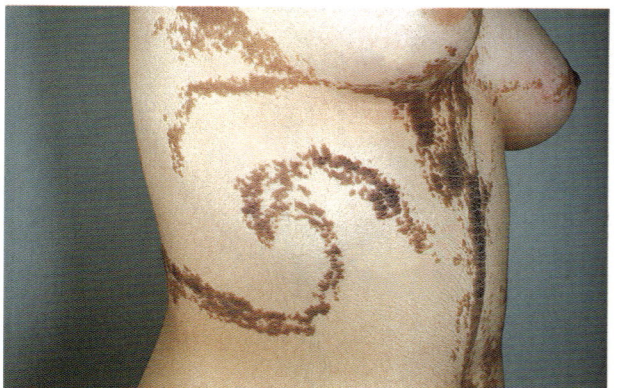

Figure 25.3

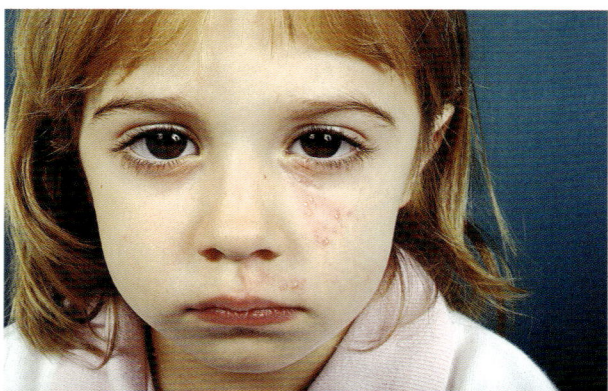

Figure 25.4

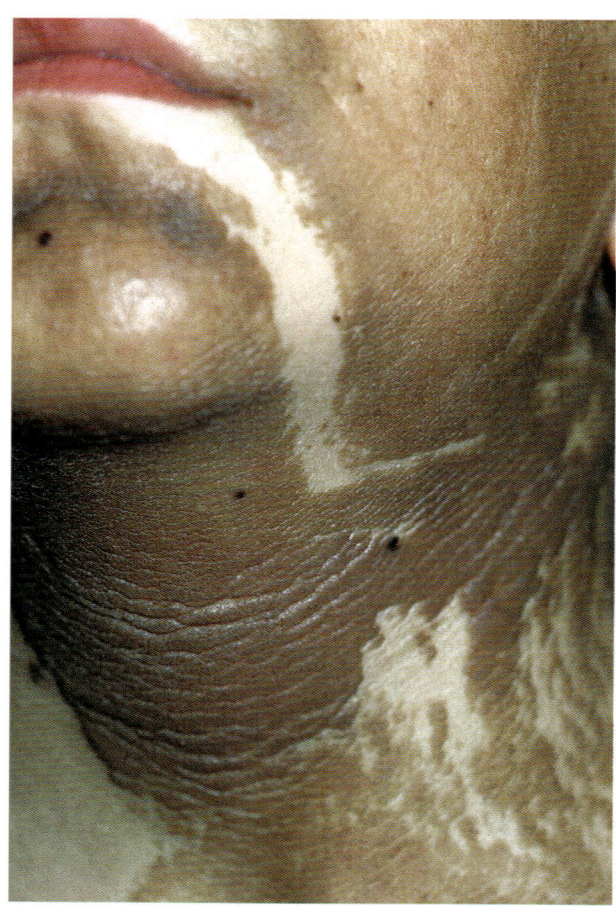

Figure 25.5

On the scalp and face the distribution may be less paradigmatic, because of the complex embryological arrangement and growth of the different tissues and structures of these areas (Figure 25.4: nevus comedonicus, Figure 25.5: nevus sebaceus). Lines tend to intersect on the face and be spiraliform on the vertex (Figures 25.6 and 25.7: scalp heterochromia, mental retardation and chromosomal abnormalities; personal observation).

The lines of Blaschko are traditionally referred to as type 1 (narrow bands as in linear epidermal nevus (Figures 25.8 and 25.13), lichen striatus and many other disorders) or, less frequently, type 2 (broad bands, as in this case with epidermolytic hyperkeratosis (Figures 25.9 and 25.13), McCune–Albright syndrome (see Chapter 19) or angora hair nevus syndrome (see Chapter 15).

Nevertheless, narrow and broad bands are not disease specific, and may be explained by:

Cutaneous mosaicism 395

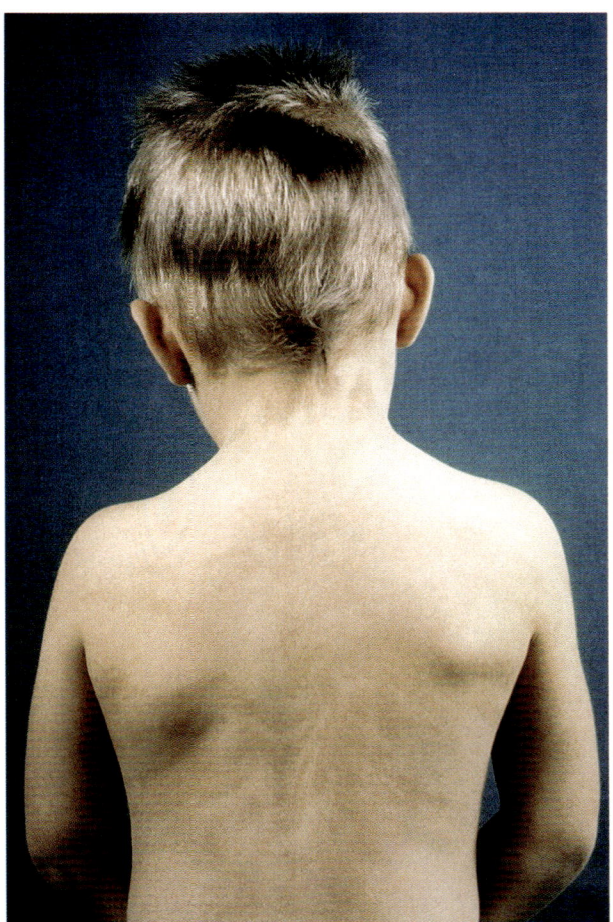

Figure 25.6

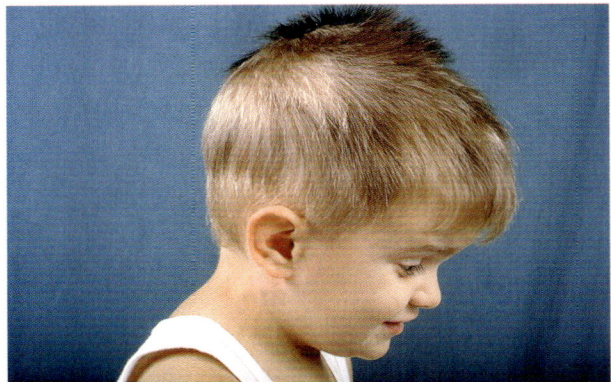

Figure 25.7

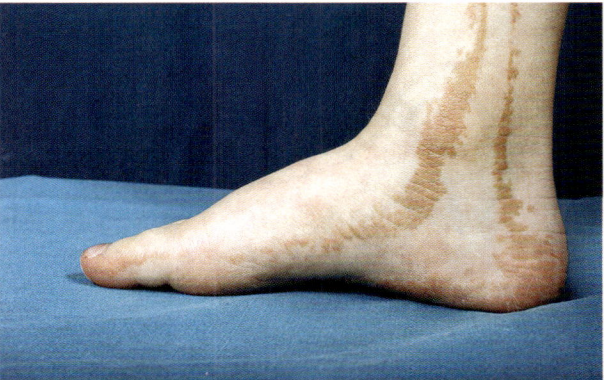

Figure 25.8

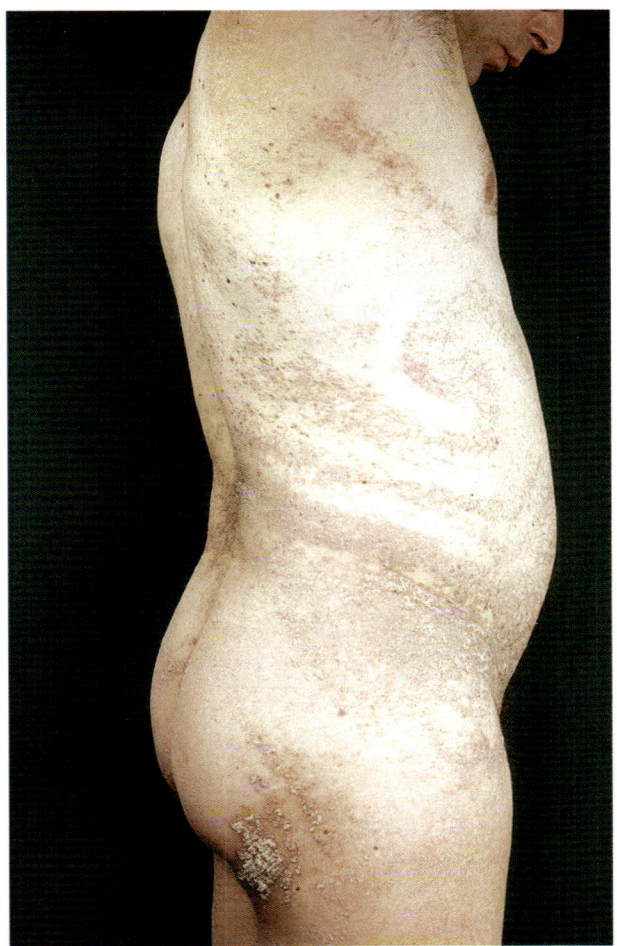

Figure 25.9

- The number of mutated cell clones originating from the posterior somites: the fewer the number of mutated cells, the thinner is the band, and the larger is the amount of the mutated population, the larger is the lesion
- The time at which the mutation occurs: an earlier mutation on the neural crest migrates first vertically and then horizontally, covering a larger area and creating a broad band; conversely, a narrow band is created by a temporally posterior mutation that does not have the time to migrate first vertically on the neural crest but is forced to migrate horizontally

This pattern seems to be followed apparently by diseases affecting keratinocytes (e.g. incontinentia

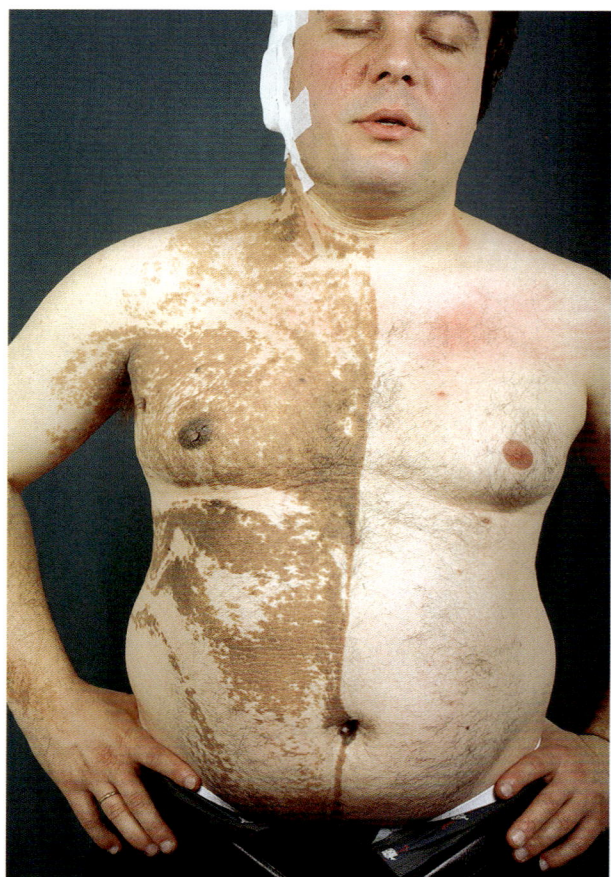

Figure 25.10

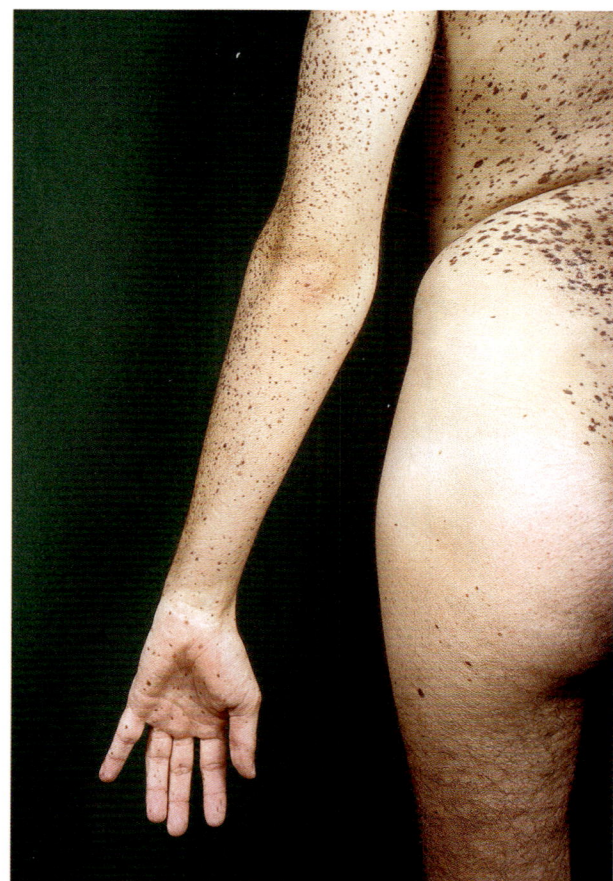

Figure 25.12

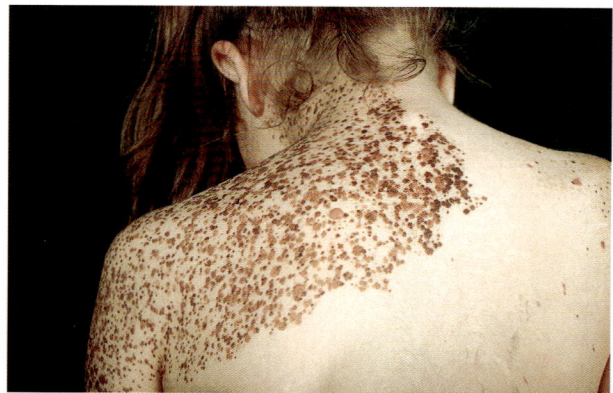

Figure 25.11

pigmenti) and melanocytes (linear melanocytic nevus), but it is not clear whether the latter is caused by a specific melanocytic mutation or by a keratinocytic mutation influencing melanocytes.

In spite of the above explanations, the terms 'zosteriform' and 'dermatomal' do not apply to cutaneous mosaicism.

Mutated lines of mosaic disease may be single, multiple, or diffuse over half the body (Figure 25.10: diffuse epidermal nevus) or the entire body (see Figure 25.1).

Checkerboard pattern

As can be seen in Figure 25.13 overleaf, this distribution may create quadrants on the back, chest and abdomen with a sharp anterior and posterior midline border. It is clearly visible that these clones of mutated cells (such as the melanocytes in speckled lentiginous nevus (SLN)) are not influenced by the elongation and rotation of the embryo, having sharp horizontal superior and inferior borders (Figure 25.11: SLN in phakomatosis pigmentokeratotica).

On the arms and legs, quadrants become elongated for obvious reasons and are no longer recognizable as and must not be confused with the linear pattern (Figure 25.12: SLN in phakomatosis pigmentokeratotica).

The checkerboard pattern is typical of SLN and phakomatosis pigmentokeratotica, but it is also visible in vitiligo (Figure 25.14), in hypo- and hyperpigmented nevi, in female carriers of X-linked hypertrichosis and in acquired post-ultraviolet radiation (UV), cutis laxa (Figure 25.15).

Cutaneous mosaicism 397

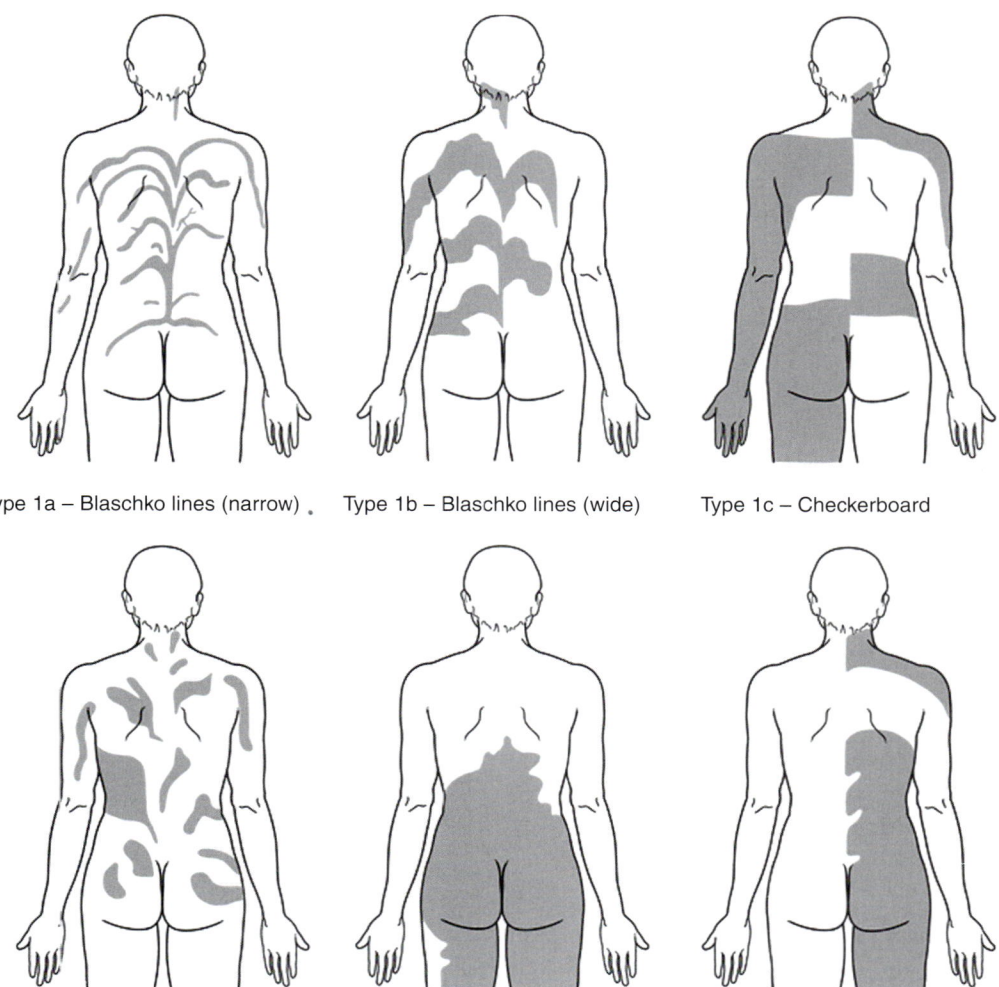

Type 1a – Blaschko lines (narrow)   Type 1b – Blaschko lines (wide)   Type 1c – Checkerboard

Type 1d – Phylloid pattern   Type 1e – Patchy pattern without midline separation   Type 1f – Lateralization pattern

Figure 25.13

'Phylloid' pattern

This pattern is visible as leaf-shaped or elongated and oval areas of hyperpigmentation in a subset of patients. It is linked almost exclusively to mosaic trisomy 13.

A few cases of phylloid-like mosaic pigmentation have been described without cytogenetic alterations.

This leaf-like formation may be explained by the presence of an interrupted linear broad-band pattern with irregular distribution and intermingled healthy cell clones, and by a rotation of the mutated cell clones that causes the particular figurated aspects and that does not respect midline separation (Figure 25.16).

Irregular patches

These are typical of giant melanocytic nevi or neurocutaneous syndromes (Figure 25.17). The borders of the lesions are irregular and figurated.

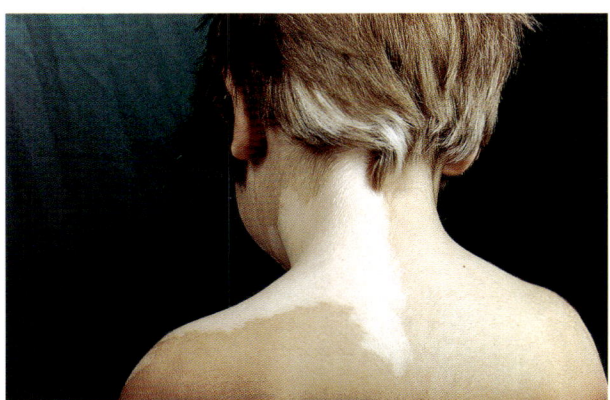

Figure 25.14

Lateralization pattern

This is typical of CHILD syndrome (Figure 25.18) (see Chapter 8). It reflects the action of ancestral lateralization genes that are well known to organize the

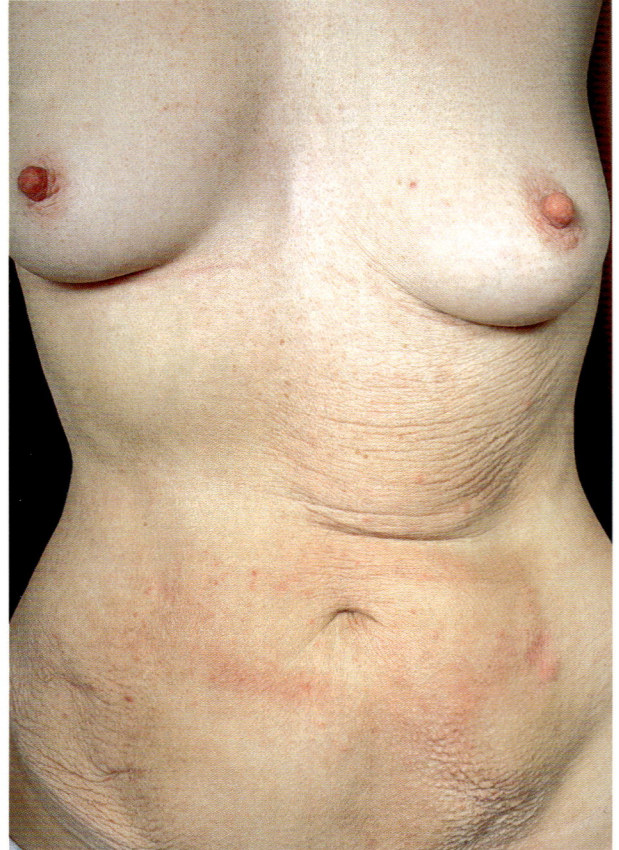

Figure 25.15

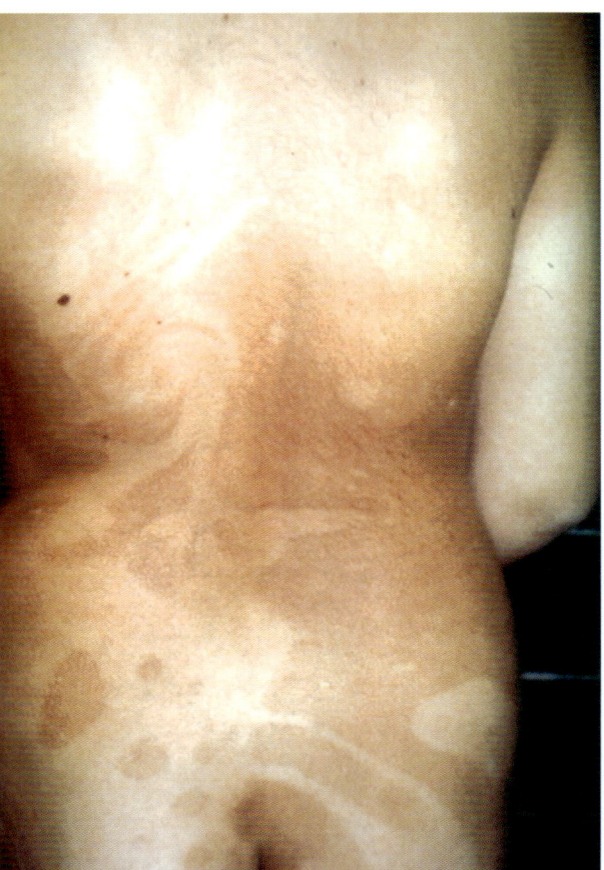

Figure 25.16

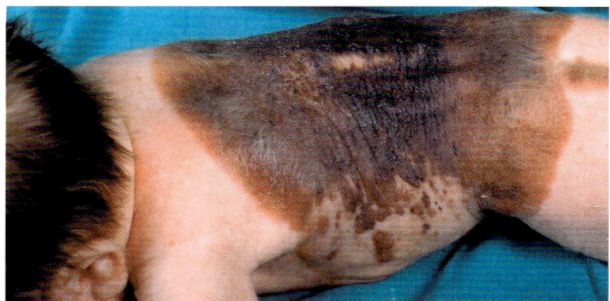

Figure 25.17

symmetry of all plants and animals. It may be that the specific mutations underlying CHILD syndrome are strictly related to the action of these genes, or the mutations are related to the time at which these genes are expressed.

The phenomenon of 'twin-spots'

Well known for many years in plants (Figure 25.19, the famous 'Happle's apple') this concept is visible in humans more frequently than expected.

Twin-spots are represented by areas of tissue that may be frequently coupled, sharing a common border (Figure 25.20: vascular twin-spot) or rarely superimposed (Figure 25.21: 'organoid' nevus and SLN in phakomatosis pigmentokeratotica), or even more rarely simply touching by a single point of contact (Figure 25.22: twin-spot of segmentary congenital vitiligo and epidermal nevus; personal observation).

They are due to two different populations of cells homozygous for a determinate trait surrounded by normal healthy heterozygous skin. Happle proposed that a mitotic recombination may give rise to two populations of stem cells that are homozygous for two different mutations, creating two skin areas with a homozygous phenotype that are, for obvious reasons, close to one another. Twin-spots have been divided by Happle into allelic and non-allelic. **Allelic twin-spotting** is represented by two homozygous populations of cells arising from mutations in the same allele (in other words affecting cells deriving from the same stem cells and originating in the same tissue) in the forms of 'duplication' and 'complete absence' of expression of the gene. The classic examples are vascular twin nevi (Figures 25.20), paired areas

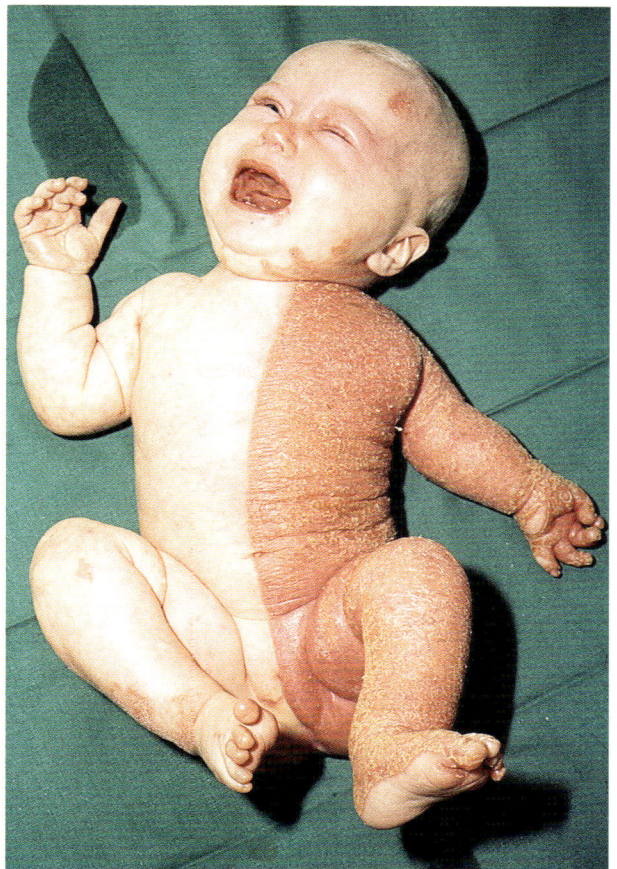

Figure 25.18

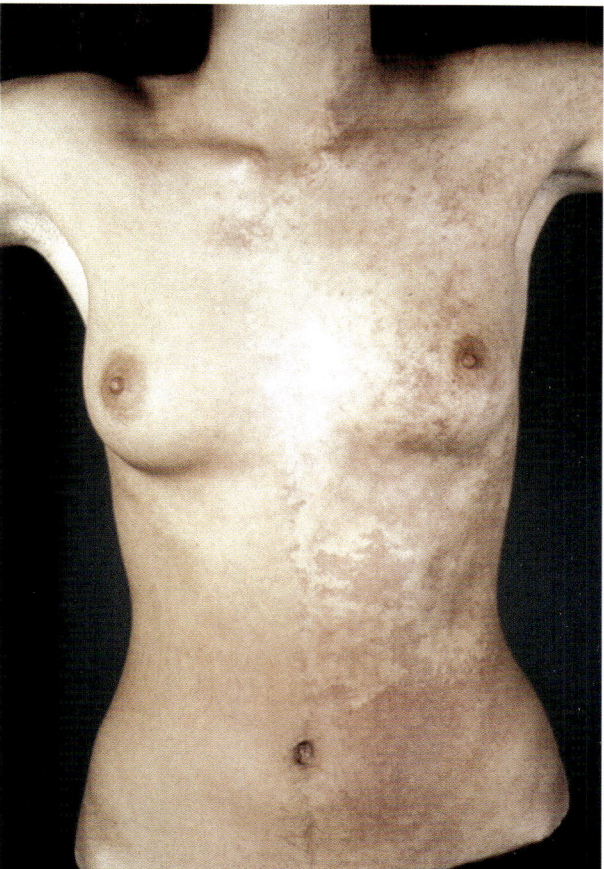

Figure 25.20

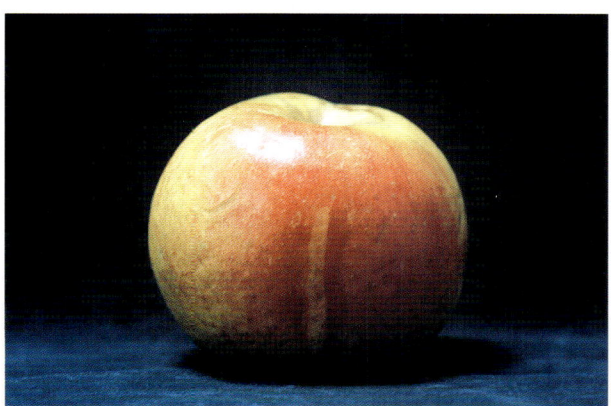

Figure 25.19

of nevus anemicus and nevus flammeus, and for hypo- and hyperpigmented nevi (Figure 25.23). The same concept also holds true for Proteus syndrome, in which areas of hypertophy may be coupled with atrophic areas.

Non-allelic twin-spotting involves two populations of cells affecting different alleles (i.e. affecting cells derived from different stem cells and originating in different tissues), and is represented by two paired areas with different phenotypes. The classic examples are phakomatosis pigmentokeratotica (see Chapter 20) and pigmentovascularis (Figure 25.24), linear epidermal nevus and contralateral vitiligo (Figure 25.22), and in recently reported 'dydymosis melorheosebacea' in which an epidermal–sebaceous nevus is related to a homolateral finding of segmental hyperostosis.

Finally, it must be remembered that mosaic vascular diseases follow a checkerboard distribution (Figures 25.26 and 25.27), (e.g. Sturge–Weber, Klippel–Trénaunay, Cobb's syndromes complex), and they should not be referred to as having a 'dermatomal' or 'zosteriform' pattern.

The dermis and fibroblasts are candidates to follow overlying epidermal diseases, as has been demonstrated by our group at the molecular level in epidermolytic hyperkeratosis, but on the other hand, lesions of dermal origin, e.g. mosaic acquired cutis laxa (mutation of elastin gene), may migrate clearly following a checkerboard pattern (Figure 25.15) or may have a less recognizable distribution, as in connective tissue nevi (see Chapter 17).

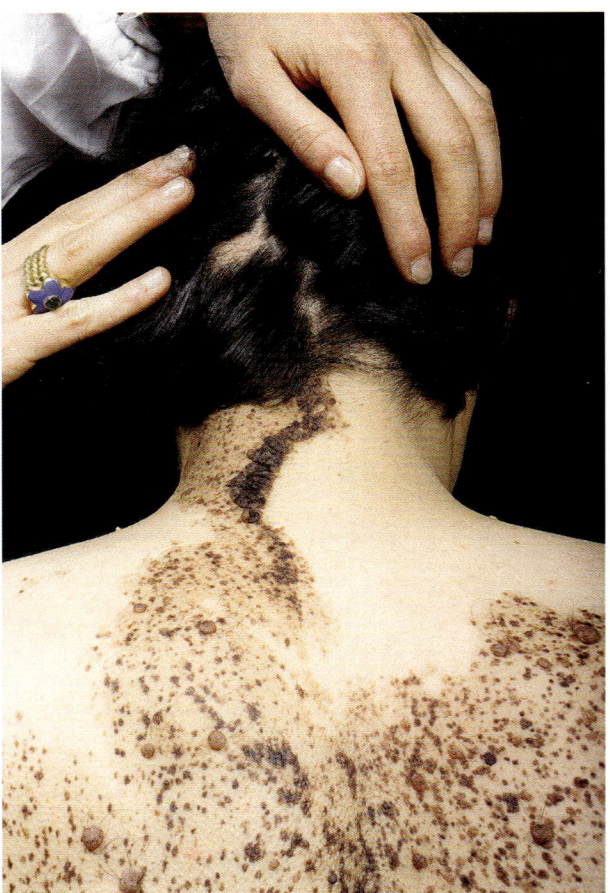

Figure 25.21

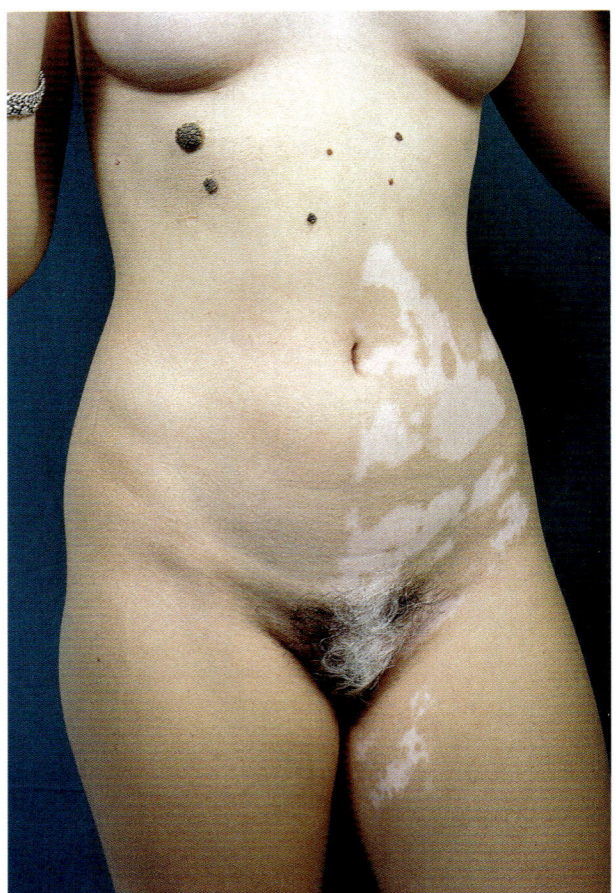

Figure 25.22

Mechanisms of inheritance of mosaicism

Usually, in medical genetics, we think in terms of the relationship between mutation and disease, and we are sure that a particular mutation is responsible for a corresponding phenotype. In mosaicism, two further parameters influence the phenotype:

- The time at which the mutation occurs, i.e. the earlier the mutation the larger the population of mutated cells involved in the embryo
- The position of the mutated clone, e.g. a somatic postzygotic mutation originating in an epidermal cell on the cephalic side of the embryo will give rise to a disease in that region

Indeed, the phenotype of a cutaneous mosaicism is determined by three factors:

- Mutation
- Time
- Position

and not exclusively by the mutation.

Mosaicism of autosomal dominant traits

Autosomal dominant lethal traits

Mosaicism can originate from lethal traits that do not allow a normal vital fetus when inherited in a classic mendelian way. These traits they are said to 'survive by mosaicism', and are visible only as a mosaic phenotype because the non-mosaic disease originating from that particular mutation is not compatible with life, and the pregnancy always results in abortion in the first weeks.

Examples of this mechanism are:

- Proteus syndrome
- Epidermal–sebaceous–organoid nevus syndrome (Schimmelpenning's)
- Phakomatosis pigmentokeratotica and pigmento-vascularis
- Encephalocraniocutaneous lipomatosis
- McCune–Albright syndrome
- Giant congenital melanocytic nevus
- Nevus comedonicus syndrome
- Sturge–Weber–Klippel–Trénaunay phenotypes
- Becker's nevus syndrome
- Speckled lentiginous nevus (SLN) syndrome

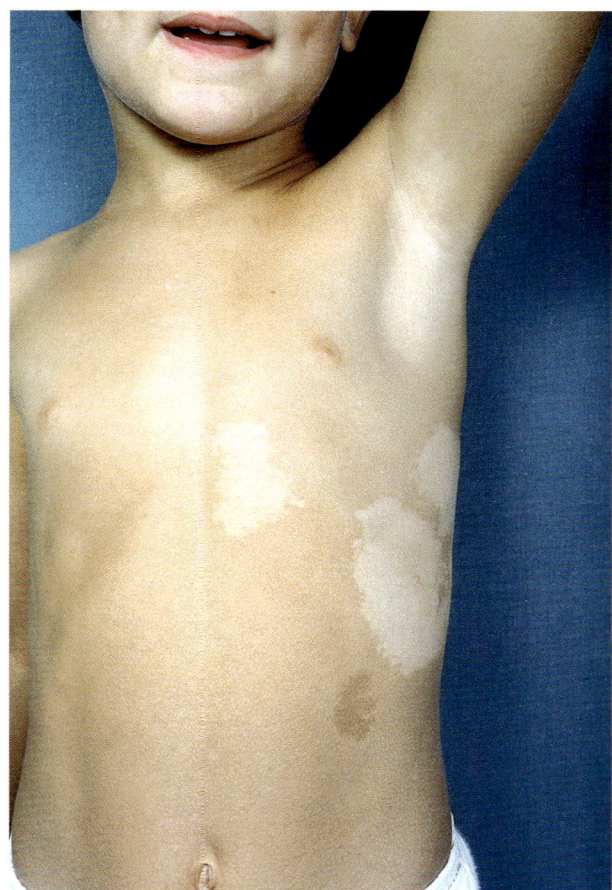

Figure 25.23

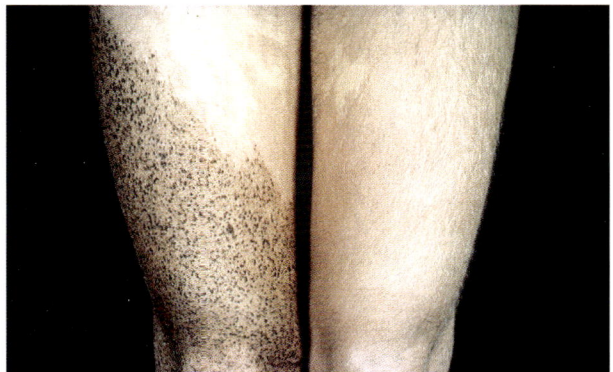

Figure 25.24

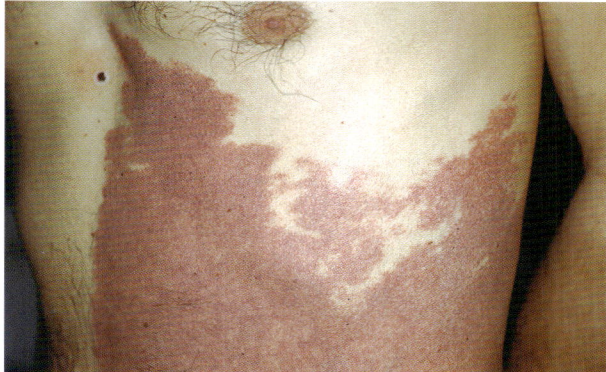

Figure 25.25

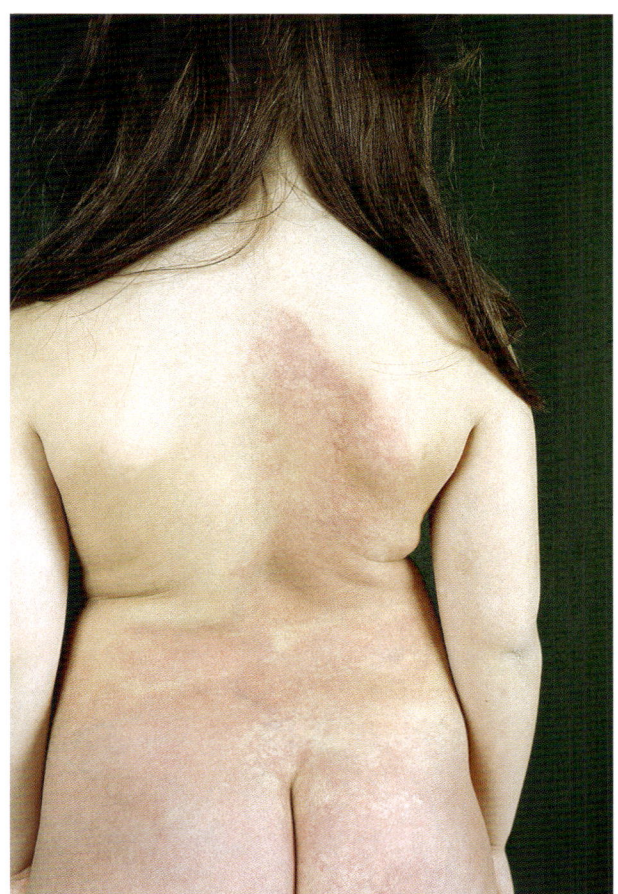

Figure 25.26

As in the best traditions, there are some exceptions to remember: for at least some of the above listed disorders, there exist some pedigrees with transmission of the trait, as occurs in Becker's nevus syndrome, Proteus syndrome and others.

Happle proposed solving this impasse by explaining the phenomenon using the 'paradominant trait inheritance theory'. Mosaic phenotypes of an autosomal dominat lethal trait (e.g. Becker's and Proteus syndromes) that occur sporadically are transmittable because a 'phenotypically silent' mutation affecting a carrier (heterozygous for the mutation) gives rise to an apparently healthy phenotype that can transmit the trait. The disease will be visible only when a second postzygotic mutation occurs by the so-called 'loss of heterozygosity' mechanism.

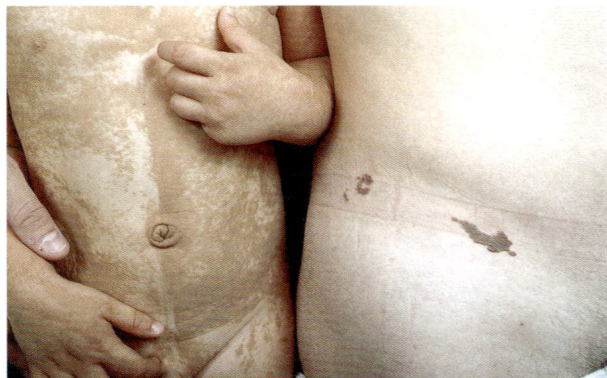

Figure 25.27

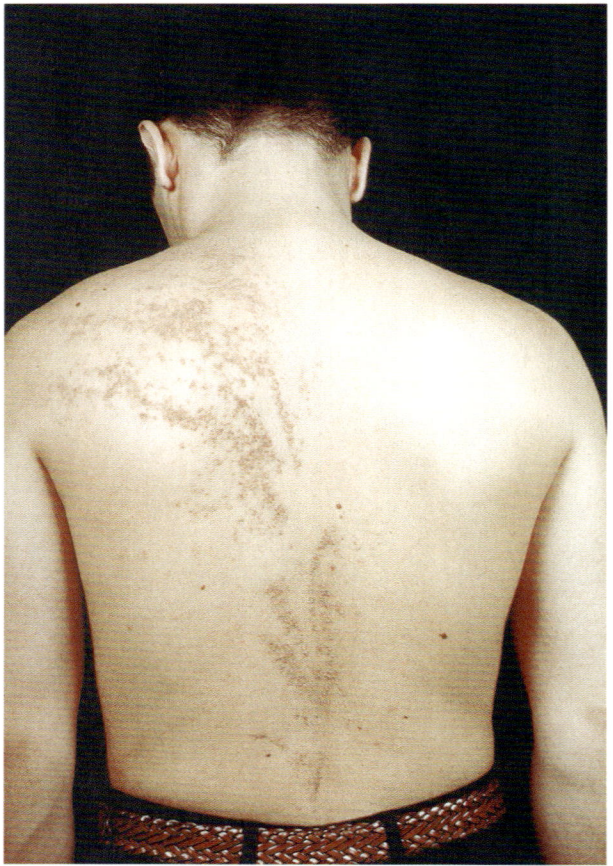

Figure 25.28

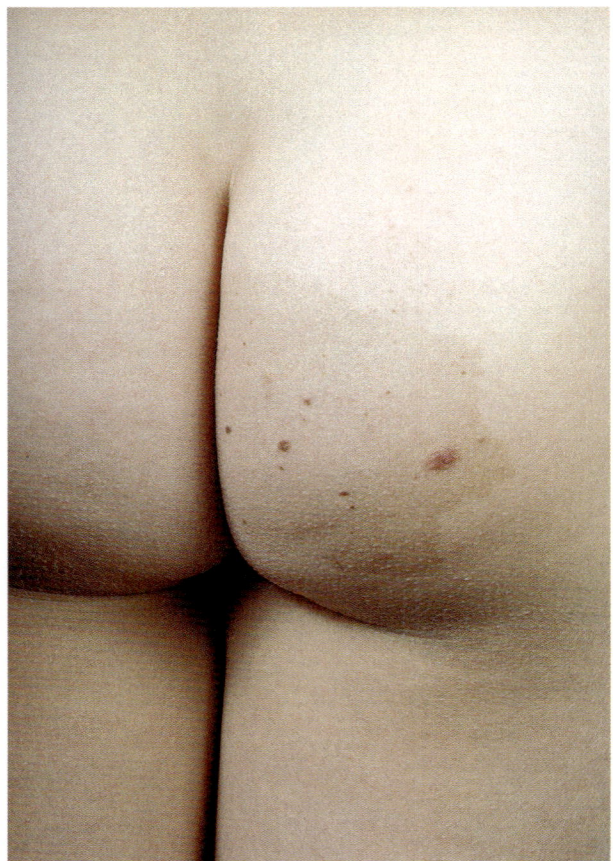

Figure 25.29

It must be noted that this phenomenon is very rare, and is reported for just a small group of diseases:

- Becker's nevus
- Proteus syndrome
- SLN
- Epidermal nevus (Figure 25.27)
- Unilateral nevoid telangiectasia
- Sturge–Weber, Klippel–Trénaunay, Cobb's phenotype complex

Autosomal dominant non-lethal traits

Non-lethal dominant traits such as Darier's disease and many others, e.g. neurofibromatosis type 1, tuberous sclerosis and epidermolytic hyperkeratosis, may be visible as a generalized classic disease or in a mosaic arrangement (Figures 25.28, 25.29 and 25.30, 25.31 and 25.32, respectively).

The disease, responding to the criteria of time and position, may be a single-strand disease, or have a more diffuse pattern or affect half of the body or the entire body, always maintaining a mosaic distribution following the Blaschko lines.

Rarely, the postzygotic mutation affects the gonads, giving rise to transmission of the trait to the offspring in the classic generalized non-mosaic phenotype (Figure 25.32).

Empirically, the more generalized the nevus the higher the chance that the gonads will be involved by the mutation, and subsequently the higher the chance to transmit the generalized disease to the offspring.

Happle proposed calling this phenomenon type 1 segmental distribution.

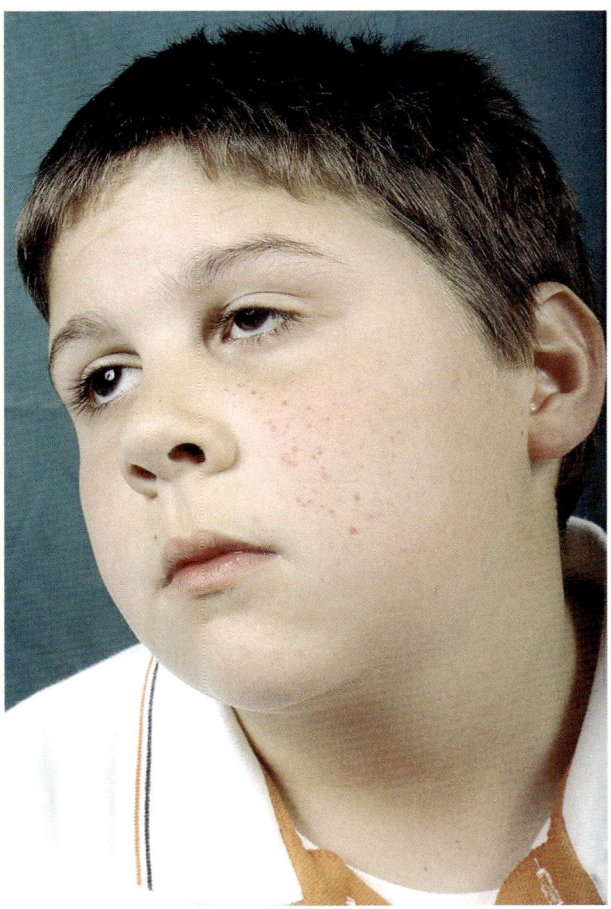

Figure 25.30

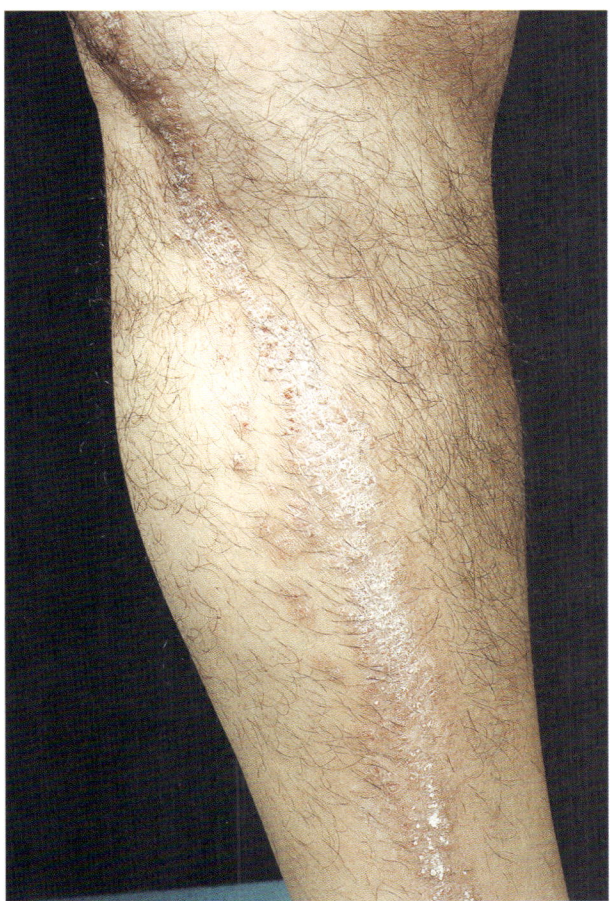

Figure 25.31

In contrast, type 2 segmental distribution is an even more rare phenomenon caused by the mechanism of loss of heterozygosity, visible in rare cases of a small group of autosomal dominant non-lethal diseases (described for Darier's disease, neurofibromatosis type 1) as 'tumeurs royales', porokeratoses, KID syndrome (see Chapter 8) and a few other diseases. The loss of the corresponding wild-type allele due to a second postzygotic mutation may give rise to a superimposed duplication of the disease that is visible phenotypically as a worsening of the symptoms in a Blaschko's lines pattern.

Autosomal recessive traits

Theoretically, autosomal recessive disease could be visible in a mosaic distribution. It must be hypothesized that two different postzygotic mutations affect the same gene in a heterozygous or even a homozygous way, giving rise to a disease visible in one of the mosaic patterns. In reality, no recessive trait has been reported in a mosaic distribution.

In contrast, this concept holds true because of the rare cases of revertant mosaicism that have been reported for autosomal recessive diseases such as junctional epidermolysis bullosa (JEB) due to mutations of the COLAXVII gene, encoding a collagenic structure known as bullous pemphigoid antigen. It has been demonstrated by Jonkman that a postzygotic mutation can erase one of the mutations causing JEB in a patient. In other words, this patient, bearing islets of normal unaffected skin in a rather irregular broad-band pattern over his left arm and palm in a heterozygous affected arrangement, suffered from a further (postzygotic) mutation that cancelled in that portion of skin the maternal inherited mutation, restoring normal unaffected skin in the areas involved by the revertant mutation (Figures 25.33 and 25.34).

X-linked trait inheritance

X-chromosome inactivation is a well-known mechanism theorized by Lyon in 1969. One of the X chromosomes (of maternal or paternal origin) is inactivated at an early stage of embryogenesis. This inactivation results in so-called 'functional mosaicism'.

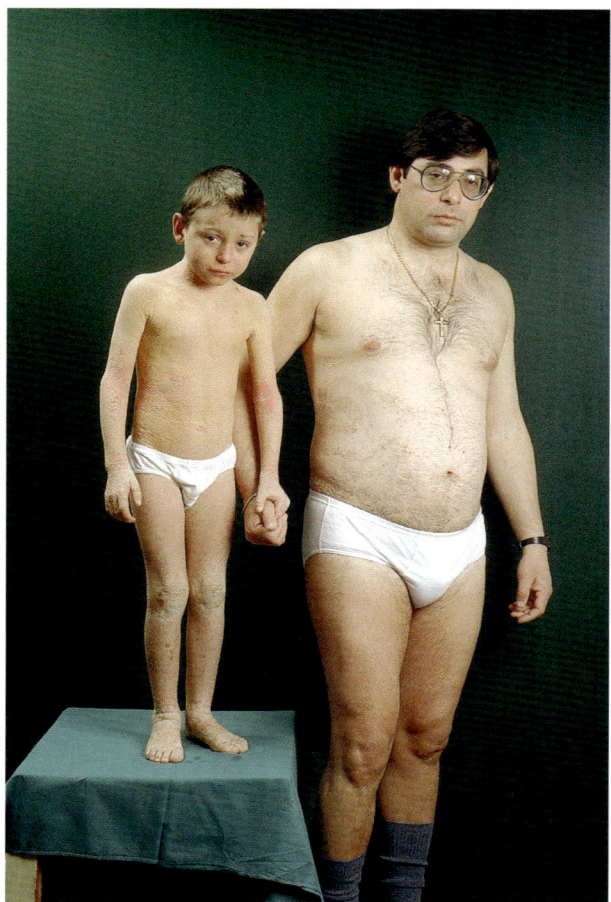

Figure 25.32

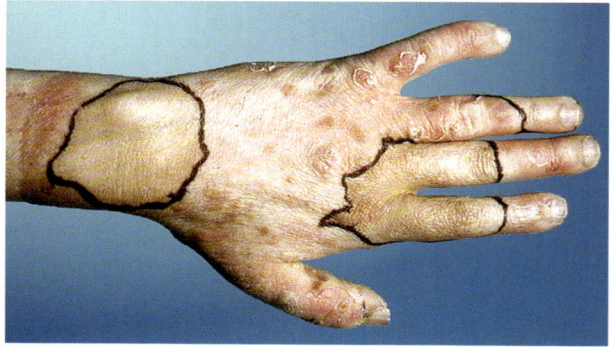

Figure 25.33

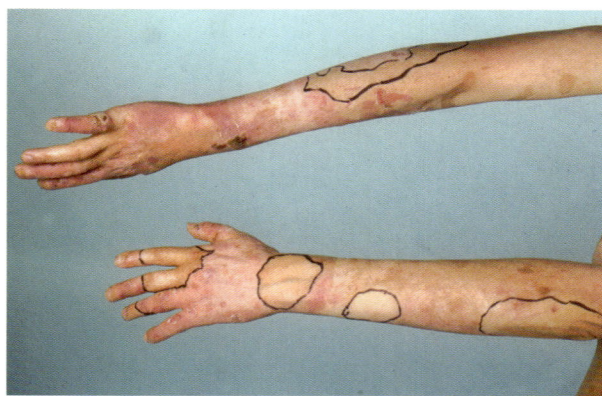

Figure 25.34

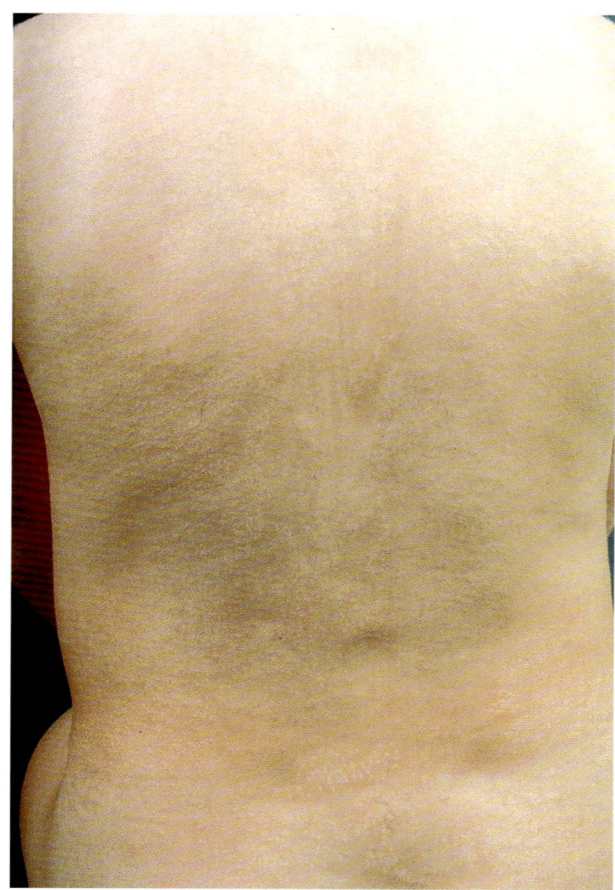

Figure 25.35

X-linked mutations can cause diseases distributed in a mosaic pattern and are classically divided into diseases that are either almost always lethal for the male fetus or non-lethal.

Lyonization may be explained by demonstration that portions of retroviral origin ('retrotransposons') are intermingled in our genome, and the X chromosome is particularly rich in such retroviral particles.

Many studies have elucidated that these parts of retroviral origin-called 'long interspersed nuclear elements' (LINE type I), are located in the proximity of Xq13 where the 'center' of X-inactivation is located. LINE I acts via a methylation–demethylation pathway giving rise to a simple on–off modulation of a cascade that can imply regulation of the classic 'random' X-inactivation and that may be involved in the mechanism of so-called

Cutaneous mosaicism

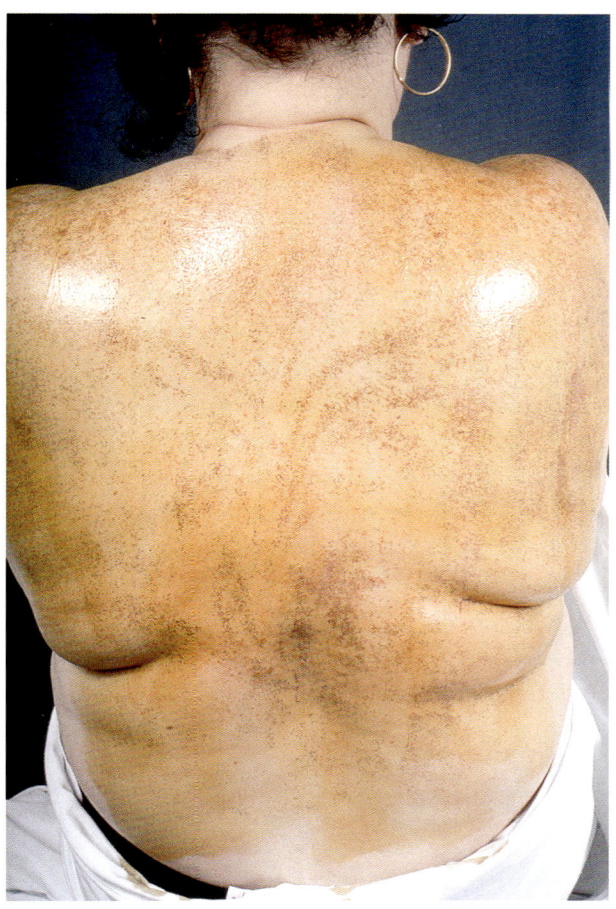

Figure 25.36

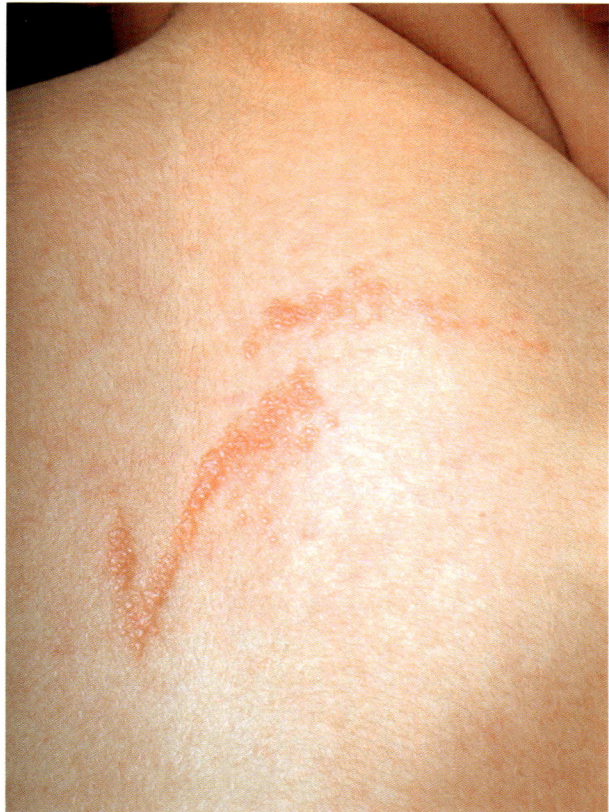

Figure 25.37

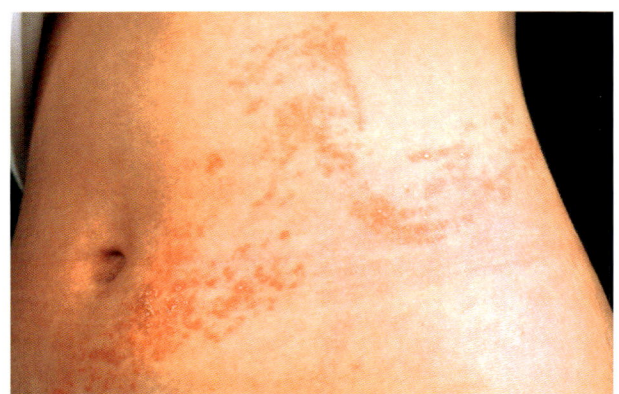

Figure 25.38

'skewed' (non-random) inactivation of the X chromosome, demonstrated in well-known diseases such as incontinentia pigmentia (IP) and Goltz's syndrome.

LINE I particles may be responsible, in other words, for the phenotype of cutaneous mosaicism due to X-linked traits as well as for the appearance of hair colors in animals, e.g. in the 'tiger-like' pattern of some boxer dogs, or in the mouse.

In the so-called lethal X-linked traits some exceptions exist: in IP and Goltz's syndrome a few males survive either by non-lethal ('hypomorphic') point mutation or by mosaicism in a fetus born from a healthy wild-type zygote.

X-linked mosaicism may have different patterns:

- Narrow bands for incontinentia pigmenti, Goltz's syndrome and hypohidrotic ectodermal dysplasia (Figure 25.35: V-shaped atrophic streaks, and Figure 25.36: starch–iodine test in a female carrier of hypohidrotic ectodermal dysplasia; same patient)
- Lateralization pattern for CHILD syndrome (Figure 25.19)
- Checkerboard pattern for X-linked hypertrichosis

Acquired cutaneous mosaicism

Owing to different stimuli, known or unknown, a cutaneous mosaicism is visible during life in a previous healthy subject. The classic example is lichen striatus (Figures 25.35 and 25.37), an inflammatory lichenoid reaction along the Blaschko lines that arises after various unknown stimuli (infectious diseases?) and that disappears with time. Lichen striatus may recur and may be multiple.

Another example of inflammatory acquired mosaicism is inflammatory linear verrucous epidermal nevus (ILVEN) and/or linear psoriasis that follows different unknown stimuli and is distributed in a narrow-band linear pattern. These lesions may persist or disappear. In such lesions, Grosshans demonstrated chromosomal abnormalities at the cytogenetic level.

A further example is acquired cutis laxa after UV exposure in a checkerboard pattern, a so far unique observation of striking appearance. In this case, lesions persisted unchanged for years (Figure 25.15).

A tentative explanation of this acquired mosaicism may be loss of heterozygosity, meaning that to develop this kind of disease both alleles must be involved, one already present at birth in a mosaic pattern but silent, and the second revealed by some triggering stimulus during life.

Retrotransposons are proposed by Happle to be responsible for the formation of acquired cutaneous mosaicism.

REFERENCES

Danarti R, Happle R. Paradominant inheritance of twin spotting: phacomatosis pigmentovascularis as a further possible example. Eur J Dermatol 2003; 13: 612

Happle R. [Phylloid hypomelanosis and mosaic trisomy 13: a new etiologically defined neurocutaneous syndrome] Hautarzt 2001; 52: 3–5. [German]

Happle R. [Segmental type 2 manifestation of autosome dominant skin diseases. Development of a new formal genetic concept] Hautarzt 2001; 52: 283–7. Review. [German]

Happle R. Dohi Memorial Lecture. New aspects of cutaneous mosaicism. J Dermatol 2002; 29: 681–92

Happle R. Transposable elements and the lines of Blaschko: a new perspective. Dermatology 2002; 204: 4–7. Review

Paller AS. Piecing together the puzzle of cutaneous mosaicism. J Clin Invest 2004; 114: 1407–9

Index

Page numbers in italics refer to plate illustrations

ABCA12 gene 43, 48
ABCC 6 gene 250
abdominal herniae, cutis laxa 248, *248*
ablepharon–macrostomy syndrome, differential
    diagnosis 359
acantholytic diseases 25–33
    acrokeratosis verruciformis 29, *29*
    Darier's disease 25–8, *25–8*
    Hailey–Hailey disease 30–1, *30–1*
    peeling skin syndrome 32–3, *32–3*
acanthosis nigricans 234, *235*, 236, 256
    and CVG 267
acne cysts, differential diagnosis 163
acne vulgaris, differential diagnosis 187
acoustic nerve neurinomas 178
acquired cutaneous mosaicism inheritance 405
acral keratoses, Cowden's syndrome 371, *372*
acro-osteolysis 333
acrochordons 367, *368*, 380, *380–1*
acrodermatitis enteropathica 334–5, *334–5*
    differential diagnosis 56, 77, 343
acrokeratoelastoidosis 89, *89*
acrokeratosis verruciformis (of Hopf) 29, *29*
    differential diagnosis 83, 89
acromegaly
    associations 267
    differential diagnosis 88
acropigmentation symmetrica of Dohi *see*
    dyschromatosis symmetrica hereditaria
acute intermittent porphyria, differential diagnosis 337
ACVRL1 gene 307
Adams–Oliver syndrome 272, *272*
    differential diagnosis 310
adenocarcinoma, Gardner syndrome 373
adnexal tumors, differential diagnosis 163
ADULT (acral-dermato-ungual-lacrimal-tooth)
    syndrome 208–10, *210*

adult progeria *see* Werner's syndrome
adult-spectrum ectodermal dysplasia
    see RAPP–Hodgkin–AEC syndrome
AEC complex 208, *208–9*
aging syndromes *see* poikilodermas and
    aging syndromes
albinisms, differential diagnosis 142
Albright's hereditary osteodystrophy 265, 266
alcohol abuse, and Launois–Bensaude syndrome 233
ALK1 gene 307, 315
alopecia
    encephalocraniocutaneous lipomatosis 363, *363*
    epidermolysis bullosa 1, 5, 7
    GAPO syndrome 364–5, *364*
    Hutchinson–Gilford syndrome 117, *118*
    incontinentia pigmenti 222, *224*
    keratoderma hereditaria mutilans 72
    KID syndrome 102, *102*
    Omenn's syndrome 345
    Oral-facial-digital syndrome (type 1) 169, *169*
    Rothmund–Thomson syndrome 113
    trichothiodystrophy 59, *60*
    see also hair diseases
alopecia areata 127–8, *127*
    differential diagnosis 146, 148
Ambras syndrome, differential diagnosis 132
AMP transcription mutations 353
amyloidosis, a CVG 267
anaphylactoid reactions, Netherton syndrome 56
anemia
    associated hair conditions 127
    hemorrhagic telangiectasia 306–7
angiofibromas, tuberous sclerosis complex 180–1, *183–4*
angiomyolipomas, tuberous sclerosis complex 181, *184–5*
angiosarcomas 110
angora hair nevus syndrome 194, *194*
anhidrotic ED *see* hypohidrotic ectodermal dysplasia

ankyloglossia 169, *169*
ankylosing spondylitis 82
annular sarcoidosis, differential diagnosis 255
aortic enlargement, Marfan's syndrome 251–2
Apert's syndrome, differential diagnosis 353
aplasia cutis 269–73, *269–73*
　associations 229, *229*, 231
　differential diagnosis 272–3, *272–3*, 310
aplasia cutis congenita, and branchio-oculofacial syndrome 356
aplastic anemia, dyskeratosis congenita 167, *168*
arachnodactyly, Marfan's syndrome 251, *251–2*
arginosuccinic aciduria, differential diagnosis 144
ARS gene 81
arthrochalasis multiplex congenita *see* Ehlers–Danlos syndromes, type VII
ATAC2 gene 31
ataxia telangiectasia 304–6, *304–6*
　differential diagnosis 111, 175, 306, 375
atherosclerosis, cerebrotendinous xanthomatosis 339
atopic dermatitis, differential diagnosis 348
atopic diathesis 54
atopic eczema, ichthyosis follicularis–atrichia–photophobia (IFAP) syndrome 125
ATP2A2 gene 26
ATP7A gene 144
atrichia with papular lesions 146–7, *147*
　differential diagnosis 126, 146
atropheoderma vermiculatum lesions 126
　differential diagnosis 129
autism, tuberous sclerosis complex 184
autosomal dominant lethal traits inheritance 400–2
autosomal dominant non-lethal traits inheritance 402–3
autosomal recessive inheritance 403

Bannayan's syndrome, differential diagnosis 176
Barber–Say syndrome 358–9, *358–9*
　differential diagnosis 132, 359
Bart's syndrome *see* epidermolysis bullosa
basal cell carcinomas
　Bazex–Dupré–Christol syndrome 383–4
　oculocutaneous albinisms 276
　Rombo syndrome 391–2, *391*
　xeroderma pigmentosum 110
　see also nevoid basal cell carcinoma syndrome
basal cell nevus syndrome *see* nevoid basal cell carcinoma syndrome
Bazex–Dupré–Christol syndrome 383–4, *384*
　differential diagnosis 369, 392
beaded hair *see* monilethrix
Beau's syndrome *see* blue rubber bleb nevus syndrome
Becker's nevus
　differential diagnosis 133
　genetics 285
Beckwith–Wiedemann syndrome, differential diagnosis 301
benign intraepithelial dyskeratosis, differential diagnosis 166

Berardinelli's syndrome *see* total lipodystrophy
BHD1 gene 381
BIDS syndrome 60–1
biliary atresia, cerebrotendinous xanthomatosis 339
binding protein (CREB) 353
Birt–Hogg–Dubé syndrome 380–1, *380–1*
Björnstad's syndrome, differential diagnosis 144
bladder diverticuli
　cutis laxa 248
　Ehlers–Danlos syndromes 239–46
Blaschko's distributions *see* lines of Blaschko
Bloch–Sulzberger syndrome *see* incontinentia pigmenti
Bloom's syndrome 374–5, *374*
　differential diagnosis 175, 306, 307, 375
blue rubber bleb nevus syndrome 312–13, *312–13*
　differential diagnosis 312
BOF syndrome *see* branchio-oculofacial syndrome
Brachmann–de Lange syndrome *see* Cornelia de Lange syndrome
Branchio-oculofacial syndrome 356–8, *356–8*
Brandt's syndrome *see* acrodermatitis enteropathica
brittle hair *see* trichothiodystrophy
broad thumb–great toe syndrome *see* Rubinstein–Taybi syndrome
Brooke–Spiegler syndrome 386–7, *386–7*
Bruch's membrane 249, *251*
Brunauer–Fuchs disease *see* striate keratoderma
bubble hair, differential diagnosis 137
bullous ichthyosiform erythroderma *see* epidermolytic hyperkeratosis
bullous impetigo, differential diagnosis 226
bullous mastocytosis, differential diagnosis 226
Buschke–Fischer–Brauer disease *see* punctate palmoplantar keratoderma
Buschke–Ollendorff syndrome 253–4, *253–4*
　associations 155, 253
butterfly telangiectases pattern 304, *304–5*
Björnstad's syndrome, and pili torti 138

C1q esterase inhibitor deficiency 348–9, *349*
C1q esterase inhibitor gene 349
cachectic dwarfism 121
cadherin mutations 84
Caenorhabditis elegans UNC-112 protein 109
café-au-lait spots
　disease associations 175, 284–5, *285*
　neurofibromatosis (type 1) 171, *171–2*, 173–4
calcium storage modulation 250
Candida infections 151
　acrodermatitis enteropathica 334–5
cardiac failure
　and Kyrle's disease 97
　see also heart defects
cardiac myxoma, Carney's complex 382–3
cardiac rhabdomyomas 185
cardiofacio-cutaneous syndrome 187–8, *187*
　differential diagnosis 188

Carney's complex 382–3, *382*
   differential diagnosis 291, 293, 380, 383
cblA/B/C/D/ genes 343
cerebro-oculo-facial-skeletal syndrome 122
cerebrotendinous xanthomatosis 339–41, *339–41*
CGI-58 gene 64
CHAND syndrome, AEC complex 208
Chediak–Higashi syndrome 349–50, *350*
   differential diagnosis 141, 276, 279
'cheveux incoiffables' *see* uncombable hair syndrome
chiasmal gliomas 172, 177
CHILD syndrome 98–9, *98–9*
   differential diagnosis 99, 101
cholestanolysis *see* cerebrotendinous xanthomatosis
chondrodysplasia punctata, differential diagnosis 384
chondroectodermal dysplasia *see* Ellis–van Creveld–Weyers acrodental dysostosis complex
Christ–Siemens–Touraine syndrome *see* hypohidrotic ectodermal dysplasia
cicatricial alopecia 328, *329*
CIE *see* congenital ichthyosiform erythroderma
'cigarette paper' scars 107
CKN1 (CSA) gene 121–2
cleft lip
   RAPP–Hodgkin–AEC syndrome 208
   Waardenburg's syndrome 283
cleft lip–palate ectodermal dysplasia syndrome 216, *216*
cleft palate, Cornelia de Lange syndrome 353
cleft tongue 169, *169*
Clouston's syndrome 217–18, *217–18*
   differential diagnosis 77, 103, 146, 218
clubbed digits
   Huriez's syndrome 79, *79*
   pachydermoperiostosis 88
   Unna–Thost palmoplantar keratoderma 71
cobblestone angiomyolipomas 181, *184–5*
cobblestone papules 25
cobblestone scales, X-linked ichthyosis 38, *38*
Cobb's syndrome 302–3, *302–3*
Cockayne's syndrome 121–2, *121*
   differential diagnosis 236, 306, 375
Coffin–Syris syndrome, differential diagnosis 354
COH1 gene 355–6
Cohen's syndrome 355–6, *355–6*
   differential diagnosis 356
COL1A1 gene 245
COL1A2 gene 245
COL3A1 gene 242, 244, 245, 246
COL5A1 gene 239, 241
COL5A2 gene 239, 241
COLAXVII gene 1, 9
cold abscesses 347
collodion babies
   CRIE 51
   Dorfman–Chanarin syndrome 63
   lamellar ichthyosis 42
   Netherton syndrome 53–4, *54*
   self-healing 40–1, *40–1*
   trichothiodystrophy 59
   X-linked dominant chondrodysplasia punctata 100
colobomas, phakomatosis pigmentokeratotica 189
colorectal cancer
   Birt–Hogg–Dubé syndrome 380–1
   Muir–Torre syndrome 369
congenital bullous autoimmune disease 14
congenital erythropoietic porphyria 332–3, *332–3*
   differential diagnosis 111, 333
congenital generalized fibromatosis, differential diagnosis 259
congenital generalized lipodystrophy *see* total lipodystrophy
congenital hemidysplasia *see* CHILD syndrome
congenital ichthyosiform erythroderma (CEI), non-bullous 42
congenital ichthyosis *see* lamellar ichthyosis
congenital livedo reticularis *see* cutis marmorata telangiectatica congenita
congenital onychodysplasia of the index finger *see* Iso–Kikuchi syndrome
congenital onychogryphosis, differential diagnosis 153
congenital reticular ichthyosiform erythroderma (CRIE) 51–2
congenital syphilis 14
congenital telangiectatic erythema *see* Bloom's syndrome
congenital temporal triangular alopecia *see* triangular alopecia
conjunctival cancer, xeroderma pigmentosum 110
conjunctivitis, CRIE 52
connective tissue nevi 253–4, *253–4*
connexin 26 (Cx26) gene 72, 103, 158
connexin 30.3 (Cx30.5) gene 66
connexin 31 (Cx31) gene 66
connexin 30 gene 217–18
Conradi–Hunermann–Happle syndrome *see* X-linked dominant chondrodysplasia punctata
corneal dyskeratosis 151
corneal dystrophy, dermochondrocorneal dystrophy 263
corneal opacity
   X-linked ichthyosis 38–9
   xeroderma pigmentosum 110
corneal ulcerations
   CRIE 52
   KID syndrome 103
   Richner–Hanhart syndrome 86, *86*
Cornelia de Lange syndrome 353–4, *354*
   differential diagnosis 353, 354
Costello's syndrome 256, *256*
   differential diagnosis 256, 267
Cowden's syndrome 371–2, *371–2*
   differential diagnosis 372, 378, 387, 392
Crandall's syndrome, and pili torti 138
CRIE *see* congenital reticular ichthyosiform erythroderma
Cronkhite–Canada syndrome, differential diagnosis 380

Cross–McKusick syndrome, differential diagnosis 276
cryptorchidism 38–9
   Cornelia de Lange syndrome 353
   LEOPARD syndrome 292
   Noonan's syndrome 179
   Rubinstein–Taybi syndrome 352
CSB gene see ERCC6 (CSB) gene
'cuirass' 48
Curth–Macklin disease see ichthyosis Curth–Macklin
cutaneomeningeal angiomatosis see Cobb's syndrome
cutaneous leiomyomatosis 261–2, *261*
cutaneous mastocytosis 260, *260*
cutaneous mosaicism 393–405
   definition 393
   inheritance mechanisms 400–5
   acquired cutaneous mosaicism 405
   autosomal dominant lethal traits 400–2
   autosomal dominant non-lethal traits 402–3
   autosomal recessive traits 403
   X-linked trait inheritance 403–5
   checkerboard patterns 396, *397*
   irregular patches 397, *398*
   lateralization pattern 397–8, *399*
   lines of Blaschko patterns 393–6
   'phylloid' pattern 397, *398*
   see also mosaic conditions
cutis laxa 247–9, *247–8*
   differential diagnosis 240, 248, 256
cutis marmorata telangiectatica congenita 308–10, *308–10*
   aplasia cutis 269
cutis tricolor 295, *295*
cutis verticis gyrata (CVG) 266–7, *266*
   differential diagnosis 267
CVG see cutis verticis gyrata
cyanosis and soft skin syndrome, differential diagnosis 392
CYLD gene 387
cylindromas, Brooke–Spiegler syndrome 386–7, *386–7*
CYP27 gene 340
cytochrome c oxidase 144

Danbolt–Closs syndrome see acrodermatitis enteropathica
Darier–White disease see Darier's disease
Darier's disease 25–8, *25–8*
   differential diagnosis 28, 29, 166, 226, 372
DDB1 gene *111*
DDB2 gene *111*
de Lange syndrome see Cornelia de Lange syndrome
De Santis–Cacchione syndrome (for XP-A) see xeroderma pigmentosum
deafness
   Clouston's disease 218
   KID syndrome 103
   LEOPARD syndrome 292
   pachyonychia congenita 151
   woolly hair 140
   xeroderma pigmentosum 111

decalvans folliculitis 220, *221*
   differential diagnosis 146
Degos' disease 389–90, *389–90*
Delleman's syndrome 273, *273*
dental deformities
   congenital erythropoietic porphyria 332, *333*
   Ehlers–Danlos type VIII syndrome 246
   GAPO syndrome 364–5, *365*
   hypohidrotic ectodermal dysplasia 204
   incontinentia pigmenti 224–5, *225*
   twenty-nail dystrophy 156
dental erosion, Papillon–Lefevre syndrome 78
dermatitis herpetiformis, associations 261
dermatochalasis see cutis laxa
dermatomycoses, differential diagnosis 50
dermochondrocorneal dystrophy 263–4, *263–4*
   differential diagnosis 264
dermolytic epidermolysis bullosa (DEB) 9–14, *10–13*
desmoglein 1 gene 153
desmoid tumors, Gardner syndrome 373
diabetes mellitus
   Kyrle's disease 97
   Launois–Bensaude syndrome 233
   lipodystrophies 235, 236
'diamond patches' depigmentation 281, *281*
dietary regimes
   low-phenylamine 86
   low-tyrosine 86
diffuse benign telangiectasia and port-wine stains complex 314–15, *314*
diffuse mastocytosis, differential diagnosis 175
diffuse palmoplantar keratoderma (PPK) see Unna–Thost palmoplantar keratoderma
digit clubbing see clubbed digits
digit loss 72–3, *72–3*, 81
DKC1 gene 167
DLX3 gene 213, 214
DNA-repair systems 62
   alpha helicase mutations 375
   germline mutations 369
   and UV irradiation 111, 122
dominant ichthyosis 35–7, *35–7*
   differential diagnosis 44
dopamine B hydroxylase 144
Dorfman–Chanarin syndrome 63–4, *63–4*
   differential diagnosis 44
Dowling–Meara EBS see epidermolytic epidermolysis bullosa (EEB)
Dowling–Degos disease see Kitamura–Dowling–Degos disease
Down's syndrome, differential diagnosis 255, 310
dwarfism, Ellis–van Creveld–Weyers acrodental dysostosis complex 214
'dredding' hair 90
DSRAD gene 296
duplication (3q) syndrome, differential diagnosis 354
dyschromatosis symmetrica hereditaria 296, *296*
dysesthesia, phakomatosis pigmentokeratotica *91*, 188

dyskeratosis congenita 166–8, *166–8*
  differential diagnosis 109, 153, 168, 375
dystopia canthorum, associations 283, *283*

eccrine spiradenoma, differential diagnosis 262
ecto-mesodermal dysplasias 227–31
  Goltz's syndrome 227–30, *227–9*
  Midas syndrome 231, *231*
ectodermal dysplasias 203–6
  cleft lip–palate 216, *216*
  Clouston's syndrome 217–18, *217–18*
  differential diagnosis 114, 124–5
  Ellis–van Creveld–Weyers acrodental
    dysostosis complex 214–15, *214–15*
  hypohidrotic ectodermal dysplasia 203–7, *203–7*
  incontinentia pigmenti 222–6, *222–5*
  pure hair–nail 220–1, *220–1*
  RAPP–Hodgkin–AEC syndrome 208–11, *208–11*
  skin fragility syndrome 219–20, *219–20*
  tricho-dento-osseous syndrome 212–13, *212*
  Witkop's syndrome 213–14, *213*
ectopic ossification, gene modulators 266
EDA (ectodysplasin) gene 206–7
EDAR gene 206–7
EDNRB gene 283
EEC syndrome *see* RAPP–Hodgkin–AEC syndrome
Ehlers–Danlos syndromes 239–47
  type (I) 239–41, *240–1*
  type (II) 241–2, *241–2*
  type (III) 242, *242*
  type (IV) 243–4, *243*
  type (V) 244
  type (VI) 245
  type (VII) 245
  type (VIII) 246
  type (IX) 246
  type (X) 247
elastin–keratinocyte interactions 98
elastosis perforans serpiginosa 255, *255*
  differential diagnosis 98, 255
Elejalde's syndrome 140–1, *141*
  differential diagnosis 279, 350
Ellis–van Creveld–Weyers acrodental dysostosis
    complex 214–15, *214–15*
encephalocraniocutaneous lipomatosis 363–4, *363–4*
  differential diagnosis 99, 176, 364
encephalotrigeminal angiomatosis
    see Sturge–Weber syndrome
enchondromatosis *see* Maffucci syndrome
endoglin gene 307, 315
epidermal nevi/nevus syndromes 192–6
  angora hair nevus syndrome 194, *194*
  Becker's nevus/syndrome 194–5, *194*
  Epidermal-sebaceous nevus syndrome 192–3, *192–3*
  nevus comedonicus syndrome 193–4, *193*
  vitamin D-resistant rickets 195, *195–6*
epidermal-melanocytic twin nevus syndrome
    see phakomatosis pigmentokeratotica

epidermal-sebaceous nevus (ESN) syndrome
    188, *188–90*, 192–3, *192–3*
  differential diagnosis 294, 364
epidermodysplasia verruciformis 385–6, *385–6*
  differential diagnosis 29
epidermoid cysts, differential diagnosis 163
epidermolysis bullosa 1–14
  differential diagnosis 14, 263
  dermolytic epidermolysis bullosa (DEB) 9–14, *10–13*
  epidermolytic epidermolysis bullosa (EEB) 1–4, *2–4*
  junctional epidermolysis bullosa (JEB) 5–9, *5–9*
epidermolytic (acantholytic) nevus 16, *18*
epidermolytic epidermolysis bullosa (EEB) 1–4, *2–4*
  differential diagnosis 220, 273
epidermolytic hyperkeratosis 15–23
  differential diagnosis 41, 43
  'classical' epidermolytic hyperkeratosis
    14, 15–18, *15–18*
  differential diagnosis 18
  ichthyosis bullosa of Siemens (IBS) 19–20, *19*
  ichthyosis Curth–Macklin 20–1, *20–1*
  'stellate' epidermolytic hyperkeratosis 22–3
epidermolytic palmoplantar keratoderma 69–70, *69–70*
  differential diagnosis 70, 74
epilepsy, tuberous sclerosis complex 183–4, 186
epiphora 167
epithelioma of Malherbe, differential diagnosis 266
ERCC2/3/4 *111*
ERCC6 (CSB) gene 121–2
eruptive vellus hair cysts *see* sebocystomatosis
erythema marginatum 348
erythrodermic ichthyosis, differential diagnosis 56
erythrodermic lamellar ichthyosis *see* lamellar ichthyosis
erythrokeratodermia variabilis 65–6, *65–6*
  differential diagnosis 56, 66
erythropoietic protoporphyria 330–1, *330–1*
  differential diagnosis 111, 331
esophageal carcinoma, Howel–Evans syndrome 376
esophageal strictures, Kindler's syndrome 108
EvC–WAD disease *see* Ellis–van Creveld–Weyers
    acrodental dysostosis complex
EVC gene 215
'exclamation point hair' 127
EYA1 gene 358

Fabry's disease 335–7, *336*
  differential diagnosis 187, 307, 336–7
facial papules
  Cowden's syndrome 371, *371*
  Muir–Torre syndrome 369, *370*
  nevoid basal cell carcinoma syndrome 367, *367–8*
  Peutz–Jeghers syndrome 378, *378–9*
  Rombo syndrome 391–2, *391*
FADS (fetal akinesia deformation syndrome)
    see restrictive dermopathy
FALDH genes 58
familial area celsi *see* alopecia areata
familial atrophic papulosis *see* Degos' disease

familial capillary malformation *see* diffuse benign
    telangiectasia and port-wine stains complex
familial hyperlipoproteinemias,
    differential diagnosis 341
familial leiomyomata *see* cutaneous leiomyomatosis
familial lipodystrophy *see* partial lipodystrophy
familial lipomatoses, differential diagnosis 176
familial reticuloendotheliosis with eosinophilia
    see Omenn's syndrome
familial subungual pterygium of nails
    see pterygium inversum of nails
familial symmetric lipomatosis
    see Launois–Bensaude syndrome
familial urticaria pigmentosa *see* cutaneous mastocytosis
Fanconi's disease, differential diagnosis 168, 306
fatty acid mutations 58
fatty tissue anomalies 233–7
    Launois–Bensaude syndrome 233–4, *233*
    partial lipodystrophy 236–7, *236*
    total lipodystrophy 234–6, *234–5*
fetal akinesia deformation syndrome (FADS)
    see restrictive dermopathy
fibrillin I encoding gene 252
fibroblastic rheumatism, differential diagnosis 264
fibromatosis hyalinica multiplex *see* juvenile
    hyaline fibromatosis
filaggrin anomalies 36
finger loss 72–3, *72–3*
'flat face', X-linked dominant
    chondrodysplasia punctata 100
flat warts, differential diagnosis 29
Flegel's disease, differential diagnosis 98
focal acral hyperkeratosis, differential diagnosis 89
focal dermal hypoplasia *see* Goltz's syndrome
follicular atrophoderma and basal cell carcinoma
    see Bazex–Dupré–Christol syndrome
follicular keratosis
    differential diagnosis 129
    pachyonychia congenita 151
folliculitis rubra *see* ulerythema ophryogenes
Fordyce angiokeratomas, differential diagnosis 337
foveal hypoplasia, oculocutaneous albinisms 275
François' syndrome *see* dermochondrocorneal dystrophy
'frog spawn' angiokeratomas 300
Fryns' syndrome, differential diagnosis 362
fucosidosis, differential diagnosis 336

galactosialidosis, differential diagnosis 337
gangliosidoses, differential diagnosis 336
gap junction-associated proteins 66, 217–18
GAPO syndrome 364–5, *364–5*
Gardner syndrome 373–4, *373*
    differential diagnosis 387
Gaucher's syndrome, differential diagnosis 58, 175
gene transcription 62
generalized cyanosis, phlebectasies and soft
    skin syndrome 322–4, *322–3*

generalized elastolysis *see* cutis laxa
genes
    ABCA(12) 43, 48
    ABCC (6) 250
    ACVRL(1) 307
    ALK(1) 307, 315
    ARS 81
    ATAC(2) 31
    ATP2A(2) 26
    ATP7A 144
    BHD(1) 381
    C1q esterase inhibitor 349
    cblA/B/C/D 343
    CGI-(58) 64
    CKN1 (CSA) 121–2
    COH(1) 355–6
    COL1A(1) 245
    COL1A(2) 245
    COL3A(1) 242, 244, 245, 246
    COL5A(1) 239, 241
    COL5A(2) 239, 241
    COLAXVII 1, 9
    connexin 26 (Cx26) 72, 103, 158
    connexion 30 (Cx 30) 217–18
    connexin 30.3 (Cx30.5) 66
    connexin 31 (Cx31) 66
    CYLD 387
    CYP(27) 340
    DDB(1) *111*
    DDB(2) *111*
    desmoglein (1) 153
    desmoplakin 84
    DKC(1) 167
    DLX(3) 213, 214
    DSRAD 296
    EDA (ectodysplasin) 206–7
    EDAR 206–7
    EDNRB 283
    endoglin 307, 315
    ERCC(2) *111*
    ERCC(3) *111*
    ERCC(4) *111*
    ERCC(6) (CSB) 121–2
    EVC 215
    EYA(1) 358
    FALDH 58
    GJB(3) 66
    GLMN 325
    GNAS(1) 265–6, 285
    HED 226
    hMSH(2) 369
    HPS 279
    hTERC (RNA telomerase) 167
    integrin a6b4 *1*, 5
    keratin 1 (K1) 17–18, 20, 22, 84
    keratin 2e (K2e) 19
    keratin 4 (K4) 166

keratin 5 (K5) 1
keratin 6 (K6) 153
keratin 9 (KRT9) 70
keratin 10 (K10) 17–18, 22
keratin 13 (K13) 166
keratin 14 (K14) 1
keratin 16 (K16) 153
keratin 17 (K17) 153
KIND1 (FlJ20116) 109
KRTHB(6/1) 134
lamin A/C 237
laminin (5) 1, 5
laminin B(1) 252
laminin 5,type XVII collagen 5
lipo-oxygenase 43
LMNA 118
LMX1B 155
loricrin 68, 77
LYST 349
lysyl hydroxylase 245
MATP 278
merlin 178–9
MITF 283
MSX(1) 214
MYO5 A 140, 142
NEMO 207, 225–6, 230
neurofibromin 173–4
NIPBL 354
NSDHL 99
OCA(1) 276
OCA(4) 278
OFD(1) 170
P 277
p(53) 386
p(63) 211
PAX(3) 283
PHYH 58
PKP(1) 220
plectin 1, 3
PRKAR1A 382
PTCH 369
PTEN 201, 372
PTPN(11) 179, 293
PTS2 receptor (PEX7) 58
PVRL(1) 216
Rab27a 142
RAG(1/2) 346
RECQ helicase 114
SLC39A(4) 334
SPINK(5) 56
SSAT 149
STRK11/LKB(1) 379
transglutaminase-1 38, 41, 43
trisomy (13) 271
TRP(1) 278
TRPS(1) 146
TSC(1) 186
TSC(2) 186
tyrosineaminotransferase (TAT) 85
uroporphyrinogen decarboxylase 328–9
VHL 303
45XO 360
XP-B 62
XP-D 62
genetic mosaicism
  background history 285
  inheritance mechanisms 400–5
  see also cutaneous mosaicism
genitalia hypertrophy, total lipodystrophy 235
genodermatoses and malignancy 367–92
  Bazex–Dupré–Christol syndrome 383–4, *384*
  Birt–Hogg–Dubé syndrome 380–1, *380–1*
  Bloom's syndrome 374–5, *374*
  Brooke–Spiegler syndrome 386–7, *386–7*
  Carney's complex 382–3, *382*
  Cowden's syndrome 371–2, *371–2*
  Degos' disease 389–90, *389–90*
  epidermodysplasia verruciformis 385–6, *385–6*
  Gardner syndrome 373–4, *373*
  Howel–Evans syndrome 376, *376*
  Muir–Torre syndrome 369–70, *370*
  multiple endocrine neoplasia syndrome
    (type 2B) 377–8, *377*
  nevoid basal cell carcinoma syndrome 367–9, *367–8*
  Peutz–Jeghers syndrome 378–80, *378–9*
  progressive mucinous histiocytosis 388–9, *388–9*
  Rombo syndrome 391–2, *391*
genodermatosis 'en cocarde'
  see erythrokeratoderma variabilis
Giedion–Gurish syndrome
  see trichorhinophalangeal syndrome
gingival hyperplasia 263, *264*
gingival hypertrophy 258, *258*
GJB3 gene 66
glaucoma, nail–patella–elbow syndrome 154
GLMN gene 325
global genome repair (GGR) system 111
glomerulonephritis, nail–patella–elbow syndrome 153
glomuvenous malformation 324–5, *324*
glucagonoma syndrome, differential diagnosis 335
GNAS1 gene 265–6, 285
Gobello's nevus syndrome 195, *195*
Goltz's syndrome 227–30, *227–29*
  associations 170, 229–30
  differential diagnosis 99, 101, 211, 226, 230, 273
Gorlin syndrome see nevoid basal cell
  carcinoma syndrome
'gothic church hyperkeratosis 74
Gottron's syndrome see symmetric progressive
  erythrokeratoderma
Gougerot–Carteaud syndrome,
  differential diagnosis 197
gout, and Launois–Bensaude syndrome 233
graft versus host disease, differential diagnosis 346

granular cell tumor, differential diagnosis 262
granuloma annulare, differential diagnosis 255
Greither's disease 74–5, *74*
Griscelli's syndrome 141–2, *142*
   differential diagnosis 140–1, 142, 279, 350
Gronblad–Strandberg syndrome
   see pseudoxanthoma elasticum
Grover's disease, differential diagnosis 28
GTPase-activating protein (GAP) family 174
Gunther's disease see congenital
   erythropoietic porphyria
gynecomastia, and pachydermoperiostosis 88

Haber's syndrome 119
Hailey–Hailey disease 30–1, *30–1*
   differential diagnosis 28, 31
hair diseases
   alopecia areata 127–8, *127*
   hypotrichosis simplex of the scalp 124–5, *124*
   ichthyosis follicularis with atrichia and
      photophobia 125–7, *125–7*
   Marie–Unna hypotrichosis 123–4, *123*
   triangular alopecia 130, *130*
   ulerythema ophryogenes 128–9
   see also alopecia; hair shaft defects; hirsutism
hair shaft defects
   atrichia with papular lesions 146–7, *147*
   Elejalde's syndrome 140–1, *141*
   Griscelli's syndrome 141–2, *142*
   keratosis follicularis spinulosa decalvans 149, *149*
   loose anagen syndrome 148, *148*
   Menkes' kinky hair syndrome 144–5, *144*
   monilethrix 134–5, *134–5*
   Netherton syndrome 55, *55*
   pili annulati 136–7, *136–7*
   pili torti 137–8, *137–8*
   trichorhinophalangeal syndrome 145–6, *145–6*
   uncombable hair syndrome 143, *143*
   woolly hair 139–40, *139*
'hairy elbows' see localized hypertrichosis
Hallopeau–Siemens DEB 9–11, *10–13*
hamartomas 182, 184
   connective tissue nevi 253, *253*
   Peutz–Jeghers syndrome 379
   Proteus syndrome 200, *201*
Happle's apple' 398, *399*
Harlequin fetus 48–9, *48–9*
Hashimoto's thyroiditis, associated conditions 127
heart defects
   Cornelia de Lange syndrome 353–4
   Costello's syndrome 256
   Ellis–van Creveld–Weyers acrodental
      dysostosis complex 214–15
   Fabry's disease 335–6
   Goltz's syndrome 229
   LEOPARD syndrome 292
   Naxos syndrome 90–1
   Noonan's syndrome 179

HED gene 226
hemangioblastoma of retina and cerebellum
   see Von Hippel–Lindau syndrome
hemangiomas
   capillary 351
   gastrointestinal 312
hemangiomatosis see Maffucci syndrome
hemiatrophy, phakomatosis pigmentokeratotica 189, *191*
hemihypotrophy, incontinentia pigmenti 225, *225*
hemophagocytic syndrome, Griscelli's syndrome 141
hemorrhagic bullae 2, *2–3*
hemorrhagic telangiectasia 306–7, *306–7*
   differential diagnosis 307, 337
hepatic vascular nodules, hemorrhagic
   telangiectasia 306–7
hepatoerythropoietic porphyria 327–9, *327–9*
hepatomegaly, total lipodystrophy 235
hepatosplenomegaly
   Griscelli's syndrome 141
   Omenn's syndrome 345
   sea-blue histiocytosis 337–8
hereditary angioedema see C1q esterase
   inhibitor deficiency
hereditary benign telangiectasia,
   differential diagnosis 307
hereditary congenital poikiloderma
   see Rothmund–Thomson syndrome
hereditary epidermal polycystic disease
   see sebocystomatosis
hereditary polymorphic light eruption,
   differential diagnosis 111
Herlitz JEB 5, *5–6*
Hermansky–Pudlak syndrome 279, *279*
   differential diagnosis 141, 276, 277, 279, 350
herniae, cutis laxa 248, *248*
herpes virus, aplasia cutis 271–2
HID see hystrix-like ichthyosis and deafness
   (HID) syndrome
hidradenitis suppurativa 151
   associations 162
hidrotic ectodermal dysplasia see Clouston's disease
Hirschsprung's malformation, associations 283, 284, 378
hirsutism 131–3
   hypertrichosis congenita 131–2, *131–2*
   localized hypertrichosis 133, *133*
hMSH2 gene 369
honeycomb hyperkeratosis 72, *72*
horseshoe kidney
   nevoid basal cell carcinoma syndrome 368
   Turner's syndrome 360
'hound dog' facies 247, *248*
Howel–Evans syndrome 376, *376*
   differential diagnosis 87, 376
HPS genes 279
hTERC (RNA telomerase) gene 167
Huriez's syndrome 79–80, *79–80*
Hutchinson–Gilford syndrome 117–19, *118*
   differential diagnosis 119, 365

hyper IgE syndrome 347–8, *347*
hyperhidrosis
   CRIE 51
   dyskeratosis congenita 167, *167*
hyperimmunoglobulinemia E syndrome
      see hyper IgE syndrome
hyperkeratosis
   dyskeratosis congenita 167, *167*
   epidermolytic *see* epidermolytic hyperkeratosis
   follicular *35–6*, 36, 42, 47
   pachyonchia congenita 151, *152*
hypertelorism, LEOPARD syndrome 292
hypertrichosis
   CRIE 51
   porphyria cutanea tarda 327, *328*
   Rubinstein–Taybi syndrome 351, *351*
hypertrichosis congenita 131–2, *131–2*
   differential diagnosis 132
hypertrichosis cubiti *see* localized hypertrichosis
hypertrichosis universalis *see* hypertrichosis congenita
hypo-anonychia congenita, differential diagnosis 155
hypoanosmy 38
hypogonadism
   dyskeratosis congenita 167
   nevoid basal cell carcinoma syndrome 368
   Noonan's syndrome 179
   Rothmund–Thompson syndrome 113
hypohidrotic ectodermal dysplasia 203–7, *203–7*
   associated conditions 138, 148
   clinical findings 203–5, *203–7*
   differential diagnosis 41, 44, 207, 211
hypomelanosis of Ito 280–1, *280–1*
hypomelanotic nevi
   associations 280
   differential diagnosis 187
hypoparathyroidism, associations 158
hypophosphatemia, organoid nevus 195
hypopigmented macules, tuberous
      sclerosis complex 180, *181–2*
hypopigmented nevus 319, *320*
hypotrichosis simplex of the scalp 124–5, *124*
hystrix-like ichthyosis and deafness
      (HID) syndrome 103

ichthyoses 35–52
   CRIE (congenital reticular ichthyosiform
      erythroderma) 51–2, *51–2*
   dominant ichthyosis 35–7, *35–7*
   harlequin fetus 48–9, *48–9*
   lamellar ichthyosis 41–7, *43–7*
   pityriasis rotunda 50, *50*
   self-healing collodion baby 40–1
   X-linked ichthyosis 38–9, *38–9*
ichthyosiform dermatosis 53–4, *53–5*
ichthyosis bullosa of Siemens (IBS) 19–20, *19*
ichthyosis Curth–Macklin 20–1, *20–1*
ichthyosis 'en confettis' *see* congenital
      reticular ichthyosiform erythroderma

ichthyosis follicularis–atrichia–photophobia
      (IFAP) syndrome 125–7, *125–7*
   differential diagnosis 103, 126, 149, 211, 384
ichthyosis hystrix 15, *17*
ichthyosis variegata *see* congenital reticular
      ichthyosiform erythroderma
ichthyosis vulgaris *see* dominant ichthyosis
idiopathic deciduous skin *see* peeling skin syndrome
IFAP syndrome *see* ichthyosis
      follicularis–atrichia–photophobia (IFAP) syndrome
ILVEN (inflammatory linear verrucous
      epidermal nevus), differential diagnosis 99
immunodeficiency disorders 345–50
   C1q esterase inhibitor deficiency 348–9, *349*
   Chediak–Higashi syndrome 349–50, *350*
   Griscelli's syndrome 141–2
   hyper IgE syndrome 347–8, *347*
   Omenn's syndrome 345–6, *345–6*
immunoglobulin deficiency, Bloom's syndrome 375
incontinentia pigmenti 222–6, *222–5*
   associations 170
   differential diagnosis 226, 362
   genetics 207, 225–6
incontinentia pigmenti acromians
      see hypomelanosis of Ito
infantile systemic hyalinosis *see* juvenile
      hyaline fibromatosis
inheritance mechanisms for mosaicism 400–5
integrin a6b4 genes *1*, 5
intestinal polyposis (generalized) type II
      see Peutz–Jeghers syndrome
Iso–Kikuchi syndrome 160, *160*
isochromosome 12p syndrome
      see Pallister–Killian syndrome

Jadassohn–Lewandowsky syndrome
      see pachyonchia congenita
Jaffé's syndrome, differential diagnosis 175
'jentigo' pattern 289, *290*
Job's syndrome *see* hyper IgE syndrome
Johansson–Blizzard syndrome 273
joint hyperextensibility
   Ehlers–Danlos type 1 syndrome 239, *241*
   Marfan's syndrome 251
junctional epidermolysis bullosa (JEB) 5–9, *5–9*
juvenile hyaline fibromatosis 258–9, *258*
   differential diagnosis 259, 264

Kallmann's syndrome *see* hypoanosmy
keloids, Ehlers–Danlos syndromes 243, *243*
keratin 1 (K1) gene 17–18, 21, 22
   (VI end domain) 71
keratin 1-associated PPK *see* Unna–Thost
      palmoplantar keratoderma
keratin 2e (K2e) gene 19
keratin 4 (K4) gene 166
keratin 5 (K5) gene 1
keratin 6 (K6) gene 153

keratin 9 (KRT9) gene 70
keratin 10 (K10) gene 17–18, 22
keratin 13 (K13) gene 166
keratin 14 (K14) gene 1
keratin 16 (K16) gene 153
keratin 17 (K17) gene 153
keratitis–ichthyosis–deafness syndrome
   see KID syndrome
keratoacanthomas, Muir–Torre syndrome 369
keratoconjunctivitis, and KID syndrome 103
keratoderma hereditaria mutilans 72–3, *72–3*
   differential diagnosis 73, 77
keratoelastoidosis marginalis, differential diagnosis 89
keratolysis exfoliativa congenita
   see peeling skin syndrome
keratosis, childhood (waxy) 196–8, *196–8*
keratosis follicularis spinulosa decalvans 149, *149*
   differential diagnosis 126, 149
keratosis multiformis idiopathica
   see pachyonychia congenita
keratosis palmoplantaris nummularis
   see painful callosities
keratosis pilaris
   associations 158
   differential diagnosis 28
keratosis pilaris atrophicans, woolly hair 140
keratosis pilaris atrophicans faciei
   see ulerythema ophryogenes
keratosis pilaris decalvans see keratosis
   follicularis spinulosa decalvans
KID syndrome 102–3, *102*
   differential diagnosis 103, 126, 149
KIND1 (FLJ20116) gene 109
Kindler's syndrome 107–9, *107–9*
   differential diagnosis 14, 80, 109, 111,
     168, 329, 331, 375, 392
kinky hair syndrome see Menkes' kinky hair syndrome
Kitamura–Dowling–Degos disease 119–20, *120*
   differential diagnosis 296
Klein–Waardenburg syndrome
   see Waardenburg's syndrome
Klippel–Trénaunay syndrome 300–1, *300–1*
   differential diagnosis 176, 201, 301, 312
Kobberling–Dunnigan syndrome
   see partial lipodystrophy
Köbner EBS 1
Koenen tumors, tuberous sclerosis complex 181–2, *185*
koilonychia, associations 158, 162, 213, *213*, 214
KRTHB6/1 genes 134
Kyrle's disease 97–8, *97*

LAMB see Carney's complex
lamellar icthyosis 42–7, *44–7*
   differential diagnosis 18, 41, 52, 58, 64
lamin A/C gene 237
laminin B1 gene 252
laminin 5 gene 1, 5
   type XVII collagen 5

Langier–Giedion syndrome
   see trichorhinophalangeal syndrome
lateralization mosaic pattern 397–8, *399*
   CHILD syndrome 98, *98–9*, 99
Laugier–Hunziker syndrome, differential diagnosis 380
Launois–Bensaude syndrome 233–4, *233*
   differential diagnosis 234
Leiner's syndrome, differential diagnosis 56, 346
leiomyomas, differential diagnosis 254
LEKTI serine protease inhibitor 56
lentigines 289, 292
lentiginous nevus see segmental lentiginosis
LEOPARD syndrome 292–3, *292–3*
   associations 158, 175
   differential diagnosis 291, 293, 380, 383
leprechaunism, differential diagnosis 236
lepromatous leprosy, differential diagnosis 88
leprosy, differential diagnosis 50
Lester's iris 154
leukemias, neurofibromatosis (type 1) 172
leukokeratoses
   dyskeratosis congenita 167, *168*
   Kindler's syndrome 108
   pachyonychia congenita 151, 153, *153*
leukonychia 158, *158*
leukoplakia, differential diagnosis 166
Lewandowsky–Lutz disease see epidermodysplasia
   verruciformis
lichen planus, differential diagnosis 166
lichen striatus, differential diagnosis 287
limb–mammary disease 210, *210–11*
   see also RAPP–Hodgkin–AEC syndrome
linear and figurated hypo/hyperpigmented
   nevi 286–8, *286–8*
   differential diagnosis 287, 362
linear hypomelanosis, differential diagnosis 226
lines of Blaschko 393–6
   examples 186, 188, *200*, *205*, 222–3,
     224, 225–6, 361, *361*
lip pseudoclefting 169, *169*
lipo-oxygenase gene 43
lipoatrophy, genetic pathways 235
lipodystrophy see partial lipodystrophy;
   total lipodystrophy
lipoid proteinosis, differential diagnosis 372
Lisch nodules 172, 177
livedo reticularis 353
LMNA gene 118
LMX1B gene 155
localized hypertrichosis 133, *133*
loose anagen syndrome 148, *148*
   differential diagnosis 148
loricrin gene 68, 77
Louis–Bar syndrome see ataxia telangiectasia
lumbar spinal defects, Cobb's syndrome 302
lupus erythematosis, differential diagnosis 390
Lutz–Miescher disease see elastosis
   perforans serpiginosa

lymphadenopathy
   Griscelli's syndrome 141
   Omenn's syndrome 345
   sea-blue histiocytosis 337–8
lymphedema 321–2, *321*
   associations 321
   differential diagnosis 321–2
lyonization 225
LYST gene 349
lysyl hydroxylase gene 245
lysyloxidase activity 144

McCune–Albright syndrome 284–5, *285*
   differential diagnosis 175
macrocephaly
   cardiofacio-cutaneous syndrome 188
   neurofibromatosis (type 1) 172
   Proteus syndrome 200
macrodactyly, Proteus syndrome 200, *201*
Madelung disease *see* Launois–Bensaude syndrome
Maffucci syndrome 311–12, *311*
   differential diagnosis 176, 201, 312, 313
Mal de Meleda 80–2, *80–1*
   differential diagnosis 73, 74, 77, 78, 82
malalignment of great toenails 157, *157*
malformative syndromes 351–5
   Barber–Say syndrome 358–9, *358–9*
   Branchio-oculofacial syndrome 356–8, *356–8*
   Cohen's syndrome 355–6, *355–6*
   Cornelia de Lange syndrome 353–4, *354*
   encephalocraniocutaneous lipomatosis 363–4, *363–4*
   GAPO syndrome 364–5, *364–5*
   Pallister–Killian syndrome 361–2, *361–2*
   Rubinstein–Taybi syndrome 351–3, *351–2*
   Turner's syndrome 359–60, *359–60*
Mantoux *see* porokeratoses
Marfan's syndrome 251–2, *251–2*
   differential diagnosis 252, 378
Margarita Island ED *see* cleft lip–palate ectodermal dysplasia syndrome
Marie–Unna hypotrichosis 123–4, *123*
   differential diagnosis 124, 125
Marinesco–Sjögren syndrome 61
mast cell growth factors 260
MATP gene 278
mauserung ridges 19, *19*
medulloblastomas, nevoid basal cell carcinoma syndrome 368
melanocytic nevi
   body hemihypotrophy 188, *190–1*
   differential diagnosis 294
   junctional EB 5–6, *7*
MELAS syndrome 287, *288*
Melkersson–Rosenthal syndrome, differential diagnosis 322, 378
MEN 2B syndrome *see* multiple endocrine neoplasia syndrome (type 2B)

Mendes da Costa's disease
   see erythrokeratoderma variabilis
Menkes' kinky hair syndrome 144–5, *144*
   differential diagnosis 62, 124
   and pili torti 138
merlin gene 178–9
metabolic diseases 327–4
   acrodermatitis enteropathica 334–5, *334–5*
   cerebrotendinous xanthomatosis 339–41, *339–41*
   congenital erythropoietic porphyria 332–3, *332–3*
   erythropoietic protoporphyria 330–1, *330–1*
   Fabry's disease 335–7, *336*
   methylmalonic aciduria 343–4, *343*
   porphyria cutanea tarda and hepatoerythropoietic porphyria 327–9, *327–8*
   prolidase deficiency 341–2, *341–2*
   sea-blue histiocytosis 337–8, *337–8*
methylmalonic aciduria 343–4, *343*
   differential diagnosis 342
Michelin tire baby 257, *257*
microbrachycephaly, Cornelia de Lange syndrome 353, *354*
microcephaly
   Cockayne's syndrome 121
   incontinentia pigmenti 223
   Rubinstein–Taybi syndrome 351, *352*
   xeroderma pigmentosum 110
microcornea 154
microphthalmia
   Goltz's syndrome 229
   Midas syndrome 231
Midas syndrome 231, *231*
mild lamellar ichthyosis, differential diagnosis 37
milia
   Bazex–Dupré–Christol syndrome 383
   Brooke–Spiegler syndrome 386, *386–7*
   differential diagnosis 163
   nevoid basal cell carcinoma syndrome 367, *368*
   oral-facial-digital syndrome (type 1) 169, *169*
Milroy–Meige–Nonne disease *see* lymphedema
Milroy's disease *see* lymphedema
MITF gene 283
mitochondrial myopathy, MELAS syndrome 287
mitral valve prolapse
   Ehlers–Danlos syndromes 239
   Marfan's syndrome 251
molluscoid tumors 239, *240*
Mongolian spots 319, *320*
monilethrix 134–5, *134–5*
   differential diagnosis 126, 134
mosaic conditions 285
   hypomelanosis of Ito 280–1
   Klippel–Trénaunay syndrome 300–1, *300–1*
   linear and figurated hypo/hyperpigmented nevi 287
   Pallister–Killian syndrome 362
   Sturge–Weber syndrome 297–9
   tuberous sclerosis complex *184*, 186
   see also cutaneous mosaicism

mosaic linear plaques, Darier's disease 25, *26*
mosaic scaling, epidermolytic (acantholytic) nevus 16, *18*
mosaic tetrasomy 12p *see* Pallister–Killian syndrome
Moulin, differential diagnosis 384
Mowat–Wilson syndrome, differential diagnosis 284
MSX proteins 213
MSX1 gene 214
mucosal lesions, Darier's disease 25–8, *25–8*
Muir–Torre syndrome 369–70, *370*
　differential diagnosis 369–70
multicentric reticulohistiocytosis, differential
　　diagnosis 264
multiple endocrine neoplasia syndrome
　　(type 2B) 377–8, *377*
multiple fibrofolliculomas
　　see Birt–Hogg–Dubé syndrome
multiple glomus tumors, differential diagnosis 313
multiple pilosebaceous cyst syndrome
　　see sebocystomatosis
multiple pterygium syndrome, differential diagnosis 360
multiple trichoepitheliomas/cylindromas
　　see Brooke–Spiegler syndrome
muscular dystrophy, and EEB 3, *4*
MYO5 A gene 140, 142
myxedema, and CVG 267
myxoid tumors, Carney's complex 382–3

Naegeli–Franceschetti syndrome 114–15, *114–15*
　differential diagnosis 115, 157
nail disorders 151–60
　Iso–Kikuchi syndrome 160, *160*
　leukonychia 158, *158*
　malalignment of great toenails 157, *157*
　nail–patella–elbow syndrome 154–5, *155*
　pachyonychia congenita 151–4, *152–3*
　pterygium inversum of nails 159, *159*
　twenty-nail dystrophy 156, *156*
nail–patella–elbow syndrome 154–5, *155*
NAME *see* Carney's complex
nasal bleeding, hemorrhagic telangiectasia 306–7
necrotic vasculitis, differential diagnosis 390
NEMO gene 207, 225–6, 230
Netherton syndrome 53–6, *53–5*
　differential diagnosis 18, 41, 44, 56, 62, 66, 346
neurinomas
　differential diagnosis 262
　neurofibromatosis (type 2) 178
neurocutaneous syndromes 171–201
　cardiofacio-cutaneous syndrome 187–8, *187*
　neurofibromatosis (type 1) 171–7
　neurofibromatosis (type 2) 178–9, *178*
　Noonan's syndrome 179–80, *180*
　papular epithelial hamartomas (PEHANA)
　　syndrome 198–9, *198–9*
　phakomatosis pigmentokeratotica 188–91, *188–91*
　tuberous sclerosis complex (TSC) 180–7, *181–5*
　waxy keratosis of childhood 196–8, *196–8*
　see also epidermal nevi/nevus syndromes

neurofibromatosis (type 1) 171–3, *171–7*
　associations 289, 290–1
　differential diagnosis 133, 175–6, 378
neurofibromatosis (type 2) 178–9, *178*
neurofibromin gene 173–4
neutral lipid storage disease
　　see Dorfman–Chanarin syndrome
nevoid basal cell carcinoma syndrome 367–9, *367–8*
　differential diagnosis 83, 175, 369
nevus anemicus 318–19, *318–19*
nevus of Cannon *see* white sponge nevus
nevus comedonicus syndrome 192, 193–4, *193*
nevus hyperpigmentosus linearis,
　　differential diagnosis 226
nevus melanoticus and nevus depigmentosus
　　see linear and figurated hypo/hyperpigmented nevi
nickel sensitivity 36
Nieman–Pick disease, differential diagnosis 338
NIPBL gene 354
non-acantholytic PPK *see* Unna–Thost
　　palmoplantar keratoderma
non-Hallopeau–Siemens DEB 9–11, *10–13*
non-Herlitz JEB 5–6, *6–8*
Noonan's syndrome 179–80, *180*
　associations 293
　differential diagnosis 179, 188, 293, 360
NSDHL gene 99
nystagmus
　cardiofacio-cutaneous syndrome 188
　Dorfman–Chanarin syndrome 64
　Goltz's syndrome 229
　Harlequin baby 48
　lamellar ichthyosis 42
　oculocutaneous albinisms 275–6, 278

obesity, Cohen's syndrome 355–6, *355*
OCA1 gene 276
OCA2 gene 277
OCA4 gene 278
occipital horn syndrome, differential diagnosis 144
ocular changes, pseudoxanthoma elasticum 249
ocular coloboma, associations 148, 165
ocular lesions
　encephalocraniocutaneous
　　lipomatosis 363–4, *363–4*
　incontinentia pigmenti 224
　trichothiodystrophy 59, *60*
　X-linked dominant chondrodysplasia punctata 101
　see also retinal abnormalities
oculocutaneous albinisms 275–8, *275–8*
　differential diagnosis 276, 277, 279
　(type I) 275–6, *275–76*
　(type II) 277, *277*
　(type III) 278, *278*
odontogenic cysts, nevoid basal cell
　　carcinoma syndrome 367–8
OFD1 gene 170
Ogna EEB subgroup 3, 4

Oley's syndrome, differential diagnosis 384
oligohydramnios, cutis laxa 248
oligophrenia, monilethrix 134
Ollier's disease 312
Olmsted's syndrome 75–7, *75–7*
   differential diagnosis 73, 77, 78, 87
Omenn's syndrome 345–6, *345–6*
   differential diagnosis 18, 41, 346
onychodystrophy, associations *102*, 195, 210, 220, *221*
optic nerve atrophy, GAPO syndrome *364*, 365
optic nerve gliomas, neurofibromatosis (type 1) 172
oral mucosa 165–70
   dyskeratosis congenita 166–8, *166–8*
   oral-facial-digital syndrome (type 1) 169–70, *169*
   white sponge nevus 165–6, *165*
oral mucosal papillomatosis, Cowden's
   syndrome 371, *371*
oral-facial-digital syndrome (type 1) 169–70, *169*
organoid nevus 195
osteo-onychodysplasia *see* nail–patella–elbow syndrome
osteochondrodystrophy, dermochondrocorneal
   dystrophy 263
osteogenesis imperfecta, associations 255
osteomas, Gardner syndrome 373
ota nevus 294, *294*

'P' gene 277
1p36.2–34 74
p53 gene 38
p63 gene 211
p63-related ectodermal dysplasia 208–11, *208–11*
   differential diagnosis 211, 273, 358
pachydermoperiostosis 88, *88*
   associations 266–7
pachyonychia congenita 151–4, *152–3*
   associations 162
   differential diagnosis 73, 77, 87, 153, 156, 166
painful callosities 87, *87*
Pallister–Killian syndrome 361
palmoplantar bullae 1–2, *2*
palmoplantar keratodermas 2, *3*, 69–91
   acrokeratoelastoidosis 89, *89*
   Clouston's disease 217, *217*
   epidermolytic palmoplantar
      keratoderma 69–70, *69–70*
   Greither's disease 74–5, *74*
   Huriez's syndrome 79–80, *79–80*
   keratoderma hereditaria mutilans 72–3, *72–3*
   Mal de Meleda 80–2, *80–1*
   Naxos syndrome 90–1, *90–1*
   Olmsted's syndrome 75–7, *75–7*
   pachydermoperiostosis 88, *88*
   painful callosities 87, *87*
   Papillon–Lefevre syndrome 77–8, *77–8*
   punctate palmoplantar keratoderma 82–3, *82–3*
   Richner–Hanhart syndrome 85–6, *85–6*
   striate keratoderma 84–5, *84*
   Unna–Thost palmoplantar keratoderma 70–1, *70–1*

Papillon–Lefevre syndrome 77–8, *77–8*
papular epithelial hamartomas (PEHANA)
   syndrome 198–9, *198–9*
   differential diagnosis 197, 199
parapsoriasis, differential diagnosis 50
Parkes–Weber syndrome 297, 298–9
partial albinism *see* piebaldism
partial albinism with immunodeficiency
   see Griscelli's syndrome
partial lipodystrophy 236–7, *236*
'party-behavior'
   Cohen's syndrome 355
   trichothiodystrophy 59
Pasini–Pierini DEB 9, *11*
Patau's syndrome, differential diagnosis 353
PAX3 gene 283
pectus carinatum 251, *252*
peeling skin syndrome 32–3, *32–3*
   differential diagnosis 33, 105
PEHANA *see* papular epithelial hamartomas
   (PEHANA) syndrome
pemphigus vulgaris, differential diagnosis 31
peptic ulcer, and pachydermoperiostosis 88
perforating dermatoses, differential diagnosis 163
Peutz–Jeghers syndrome 378–80, *378–9*
   differential diagnosis 291, 293, 380, 383
phakomas (retina) 185
phakomatosis pigmentokeratotica 188–91, *188–91*
   differential diagnosis 190, 295, 320
phakomatosis pigmentovascularis 319–20, *319–20*
   differential diagnosis 190, 295, 320
pheochromocytomas 377
photosensitivity
   Cockayne's syndrome 121–2
   congenital erythropoietic porphyria 332–3
   dyschromatosis symmetrica hereditaria 296
   erythropoietic protoporphyria 330–1
   ichthyosis follicularis–atrichia–photophobia
      (IFAP) syndrome 125–6
   Kindler's syndrome 107
   oculocutaneous albinisms 275–6
   Rothmund–Thomson syndrome 113–14
   trichothiodystrophy 61, 62
   xeroderma pigmentosum 110–11
   see also UV light exposure
'phylloid' mosaic pattern 287, 397, *398*
phytanic acid deficiency *see* Refsum syndrome
phytanoil-CoA hydroxylase (PHYH) gene 58
PIBIDS syndrome 61
piebaldism 281–2, *281–2*
pigmentation disorders 275–96
   cutis tricolor 295, *295*
   dyschromatosis symmetrica hereditaria 296, *296*
   Hermansky–Pudlak syndrome 279, *279*
   hypomelanosis of Ito 280–1, *280–1*
   LEOPARD syndrome 292–3, *292–3*
   linear and figurated hypo/hyperpigmented
      nevi 286–8, *286–8*

McCune–Albright syndrome 284–5, *285*
oculocutaneous albinisms 275–8, *275–8*
ota nevus 294, *294*
piebaldism 281–2, *281–2*
segmental lentiginosis 289–91, *289–91*
Waardenburg's syndrome 283–4, *283*
pili annulati 136–7, *136–7*
  differential diagnosis 137
pili torti 137–8, *137–8*
  associations 158
  differential diagnosis 137, 138
pili triangulari et canaliculi *see* uncombable
    hair syndrome
pincer nails 151, *152*
pityriasis alba, differential diagnosis 50
pityriasis rotunda 50, *50*
pityriasis rubra pilaris 104–5, *104–5*
  differential diagnosis 105, 153
PKP1 gene 220
plakoglobin 91
plakophilin 1 gene 220
plectin 1, 3, 91
plexiform tumors 171, 173, *173*, *174*
'plucked-chicken skin' plaques 249, *250*
poikilodermas and aging syndromes 107–22
  Cockayne's syndrome 121–2, *121*
  Hutchinson–Gilford syndrome 117–19, *118*
  Kindler's syndrome 107–9, *107–9*
  Kitamura–Dowling–Degos disease 119–20, *120*
  Naegeli–Franceschetti syndrome 114–15, *114–15*
  Rothmund–Thomson syndrome 113–14, *113*
  Werner's syndrome 116–17, *116*
  xeroderma pigmentosum 110–12, *110–12*
polyostotic fibrous dysplasia
    see McCune–Albright syndrome
porokeratoses 93–6, *93–6*
porokeratosis, differential diagnosis 95
porokeratosis of Mibelli, differential diagnosis 255, 337
porokeratotic eccrine ostial and dermal
    duct nevus 194
porphyria cutanea tarda and hepatoerythropoietic
    porphyria 327–9, *327–9*
porphyrias
  acute intermittent 337
  differential diagnosis 375
  mixed 329
  see also individual conditions
port wine stains
  diffuse benign telangiectasia complex 314–15, *314*
  Klippel–Trénaunay syndrome 300–1, *300*
  Proteus syndrome 200
  Sturge–Weber syndrome 297–9, *297–9*
Prader–Willi syndrome, differential diagnosis 356
primary lymphedema *see* lymphedema
PRKAR1A gene 382
progeria *see* Hutchinson–Gilford syndrome
progressive mucinous histiocytosis 388–9, *388–9*
progressive osseous heteroplasia 264–6, *265*

prolidase deficiency 341–2, *341–2*
Proteus syndrome 200–1, *200–1*
  differential diagnosis 176, 190, 201, 301, 322, 364
proto-oncogene *c-kit* mutations 282
prurigo, Hallopeau–Siemens DEB 11, *13*
pseudomonilethrix, and pili torti 138
pseudoxanthoma elasticum 249–51, *250–1*
  differential diagnosis 240, 251
psoriasis, differential diagnosis 105, 153
PTCH gene 369
PTEN gene 201, 372
PTPN11 gene 179, 293
PTS2 receptor (PEX7) gene 58
pulmonary failure, sea-blue histocytosis 337–8
pulmonary stenosis
  cardiofacio-cutaneous syndrome 188
  neurofibromatosis (type 1) 172
pulmonary infections, hemorrhagic telangiectasia 306–7
punctate palmoplantar keratoderma 82–3, *82–3*
punctate porokeratosis, differential diagnosis 83
pure hair–nail ectodermal dysplasias 220–1, *220–1*
putrescin accumulation 149
PVRL1 gene 216
pyloric atresia, junctional EB 7, *9*
pyogenic infections 17

Rab27a gene 142
Rabson–Mendenhall syndrome, differential diagnosis 236
RAG1/2 genes 346
'rail sleeper' hyperpigmentation 222, *223*
RAPP–Hodgkin–AEC syndrome 208–11, *208–11*
  differential diagnosis 211, 273, 358
ras oncogene activity 174
recessive dystrophic EB 1, 9–14, *10–13*
recessive ichthyosis *see* lamellar ichthyosis
RECQ helicase gene 114
Reed's syndrome 261
Refsum syndrome 58–9, *59*
renal abnormalities, Turner's syndrome 360
renal acidosis, and Launois–Bensaude syndrome 233
renal angiolipomas 185
renal calculi, associations 158
renal dysplasia, nail–patella–elbow syndrome 154
renal failure
  Fabry's disease 335–7
  Kyrle's disease 97
Rendu–Osler syndrome *see* hemorrhagic telangiectasia
restrictive dermopathy 262–3, *262–3*
  differential diagnosis 48, 263
reticulohistiocytosis, differential diagnosis 338
retinal abnormalities, Sturge–Parkes–Weber complex 298
retinal angiomas, Von Hippel–Lindau syndrome 303
rhabdomyomas 185
Richner–Hanhart syndrome 85–6, *85–6*
  differential diagnosis 87
rickets, epidermal nevi 195–6
ringed chromosome disease, differential diagnosis 175
ringed hair *see* pili annulati

RNA processing mutations 167, 296
Rombo syndrome 391–2, *391*
   differential diagnosis 384, 392
Rosselli–Giulienetti syndrome
   see cleft lip–palate ectodermal dysplasia syndrome
Rothmund–Thomson syndrome 113–14, *113*
   differential diagnosis 109, 111, 119, 168, 306
Rubinstein–Taybi syndrome 351–3, *351–52*

Sabonis' syndrome 60
Schimmelpenning syndrome
   see epidermal-sebaceous nevus syndrome
schizophrenia
   cutis verticis gyrata 266
   tuberous sclerosis complex 183–4
Schop–Schulz–Passarge syndrome,
   differential diagnosis 78, 80
schwannomas, neurofibromatosis (type 2) 178
schwannomatosis, differential diagnosis 179
sclerodactyly 79
scleroderma, differential diagnosis 237, 266
scleromalacia perforans 333, *333*
sclerotylosis *see* Huriez's syndrome
scrotal tongue 234, *235*, 283, *283*, 371, 383
sea-blue histiocytosis 337–8, *337–8*
sebaceous gland tumors, Muir–Torre
   syndrome 369, *370*
sebocystomatosis 161–3, *161–3*
   associations 151
   differential diagnosis 163, 234
seborrheic alopecia, differential diagnosis 130
seborrheic dermatitis, differential diagnosis 28, 105
secretan's syndrome, differential diagnosis 322
segmental lentiginosis 289–91, *289–91*
   associations 289, 290–1
   differential diagnosis 291
Seip–Lawrence syndrome *see* total lipodystrophy
self-healing collodion baby 40–1, *40–51*
   differential diagnosis 41, 43
Setleis disease 273, *273*
shagreen patches, tuberous sclerosis
   complex 181, *184*, 253
Shah–Waardenburg syndrome
   see Waardenburg's syndrome
'Siamese cat' pattern 276
sideremia 328
Silver–Russell syndrome, differential diagnosis 175
'silvery' hair 140–2, *141–2*
Simian crease, Rubinstein–Taybi syndrome 351
Sjögren–Larsson syndrome 57–8, *57*
   differential diagnosis 62
skull defects and ulcerations, aplasia
   cutis 269–70, *269–71*
SLC39A4 gene 334
SLURP-1 protein 81
solar keratoses 110
solitary osteoma cutis, differential diagnosis 266
Sotos syndrome, and CVG 267

speckled lentiginous nevus (SLN) 188, *190*, 319, *319*
   differential diagnosis 294
   epidermal nevi 195, *195–6*
sphenoid displacement, neurofibromatosis (type 1) 172
sphingolipid storage 336
spina bifida, differential diagnosis 303
SPINK5 gene 56
spiradenomas 386
spun-glass hair *see* uncombable hair syndrome
squamous cell carcinoma
   dyskeratosis congenita 167
   epidermodysplasia verruciformis 385
   Hallopeau–Siemens DEB 11, *13*
   Huriez's syndrome 79
   KID syndrome 103
   Kindler's syndrome 108–9
   oculocutaneous albinisms 276
   pachydermoperiostosis 88
   porokeratosis 95
   Rothmund–Thomson syndrome 113–14
SSAT gene 149
staphylococcal abscess syndrome
   see hyper IgE syndrome
steatocystoma multiplex *see* sebocystomatosis
steely hair syndrome *see* Menkes' kinky hair syndrome
'stellate' epidermolytic hyperkeratosis 22–3, *22–3*
steroid sulfatase enzyme deficiency 38
sterol biosynthesis 101
stippled epiphyses 100, *100*
strabismus
   Cohen's syndrome 355
   Goltz's syndrome 229
   oculocutaneous albinisms 275
   Rubinstein–Taybi syndrome 352
striate keratoderma 84–5, *84*
STRK11/LKB1 gene 379
Sturge–Weber syndrome 297–9, *297–9*
Sugio–Kajii syndrome
   see trichorhinophalangeal syndrome
sulfur-deficient brittle hair syndrome
   see trichothiodystrophy
superoxide dismutase activity 144
symmetric progressive erythrokeratoderma 67–8
syndactyly
   monilethrix 134
   oral-facial-digital syndrome (type 1) 169
syndromic ichthyoses 53–64
   differential diagnosis 44, 58
   Netherton syndrome 53–6, *53–5*
   Refsum syndrome 58–59, *59*
   trichothiodystrophy 59–63, *60–2*
systemic lupus erythematosus, differential diagnosis 306

Tay's syndrome 61
telangiectases, butterfly pattern 304, *304–5*
tetrasomy 12p 362
TFIIH factor complex 62
thrombocytopenia, sea-blue histiocytosis 338

thyroid carcinomas, medullary 377–8
thyroid gland lesions, Cowden's syndrome 371–2
tinea versicolor, differential diagnosis 50
Torre syndrome *see* Muir–Torre syndrome
total lipodystrophy 234–6, *234–5*
    differential diagnosis 236
Touraine–Solente–Gole syndrome
    see pachydermoperiostosis
transcription-coupled repair (TCR) system 111
transglutaminase-1 gene mutations 38, 40–1, 43
tretinoin 166
triangular alopecia 130, *130*
trichilemmal cysts, differential diagnosis 163
tricho-dento-osseous syndrome 212–13, *212*
trichorhinophalangeal syndrome 145–6, *145–6*, 170
trichorrhexis invaginata 55, *55*
trichothiodystrophy 59–63, *60–2*
    differential diagnosis 58, 62, 211
    pili torti 138
trichotillomania, differential diagnosis 148
trisomy 13 syndrome, differential diagnosis 353
trisomy 13 gene 271
TRP1 gene 278
TRPS *see* trichorhinophalangeal syndrome
TRPS1 gene 146
TSC *see* tuberous sclerosis complex
TSC1/2 genes 186
tuberin 186
tuberous sclerosis complex (TSC) 180–7, *181–5*
    differential diagnosis 175, 187, 370, 372, 387
'tumeurs royales' 171, *174–5*
tumor necrosis factor-mediated aptosis 207, 225–6
Turcot's syndrome, differential diagnosis 374
Turner's syndrome 359–60, *359–60*
    differential diagnosis 175, 179, 360
turricephalic vault 187
'twin-spot' phenomenon 188–9, 295, 318,
    320, 398–9, *399–402*
    allelic 398
    classical examples 398–9, *399*, *401*
    non-allelic *398*, 399, *401–2*
twisted hair *see* pili torti
tylosis carcinoma *see* Howel–Evans syndrome
tyrosinase modulating activity 144, 276, 277
tyrosinase albinism *see* oculocutaneous albinisms
tyrosine kinase receptor mutations 378
tyrosine aminotransferase (TAT) gene 86
tyrosinemia type II *see* Richner–Hanhart syndrome

ulerythema ophryogenes 125, *126*, 128–9, *128–9*, 179, 383
    differential diagnosis 129
ultraviolet-sensitivity syndrome 122
uncombable hair syndrome 143, *143*
    differential diagnosis 143, 148
unilateral nevoid and generalized 'essential'
    telangiectasia 315–18
Unna–Thost palmoplantar keratoderma 70–1, *70–1*
    differential diagnosis 70, 71, 74

unusual face/atrophic skin/hirsutism
    syndrome *see* Barber–Say syndrome
urethral duplication, nail–patella–elbow syndrome 154
uroporphyrinogen decarboxylase gene 328–9
uroporphyrinogen III co-synthetase gene 333
urticaria pigmentosa 260, *260*
uterine leiomyomata, associations 261
UV light exposure
    Bloom's syndrome 375
    epidermodysplasia verruciformis 385–6
    segmental lentiginosis 290–1
    and X-linked ichthyosis 38
    see also photosensitivity

vascular disorders 297–325
    ataxia telangiectasia 304–6, *304–6*
    blue rubber bleb nevus syndrome 312–13, *312–13*
    Cobb's syndrome 302–3, *302–3*
    complex of Sturge–Parkes–Weber/Klippel–Trénaunay/
        Cobb's syndromes 297
    cutis marmorata telangiectatica
        congenita 308–10, *308–10*
    diffuse benign telangiectasia and port-wine
        stains complex 314–15, *314*
    generalized cyanosis, phlebectasies
        and soft skin syndrome 322–4, *322–3*
    glomuvenous malformation 324–5, *324*
    hemorrhagic telangiectasia 306–7, *306–7*
    Klippel–Trénaunay syndrome 300–1, *300–1*
    lymphedema 321–2, *321*
    Maffucci syndrome 311–12, *311*
    nevus anemicus 318–19, *318–19*
    phakomatosis pigmentovascularis 319–20, *319–320*
    Sturge–Weber syndrome 297–9, *297–9*
    unilateral nevoid and generalized 'essential'
        telangiectasia 315–18, *315–18*
    Von Hippel–Lindau syndrome 303–4, *304*
V(D)J recombinase activity 346
VHL gene 303
vitamin D-resistant rickets 195
vitiligo
    associated hair conditions 127
    differential diagnosis 281, 282, 284, 296, 319
Vohwinkel's syndrome *see* keratoderma
    hereditaria mutilans
Von Hippel–Lindau syndrome 303–4, *304*
Von Recklinghausen's disease
    see neurofibromatosis type 1
Vörner's disease *see* epidermolytic
    palmoplantar keratoderma

Waardenburg's syndrome 283–4, *283*
    differential diagnosis 282, 284
'watch glass' nails 88
Watson syndrome 172, 175
    differential diagnosis 188, 293
waxy keratosis of childhood 196–8, *196–8*
Weary's syndrome *see* Kindler's syndrome

webbed neck, Turner's syndrome 359, *359*
Weber–Cockayne EBS 1
Werner's syndrome 116–17, *116*
   differential diagnosis 80, 116
white forelocks 282, *282*
white macules
   CRIE 51
   Rothmund–Thomson syndrome 113, *113*
white nails, leukonychia 158, *158*
white sponge nevus 165
whorled hypermelanosis, differential diagnosis 226
whorled nevoid hyperhypomelanosis
      see linear and figurated hypo/hyperpigmented nevi
Winchester's syndrome, differential diagnosis 259
Wiskott–Aldrich syndrome, differential diagnosis 348
Witkop's syndrome 213–14, *213*
Wolff–Parkinson–White arrhythmias 185
woolly hair 139–40, *139*

X-linked dominant chondrodysplasia
      punctata 100–1, *100–1*
   differential diagnosis 99

X-linked ichthyosis 38–9, *38–9*
   differential diagnosis 38, 58, 62
X-linked trait inheritance 403–5
xanthogranulomas, juvenile 171, *176*
xeroderma pigmentosum 110–12, *110–12*, 122
   differential diagnosis 61, 109, 114, 375, 383, 392
xerosis, Marfan's syndrome 251
xerostomia, Harlequin baby 48
45XO gene 360
XO syndrome *see* Turner's syndrome
XP-B genes 62
XP-D genes 62

YAG (yttrium–aluminum–garnet) 163

zinc absorption defects, acrodermatitis
      enteropathica 334–5
zinc finger homeobox B gene 284
Zinsser–Cole–Engman syndrome
   see dyskeratosis congenita
Zlotogora–Ogur syndrome *see* cleft lip–palate
      ectodermal dysplasia syndrome